NUTRITION AND FUNCTIONAL FOODS FOR HEALTHY AGING

NUTRITION AND FUNCTIONAL FOODS FOR HEALTHY AGING

Edited by

RONALD ROSS WATSON

University of Arizona, Mel and Enid Zuckerman College of Public Health, and School of Medicine, Arizona Health Sciences Center, Tucson, AZ, United States

ELSEVIER

ACADEMIC PRESS

An imprint of Elsevier

elsevier.com

Academic Press is an imprint of Elsevier
125 London Wall, London EC2Y 5AS, United Kingdom
525 B Street, Suite 1800, San Diego, CA 92101-4495, United States
50 Hampshire Street, 5th Floor, Cambridge, MA 02139, United States
The Boulevard, Langford Lane, Kidlington, Oxford OX5 1GB, United Kingdom

Notices
Knowledge and best practice in this field are constantly changing. As new research and experience broaden our understanding, changes in research methods, professional practices, or medical treatment may become necessary.

Practitioners and researchers must always rely on their own experience and knowledge in evaluating and using any information, methods, compounds, or experiments described herein. In using such information or methods they should be mindful of their own safety and the safety of others, including parties for whom they have a professional responsibility.

To the fullest extent of the law, neither the Publisher nor the authors, contributors, or editors, assume any liability for any injury and/or damage to persons or property as a matter of products liability, negligence or otherwise, or from any use or operation of any methods, products, instructions, or ideas contained in the material herein.

British Library Cataloguing-in-Publication Data
A catalogue record for this book is available from the British Library

Library of Congress Cataloging-in-Publication Data
A catalog record for this book is available from the Library of Congress

ISBN: 978-0-12-805376-8

For Information on all Academic Press publications visit our website at https://www.elsevier.com/books-and-journals

Publisher: Nikki Levy
Acquisition Editor: Megan Ball
Editorial Project Manager: Billie Jean Fernandez
Production Project Manager: Caroline Johnson
Designer: Victoria Pearson

Typeset by MPS Limited, Chennai, India

Contents

5. Appetite Regulation in Healthy Aging

STIJN SOENEN AND IAN CHAPMAN

6. Human Microbiome and Aging

SEEMA JOSHI AND MELISSA NAVINSKEY

7. Fibromyalgia Syndrome: Role of Obesity and Nutrients

MANISHA J. OZA, MAYURESH S. GARUD, ANIL BHANUDAS GAIKWAD AND YOGESH A. KULKARNI

8. Aging and Gait

KUNAL SINGHAL AND JEFFREY B. CASEBOLT

9. Assessment of Nutritional Status in the Elderly

TERESA KOKOT, EWA MALCZYK, EWA ZIÓŁKO, MAŁGORZATA MUC-WIERZGOŃ AND EDYTA FATYGA

10. Eating Capability Assessments in Elderly Populations

LAURA LAGUNA, ANWESHA SARKAR AND JIANSHE CHEN

II

NUTRIENTS (VITAMINS AND MINERALS) IN HEALTH IN AGING ADULTS

11. Healthy Food Choice and Dietary Behavior in the Elderly

CHRISTINE BROMBACH, MARIANNE LANDMANN, KATRIN ZIESEMER, SILKE BARTSCH AND GERTRUD WINKLER

12. Vitamin D and Diabetes in Elderly People

NICOLA VERONESE, ENZO MANZATO AND GIUSEPPE SERGI

13. Vitamin D and the Elderly Orthopedic Patient

GERRIT STEFFEN MAIER, ANDREAS ALOIS KURTH, KONSTANTIN HORAS, KRISTINA KOLBOW, JÖRN BENGT SEEGER, KLAUS EDGAR ROTH, DJORDJE LAZOVIC AND UWE MAUS

14. Vitamins and Minerals in Older Adults: Causes, Diagnosis, and Treatment of Deficiency

JENNIFER DOLEY

15. The Role of B Group Vitamins and Choline in Cognition and Brain Aging

FRANCESCO BONETTI, GLORIA BROMBO AND GIOVANNI ZULIANI

16. Vitamin B_{12} Deficiency in the Elderly

CHIT WAI WONG

17. Vitamin E Isoform-Specific Functions in Allergic Inflammation and Asthma

JOAN M. COOK-MILLS

III

DIETARY SUPPLEMENTS AND HERBS, FUNCTIONAL FOODS, IN HEALTH IN AGING ADULTS

18. Polyphenols and Intestinal Health

KRISTINA B. MARTINEZ, JESSICA D. MACKERT AND MICHAEL K. MCINTOSH

19. Nootropics, Functional Foods, and Dietary Patterns for Prevention of Cognitive Decline

FRANCESCO BONETTI, GLORIA BROMBO AND GIOVANNI ZULIANI

20. Chalcones Target the Tumor Necrosis Factor–Related Apoptosis-Inducing Ligand (TRAIL) Signaling Pathway for Cancer Chemoprevention

MAŁGORZATA KŁÓSEK, ANDRZEJ KAROL KUROPATNICKI, EWELINA SZLISZKA, ILONA KORZONEK-SZLACHETA AND WOJCIECH KRÓL

21. Anti-inflammatory Dietary Ingredients, Medicinal Plants, and Herbs Exert Beneficial Health Effects in Aging

KIRAN S. PANICKAR AND DENNIS E. JEWELL

22. Calorie Restriction Mimetics From Functional Foods: Impact on Promoting a Healthy Life Span

WAI YAN SUN AND YU WANG

23. Nutraceuticals for Healthy Skin Aging

ELAINE CRISTINA FARIA ABRAHÃO MACHADO, LETÍCIA AMBROSANO, RENAN LAGE, BEATRICE MARTINEZ ZUGAIB ABDALLA AND ADILSON COSTA

27. Cellular and Physiological Effects of Arginine in Seniors

VANCE L. ALBAUGH, MELISSA K. STEWART AND ADRIAN BARBUL

28. Late-Onset Caloric Restriction Alters Skeletal Muscle Metabolism: Mechanisms from Animal and Human Studies

CHIAO-NAN CHEN

29. Healthy Foods for Healthy Aging: The Case for Protein

KAREN S. KUBENA AND W. ALEX MCINTOSH

List of Contributors

Beatrice Martinez Zugaib Abdalla ABC School of Medicine, Santo Andre, SP, Brazil

Vance L. Albaugh Vanderbilt University School of Medicine, Nashville, TN, United States

Letícia Ambrosano Catholic University of Campinas, Campinas, SP, Brazil

Adrian Barbul Vanderbilt University School of Medicine, Nashville, TN, United States

Silke Bartsch Pädagogische Hochschule Karlsruhe, Karlsruhe, Germany

Francesco Bonetti University of Ferrara, Ferrara, Italy

Christine Brombach ZHAW, Zurich University of Applied Sciences, Wädenswil, Switzerland

Gloria Brombo University of Ferrara, Ferrara, Italy

Jeffrey B. Casebolt West Texas A&M University, Canyon, TX, United States

Thomas W. Castonguay University of Maryland, College Park, MD, United States

Ian Chapman Royal Adelaide Hospital, Adelaide, SA, Australia

Chiao-nan Chen Chang Gung University, Taoyuan, Taiwan

Jianshe Chen Zhejiang Gongshang University, Hangzhou, China

Jake Alexander Clor Wayne State University, Detroit, MI, United States

Joan M. Cook-Mills Northwestern University, Chicago, IL, United States

Adilson Costa Catholic University of Campinas, Campinas, SP, Brazil

Jennifer Doley Carondelet St. Mary's Hospital, Tucson, AZ, United States

Edyta Fatyga Medical University of Silesia in Katowice, Katowice, Poland

Maria Pontes Ferreira Wayne State University, Detroit, MI, United States

Anil Bhanudas Gaikwad Birla Institute of Technology and Science, Pilani, Rajasthan, India

Mayuresh S. Garud Shobhaben Pratapbhai Patel School of Pharmacy & Technology Management, SVKM's NMIMS, Mumbai, Maharashtra, India

Konstantin Horas Julius-Maxilians-University, Würzburg, Germany

Samantha Hudgins University of Maryland, College Park, MD, United States

Sebastian Huhn Max Planck Institute for Human Cognitive and Brain Sciences, Leipzig, Germany; University of Leipzig, Leipzig, Germany

Dennis E. Jewell Hill's Pet Nutrition Center, Topeka, KS, United States

Seema Joshi Dwight D. Eisenhower Veterans Affairs Medical Center, Leavenworth, KS, United States

Teresa Juarez-Cedillo Mexican Institute of Social Security, Mexico City, Mexico; National Autonomous University of Mexico, Mexico City, Mexico

Małgorzata Kłósek Medical University of Silesia, Katowice, Poland

Teresa Kokot Medical University of Silesia in Katowice, Katowice, Poland

Kristina Kolbow Carl-von-Ossietzky-University, Oldenburg, Germany

Ilona Korzonek-Szlacheta Medical University of Silesia, Katowice, Poland

Wojciech Król Medical University of Silesia, Katowice, Poland

Karen S. Kubena Texas A&M University, College Station, TX, Unites States

Yogesh A. Kulkarni Shobhaben Pratapbhai Patel School of Pharmacy & Technology Management, SVKM's NMIMS, Mumbai, Maharashtra, India

Andrzej Karol Kuropatnicki Pedagogical University of Krakow, Krakow, Poland

Andreas Alois Kurth Themistocles Gluck Hospital, Ratingen, Germany

Renan Lage Catholic University of Campinas, Campinas, SP, Brazil

Laura Laguna University of Leeds, Leeds, United Kingdom

Marianne Landmann Friedrich-Schiller-University Jena, Jena, Germany

Djordje Lazovic Carl-von-Ossietzky-University, Oldenburg, Germany

Guillermo López-Lluch Universidad Pablo de Olavide, Sevilla, Spain

Elaine Cristina Faria Abrahão Machado Catholic University of Campinas, Campinas, SP, Brazil

Jessica D. Mackert UNC-Greensboro, Greensboro, NC, United States

Gerrit Steffen Maier Carl-von-Ossietzky-University, Oldenburg, Germany

Ewa Malczyk University of Applied Sciences, Nysa, Poland

Enzo Manzato University of Padova, Padova, Italy; National Research Council, Padova, Italy

Kristina B. Martinez University of Chicago, Chicago, IL, United States

Uwe Maus Carl-von-Ossietzky-University, Oldenburg, Germany

Ruben Maya-Luevano Wayne State University, Detroit, MI, United States

Michael K. McIntosh UNC-Greensboro, Greensboro, NC, United States

W. Alex McIntosh Texas A&M University, College Station, TX, Unites States

Małgorzata Muc-Wierzgoń Medical University of Silesia in Katowice, Katowice, Poland

Melissa Navinskey Dwight D. Eisenhower Veterans Affairs Medical Center, Leavenworth, KS, United States

Manisha J. Oza Shobhaben Pratapbhai Patel School of Pharmacy & Technology Management, SVKM's NMIMS, Mumbai, Maharashtra, India; SVKM's Dr. Bhanuben Nanavati College of Pharmacy, Mumbai, Maharashtra, India

Kiran S. Panickar Hill's Pet Nutrition Center, Topeka, KS, United States

Klaus Edgar Roth Johannes-Gutenberg-University, Mainz, Germany

Anwesha Sarkar University of Leeds, Leeds, United Kingdom

Jörn Bengt Seeger Justus-Liebig-University, Giessen, Germany

Giuseppe Sergi University of Padova, Padova, Italy

Kunal Singhal University of Tennessee Health Science Center, Memphis, TN, United States

Stijn Soenen Royal Adelaide Hospital, Adelaide, SA, Australia

Adele Sparavigna Clinical Research and Bioengineering Institute, Monza, Italy

Melissa K. Stewart Vanderbilt University School of Medicine, Nashville, TN, United States

Wai Yan Sun The University of Hong Kong, Hong Kong, China

Ewelina Szliszka Medical University of Silesia, Katowice, Poland

Nicola Veronese University of Padova, Padova, Italy

Prabhakar Vissavajjhala Sugen Life Sciences Pvt Ltd, Tirupati, Andhra Pradesh, India

Yu Wang The University of Hong Kong, Hong Kong, China

Gertrud Winkler Albstadt-Sigmaringen University, Sigmaringen, Germany

A. Veronica Witte Max Planck Institute for Human Cognitive and Brain Sciences, Leipzig, Germany; University of Leipzig, Leipzig, Germany

Chit Wai Wong Caritas Medical Centre, Kowloon, Hong Kong

Katrin Ziesemer University of Konstanz, Konstanz, Germany

Ewa Ziółko Medical University of Silesia in Katowice, Katowice, Poland

Giovanni Zuliani University of Ferrara, Ferrara, Italy

Preface

Section I: Overview Health and Aging. In some countries, longevity continues to increase as it did in the 20th century. How to maximize this through personal choice and medical advice is vital. Vissavajjhala provides an overview of the role of nutrients in this process. Then specific organs are reviewed. Sparavigna investigates the function of the skin and appearance. Juarez-Cedillo notes the changes in nutritional needs in seniors. Castonguay searches the literature for hypothalamic control of appetite through sugars and glucocorticoids. Then Soenen further expands on regulation of appetite in the healthy elderly. Oza et al. describe fibromyalgia syndrome though nutrient intake and obesity in seniors. It is important to know what nutrients to assess, which Kotot and coworkers review.

Section II: Nutrients (Vitamins and Minerals) in Health in Aging Adults. Specific vitamins appear to play important functions in the aging process and may need supplementation. Veronese, Manzato, and Sergi evaluate vitamin D and diabetes because of vitamin D's reputation for enhancing health. Maier and coworkers expand this review with a discussion of vitamin D in orthopedic patients. Doley reviews the arena of vitamins and minerals related to the causes and treatment of their deficiency in elderly patients. Then Bonetti and coauthors further expand and focus on B vitamins and choline in brain function and cognition. Wong supports the role of vitamin deficiency as a problem for seniors by describing vitamin B12 deficiency in older adults. Finally, Cook-Mills reviews vitamin E isoform-specific function in allergic inflammation and asthma.

Section III: Dietary Supplements and Herbs, Functional Foods, in Health in Aging Adults. Martinez and coauthors review health of the colon as modified by age and polyphenols. Bonetti et al. review cognitive decline in the elderly, especially as modified by nootropics, functional foods, and diet as therapies. Klosek and authors described the use chalcones as modified by tumor necrosis factor treatment of cancer chemoprevention. Sun reviews calorie restriction mimetics from functional foods. The review further can therefore lengthen the life span, which is also reviewed. Huhn and Witte describe the grape extract resveratrol to prevent and treat mental decline in cognitive diseases. Maya-Luevano and Ferreira review dietary extracts on sexual function in aging using native plant materials from North America.

Section IV. Protein and Energy in Health and Growth of Elderly. López-Lluch reviews coenzyme Q10, which plays a role in energy metabolism as related to aging, and reduced exercise. Albaugh reviews the amino acid arginine and its effects on the bodily activities as well as cell function in older adults. Finally, Kubena reviews foods high and low in cholesterol and their effect on healthy aging and accelerated decline.

Acknowledgments

The work of Dr. Watson's editorial assistant, Bethany L. Stevens, was critical to the successful completion of the book in communicating with authors and working on their manuscripts. The support of Billie Jean Fernandez is also very much appreciated. Support for Ms. Stevens's and Dr. Watson's work was graciously provided by Natural Health Research Institute (www.naturalhealthresearch.org). This independent, not-for-profit organization supports science-based research on natural health and wellness. It is committed to informing the public about scientific evidence on the usefulness and cost-effectiveness of diet, supplements, and healthy lifestyles to improve health and wellness and reduce disease. Finally, the work of librarian of the Arizona Health Science Library, Mari Stoddard, was vital and very helpful in identifying key researchers who participated in the book.

P A R T I

OVERVIEW HEALTH AND AGING

CHAPTER

1

Impact of Nutrition on Healthy Aging

Prabhakar Vissavajjhala

Sugen Life Sciences, Pvt Ltd, Tirupati, Andhra Pradesh, India

INTRODUCTION

Aging is a continuous, unidirectional phenomenon for any system; in a real sense, it refers to all of the changes that occur during a system's entire existence. However, *biological aging* is often perceived as the changes that occur toward *senility*, or the declining phase of an individual. *Growth* and *development* are the terms often used to denote the changes occurring from inception to an organism's early phases, but these are also part of aging. Metaphorically, if the human body is similar to an automobile, the best performance of the body or vehicle is mostly based on maintenance through timely inputs of appropriate fuel as measured both quantitatively and qualitatively. Besides providing energy, ideally the fuel does not generate or produces only minimal harmful residues or effects and lets the body or vehicle function smoothly over a long period of time with a sense of well-being. Such a scenario for humans may be best termed *healthy aging*. This serves as the basis not only of healthy growth and development during an individual's earliest phases but also for a feeling of wellness during senility, where the fuel in question is nothing but nutritious food. In practice, healthy aging for humans depends on eating right, which often also means avoiding the wrong types of foods.

Though inborn genetic defects profoundly affect an individual's health and wellness, in general they may not be frequent. Obviously, for humans the impact of food for healthy development and survival has been of paramount interest, especially in the wake of recent alarming global trends in the numbers of overweight and obese adults and adolescents. When high caloric intake and inadequate nutrient variety and density coincide with sedentary lifestyles, the results have included diet-induced metabolic syndrome and adverse consequences on health such as insulin resistance, type 2 diabetes, cardiovascular complications, inflammation, inflammatory diseases, and some types of cancer. In addition, such situations often necessitate pharmacological intervention, which add to both social and economic burdens on countries all over the world. How a variety of foods that include diverse nutrients can address issues of metabolic syndrome has been recently reviewed (Vissavajjhala, 2014), but this chapter provides a simplified overview, highlighting the enormity of the impact of dietary fiber (DF), prebiotics, and probiotics specifically in conjunction with gastrointestinal (GI) tract and gut microbiota on humans for healthy development that continues even as individuals age.

DIETARY FIBER

DF or *roughage* is defined as the "undigested plant material that animals/humans may ingest." Chemically, DF consists of nonstarch polysaccharides such as arabinoxylans, cellulose, and hemicellulose and many other plant components such as resistant starch (RS), resistant dextrins, inulin, lignin, chitins, pectins, β-glucans, and oligosaccharides. Based on its physical properties, DF has both water-soluble and water-insoluble components (Slavin, 2013).

While all plant foods contain some DF, some are richer in specific ones. *Soluble fiber* is found in varying quantities in all plant foods, including oatmeal, rye, chia, barley, nuts, beans, lentils, some fruits (including figs, avocado,

Nutrition and Functional Foods for Healthy Aging.
DOI: http://dx.doi.org/10.1016/B978-0-12-805376-8.00001-0

plums, prunes, berries, ripe bananas, the skin of apples, quinces, and pears), certain vegetables such as broccoli and Jerusalem artichokes, root tubers and root vegetables such as sweet potatoes and onions, psyllium seed husks, and flax seeds. Sources of *insoluble fiber* include whole grain foods, including whole wheat, corn bran, and brown rice; legumes such as beans and peas, nuts, and seeds; potato skins; lignans; vegetables such as cauliflower, zucchini, celery, carrots, and cucumbers; and some fruits, including avocado, unripe bananas, the skins of some fruits such as kiwis, grapes, and tomatoes (Spiller, 2001).

GI AND GUT MICROBIOTA

A plethora of microbial populations develop in humans, the distribution of which include the skin, the oral and nasal cavities, and the urogenital, respiratory, and GI tracts. They are colonized by an enormous variety of bacteria, archaea, fungi, and viruses that form a community collectively known as the *human microbiome* or *microbiota*. Among them, the key player in host health, and working in conjunction with DF, is the *commensal GI* or *gut microbial population*, which comprises more than 1000 different species contributing more than 3.3 million microbial genes to the human GI tract. In fact, the human acquisition of certain vitamins such as B and K and antibiotics is only possible because commensal bacteria are present in the digestive tract.

Mechanisms of Health Benefits

Though human food may contain a variety of carbohydrates and polysaccharides in the form of plant material (cell walls and storage polymers), animal connective tissue, food additives, and microbial and fungal products, the digestion of carbohydrates in humans is confined only to starch, lactose, and sucrose (El Kaoutari et al., 2013) because of indigenous limitations. Human gut microbiota compensate for the lack of necessary enzymatic entities in the host genetic makeup to act on DF components and generate microbial metabolites that result in health benefits for the host. While soluble components of DF are readily fermented by microbiota in the colon and result in gases and physiologically active by-products, most of the insoluble components of DF are metabolically inert (e.g., lignin), may be fermented (e.g., RS), or are incompletely fermented (e.g., cellulose) in the large intestine. Due to their physical presence and ability to absorb water, insoluble DF increases fecal mass (called bulking), eases defecation, and minimizes constipation. Bulking also aids in diluting toxins, reducing intracolonic pressure, shortening fecal transit time, and increasing defecation frequency.

Short-chain fatty acids (SCFAs) contain fewer than six carbons: in general, formate (C1), acetate (C2), propionate (C3), butyrate (C4), and valerate (C5) are produced as microbial metabolites in the colon, playing critical roles both locally (GI level) and systemically, influencing host health and immunity. These will be highlighted in later sections.

Diversity of Gut Microbiota

The complexities and variability of adult gut microbial populations have become increasingly evident in recent years and led to the establishment of the Human Microbiome Project (HMP) (http://www.hmpdacc.org/). Owing to the burgeoning technological advances in genomic DNA sequencing, the emergence of metagenomics—the study of collective genomes of the members of microbial community in the human gut—has vastly increased human awareness of gut microbiota. The study involves cloning and analyzing the genomes without culturing the organisms in the community, offering the opportunity to describe the diverse microbial inhabitants, many of which cannot be cultured (Ursell et al., 2012).

Humans may have 10^{14} microbes—i.e., 10 times more than the eukaryotic cells in the human body—existing as commensal colonies and often playing critical roles in human health and disease (Koboziev et al., 2014). The intricate microbiome includes mostly bacteria, which live with commensal (not harmful) or symbiotic (mutually beneficial) or dysbiotic (potentially harmful or pathogenic) characteristics in relation to the host. Hence, imbalances of gut microbiota may lead to a number of pathologies such as obesity, types 1 and 2 diabetes, inflammatory bowel disease, colorectal cancer, and chronic inflammation (inflammaging) and immunosenescence in the elderly (Brown et al., 2012).

The mammalian microbiota are highly variable with several dominant bacterial phyla: Firmicutes (e.g., *Lactobacillus, Clostridium*), *Bacteroidetes* (some commensals such as *Bacteroides ovatus* and some pathogenics such as *Bacteriodes fragilis* and *Bidens vulgatus*), Actinobacteria (e.g., the genera *Bifidobacteria* and *Streptomyces*), and Proteobacteria (e.g., *Escherischia coli* and *Pseudomonas* species) (Dethlefsen et al., 2007; Zoetendal et al., 2006). Firmicutes and

Bacteroides account for more than 90% of the bacterial population in the colon (Ley et al., 2008), while Actinobacteria and Proteobacteria (which includes members of the family Enterobacteriaceae) are scarcely present (<1–5%) (Eckburg et al., 2005).

Factors Influencing Gut Microbiota

Apart from host genetics, numerous factors such as premature delivery, mode of delivery, antibiotic usage, and diet can play important roles in how the intestinal microbiota of infants are shaped (Conlon and Bird, 2015). Microbes colonize the human gut during or shortly after birth. The fact that babies delivered naturally have higher gut bacterial counts at 1 month of age than those delivered by cesarean section (Huurre et al., 2008) suggests that gut colonization by microbes begins during and is enhanced by natural birth. The growth and development of a robust gut microbiota is important for the development of the individual's immune system (Kelly et al., 2007) and continues during breast-feeding, a stage that seems to be crucial for an individual's long-term health. The microbiotic diversity of breast-fed infants has been reported to be better than infants fed on formula food (Le Huerou-Luron et al., 2010). Oligosaccharides present in breast milk promote the growth of *Lactobacillus* and *Bifidobacterium*, which dominate the infant gut (Harmsen et al., 2000), strengthen or promote the development of the immune system, and may help prevent conditions such as eczema and asthma (Arslanoglu et al., 2008).

Prebiotics

Following the pioneering effort by Gibson and Roberfroid (1995), the prebiotic concept has been refined and redefined many times. *Prebiotics* are defined as "selectively fermented ingredients that result in specific changes, in the composition and/or activity in the GI microbiota, thus conferring benefit/s upon host health" (Gibson et al., 2010).

Inulin-type fructans, fructooligosaccharides (FOS), and galactooligosaccharides (GOS) (nondigestible short-chain carbohydrates) are the quintessential prebiotics that typically target the *Bifidobacterium* and *Lactobacillus* groups. Inulin and FOS occur naturally in various foods, including cereals, fruits, and vegetables, so they are ubiquitous in most diets.

Probiotics

Probiotics are defined as live microorganisms that confer a health benefit to their host when administered in adequate quantities. The most commonly consumed probiotics belong to the genera *Lactobacillus* and *Bifidobacterium*. Probiotics may improve host health by augmenting immune function, which occurs through reinforcing the mucosal barrier function, reducing the mucosal transfer of luminal organisms and metabolites to the host, increasing mucosal antibody production, strengthening epithelial integrity, and empowering the antagonism of pathogenic microorganisms. However, the results of studies in humans are varied, most likely due to methodological discrepancies (such as dose and duration of probiotic administration, sampling regimens, and microbiological techniques) and differences in host cohorts (age, health status). It is clear from *in vivo* studies in humans and animal models that probiotic efficacy in promoting health is strain dependent rather than species or genus specific (Floch et al., 2011; Khani et al., 2012).

THE ROLE OF SCFAs IN HEALTH AND DISEASE

The SCFAs (especially acetate, propionate, and butyrate) are the end products of gut microbial activity on DF and prebiotics and have been known for a few decades as playing a role in health and disease. Studies have been gaining momentum of late in exploring and expanding the scope and opportunity of investigation. The highest concentrations of SCFAs are in the colon following a meal. While SCFAs exert their effects locally in colon cells, they are as well transported and act systemically through their receptors. SCFAs are weak acids ($pK_a \sim 4.8$) and help lower the pH within the colon, thereby inhibiting the growth and activity of pathogenic bacteria. SCFAs can act independently of their receptors to modulate histone acetylation and cell proliferation.

The Antitumorigenic Effects of SCFAs

SCFAs, especially butyrate, exhibit strong antitumorigenic properties, inhibit cell proliferation, and induce differentiation and apoptosis in a variety of cell lines, including human colorectal cancer cell lines HCT-116 and HT-29

(Hinnebusch et al., 2002). Indeed, SCFAs have been shown to confer protection from the development of colorectal cancer. While propionate and butyrate significantly inhibit cell proliferation, acetate has little or no effect. Both propionate and butyrate have been shown to induce apoptosis *in vitro* (Fung et al., 2011).

Modulation of Histone Acetylation by SCFA

Epigenetic mechanisms—histone acetylation by histone acetyl transferases (MacDonald and Howe, 2009) and deacetylation by histone deacetylases (HDACs) (Seto and Yoshida, 2014)—can regulate and modulate gene expression. SCFA metabolites produced by microbiota inhibit HDAC activity, modulating gene expression in target cells (Grunstein, 1997). Mechanistically, SCFAs function as noncompetitive inhibitors of HDACs, effectively both *in vitro* and *in vivo* (Cousens et al., 1979). Butyrate is the most potent inhibitor of HDACs, achieving 80% inhibition of calf thymus HDAC1/2 *in vitro*; propionate and valerate are the next most efficacious with a 60% inhibition *in vitro*. It has been shown that butyrate and propionate specifically inhibit HDAC1 and HDAC3 (Huber et al., 2011). Butyrate induces histone hyperacetylation in both normal and cancerous cell lines (Aoyama et al., 2010; Khan and Jena, 2014; Kim et al., 2007; Li and Li, 2006; Wu et al., 2012), not due to acetylation *per se* but to HDAC inhibition, which in turn increases the half-life of histone acetyl groups (Cousens et al., 1979). Though SCFAs are reported to exert HDAC inhibition directly after entering colonocytes through a transporter—SLC5A8 (Singh et al., 2010)—there is also evidence that an SCFA receptor can mediate HDAC inhibition (Wu et al., 2012).

Butyrate, while inhibiting adipogenic differentiation, may enhance osteogenic differentiation from mouse adipose-derived mesenchymal stromal cells, making it a promising alternative for autologous skeletal tissue engineering through HDAC inhibition (Xu et al., 2009).

Receptors of SCFAs

Extraintestinal or systemic effects of SCFAs involve SCFA receptors. Of the four identified, three are G protein–coupled receptors (GPRs) (−41, −43, and −109a) and an olfactory receptor (OLFR78).

GPR41 (Free Fatty Acid Receptor 3: FFAR3)

Both GPR41/FFAR3 and GPR43/FFAR2, which had previously remained orphans (their endogenous ligands were not known), were deorphanized to be receptors for SCFAs (Brown et al., 2003; Le Poul et al., 2003).

GPR41 is found coupled to the G_i of G proteins (Brown et al., 2003) and is most responsive to propionate (EC_{50} 12 μM; Le Poul et al., 2003), although other SCFAs such as formate, acetate, butyrate, and isobutyrate also elicit varying degrees of activation. GPR41 is expressed in a variety of tissues and cell types, including the colon, kidneys, sympathetic nervous system, and blood vessels (Xiong et al., 2004; Tazoe et al., 2009), where they respond to microbiota-generated SCFAs to mediate the host's physiological responses. GPR41 has been implicated as having a role in inhibiting cell proliferation and inducing apoptosis (Kimura et al., 2001), energy homeostasis (Inoue et al., 2014), T-cell differentiation, and immunity (Kim et al., 2014).

GPR43 (Free Fatty Acid Receptor 2: FFAR2)

Though GPR43/FFAR2 is responsive to propionate (EC_{50} 300 μM; Le Poul et al., 2003), it can also be activated by acetate, and butyrate is found to be the strongest of the three ligands (Le Poul et al., 2003). While GPR41 couples only to G_i, GPR43 is found coupled to both the G_i and G_q of G proteins (Brown et al., 2003; Le Poul et al., 2003). GPR43 is expressed mainly in vasculature and immune cells, including lymphocytes, neutrophils, monocytes, and peripheral blood mononuclear cells (Karaki et al., 2006; Kimura et al., 2001; Tazoe et al., 2009; Xiong et al., 2004). SCFAs regulate the expression of cytokines and chemokines in both cultured intestinal epithelial cells and in mice via the activation of GPR43. GPR43-deficient mice have extensive dysregulation of inflammatory responses, showing excessive inflammation in models of colitis, arthritis, and asthma (Maslowski et al., 2009). GPR43-deficient mice exhibit obesity. GPR43 activation by SCFAs promotes glucagon-like peptide-1 (GLP-1) secretion in the gut, increasing insulin sensitivity and suppressing fat accumulation in adipose tissue (Kimura et al., 2013).

GPR109a

Initially, GPR109a was determined to be a niacin receptor and was subsequently found to be responsive to β-D-hydroxybutyrate as well as butyrate (Taggart et al., 2005) but not to acetate or propionate. GPR109a is expressed in colon epithelial cells proportionately to gut microbiota (Cresci et al., 2010). Activation of GPR109a by butyrate suppresses carcinogenesis (Singh et al., 2014).

OLFR78

OLFR78 has been deorphanized to be a receptor for SCFAs (Pluznick et al., 2013). OLFR78 responds to acetate and propionate (EC_{50} 2.35 mM and 920 μM, respectively) but not to butyrate. While OLFR78, GPR41, and GPR43 all localize to blood vessels, OLFR78, also localizes to a specialized renal vessel (afferent arteriole) where renin is stored and secreted. Both OLFR78 and GPR41 play SCFA-activated roles to modulate blood pressure (Pluznick et al., 2013).

Systemic Effects of SCFAs

At extraintestinal level, butyrate exerts potentially useful effects on many conditions, including hemoglobinopathies, metabolic diseases, hypercholesterolemia, insulin resistance, and ischemic stroke. Majority of these are related to its potent regulatory effects on gene expression. The wide spectrum of positive effects exerted by butyrate suggests a high potential therapeutic use in human medicine (Canani et al., 2011).

SCFAs: Energy Metabolism and Feeding Behavior

SCFAs are the main energy sources for gut cells and as such play a central role in the physiology and metabolism of these cells, including proliferation, differentiation, apoptosis, mucin production, and lipid metabolism (Roy et al., 2006). Administration of butyrate decreases plasma glucose and increases insulin levels in diabetic rats as a result of cell proliferation in the pancreatic islets (Khan and Jena, 2014).

Butyrate enhances fatty acid oxidation and thermogenesis by increasing the expression of peroxisome proliferator-activated receptor-γ coactivator-1α (PGC-1α) and the phosphorylation of adenosine-monophosphate–activated kinase in muscle and liver tissues, and the expression of PGC-1α and mitochondrial uncoupling protein-1 in brown adipose tissues (Donohoe et al., 2011). Propionate and butyrate activate intestinal gluconeogenesis via a gut–brain neural circuit, thereby promoting metabolic benefits on body weight and glucose control (De Vadder et al., 2014). Acetate reduces appetite by changing the expression profiles of appetite-regulating neuropeptides in hypothalamus through activation of TCA cycle in mice (Frost et al., 2014).

Propionate significantly increased the release of anorectic, postprandial plasma peptide YY, and GLP-1 from colonic cells in human primary culture. In overweight human subjects, it significantly reduced the energy intake, weight gain, intraabdominal adipose tissue distribution, and intrahepatocellular lipid content and prevented deterioration in insulin sensitivity (Chambers et al., 2014). Butyrate and propionate were shown to protect against diet-induced obesity and regulated gut hormones in mice (Lin et al., 2012). The oral administration of acetate improved glucose tolerance and suppressed obesity in diabetic rat models (Yamashita et al., 2007).

As various studies point toward propionate's hypophagic and hypocholesterolemic effects in humans, it may act as an important factor in the amelioration of obesity, a lifestyle disease arising due to energy imbalance. Thus, propionate along with acetate may also be involved in the regulation of adipogenesis, and adipokine release may depress appetite and combat the obesity epidemic (Arora et al., 2011).

SCFAs and Gut–Brain Axis Communication

The gut–brain axis is a bidirectional communication system between the central nervous system (CNS) and the GI tract. Regulation of the microbiota–brain–gut axis is essential for maintaining homeostasis, including that of the CNS. A number of approaches have been used to probe this axis, including the use of germ-free animals, probiotic agents, antibiotics, or animals exposed to pathogenic bacterial infections. Together, it is clear that the gut microbiota can be a key regulator of mood, cognition, pain, and obesity. Understanding microbiota–gut–brain communications is an exciting but challenging area of research that may contribute new insights into individual variations in cognition, personality, mood, sleep, and eating behavior and how they contribute to a range of neuropsychiatric diseases ranging from affective disorders to autism and schizophrenia. Finally the concept of psychobiotics, bacteria-based interventions with mental health benefits, is an emerging new field (Burokas et al., 2015).

SCFAs and Immunity

At the intestinal level, butyrate plays a regulatory role on transepithelial fluid transport, ameliorates mucosal inflammation and oxidative status, reinforces the epithelial defense barrier, and modulates visceral sensitivity and intestinal motility.

In mammals, besides their function as energy sources for epithelial cells, SCFAs are also potential immunostimulatory molecules (Kim et al., 2014; Shapiro et al., 2014), show improved lymphocyte function (Belkaid et al., 2013), and have immune-related effects resulting from their binding to the GPRs (Louis et al., 2014). GPR43 recognizes acetate, propionate, and butyrate and is highly expressed in neutrophils, macrophages, and monocytes. In contrast, GPR41 expression is low or undetectable in the same cells (Brestoff and Artis, 2013). GPR43 stimulation by SCFAs is necessary for the normal resolution of inflammatory responses in mice. Other immune-regulation activities of SCFAs include the inhibition of HDACs (Chang et al., 2014), regulation of autophagy (Donohoe et al., 2011), regulation of T-cell differentiation (Kim et al., 2014), and stimulation of heat shock protein production (Ren et al., 2001). Although the full spectrum of molecular mechanisms and the functioning of immune cells remains far from known, it is clear that SCFAs do play a central role in immunity of mammals.

Gut microbiota, via HDAC inhibition elicited by SCFA, affect the balance between pro- and antiinflammatory mechanisms (Arpaia et al., 2013). Propionate and butyrate inhibit production of tumor necrosis factor-α and nuclear factor-κB in neutrophils, thereby showing antiinflammatory effects (Vinolo et al., 2011).

ONGOING AND FUTURE DIRECTIONS

Although most studies of SCFAs show beneficial effects, more human *in vivo* studies are necessary to contribute to our current understanding of SCFA-mediated effects on colonic function in health and disease (Hamer et al., 2008).

All established prebiotics to date are carbohydrates, including inulin-type fructans and GOS. While other dietary carbohydrates also qualify as prebiotics, the interindividual variability in the microbial response to RS suggests successful dietary interventions with RS need to be personalized (Tremaroli and Backhed, 2012). Similarly the relation between various indigestible carbohydrates and their catalyzing bacteria for human health benefits should be explored (Martens et al., 2014).

Other than carbohydrates, cocoa flavanols may also function as prebiotics. They increase the relative abundance of *Bifidobacterium* and *Lactobacillus* at the expense of potentially pathogenic bacteria, notably the *Clostridium histolyticum* group (Martin et al., 2012). The other emerging potential prebiotics are seaweeds and microalgae (De Jesus Raposo et al., 2016).

The current concept of prebiotics should be revamped and broadened beyond *Bifidobacterium* and *Lactobacillus*, as these genera alone may not include all the important contributors to host health (Conlon et al., 2012). Emerging candidates include butyrate-producing bacterial groups related to *Eubacterium rectale/Roseburia* spp. and *Faecalibacterium prausnitzii*. Populations of *F. prausnitzii* are reported to be decreased in Crohn's disease, while populations of *Roseburia* relatives appear to be particularly sensitive to diet composition in human volunteer studies (Louis and Flint, 2009). Gut microbiota in older human subjects is reported to be least optimal for healthy aging (O'Connor et al., 2014). Cohort studies in Europe and China, despite the ethnic and dietary differences, revealed that patients with type 2 diabetes had a lower proportion of butyrate-producing and a larger proportion of nonbutyrate-producing *Clostridiales* (Karlsson et al., 2013; Tilg and Moschen, 2014).

While strategies for the microencapsulated delivery of bacteria (Cook et al., 2012) and the selective manipulation of microbiota (Montalban-Arques et al., 2015) have been reported, another attempt to modulate gut bacteria is fecal microbiota transplantation (Xu et al., 2015). Nevertheless, our current understanding of the intestinal ecosystem is still insufficient, as impacts of human virus and bacteriophages (virus infecting gut bacteria) also need to be taken into account for human health and disease. Further research efforts are needed to explore the scope of these potential aspects.

References

Aoyama, M., Kotani, J., Usami, M., 2010. Butyrate and propionate induced activated or non-activated neutrophil apoptosis via HDAC inhibitor activity but without activating GPR-41/GPR-43 pathways. Nutrition 26, 653–661.

Arora, T., Sharma, R., Frost, G., 2011. Propionate. Anti-obesity and satiety enhancing factor? Appetite 56, 511–515.

Arpaia, N., Campbell, C., Fan, X., Dikiy, S., van der Veeken, J., de Roos, P., et al., 2013. Metabolites produced by commensal bacteria promote peripheral regulatory T-cell generation. Nature 504, 451–455.

Arslanoglu, S., Moro, G.E., Schmitt, J., Tandoi, L., Rizzardi, S., Boehm, G., 2008. Early dietary intervention with a mixture of prebiotic oligosaccharides reduces the incidence of allergic manifestations and infections during the first two years of life. J. Nutr. 138, 1091–1095.

Belkaid, Y., Bouladoux, N., Hand, T.W., 2013. Effector and memory T cell responses to commensal bacteria. Trends Immunol. 34, 299–306.

Brestoff, J.R., Artis, D., 2013. Commensal bacteria at the interface of host metabolism and the immune system. Nat. Immunol. 14, 676–684.

Brown, A.J., Goldsworthy, S.M., Barnes, A.A., Eilert, M.M., Tcheang, L., Daniels, D., et al., 2003. The orphan G protein-coupled receptors GPR41 and GPR43 are activated by propionate and other short chain carboxylic acids. J. Biol. Chem. 278, 11312–11319.

Brown, K., DeCoffe, D., Molcan, E., Gibson, D.L., 2012. Diet-induced dysbiosis of the intestinal microbiota and the effects on immunity and disease. Nutrients 4, 1095–1119.

Burokas, A., Moloney, R.D., Dinan, T.G., Cryan, J.F., 2015. Microbiota regulation of the mammalian gut-brain axis. Adv. Appl. Microbiol. 91, 1–62.

Canani, R.B., Costanzo, M.D., Leone, L., Pedata, M., Meli, R., Calignano, A., 2011. Potential beneficial effects of butyrate in intestinal and extraintestinal diseases. World J. Gastroenterol. 17, 1519–1528.

Chambers, E.S., Viardot, A., Psichas, A., Morrison, D.J., Murphy, K.G., Zac-Varghese, S.E., et al., 2014. Effects of targeted delivery of propionate to the human colon on appetite regulation, body weight maintenance and adiposity in overweight adults. Gut 64, 1744–1754.

Chang, P.V., Hao, L., Offermanns, S., Medzhitov, R., 2014. The microbial metabolite butyrate regulates intestinal macrophage function via histone deacetylase inhibition. Proc. Natl. Acad. Sci. U.S.A. 111, 2247–2252.

Conlon, M.A., Bird, A.R., 2015. The impact of diet and lifestyle on gut microbiota and human health. Nutrients 7, 17–44.

Conlon, M.A., Kerr, C.A., McSweeney, C.S., Dunne, R.A., Shaw, J.M., Kang, S., et al., 2012. Resistant starches protect against colonic DNA damage and alter microbiota and gene expression in rats fed a western diet. J. Nutr. 142, 832–840.

Cook, M.T., Tzortzis, G., Charalampopoulos, D., Khutoryanskiy, V.V., 2012. Microencapsulation of probiotics for gastrointestinal delivery. J Control. Release 162, 56–67.

Cousens, L.S., Gallwitz, D., Alberts, B.M., 1979. Different accessibilities in chromatin to histone acetylase. J. Biol. Chem. 254, 1716–1723.

Cresci, G.A., Thangaraju, M., Mellinger, J.D., Liu, K., Ganapathy, V., 2010. Colonic gene expression in conventional and germ-free mice with a focus on the butyrate receptor GPR109A and the butyrate transporter SLC5A8. J. Gastrointest. Surg. 14, 449–461.

De Jesus Raposo, M.F., de Morais, A.M., de Morais, R.M., 2016. Emergent sources of prebiotics: seaweeds and microalgae. Marine Drugs 14, 27. http://dx.doi.org/10.3390/md14020027.

Dethlefsen, L., McFall-Ngai, M., Relman, D.A., 2007. An ecological and evolutionary perspective on human-microbe mutualism and disease. Nature 449, 811–818.

De Vadder, F., Kovatcheva-Datchary, P., Goncalves, D., Vinera, J., Zitoun, C., Duchampt, A., et al., 2014. Microbiota-generated metabolites promote metabolic benefits via gut-brain neural circuits. Cell 156, 84–96.

Donohoe, D.R., Garge, N., Zhang, X., Sun, W., O'Connell, T.M., Bunger, M.K., et al., 2011. The microbiome and butyrate regulate energy metabolism and autophagy in the mammalian colon. Cell Metab. 13, 517–526.

Eckburg, P.B., Bik, E.M., Bernstein, C.N., Purdom, E., Dethlefsen, L., Sargent, M., et al., 2005. Diversity of the human intestinal microbial flora. Science 308, 1635–1638.

El Kaoutari, A., Armougom, F., Gordon, J.I., Raoult, D., Henrissat, B., 2013. The abundance and variety of carbohydrate-active enzymes in the human gut microbiota. Nat. Rev. Microbiol. 11, 497–504.

Floch, M.H., Walker, W.A., Madsen, K., Sanders, M.E., Macfarlane, G.T., Flint, H.J., et al., 2011. Recommendations for probiotic use—2011 update. J. Clin. Gastroenterol. 45, S168–S171.

Frost, G., Sleeth, M.L., Sahuri-Arisoylu, M., Lizarbe, B., Cerdan, S., Brody, L., et al., 2014. The short-chain fatty acid acetate reduces appetite via a central homeostatic mechanism. Nat. Commun. 5, 3611. http://dx.doi.org/10.1038/ncomms4611.

Fung, K.Y., Brierley, G.V., Henderson, S., Hoffmann, P., McColl, S.R., Lockett, T., et al., 2011. Butyrate-induced apoptosis in HCT116 colorectal cancer cells includes induction of a cell stress response. J. Proteome Res. 10, 1860–1869.

Gibson, G.R., Roberfroid, M.B., 1995 Dietary modulation of the human colonic microbiota—introducing the concept of prebiotics. J. Nutr. 125, 1401–1412.

Gibson, G.R., Scott, K.P., Rastall, R.A., Tuohy, K.M., Hotchkiss, A., Dubert-Ferrandon, A., et al., 2010. Dietary prebiotics: current status and new definition. Food Sci. Technol. Bull. Funct Foods 7, 1–19.

Grunstein, M., 1997. Histone acetylation in chromatin structure and transcription. Nature 389, 349–352.

Hamer, H.M., Jonkers, D., Venema, K., Vanhoutvin, S., Troost, F.J., Brummer, R.J., 2008. Review article: the role of butyrate on colonic function. Aliment. Pharmacol. Ther. 27, 104–119.

Harmsen, H.J., Wildeboer-Veloo, A.C.M., Raangs, G.C., Wagendorp, A.A., Klijn, N., Bindels, J.G., et al., 2000. Analysis of intestinal flora development in breast-fed and formula-fed infants by using molecular identification and detection methods. J. Pediatr. Gastroenterol. Nutr. 30, 61–67.

Hinnebusch, B.F., Meng, S., Wu, J.T., Archer, S.Y., Hodin, R.A., 2002. The effects of short-chain fatty acids on human colon cancer cell phenotype are associated with histone hyperacetylation. J. Nutr. 132, 1012–1017.

Huber, K., Doyon, G., Plaks, J., Fyne, E., Mellors, J.W., Sluis-Cremer, N., 2011. Inhibitors of histone deacetylases: correlation between isoform specificity and reactivation of HIV type 1 (HIV-1) from latently infected cells. J. Biol. Chem. 286, 22211–22218.

Huurre, A., Kalliomaki, M., Rautava, S., Rinne, M., Salminen, S., Isolauri, E., 2008. Mode of delivery—Effects on gut microbiota and humoral immunity. Neonatology 93, 236–240.

Inoue, D., Tsujimoto, G., Kimura, I., 2014. Regulation of energy homeostasis by GPR41. Front. Endocrinol. (Lausanne) 5, 81. http://dx.doi.org/10.3389/fendo.2014.00081.

Karaki, S., Mitsui, R., Hayashi, H., Kato, I., Sugiya, H., Iwanaga, T., et al., 2006. Short-chain fatty acid receptor, GPR43, is expressed by enteroendocrine cells and mucosal mast cells in rat intestine. Cell Tissue Res. 324, 353–360.

Karlsson, F.H., Tremaroli, V., Nookaew, I., Bergstrom, G., Behre, C.J., Fagerberg, B., et al., 2013. Gut metagenome in European women with normal, impaired and diabetic glucose control. Nature 498, 99–103.

Kelly, D., King, T., Aminov, R., 2007. Importance of microbial colonization of the gut in early life to the development of immunity. Mutat. Res. 622, 58–69.

Khan, S., Jena, G.B., 2014. Protective role of sodium butyrate, a HDAC inhibitor on beta-cell proliferation, function and glucose homeostasis through modulation of p38/ERK MAPK and apoptotic pathways: study in juvenile diabetic rat. Chem. Biol. Interact. 213, 1–12.

Khani, S., Hosseini, H.M., Taheri, M., Nourani, M.R., Imani Fooladi, A.A., 2012. Probiotics as an alternative strategy for prevention and treatment of human diseases: a review. Inflamm. Allergy Drug Targets 11, 79–89.

Kim, C.H., Park, J., Kim, M., 2014. Gut microbiota-derived short-chain fatty acids, T cells, and inflammation. Immune Netw. 14, 277–288.

Kim, H.J., Rowe, M., Ren, M., Hong, J.S., Chen, P.S., Chuang, D.M., 2007. Histone deacetylase inhibitors exhibit anti-inflammatory and neuroprotective effects in a rat permanent ischemic model of stroke: multiple mechanisms of action. J. Pharmacol. Exp. Ther. 321, 892–901.

Kimura, M., Mizukami, Y., Miura, T., Fujimoto, K., Kobayashi, S., Matsuzaki, M., 2001. Orphan G protein-coupled receptor, GPR41, induces apoptosis via a p53/Bax pathway during ischemic hypoxia and reoxygenation. J. Biol. Chem. 276, 26453–26460.

Kimura, I., Ozawa, K., Inoue, D., Imamura, T., Kimura, K., Maeda, T., et al., 2013. The gut microbiota suppresses insulin-mediated fat accumulation via the short-chain fatty acid receptor GPR43. Nat. Commun. 4, 1829. http://dx.doi.org/10.1038/ncomms2852.

Koboziev, I., Webb, C.R., Furr, K.L., Grisham, M.B., 2014. Role of the enteric microbiota in intestinal homeostasis and inflammation. Free Radic. Biol. Med. 68, 122–133.
Le Huerou-Luron, I., Blat, S., Boudry, G., 2010. Breast- v. formula-feeding: impacts on the digestive tract and immediate and long-term health effects. Nutr. Res. Rev. 23, 23–36.
Le Poul, E., Loison, C., Struyf, S., Springael, J.Y., Lannoy, V., Decobecq, M.E., et al., 2003. Functional characterization of human receptors for short chain fatty acids and their role in polymorphonuclear cell activation. J. Biol. Chem. 278, 25481–25489.
Ley, R.E., Hamady, M., Lozupone, C., Turnbaugh, P.J., Ramey, R.R., Bircher, J.S., et al., 2008. Evolution of mammals and their gut microbes. Science 320, 1647–1651.
Li, R.W., Li, C., 2006. Butyrate induces profound changes in gene expression related to multiple signal pathways in bovine kidney epithelial cells. BMC Genom. 7, 234247. http://dx.doi.org/10.1186/1471-2164-7-234.
Lin, H.V., Frassetto, A., Kowalik Jr., E.J., Nawrocki, A.R., Lu, M.M., Kosinski, J.R., et al., 2012. Butyrate and propionate protect against diet-induced obesity and regulate gut hormones via free fatty acid receptor 3-independent mechanism. PLoS ONE 7, e35240. http://dx.doi.org/10.1371/journal.pone.0035240.
Louis, P., Flint, H.J., 2009. Diversity, metabolism and microbial ecology of butyrate-producing bacteria from the human large intestine. FEMS Microbiol. Lett. 294, 1–8.
Louis, P., Hold, G.L., Flint, H.J., 2014. The gut microbiota, bacterial metabolites and colorectal cancer. Nat. Rev. Microbiol. 12, 661–672.
MacDonald, V.E., Howe, L.J., 2009. Histone acetylation: where to go and how to get there. Epigenetics 4, 139–143.
Martens, E.C., Kelly, A.G., Tauzin, A.S., Brumer, H., 2014. The devil lies in the details: how variations in polysaccharide fine-structure impact the physiology and evolution of gut microbes. J. Mol. Biol. 426, 3851–3865.
Martin, F.P.J., Montoliu, I., Nagy, K., Moco, S., Collino, S., Guy, P., et al., 2012. Specific dietary preferences are linked to differing gut microbial metabolic activity in response to dark chocolate intake. J. Proteome Res. 11, 6252–6263.
Maslowski, K.M., Vieira, A.T., Ng, A., Kranich, J., Sierro, F., Yu, D., et al., 2009. Regulation of inflammatory responses by gut microbiota and chemoattractant receptor GPR43. Nature 461, 1282–1286.
Montalban-Arques, A., De Schryver, P., Bossier, P., Gorkiewicz, G., Mulero, V., Gatlin, D.M., et al., 2015. Selective manipulation of the gut microbiota improves immune status in vertebrates. Front. Immunol. 6, 512. http://dx.doi.org/10.3389/fimmu.2015.00512.
O'Connor, E.M., O'Herlihy, E.A., O'Toole, P.W., 2014. Gut microbiota in older subjects: variation, health consequences and dietary intervention prospects. Proc. Nutr. Soc. 73, 441–451.
Pluznick, J.L., Protzko, R.J., Gevorgyan, H., Peterlin, Z., Sipos, A., Han, J., et al., 2013. Olfactory receptor responding to gut microbiota-derived signals plays a role in renin secretion and blood pressure regulation. Proc. Natl. Acad. Sci. U.S.A. 110, 4410–4415.
Ren, H., Musch, M.W., Kojima, K., Boone, D., Ma, A., Chang, E.B., 2001. Short-chain fatty acids induce intestinal epithelial heat shock protein 25 expression in rats and IEC 18 cells. Gastroenterology 121, 631–639.
Roy, C.C., Kien, C.L., Bouthillier, L., Levy, E., 2006. Short-chain fatty acids: ready for prime time? Nutr. Clin. Pract. 21, 351–366.
Seto, E., Yoshida, M., 2014. Erasers of histone acetylation: the histone deacetylase enzymes. Cold Spring Harb. Perspect. Biol. 6, a018713. http://dx.doi.org/10.1101/cshperspect.
Shapiro, H., Thaiss, C.A., Levy, M., Elinav, E., 2014. The cross talk between microbiota and the immune system: metabolites take center stage. Curr. Opin. Immunol. 30, 54–62.
Singh, N., Gurav, A., Sivaprakasam, S., Brady, E., Padia, R., Shi, H., et al., 2014. Activation of Gpr109a, receptor for niacin and the commensal metabolite butyrate, suppresses colonic inflammation and carcinogenesis. Immunity 40, 128–139.
Singh, N., Thangaraju, M., Prasad, P.D., Martin, P.M., Lambert, N.A., Boettger, T., et al., 2010. Blockade of dendritic cell development by bacterial fermentation products butyrate and propionate through a transporter (Slc5a8)-dependent inhibition of histone deacetylases. J. Biol. Chem. 285, 27601–27608.
Slavin, J., 2013. Fiber and prebiotics: mechanisms and health benefits. Nutrients 5, 1417–1435.
Spiller, G.A. (Ed.), 2001. CRC Handbook of Dietary Fiber in Human Nutrition, third ed. CRC Press. Print ISBN: 978-0-8493-2387-4. eBook ISBN: 978-1-4200-3851-4.
Taggart, A.K., Kero, J., Gan, X., Cai, T.Q., Cheng, K., Ippolito, M., et al., 2005. (D)-Beta-hydroxybutyrate inhibits adipocyte lipolysis via the nicotinic acid receptor PUMA-G. J. Biol. Chem. 280, 26649–26652.
Tazoe, H., Otomo, Y., Karaki, S., Kato, I., Fukami, Y., Terasaki, M., et al., 2009. Expression of short-chain fatty acid receptor GPR41 in the human colon. Biomed. Res. 30, 149–156.
Tilg, H., Moschen, A.R., 2014. Microbiota and diabetes: an evolving relationship. Gut 63, 1513–1521.
Tremaroli, V., Backhed, F., 2012. Functional interactions between the gut microbiota and host metabolism. Nature 489, 242–249.
Ursell, L.K., Metcalf, J.L., Parfrey, L.W., Knight, R., 2012. Defining the human microbiome. Nutr. Rev. 70, S38–S44.
Vinolo, M.A., Rodrigues, H.G., Hatanaka, E., Sato, F.T., Sampaio, S.C., Curi, R., 2011. Suppressive effect of short-chain fatty acids on production of proinflammatory mediators by neutrophils. J. Nutr. Biochem. 22, 849–855.
Vissavajjhala, P., 2014. Importance of food and nutrients as medicine for health and wellness-An overview. Indian J. Agric. Biochem. 27, 93–103.
Wu, J., Zhou, Z., Hu, Y., Dong, S., 2012. Butyrate-induced GPR41 activation inhibits histone acetylation and cell growth. J Genet. Genomics 39, 375–384.
Xiong, Y., Miyamoto, N., Shibata, K., Valasek, M.A., Motoike, T., Kedzierski, R.M., et al., 2004. Short-chain fatty acids stimulate leptin production in adipocytes through the G protein-coupled receptor GPR41. Proc. Natl. Acad. Sci. U.S.A. 101, 1045–1050.
Xu, Y., Hammerick, K.E., James, A.W., Carre, A.L., Leucht, P., Giaccia, A.J., et al., 2009. Inhibition of histone deacetylase activity in reduced oxygen environment enhances the osteogenesis of mouse adipose-derived stromal cells. Tissue Eng. Part A 15, 3697–3707.
Xu, M.Q., Cao, H.L., Wang, W.Q., Wang, S., Cao, X.C., Yan, F., et al., 2015. Fecal microbiota transplantation broadening its application beyond intestinal disorders. World J. Gastroenterol. 21, 102–111.
Yamashita, H., Fujisawa, K., Ito, E., Idei, S., Kawaguchi, N., Kimoto, M., et al., 2007. Improvement of obesity and glucose tolerance by acetate in type 2 diabetic Otsuka Long-Evans Tokushima fatty (OLETF) rats. Biosci. Biotechnol. Biochem. 71, 1236–1243.
Zoetendal, E.G., Vaughan, E.E., De Vos, W.M., 2006. A microbial world within us. Mol. Microbiol. 59, 1639–1650.

CHAPTER

2

Aging and the Recovery of Skin Function and Appearance

Adele Sparavigna

Clinical Research and Bioengineering Institute, Monza, Italy

INTRODUCTION

Aging can be defined as a physiological process characterized by a continuous and irreversible loss of homeostasis that involves the whole body. With the progressive increase of life expectancy in developed countries, the prevalence of aging-related diseases is increasing, making it necessary to implement specific preventive strategies. The leading role of diet in maintaining health throughout the human life cycle has been well established by a multitude of scientific papers from different medical disciplines. The effects of an unbalanced diet can be detected at different levels: diets rich in saturated fats, cholesterol, and animal protein or high in salt and sugar can not only increase metabolic and cardiovascular disease risk but also contribute to the accumulation of oxidative and inflammatory responses, increasing the production of free radicals that damage all cellular constituents and lead to an acceleration in the aging process. Skin, as an integral part of the system, is affected by these responses. Wrinkles, atrophy, gray spots, and loss of hydration and elasticity are the most visible signs. To understand how diet contributes to the maintenance of skin health is particularly relevant because skin aging is determined by the combined influences of intrinsic factors (chronological, hormonal, and genetic) and extrinsic ones that can be divided in behavioral factors such as sun exposure (responsible for photoaging), cigarette smoking, diet, alcohol drinking, drug abuse, and environmental factors such as pollution, weather, and humidity.

The correlation between diet and skin health was recently well established for several skin diseases. Examples include acne (especially for milk and dairy products, which have been correlated in several studies with more severe diseases) (Melnik, 2015), atopic dermatitis (which improves with the intake of essential fatty acids and certain probiotics) (Mohajeri and Newman, 2014), and psoriasis (which is significantly correlated with metabolic syndrome) (Voiculescu et al., 2014). Correcting poor and unbalanced nutrition undoubtedly improves skin health, but what is not yet entirely clear is what substances can improve skin health and appearance and counteract skin aging in a targeted manner for a person who is well nourished. Thanks to the analysis of recent scientific literature and my personal experience as a dermatologist and researcher, I will try to investigate these issues, focusing on the traditional feeding practices of Italy, my home country, which are most famously represented by the Mediterranean diet.

SKIN AGING

As far as skin is concerned, the aging phenomenon is caused by exogenous and endogenous factors. Ultraviolet (UV) radiation exposure is the main exogenous factor responsible for aging in the skin, especially in fair-skinned Caucasian subjects and exerts its effect predominantly through the accumulation of free radicals in the tegument.

Nutrition and Functional Foods for Healthy Aging.
DOI: http://dx.doi.org/10.1016/B978-0-12-805376-8.00002-2

Smoking, pollution, sleep deprivation, and poor nutrition are other exogenous factors that promote skin aging. The difference between the two types of skin aging—exogenous and endogenous—can be observed by comparing UV-protected and UV-exposed sites. Endogenously aged skin displays epidermal and dermal atrophy, a reduced extracellular matrix (collagen, elastin fibers, and glycosaminoglicans), and marked vascular changes. Skin functions are impaired: thermoregulation, glandular function, wound healing, the epidermal barrier, and melanogenesis are all diminished. Exogenous aging also displays thickened stratum corneum, the aggregation of abnormal elastic fibers in the dermis (solar elastosis), and deep altered production and distribution of melanin, which leads to uneven pigmentation.

DIET AND SKIN AGING

The contribution of diet to how skin ages remains largely unclear. While skin scientists know what skin diseases and impairments can occur because of most nutritional deficiencies (e.g., vitamins E and C, carotenoids, and polyunsaturated fatty acids), we miss studies that precisely correlate the signs of aging with qualitative and quantitative nutrient intakes (Draelos, 2013) We do not know to what extent a "good diet"—which is hard to define—or a supplemented diet can contribute to successful skin aging. Cosgrove et al. (2007) evaluated the associations between nutrient intakes and the appearance of aging skin using data from the first National Health and Nutrition Examination Survey conducted in the United States between 1971 and 1974. Clinical dermatological examinations were conducted of 4025 women ages 40–75 years and data were gathered for their dietary habits and other variables (e.g., body mass index, race, energy intake, physical activity, and smoking). The authors found that higher intakes of vitamin C and linoleic acid and lower intakes of fats and carbohydrates were associated with better skin aging appearance (fewer wrinkles, less senile dryness, and less skin atrophy) independently of other factors known to affect skin aging. This study is different from many others in the literature because it examined nutrient intakes from food rather than from nutritional supplements or topically applied nutrients. Nevertheless, no direct conclusion about nutrients and skin aging appearance could be determined. Significant dietary changes have occurred in the past 30 years, however, and the use of facial cosmetics has seen a tremendous increase. For these reasons, studying the relationship between dietary attitudes and skin aging has become even more complicated. On one side is the structural and biochemical complexity of aging in skin and its appendages; on the other side is the extreme variability of genetic, physiological, and pathological factors as well as environment and behavior. All of these affect our knowledge in this field. Until we have at our disposal techniques to make in vivo measurements of the different nutrients in the skin (this can only be considered science fiction now), it will be almost impossible to accurately evaluate the effect of single or grouped dietary constituents on skin aging. Anyway, although science and common sense suggest that a healthy diet such as the Mediterranean diet with its emphasis on fresh fruits and vegetables, nuts, fish, olive oil, and integral cereals may improve aging in general and skin appearance in particular, many challenges remain in designing and running nutritional research (Draelos, 2013). If we look at the aging phenomenon on a biological basis, we may be able to better predict how nutritional factors can affect it. Up to now, the main mechanisms causing aging of tissue and organs are as follows:

- Oxidative stress
- Nonenzymatic glycation products
- Sex hormone imbalance
- Telomere shortening

In this chapter we will analyze each of these mechanisms and their correlations with dietary habits.

Oxidative Stress and Chronic Inflammation

Reactive oxygen species (ROS) are essential to life. We breathe oxygen, and properly generated ROS has beneficial protective and antiaging effects on cells. Nevertheless, ROS production from several sources in our everyday lives such as UV exposure, inflammation, stress, pollution, and smoking leads to an excess of free radicals that hurt the chemical stability of cellular structures. This is why cells have their own intrinsic antioxidative enzyme systems such as superoxide dismutase that are able to neutralize ROS by taking a free electron from another source. Vitamins A, C, and E and polyphenols all exert strong antioxidation effects and work synergistically. A fundamental strategy for enhancing skin protection from oxidative stress is to support the endogenous antioxidant system via the antioxidants normally present in the skin. Since these antioxidants work in a complex harmony, a permanent intake of isolated antioxidants is not physiologically as effective as consuming a diet rich in fruits and vegetables; this remains the healthiest and safest way to maintain youthful and healthy skin.

A vast literature has been produced over the past decades about the role of antioxidants in a balanced diet. Even more detailed recent studies directly correlate dietary intake of antioxidants with skin protection: resveratrol has been demonstrated to attenuate skin atrophy induced by oxidative damage (Watanabe et al., 2015), and cocoa (Karim et al., 2014) and green tea polyphenols (Roh et al., 2015) confer protective effects on skin against UV-induced acceleration of skin aging. So far, a variety of phytomolecules derived in particular from polyphenols, triterpenes, and sterol classes have demonstrated a promising activity on skin aging. Among them, carnosic acid, curcuglicoside, curcumin, glycyrrizic acid, and extracts and pure compounds from Fabaceae, Asteraceae, and Zingiberaceae appear most interesting (Tundis et al., 2015). In particular, maslinic acid found in olive oil is a natural triterpene that has protective effects against chronic inflammatory diseases through its modulation of arachidonic acid metabolism (Yap and Lim, 2015).

Nonenzymatic Glycation Products

Nonenzymatic glycation was first diagnosed and described in diabetic patients as leading to the accumulation of advanced glycation end (AGE) products in several tissues and organs. AGEs have been associated with end-stage renal disease, chronic obstructive pulmonary disease, atherosclerosis, and connective tissue impairment. The term *glycation* has emerged in recent years to describe one of the most important aging factors for human tissues and organs (Simm et al., 2015); it now commonly refers to the nonenzymatic process of proteins, lipids, and nucleic acids covalently bonding to the sugar molecules glucose and fructose. Glycation occurs at random molecular sites and generally results in the inhibition of the target molecule's functions. Immunostaining has demonstrated the presence of glycation in aged skin and resulting structural, morphological, and functional impairments. Glucose and fructose play a critical role in glycation, but foods containing glycated proteins also provide further exogenous AGEs to an organism. Barbecued meats, toasted bread, dark-colored soft drinks, and donuts contain high levels of AGEs. Now we know that grilling, frying, and roasting methods produce higher levels of AGEs in cooked food. Orally consumed and endogenous AGEs are proinflammatory and accumulate on nucleic acids, proteins, and lipids. Fortunately, dietary habits can reduce AGEs in the body. First, a diet should contain low levels of monosaccharides, which are responsible for the glycation phenomenon. Water-based cooking methods such as boiling and streaming produce a logarithmically lower amount of AGEs. Several aromatic herbs and spices are believed to be able to reduce the endogenous production of AGEs: cinnamon, oregano, cloves, ginger, garlic, α-lipoic acid, carnitine, flavonoids, resveratrol, vitamins, zinc, and manganese. Furthermore, since glycation is accelerated in the presence of an ROS, the intake of antioxidants is able to limit the production of endogenous AGEs (Draelos, 2013).

Sex Hormone Imbalances

Some of the changes that affect aging skin in menopausal women occur as a consequence of estrogen deficiency. The mechanisms involved seem to originate from the dermal and epidermal reduction of cellularity, collagen quantity, and skin thinning. This mechanism is responsible for a total cumulative loss of about 30% of skin thickness in the first 5 years after menopause. Keratinocytes and dermal fibroblasts exhibit receptors for sexual hormones, which is why we observe collagen and glycosaminoglycans deficiency after menopause. The role of estrogens in maintaining dermal thickness is demonstrated by the fact that orally administrated isoflavone-rich soy extract during six consecutive months causes significant increases in epithelial and dermal thickness (Accorsi-Neto et al., 2009). Since estrogen therapy is not always feasible due to its side effects and contraindications, phytormones in the diet represent a natural and valid alternative to hormonal therapy after menopause. Although phytoestrogens are nonsteroidal substances, they have a heterocyclic phenolic composition that shows structural similarities to the estrogens. Of particular interest is their higher affinity for the β subtype of the estrogen receptor that is present in bones, skin, and the cardiovascular system (all the organs suffering from estrogen deprivation after menopause) while having reduced or even antagonist effects on the α subtype of the estrogen receptor (found in the uterus and breast, which are at higher risk of cancerization after estrogen stimulation). This is why phytoestrogens are considered selective estrogen receptor modulators and are widely used to treat menopause estrogen deficiency. Soy isoflavones—in particular, genistein—are the best studied phytoestrogens (Nagaraju et al., 2013). Anyway, while soy is very abundant in many Asian diets, it is not characteristic of the Mediterranean diet, which helps explain why not all Western women are able to tolerate it. Also allergies to soy are more frequent in Western countries (Cordle, 2004). Other vegetables contain many other natural sources of phytoestrogens (Agradi et al., 2006). Species belonging to the Leguminosae, Apiaceae, Graminaceae, Iridaceae, Chenopodiaceae, Cruciferae (or Brassicaceae), and Solanaceae families provide significant amounts of phytoestrogens. Among the species from these families are such widely consumed foods such as beans and other legumes, tomatoes, cabbage, carrots, and some cereals. When supported by proper cooking practices as in the Mediterranean tradition, vegetable foods rich in phytoestrogens can help maintain healthy and young skin.

Telomere Shortening

Telomeres are DNA–protein complexes at the end of chromosomes that protect the genetic material and promote chromosomal stability. Telomeres shorten with time because they cannot replicate completely each time the cell divides; for that reason, they may be the most powerful biological clock yet elucidated. Furthermore, it has been demonstrated that being overweight, stressed, and sedentary accelerates the shortening of telomeres (Epel, 2012). Progressive shortening of telomeres leads to senescence, apoptosis, and oncogenic transformation of somatic cells that affect an individual's health and lifespan. Shorter telomeres have also been associated with increased skin aging (Kosmadaki and Gilchrest, 2004; Masood, 2011).

Telomere length positively correlates with the dietary intake of fiber and negatively associates with waist circumference. A diet rich in antioxidant omega-3 fatty acids and vitamins C and E, and beta-carotene is associated with a reduced rate of telomere shortening. Antioxidants are known to protect telomeric DNA from oxidative damage caused by extrinsic and intrinsic DNA damaging agents. Reduced protein intake also seems to increase cell longevity. Of notable interest is that improved nutrition, increased exercise, and better stress management might also booster the enzyme telomerase, which directs the replication of telomeres and adds telomeric repeat sequences to the chromosomal DNA ends.

THE MEDITERRANEAN DIET

The Mediterranean diet was studied for the first time in a systematic and scientific way by American scientist Ancel Keys, who demonstrated the influence of diet on longevity and health. This analysis involved some Mediterranean countries in the 1950s following the austere times in the wake of World War II, which were characterized by a physically active lifestyle and a frugal diet based mostly on vegetable products (Monteagudo et al., 2015). The Mediterranean coast is characterized by great ethnic, cultural, religious, economic, and political differences that may have influenced the quantity and quality of food. Nevertheless, these countries traditionally share the availability of the same foods derived from agriculture, herding, and fishing. Some studies widely accepted by the scientific community showed that in the early 1960s in these geographical areas, life expectancy was almost the highest in the world and that the incidence of heart disease, some cancers, and other chronic diseases related to diet was among the lowest in the world. This occurred despite high smoking, low socioeconomic levels, and a shortage of health care. It is significant that this diet is common where olive trees are traditionally grown; one accepted definition of this nutritional pattern relates to diet practiced in Mediterranean areas dominated by olive trees (Keys, 1980).

The characteristics of the Mediterranean diet are abundant fruits, vegetables, wholemeal bread and cereals, legumes, nuts, and seeds, all of them fresh, natural, seasonal, and locally sourced. Olive oil is the principal source of fat, daily servings of fresh fruit are used as dessert, and refined sugars or honey are consumed only a few times a week. Dairy products (principally cheese and yogurt) are consumed daily in moderate amounts, as are fish and poultry. Only a few eggs (0–4) are consumed per week; red meat is eaten in modest amounts; and wine, generally red, is also consumed in modest amounts, generally during the meal (Pitsavos et al., 2005). Numerous studies over several decades confirmed that the Mediterranean diet can reduce the risk of cardiovascular and metabolic disease and improve cognitive health (Davis et al., 2015), but what about skin health?

Recent publications regarding the correlation between eating habits and skin cancer have demonstrated that the Mediterranean diet may contribute to lower rates of skin cancers despite high levels of solar radiation in Mediterranean countries (Fortes et al., 2008; Malagoli et al., 2015; Shapira, 2010). Taking into account what we learned from the scientific literature and what has been explained in this chapter, the correspondence between the Mediterranean diet and good dietary habits based on potentiating antiaging mechanisms in the skin is quite high (Fig. 2.1).

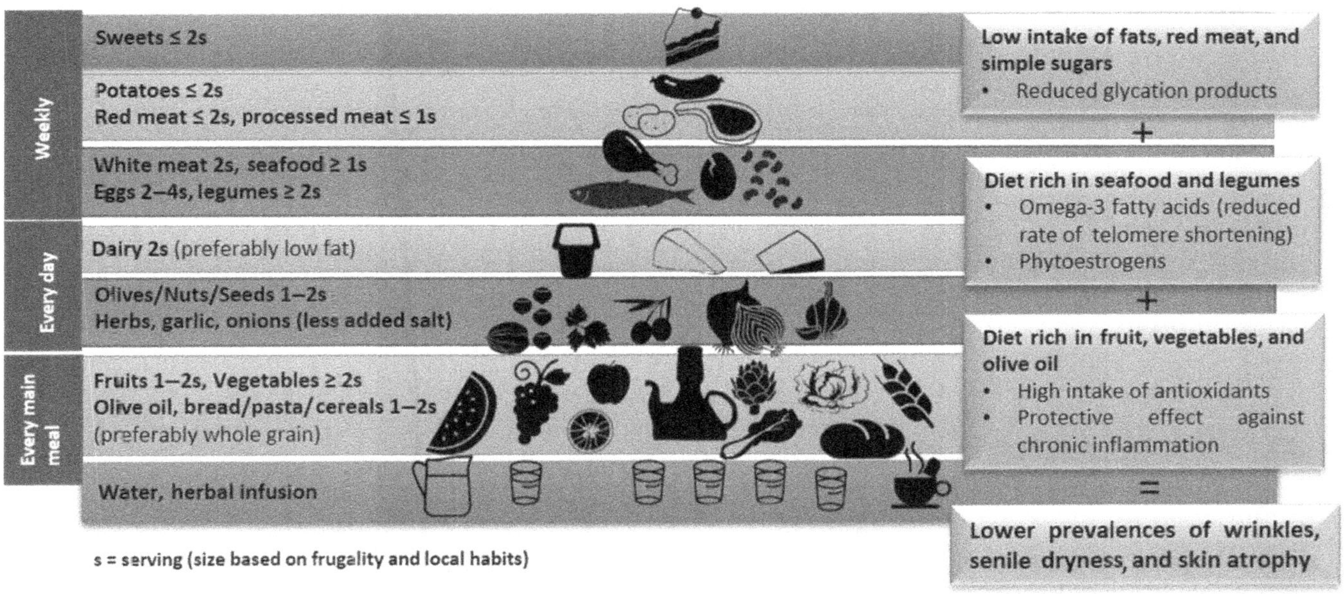

FIGURE 2.1 Skin Mediterranean diet pyramid. *Adapted from Dernini, S., Berry, E.M., 2015. Mediterranean diet: from a healthy diet to a sustainable dietary pattern. Front. Nutr. 2: 1 (Dernini and Berry, 2015).*

References

Accorsi-Neto, A., Haidar, M., Simões, R., Simões, M., Soares-Jr, J., Baracat, E., 2009. Effects of isoflavones on the skin of postmenopausal women: a pilot study Clinics 64 (6), 505–510

Agradi, E., Vegeto, E., Sozzi, A., Fico, G., Regondi, S., Tomè, F., 2006. Traditional healthy Mediterranean diet: estrogenic activity of plants used as food and flavoring agents. Phytother. Res. 20 (8), 670–675.

Cordle, C.T., 2004. Soy protein allergy: incidence and relative severity. J. Nutr. 134 (5), 1213S–1219S.

Cosgrove, M.C., Franco, O.H., Granger, S.P., Murray, P.G., Mayes, A.E., 2007. Dietary nutrient intakes and skin-aging appearance among middle-aged American women. Am. J. Clin. Nutr. 86, 1225–1231.

Davis, C., Bryan, J., Hodgson, J., Murphy, K., 2015. Definition of the Mediterranean diet: a literature review. Nutrients 7 (11), 9139–9153.

Dernini, S., Berry, E.M., 2015. Mediterranean diet: from a healthy diet to a sustainable dietary pattern. Front. Nutr 2, 1.

Draelos, Z.D., 2013. Aging skin: the role of diet: facts and controversies. Clin. Dermatol. 31, 701–706.

Epel, E., 2012. How "reversible" is telomeric aging? Cancer Prev. Res. (Phila) 5, 1163–1168.

Fortes, C., Mastroeni, S., Melchi, F., Pilla, M.A., Antonelli, G., Camaioni, D., et al., 2008. A protective effect of the Mediterranean diet for cutaneous melanoma Int. J. Epidemiol. 37 (5), 1018–1029.

Karim, A.A., Azlan, A., Ismail, A., Hashim, P., Abd Gani, S.S., Zainudin, B.H., et al., 2014. Phenolic composition, antioxidant, anti-wrinkles and tyrosinase inhibitory activities of cocoa pod extract. BMC Complement Altern. Med. 7, 14–381.

Keys, A.B., 1980. Seven Countries: A Multivariate Analysis of Death and Coronary Heart Disease. Harvard University Press, Cambridge, MA, 0-674-80237-3.

Kosmadaki, M.G., Gilchrest, B.A., 2004. The role of telomeres in skin aging/photoaging. Micron 35 (3), 155–159.

Malagoli, C., Malavolti, M., Agnoli, C., Crespi, C.M., Fiorentini, C., Farnetani, F., et al., 2015. Diet quality and risk of melanoma in an Italian population. J. Nutr. 145 (8), 1800–1807.

Masood, A.S., 2011. Telomeres, lifestyle, cancer, and aging. Curr. Opin. Clin. Nutr. Metab. Care. 14 (1), 28–34.

Melnik, B.C., 2015. Linking diet to acne metabolomics, inflammation, and comedogenesis: an update. Clin. Cosmet. Investig. Dermatol. 15 (8), 371–388.

Mohajeri, S., Newman, S.A., 2014. Review of evidence for dietary influences on atopic dermatitis. Skin Therapy Lett 19 (4), 5–7.

Monteagudo, C., Mariscal-Arcas, M., Rivas, A., Lorenzo-Tovar, M.L., Tur, J.A., Olea-Serrano, F., 2015. Proposal of a Mediterranean diet serving score. PLoS One 10 (6), e0128594.

Nagaraju, G.P., Zafar, S.F., El-Rayes, B.F., 2013. Pleiotropic effects of genistein in metabolic, inflammatory, and malignant diseases. Nutr. Rev. 71 (8), 562–572.

Pitsavos, C., Panagiotakos, D.B., Tzima, N., Chrysohoou, C., Economou, M., Zampelas, A., et al., 2005. Adherence to the Mediterranean diet is associated with total antioxidant capacity in healthy adults: the ATTICA study. Am. J. Clin. Nutr. 82 (3), 694–699.

Roh, E., Kim, J.E., Kwon, J.Y., Park, J.S., Bode, A.M., Dong, Z., et al., 2015. Molecular Mechanisms of green tea polyphenols with protective effects against skin photoaging. Crit. Rev. Food Sci. Nutr. 26, 0.

Shapira, N., 2010. Nutritional approach to sun protection: a suggested complement to external strategies. Nutr. Rev. 68 (2), 75–86.

Simm, A., Müller, B., Nass, N., Hofmann, B., Bushnaq, H., Silber, R.E., et al., 2015. Protein glycation-between tissue aging and protection. Exp. Gerontol. 68, 71–75

Tundis, R., Loizzo, M.R., Bonesi, M., Menichini, F., 2015. Potential role of natural compounds against skin aging. Curr. Med. Chem. 22 (12), 1515–1538.

Voiculescu, V.M., Lupu, M., Papagheorghe, L., Giurcaneanu, C., Micu, E., 2014. Psoriasis and Metabolic Syndrome—scientific evidence and therapeutic implications. J. Med. Life 7 (4), 468–471.

Watanabe, K., Shibuya, S., Ozawa, Y., Izuo, N., Shimizu, T., 2015. Resveratrol Derivative-rich melinjo seed extract attenuates skin atrophy in sod1-deficient mice. Oxid. Med. Cell Longev. 2015, 391075.

Yap, W.H., Lim, Y.M., 2015. Mechanistic perspectives of maslinic acid intargeting inflammation. Biochem. Res. Int. http://dx.doi.org/10.1155/2015/279356.

CHAPTER

3

Changes in Nutritional Needs With Aging

Teresa Juarez-Cedillo[1,2]

[1]Mexican Institute of Social Security, Mexico City, Mexico [2]National Autonomous University of Mexico, Mexico City, Mexico

INTRODUCTION

Aging brings physiological, physical, mental, social, and environmental changes that can negatively impact the nutritional status of the elderly population regardless of medical conditions or lifestyles. Knowing the causes of changing nutritional needs and dietary preferences is needed to understand a patient's nutritional status. To meet their nutritional needs, more than just diet must be considered. Although there is no uniformly accepted definition of malnutrition in the elderly, common indicators include involuntary weight loss, abnormal body mass index (BMI) (Leonard and Ulijaszek, 2002), specific vitamin deficiencies, and decreased dietary intake (Reuben et al., 2004). Even though older persons are particularly vulnerable to malnutrition, attempts to provide them with adequate nutrition often encounter practical problems. First, nutritional requirements for the aging are not well defined. Since both lean body mass and basal metabolic rate decline with age, an older person's energy requirement per kilogram of body weight is also reduced. Understanding that diet and nutrition play an important role in maintaining health, preventing disease, and functioning (WHO, 2003), this chapter reviews the changing nutritional needs of aging, diagnostic evaluation, and management of elderly patients and offers guidelines for the prevention of disabilities related to nutritional needs.

AGE-RELATED CHANGES AFFECT NUTRITION

As people age, multiple changes affect an individual's nutritional status. The main body composition changes are a loss of fat free mass and fat mass from muscles, organ tissues, skin, and bone (Hebuterne et al., 2001). This change in the body composition leads to a decrease in basal metabolic rate, which translates into a lower requirement for other nutrients (Olson et al., 1989). Hence, an approximate doubling of body fat between ages 20 and 50 has been observed (Perissinotto et al., 2002; Roberts and Dallal, 1998). Some authors have determined that fat increases at a rate >7.5% per decade in both genders (Hughes et al., 2002) and that older subjects have a mean of fat tissue 7 kg higher than younger ones (Piers et al.,1998). The basal metabolism or energy requirements for the elderly diminish by about 100 kcal/day per decade. For some seniors, it may be difficult to meet daily micronutrient requirements with this reduced caloric intake (Morley, 1997; Compher et al., 1998).

Age-related changes to the gastrointestinal tract may affect oral intake, but it is unclear if these normal physiological changes themselves contribute to decreased food intake (Westenhoefer, 2005). Oral and dental issues, esophageal motility, and atrophic gastritis may also affect nutritional status. The latter may be implicated in impaired vitamin B_{12} and iron adsorption (Wells and Dumbrell, 2006).

Nutrition and Functional Foods for Healthy Aging.
DOI: http://dx.doi.org/10.1016/B978-0-12-805376-8.00003-4

In addition to gastrointestinal physiological changes, renal function declines with age. This decreases responsiveness to antidiuretic hormones, which often results in an increased risk of dehydration in older patients and may also affect vitamin D adsorption (Compher et al., 1998).

It is well known that aging is associated with a gradual decline in energy requirements, a reduction in the basal metabolic rate, and a physiological diminution in food intake (Zafon, 2007). Recent studies has revealed the existence of genes involved with hormonal signals that play an important role in the regulator of energy metabolism, including fat storage (Cheng et al., 2004). Hence, genetic approaches provide a direct demonstration that aging is related to a metabolic reorganization of adipose tissue. The aforementioned ideas are consistent with the concept that aging is associated with a shift away from energy use toward energy storage. Other points to consider are the changes related to diseases common in older persons.

CHANGES IN NUTRITIONAL NEEDS

Many older adults face changes that can affect their food intake and nutritional status. Many need fewer calories to maintain their weight but still need the same amounts of vitamins and minerals as they did when they were younger (DH, 1991; Roberts and Dallal, 2005).

Consuming a diet that meets nutrition requirements without exceeding energy requirements poses an additional challenge for older adults and requires limiting discretionary energy intake. Recent evidence on dietary trends is concerning. The usual intake for a large percentage of older adults ages 51–70 was below the minimum recommended amounts, especially for nutrient-rich food groups. More than 90% of persons 51–70 years old and >80% of persons 71 and older had intakes of empty energy that exceeded the discretionary energy allowances (Krebs-Smith et al., 2010).

The dietary fiber intake of older adults is lower than recommended levels (Food and Nutrition and Institute of Medicine, 2005). In addition to providing nutrients such as vitamins, minerals, and antioxidants, fiber provides benefits such as improved gastric motility, improved glycemic control, and reduced cholesterol. About 60% of calories should come from carbohydrates, with emphasis on complex carbohydrates. Vegetables, fruits, grain products, cereals, seeds, legumes, and nuts are all sources of dietary fiber. Foods low in fiber are frequently inferior in nutrient composition and contribute to discretionary energy intake, thereby decreasing the nutrient density of the diet and placing older adults at risk of malnutrition and obesity. For this reason, is very important that when making recommendations regarding the fiber content in the diet of an older adult, fluid intake must be appropriately assessed and guidelines for adequate fluid should accompany those for dietary fiber (Food and Nutrition and Institute of Medicine, 2005).

Water is the most important of all nutrients and serves many essential functions. Adequate water intake reduces stress on kidney function, which tends to decline with age. Adequate fluid intake also eases constipation. With the aging process, the ability to detect thirst declines, so it is not advised to wait to drink water until one is thirsty. The kidneys' decreased ability to concentrate urine, blunted thirst sensation, endocrine changes in functional status, alterations in mental status and cognitive abilities, adverse effects of medications, and mobility disorders are commonly reported risk factors for dehydration in older adults. Individuals should be sure to drink plenty of water, juice, milk, and coffee or tea to stay properly hydrated. The equivalent to eight glasses of fluid should be consumed every day (Amella, 2007). Dehydration, a form of malnutrition, is a major problem in older adults, especially persons aged 85 and older and institutionalized older adults (Food and Nutrition and Institute of Medicine, 2005). Regular consumption of high-quality proteins can be challenging for older adults with physical and environmental limitations (Chernoff, 2004). The question of whether or not dietary protein needs change with advancing age is subject to scientific debate. Studies suggest that 0.8 g of dietary protein per kilogram of body weight daily is adequate to meet minimum dietary needs. Although a protein intake moderately greater than that amount may be beneficial to enhance muscle protein anabolism and reduce progressive loss of muscle mass with age. Some experts suggest that a protein intake of 1.0 g to 1.6 g/kg daily is safe and adequate to meet the needs of healthy older adults. Aging does not impair the ability to synthesize muscle protein after consumption of foods rich in high-quality protein or a high-quality protein meal and resistance exercise. Therefore, some experts now recommend that older adults consume between 25 and 30 g high-quality protein at each meal. For many older adults, this primarily means including a high-quality protein source at each meal throughout the day as recommended in the US Department of Agriculture's MyPlate food guidance system (Tholking et al., 2011; Bernstein et al., 2012).

USING SUPPLEMENTS

Although little research has been conducted on micronutrient requirements in the elderly, certain key nutrients demand attention (Rand et al., 2003). Among the micronutrients, the significant ones associated with deficiencies in the elderly include vitamins A, B_{12}, C, and D and calcium, iron, zinc, and other trace minerals.

Vitamin B_{12} is a nutrient of interest in the old primarily because the consumption of foods rich in this nutrient decreases with age (Wakimoto and Block, 2001). An estimated 6–15% of older adults have a vitamin B_{12} deficiency, and approximately 20% are estimated to have marginal status. The atrophic gastritis is a severe impediment to the transport and release of vitamin B_{12}. The production of gastric acid is necessary to digest food rich in vitamin B_{12} such as animal protein. The vitamin B_{12} requirements that are not met through diet can be met with supplements that contain crystalline vitamin B_{12}, although there is still a limited bioavailability (Olson et al., 1989). For elderly adults, the recommendation to meet vitamin B_{12} needs is through foods fortified with B_{12} or that naturally contain B_{12}. The primary source of vitamin B_{12}, is expensive, difficult to chew, and has been associated with elevated blood lipids. Further research is needed to investigate the efficacy and benefits of fortification of foods with vitamin B_{12} in older adults (Green, 2009).

It has been suggested that dietary vitamin A be obtained from an increased intake of carotenoids, including β-carotene among others. Compromised hepatic function may contribute to an increased risk of toxicity, particularly in those who are using supplements or eating fortified foods. Vitamin A has many roles in the maintenance of health; it is important to maintain normal vision, for cell differentiation, efficient immune function, and genetic expression. Vitamin A recommendations for older adults have been lowered from previous editions of the recommended daily amounts. Current suggested levels are 700 μg retinol activity equivalents (RAEs) for women and 900 μg RAE for men. Some researchers have recommended that these recommendations be set at even lower levels because, although the vitamin A intake for many older adults is below current recommendations, their vitamin A levels remain normal (Bjelakovic et al., 2014).

Vitamin D and Calcium

Among their numerous benefits, adequate vitamin D and calcium are best known for their crucial role in the prevention and delay of the progression of osteoporosis. Older adults are at high risk of vitamin D inadequacy because of limited sources of vitamin D in the diet (fortified milk, fatty fishes), less exposure to sunlight, a decreased capacity to synthesize vitamin D in the skin even when exposure to sunlight is plentiful, and a decreased capacity of the kidneys to convert vitamin D into its active form (Nieves, 2003). There are two primary sources of vitamin D: diet and skin. Dietary sources of vitamin D are fatty fishes and fortified dairy products. Skin as a source for vitamin D precursor may be helpful for those who live in temperate climates, but for those who live in warmer areas fear of skin cancer is an impediment to activating vitamin D precursors. In addition, the vitamin D precursor found in skin decreases with age. Adequate intake of calcium and vitamin D are difficult to achieve from food alone. Historically, calcium and vitamin D from dietary or supplement sources have been the major therapeutic focus for bone health. The ability of the kidney and liver to hydroxylate vitamin D precursors is affected by age, thereby suggesting that the vitamin D requirements might be higher than have been recommended (Shiue, 2016). Other nutrients such as protein, vitamins A and K, magnesium, and phytoestrogens are also involved in bone health, and research continues to expand the understanding of the roles of these nutrients in the bone health of older adults (Kitchin and Morgan, 2003; Nieves, 2003).

Iron is a mineral naturally present in many foods and added to some food products and available as a dietary supplement. Iron is an essential component of hemoglobin, an erythrocyte protein that transfers oxygen from the lungs to the tissues (Wessling-Resnick, 2014). As a component of myoglobin, a protein that provides oxygen to muscles, iron supports metabolism (Aggett, 2012). Iron is also necessary for the growth, development, normal cellular functioning, and synthesis of some hormones and connective tissue (Aggett, 2012; Murray-Kolbe et al., 2010).

Dietary iron has two main forms: heme and nonheme (Wessling-Resnick, 2014). Plants and iron-fortified foods contain nonheme iron only, whereas meat, seafood, and poultry contain both heme and nonheme iron (Aggett, 2012). Heme iron, which is formed when iron combines with protoporphyrin IX, contributes about 10–15% of total iron intake in Western populations (Aggett, 2012; Food and Nutrition and Institute of Medicine, 2005).

Most of the 3–4 g of elemental iron in adults is in hemoglobin (Aggett, 2012). Much of the remaining iron is stored in the form of ferritin or hemosiderin (a degradation product of ferritin) in the liver, spleen, and bone marrow or is located in myoglobin in muscle tissue (Wessling-Resnick, 2014). Humans typically lose only small amounts of iron in urine, feces, the gastrointestinal tract, and skin (Drakesmith and Prentice, 2012). Needs for iron in older males revert to the same levels as those for adult males: 10 mg/day (Garry et al., 2000; Fleming et al., 2002).

Zinc has been recognized as an essential mineral with a role in many enzymes, gene expression, and immune function, among other physiological functions. Marginal intake of dietary zinc will lead to lower physiologic zinc levels, but the real challenge may be factors that inhibit or interfere with zinc absorption. Consequences of poor zinc status may include reduced immune function, dermatitis, loss of taste acuity, and impaired wound healing. Zinc supplementation may contribute to a reversal of symptoms in individuals who are zinc deficient. In individuals who have adequate zinc status, however, supplementation will not improve their conditions (Beckett and Ball, 2015).

Copper is a trace mineral that is part of several enzymes and proteins that are essential for the body to adequately use iron. Lower copper intake has been implicated with other variables such as heightened cholesterol and in some studies as a possible risk factor for cardiovascular disease. Due to the difficulty in measuring copper status, the many factors such as zinc, carbohydrate, and vitamin C intake that affect copper bioavailability remain unknown (Wu et al., 2002). Copper is widely distributed in a variety of foods and is relatively accessible if a diet with variety is consumed in adequate amounts. Estimated average requirements for copper for adults to age 70 have been established at 700 μg/day (Arredondo and Núñez, 2005).

There is little specific information regarding micronutrient requirements for elderly. It seems that the metabolic changes that occur with aging would have some impact on vitamin, mineral, but there is a clear need for future research to elucidate these nutrient needs.

ASSESSING NUTRITIONAL STATUS

A comprehensive assessment of nutritional status includes anthropometric measurements, laboratory values, physical exam, and patient history. Anthropometric measures include height, weight, BMI, body fat measurement, and muscle mass measurement. Laboratory values should include albumin, retinal-binding prealbumin, transferring, complete blood count, serum folate, vitamin B_{12}, and cholesterol. A diet history is helpful if there is good 24-h recall or if a food record for 3 days leading up to the exam can be completed.

The elderly are vulnerable to a number of nutritional risks because of associated multiple pathologies and the frequent changes in body composition and nutritional needs they undergo. Furthermore, nutritional assessment in the elderly is especially difficult because many of the signs of malnutrition are also associated with aging. Recently, rapid-application scales have appeared for the purpose of allowing nutritional assessment in geriatrics; these instruments can be classified according to their objective and scope of application.

Nutritional Screening Initiative, Level I and II Screening

This set of instruments is well suited to community screening. It incorporates a simple nomogram to determine BMI and a questionnaire of laboratory data (albumin and serum cholesterol), clinical characteristics, eating habits, living environment, and mental and cognitive states. Level II adds skinfold measurements and biochemical indicators. The objective of these instruments is to estimate the magnitude and causes of malnutrition (Montorio and Lázaro, 1996). The questionnaire, applied separately, can be used as an indicator of high, medium, or low risk of malnutrition.

Mini Nutritional Assessment

This questionnaire was created for the elderly population and can be applied in cases of ambulatory or hospitalized care. It qualifies the condition of a malnourished patient, the risk of malnutrition, and the general nutritional status. It can be performed in approximately 10 min with a total possible score of 30 points. A score above 23.5 classifies the individual as well fed; scores between 17 and 23.5 indicate a situation of risk, in spite of no evidence of loss or biochemical alteration; and scores below 17 express a situation of malnutrition (Guigoz et al., 1996).

Mini Nutritional Assessment–Short Form

This abbreviated form was created to reduce the time of administration to 10 min without losing diagnostic power and thus simplifying and generalizing implementation in clinical practice. Among its characteristics, the following stand out: good correlation with the mini nutritional assessment (MNA), adequate sensitivity and specificity, and good internal consistence. This form presents false positives when compared with customary dietary assessment due to the fact that it detects not only malnourished individuals but also those at risk of malnutrition. This version consists of six questions that can be effectively asked in approximately 3 min. The questionnaire should be used in two phases: (1) filling out the short form and if a risk of malnutrition is detected (score lower than or equal to 11 points), then (2) the entire questionnaire is administered (Rubenstein et al., 2001).

Malnutrition Universal Screening Tool

Initially, this tool was developed for noninstitutionalized individuals, but currently its use has been validated in various contexts, including the hospital environment, external consultation, and home residences (Stratton et al., 2004). Its limitations include not incorporating any measure of functionality and a focus on acute disease.

Subjective Global Assessment

This method was designed by Detsky et al. (1987) to estimate nutritional status through clinical history and physical exploration. It has greater sensitivity and specificity than assessment with measurements of albumin, transferrin, cutaneous sensitivity, anthropometry, height creatinine, and the prognostic nutritional index. The subjective global assessment (SGA) can be used to determine which patients require nutritional intervention and which would benefit from intensive nutritional support.

The data obtained from the clinical history include the evolution of weight, current dietary intake in relation to customary dietary intake, digestive symptoms present in the preceding 2 weeks, functional capacity, and metabolic requirements. Within the scope of the physical examination are evaluations of loss of subcutaneous fat and musculature and the presence of edema or ascites. Each element is evaluated as light, moderate, or severe, and patients are classified into three groups: adequate nutritional status, suspicion of malnutrition or moderate malnutrition, and severe malnutrition.

Laboratory tests based on blood and urine can be important indicators of nutritional status, but they are influenced by nonnutritional factors as well. Lab results can be altered by medications, hydration status, and disease states.

Clinical data provide information about an individual's medical history, including acute and chronic illness and diagnostic procedures, therapies, or treatments that may increase nutrient needs or induce malabsorption (Older Americans Act, 2016).

CONCLUSION

There is little specific information regarding micronutrient requirements for the elderly. One challenge in defining nutritional needs is the heterogeneity of elderly adults. To understand the dietary needs of the older adult, it is important to know what the basic requirements of the healthy older adult are and whether the metabolic changes that occur with aging will have some impact on a vitamin or mineral. For this reason, there is a clear need for future research to elucidate these nutrient needs. A comprehensive assessment must include a lot more than just basic nutritional assessment and should consider the person's overall physical, mental, and psychosocial status. This will lead to a better understanding of how to realistically meet the nutritional needs of older adults compounded by the likelihood of multiple chronic conditions, the use of many prescriptions, and the variable quality of nutritional intake associated with limited income, disability, and institutionalization.

References

Aggett, P.J., 2012. Iron. In: Erdman, J.W., Macdonald, I.A., Zeisel, S.H. (Eds.), Present Knowledge in Nutrition, 10th ed. Wiley-Blackwell, Washington, DC, pp. 506–520.

Amella, E.J., 2007. Assessing nutrition in older adults. Try This: Best Practices in Nursing Care to Older Adults. Retrieved from www.hartfordign.org/publications/trythis/issue_9.pdf.

Arredondo, M., Núñez, M.T., 2005. Iron and copper metabolism. Mol. Aspects Med. 26, 313–327.

Beckett, J.M., Ball, M.J., 2015. Zinc status of northern Tasmanian adults. J. Nutr. Sci. 20 (4), e15.

Bernstein, M., Munoz, N., Academy of Nutrition, Dietetics, 2012. Position of the Academy of Nutrition and Dietetics: food and nutrition for older adults: promoting health and wellness. J. Acad. Nutr. Diet. 112 (8), 1255–1277.

Bjelakovic, G., Nikolova, D., Gluud, C., 2014. Antioxidant supplements and mortality. Curr. Opin. Clin. Nutr. Metab. Care 17, 40–44.

Cheng, C., Graziani, C., Diamond, J.J., 2004. Cholesterol-lowering effect of the Food for Heart Nutrition Education Program. J. Am. Diet. Assoc. 104, 1868–1872.

Chernoff, R., 2004. Protein and older adults. J. Am. Coll. Nutr. 23, 627s–630s.
Compher, C., Kim, J.N., Bader, J.G., 1998. Nutritional requirements of an aging population with emphasis on subacute care patients. AACN Clin. Issues 9, 441–450.
Detsky, A.S., Mc Laughlin, J.R., Baker, J.P., Johnson, N., Whittaker, S., Mendelson, R.A., et al., 1987. What is subjective global assessment of nutritional status? J. Parenter. Enteral. Nutr. 11, 8–13.
DH (Department of Health), 1991. Dietary Reference Values for food energy and nutrients for the United Kingdom. Report of the Panel on Dietary Reference Values of the Committee on Medical Aspects of Food Policy. HMSO, London, UK.
Diet, Nutrition and the Prevention of Chronic Diseases. Geneva: World Health Organization; 2003. WHO Technical Report Series, No. 916.
Drakesmith, H., Prentice, A.M., 2012. Hepcidin and the Iron-Infection Axis. Science 338, 768–772.
Fleming, D.J., Tucker, K.L., Jacques, P.F., Dallal, G.E., Wilson, P.W., Wood, R.J., 2002. Dietary factors associated with the risk of high iron stores in the elderly Framingham Heart Study Cohort. Am. J. Clin. Nutr. 76, 1375–1384.
Food and Nutrition Board, Institute of Medicine, 2005. Dietary Reference Intakes for Energy, Carbohydrate, Fiber, Fat, Fatty Acids, Cholesterol, Protein and Amino Acids (Macronutrients). National Academies Press, Washington, DC.
Garry, P.J., Hunt, W.C., Baumgartner, R.N., 2000. Effects of iron intake on iron stores in elderly men and women: longitudinal and cross-sectional results. J. Am. Coll. Nutr. 19, 262–269.
Green, R., 2009. Is it the time for vitamin B-12 fortification? What are the questions? Am. J. Clin. Nutr. 89, 712s–716s.
Guigoz, Y., Vellas, B.J., Garry, P.J., 1996. Assessing the nutritional status of the elderly. The Mini Nutritional Assessment as part of the geriatric evaluation. Nutr. Rev. 54, 59–65.
Hebuterne, X., Bermon, S., Schneider, S.M., 2001. Ageing and muscle: the effects of malnutrition, renutrition, and physical exercise. Curr. Opin. Clin. Nutr. Met. Care 4295–300, 300.
Hughes, V.A., Frontera, W.R., Roubenoff, R., Evans, W.J., Fiatarone Singh, M.A., 2002. Longitudinal changes in body composition in older men and women: role of body weight change and physical activity. Am. J. Clin. Nutr. 76, 473–481.
Kitchin, B., Morgan, S., 2003. Nutritional considerations in osteoporosis. Curr. Opin. Rheumatol. 15, 476–480.
Krebs-Smith, S.M., Guenther, P.M., Subar, A., Kirkpatrick, S.I., Dodd, K.W., 2010. Americans do not meet federal dietary recommendations. J. Nutr. 140, 1832–1838.
Leonard, W.R., Ulijaszek, S.J., 2002. Energetics and evolution: an emerging research domain. Am. J. Hum. Biol. 14, 547–550.
Montorio, I.C., Lázaro, S.H., 1996. Instrumentos de evaluación funcional en la edad avanzada: Un análisis bibliométrico. Rev. Esp. Geriatr. Gerontol. 31, 45–54.
Morley, J.E., 1997. Anorexia of aging: physiologic and pathologic. Am. J. Clin. Nutr. 66, 760–773.
Murray-Kolbe, L.E., Beard, J., 2010. Iron. In: Coates, P.M., Betz, J.M., Blackman, M.R. (Eds.), Encyclopedia of Dietary Supplements, 2nd ed. Informa Healthcare, London and New York, pp. 432–438.
Nieves, J.W., 2003. Calcium, vitamin D, and nutrition in elderly adults. Clin. Geriatr. Med. 19, 321–335.
Older Americans Act. US Department of Health and Human Services Administration on Aging website. http://www.aoa.gov/AoARoot/AoA_Programs/OAA/index.aspx. Accessed February 1, 2016.
Olson J.A. Vitamin A. In: Rucker RB, Suttie JW, McCormick DB, Machlin Penfold P and Crowthwe S., 1989. Causes and management of neglected diet in the elderly 1:20-2.
Perissinotto, E., Pisent, C., Sergi, G., Grigoletto, F., Enzi, G., 2002. Anthopometric measurements in the elderly: age and gender differences. Br. J. Nutr. 87, 177–186.
Piers, L.S., Soares, M.J., McCormack, L.M., O'Dea, K., 1998. Is there evidence for an age-related reduction in metabolic rate? J. Appl. Physiol. 85, 2196–2204.
Rand, W.M., Pellett, P.L., Young, V.R., 2003. Meta-analysis of nitrogen balance studies for estimating protein requirements in healthy adults. Am. J. Clin. Nutr. 77, 109–127.
Reuben, D.B., Herr, K.A., Pacala, J.T., Pollock, B.G., Potter, J.F., Semla, T.P., 2004. Geriatrics at Your Fingertips. Blackwell Publishing, Malden, MA.
Roberts, S.B., Dallal, G.E., 1998. Effects of age on energy balance. Am. J. Clin. Nutr. 68 (Suppl.), 975S–979S.
Roberts, S.B., Dallal, G.E., 2005. Energy requirements and aging. Public Health Nutr. 8, 1028–1036.
Rubenstein, L.Z., Harker, J.O., Salva, A., Guigoz, Y., Vellas, B., 2001. Screening for undernutrition in geriatric practice: developing the short-form mini nutritional assessment (MNA-SF). J. Gerontol. A Biol. Sci. Med. Sci. 56, M366–M372.
Rucker, R.B., Suttie, J.W., McCormick, D.B., Machlin, L.J., 2001. The Handbook of Vitamins. Marcel Dekker, New York. 1–50.
Shiue, I., 2016. Cold homes are associated with poor biomarkers and less blood pressure check-up: English Longitudinal Study of Ageing, 2012-2013. Environ. Sci. Pollut. Res. Int. 23, 7055–7059.
Stratton, R.J., Hackston, A., Longmore, D., Dixon, R., Price, S., Stroud, M., et al., 2004. Malnutrition in hospital outpatients and inpatients: prevalence, concurrent validity and ease of use of the "malnutrition universal screening tool" (MUST) for adults. Br. J. Nutr. 92, 799–808.
Tholking, M.M., Mellowspring, A.C., Eberle, S.G., Lamb, R.P., Myers, E.S., Scribner, C., et al., 2011. American Dietetic Association: standards of practice and standards of professional performance for registered dietitians (competent, proficient, and expert) in disordered eating and eating disorders (DE and ED). J. Am. Diet. Assoc. 111, 1242–1249. e37.
Wakimoto, P., Block, G., 2001. Dietary intake, dietary patterns, and changes with age: an epidemiological perspective. J. Gerontol. Series AMed Sci 56A, 65–80.
Wells, J.L., Dumbrell, A.C., 2006. Nutrition and aging: assessment and treatment of compromised nutritional status in frail elderly patients. Clin. Interv. Aging 1, 67–79.
Wessling-Resnick, M., 2014. Iron. In: Ross, A.C., Caballero, B., Cousins, R.J., Tucker, K.L., Ziegler, R.G. (Eds.), Modern Nutrition in Health and Disease, 11th ed. Lippincott Williams & Wilkins, Baltimore, MD, pp. 176–188.
Westenhoefer, J., 2005. Age and gender dependent profile of food choice. Forum. Nutr. 57, 44–51.
Wu, K., Willett, W.C., Fuchs, C.S., Colditz, G.A., Giovannucci, E., 2002. Calcium intake and risk of colon cancer in women and men. J. Natl. Cancer Inst. 94, 437–446.
Zafon, C., 2007. Oscillations in total body fat content through life: an evolutionary perspective. Obes. Rev. 8 (6), 525–530.

CHAPTER

4

Sugars, Glucocorticoids, and the Hypothalamic Controls of Appetite

Thomas W. Castonguay and Samantha Hudgins

University of Maryland, College Park, MD, United States

OVERVIEW

The obesity epidemic that we are experiencing in the United States is a crisis that affects all Americans. In general, obesity does not discriminate among ages, races, classes, or genders. In 1985, the rate of obesity across our country was less than 14% but by 2014 the rate was 35% (Ogden et al., 2014). Furthermore, obesity is quickly becoming a leading cause of major health problems and death. The research community, along with policy makers and health-care officials are grappling to find the causes of this sudden increase in Americans' girth. Several researchers have targeted sugar—in particular, high-fructose corn syrup (HFCS)—as a potential accomplice in the obesity epidemic. Supporters have pointed out that fructose has become more prevalent in our diets over the past century. In 1900, the average fructose intake was 15 g/day. Fructose was consumed mainly through fruits and vegetables, which have the added benefit of fiber (Bray, 2010). However, as of 2010, fructose consumption had risen to 73 g/day and was being consumed in highly processed forms.

This research is further complicated by the varied forms of sugar in today's Western diet. Sucrose, more commonly known as table sugar, is a disaccharide composed of a fructose molecule bonded to a glucose molecule. As a consequence, 50% of sucrose is fructose. HFCS is derived from corn sugar rich in glucose; the corn sugar is processed to increase fructose concentrations, which results in the much sweeter HFCS. Interestingly, HFCS can be produced to different sweetness by increasing the fructose concentrations. The most commonly used form of HFCS is 45% fructose followed by the less common 85% fructose. Therefore, HFCS is erroneously targeted as the sole cause of obesity. Rather, we believe fructose containing sugars, specifically in processed foods, may be the culprit of sugar-induced obesity. Further, while glucose and fructose are not typically used to sweeten foods and beverages alone, researchers still use the individual monosaccharides as treatment to better understand the molecular contributions of each sugar component.

One particularly attractive hypothesis linking obesity to fructose consumption is that increased fructose intake can disrupt normal liver metabolism and lead to an increase in hepatic lipogenesis. We will subsequently refer to this link as the *hepatic lipogenesis hypothesis*. A second but equally attractive hypothesis that links obesity to fructose is that monosaccharides quickly induce increases in both hepatic and adipose intracellular glucocorticoids that then promote increased fat accumulation. Finally, a third line of research that links obesity to fructose intake comes from recent findings from our laboratory that overnight access to fructose suppresses hypothalamic peptides that are involved with the regulation of normal hunger and satiety. In this chapter, we will review the data from inquiries into each set of experiments that link the intake of sugar—fructose in particular—to physiological conditions that favor the development of excess body fat. The review presented here is not exhaustive but puts our contributions in context so as to make the point that there is no one simple answer to the question, "How does an increase in sugar consumption promote obesity?"

Nutrition and Functional Foods for Healthy Aging.
DOI: http://dx.doi.org/10.1016/B978-0-12-805376-8.00004-6

THE LIPOGENESIS HYPOTHESIS

The Metabolism of Fructose

Fructose can alter normal lipid metabolism in the liver in part by generating unregulated surges of pyruvate. Pyruvate enters the mitochondria via pyruvate dehydrogenase and forms acetyl coenzyme A (acetyl-CoA) that acts as a carbon source for three different pathways: the citric acid cycle, lipogenesis, and the formation of ketone bodies. In the lipogenic pathway, acetyl-CoA is shuttled across the mitochondrial membrane as citrate and is then restored back to acetyl-CoA in the mitochondrial cytosol via ATP citrate lyase. Here acetyl-CoA provides a substrate for the production of long-chain fatty acids facilitated by fatty acid synthase (Bar-On and Stein, 1968). Rats that have been fed 63% fructose for 24–48h and then fasted developed liver steatosis (Castro et al., 2011; Castro et al., 2013). Leptin production drops by 20–30% when normal weight female subjects consumed 30% caloric intake from a fructose-sweetened beverage compared to a glucose-sweetened beverage (Stanhope et al., 2008). Havel and Stanhope later hypothesized that the leptin reduction observed following fructose consumption can be attributed to the absence of an insulin response that stimulates leptin production. As a result, the leptin reduction observed during fructose consumption may lead to increased energy intake or decreased energy expenditure or both and subsequent weight gain.

In summary, short-term exposure to dietary fructose, as opposed to glucose, can result in marked increases in several enzymes that in turn can lead to metabolic dysfunction in rats and humans. The increases in gene expression such as those already noted as well as a lack of key regulatory steps in initial fructose metabolism favors de novo lipogenesis (synthesis of triglycerides) in the liver. As a consequence, an overproduction of very-low-density lipoproteins (VLDLs) and triglycerides are released into circulation, leading to hypertriglyceridemia (HTG). In contrast, glucose does not directly increase the gene expression that facilitates de novo lipogenesis; instead, it is insulin that is lipogenic. Thus, sugars like sucrose and HFCS stimulate lipogenesis through dual mechanisms. However, glucose alone may be able to spare a massive unregulated surge of metabolites that favor lipid production due to the singular effect of insulin.

APOC3 and Hypertriglyceridemia

Large amounts of fructose in the diet can lead to HTG in both humans and laboratory rodents (Bocarsly et al., 2010; Teff et al., 2004; Teff et al., 2009). There are several plausible mechanisms that link fructose to HTG. We have recently examined the role of apolipoprotein C-III (APOC3) in promoting HTG in less than 24h (Castonguay and Campbell, 2014). A lipoprotein, APOC3 is expressed in the liver of humans and rodents and is one of the most abundant apolipoproteins in plasma, with an average concentration of about 12mg/dL. Plasma APOC3 concentrations are positively correlated to plasma triglycerides and VLDL triglycerides. In addition, transgenic mice that overexpress the APOC3 gene exhibit hyperlipidemia. Conversely, mice with suppressed APOC3 were protected from hyperlipidemia (Jong et al., 1999).

We tested various types of fructose-containing sugars (fructose, sucrose, and HFCS) with the intent of replicating our earlier observations that overnight access to fructose can promote HTG as well as examine the role of APOC3 in promoting HTG (Castonguay and Campbell, 2014). Briefly, 40 rats were randomly assigned to five weight-matched groups ($n = 8$). Rats assigned to the first group were given ad libitum access to control diet (Harlan rodent diet 7012). Rats assigned to the remaining four groups had ad libitum access to the control diet as well as ad libitum access to one of the following solutions: 16% weight/volume (w/v) fructose, 16% w/v glucose, or 16% w/v sucrose. Presented in Table 4.1 is a comparison of several measured endpoints. Note that only the rats that were fed fructose containing sugars differed from controls in circulating triglycerides under our experimental conditions.

Since pure fructose is the most lipogenic of all the sugars, consumption of pure fructose was expected to elicit the greatest perturbation in APOC3 messenger RNA (mRNA) and protein. This was not the case. We found that sucrose- and glucose-fed groups had similar significant positive fold changes in APOC3 gene expression at 2.68 and 2.59, respectively, when compared to controls. Interestingly, HFCS had a positive fold change of 2.40 but failed to differ significantly from controls. Fructose consumption elicited a negative fold change at 0.86 but again this difference was not statistically significant different from control. Refer to Fig. 4.1.

Contrary to other studies that suggest APOC3 is responsible for HTG, we believe that there may be an alternative mechanism to elicit HTG in 24h or less that has not yet been identified. This result suggests that the ratio of other lipoproteins to APOC3 may be the key to understanding how fructose consumption results in HTG. Clearly, more research is needed.

TABLE 4.1 Average Insulin, Triglycerides, Glucose, and APOC3 in Plasma Following 24-h Sugar Access

Group	Insulin (ng/mL)	Triglycerides (mg/dL)	Glucose (mg/dL)	APOC3 (ng/mL)
Control	$4.2^{a} \pm 0.6$	$73.4^{c} \pm 20.7$	$150.0^{a} \pm 2.0$	$321.9^{a} \pm 53.7$
Fructose	$4.5^{a} \pm 0.9$	$311.6^{a} \pm 41.6$	$155.7^{a} \pm 2.9$	$412.7^{a} \pm 87.4$
Glucose	$4.4^{a} \pm 1.1$	$132.1^{bc} \pm 20.6$	$147.2^{a} \pm 3.4$	$208.4^{a} \pm 57.0$
HFCS	$4.2^{a} \pm 0.9$	$286.2^{a} \pm 31.6$	$148.8^{a} \pm 3.6$	$243.9^{a} \pm 64.4$
Sucrose	$4.5^{a} \pm 0.7$	$257.4^{ab} \pm 30.3$	$149.9^{a} \pm 2.1$	$333.8^{a} \pm 71.1$

Taken from Castonguay, T.W., Campbell, E.S., 2014. Fructose intake and circulating triglycerides: an examination of the role of APOC3. J. Diabetes Obesity 1, 1–7.

Group means ± SEM are presented here for plasma insulin, triglycerides, glucose, and APOC3. Superscripts with different letters indicate a significant difference at the $p < .05$ level. Refer to Campbell and Castonguay (2014) for further details.

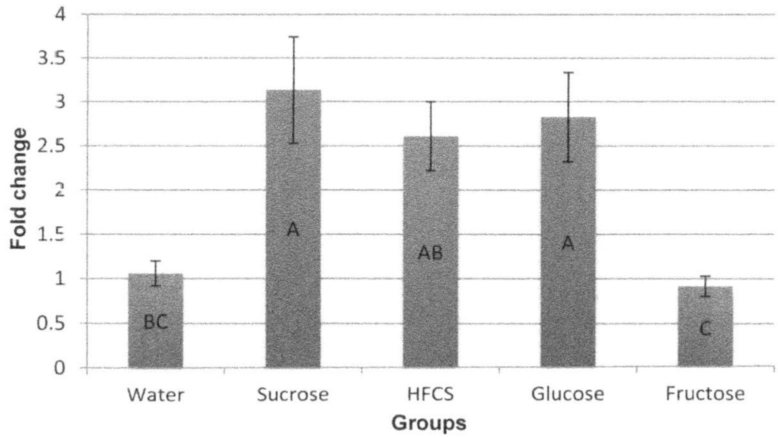

FIGURE 4.1 APOC3 mRNA gene expression. Only the glucose containing sugars sucrose, HFCS, and glucose were able to significantly increase the mRNA expression of APOC3. *Source: Taken from Campbell et al., 2014. Taken from Castonguay, T.W., Campbell, E.S., 2014. Fructose Intake and Circulating Triglycerides: An Examination of the Role of APOC 3 Journal of Diabetes and Obesity 1, 1–7.*

Sugar and the HSD Hypothesis

Fifty years of research has made it clear that glucocorticoids are involved in obesity, including diet-induced obesity. For review, see London and Castonguay (2009). Although elevated circulating corticosterone is not a defining characteristic of all obesities, the steroid nevertheless plays a critical role in its etiology. One plausible hypothesis that links corticosteroids to obesity is a dysregulation of local intracellular levels of active steroid via 11β-hydroxysteroid dehydrogenase type 1 (11β-HSD-1) activity (London et al., 2007). Results from our laboratory point to both sucrose and fructose as particularly effective dietary components that are capable of altering 11β-HSD-1 mRNA and at the same time promote increased adiposity. Our preliminary inquiries suggest that nicotinamide adenine dinucleotide phosphate (NADPH) is an essential donor in the oxidoreductase activity of 11β-HSD-1.

Furthermore, fructose contributes to lipogenesis not only through unregulated Acetyl-CoA production but also through the unregulated production of glucose-6-phosphate (G6P). At lower concentrations, G6P would typically enter glycolysis; however, marked increases stimulate NADPH production through the pentose phosphate pathway as evidenced by increased H6PDH mRNA in the liver of sugar-fed rats. As the hydrogen donor to 11β-HSD-1 oxo-reductase activity, increased NADPH production results in aberrant 11β-HSD-1 activity that supports lipogenesis. Perhaps this dual effect accounts for why access to glucose fails to promote comparable levels of obesity. Dietary glucose is subject to tighter metabolic regulation.

The HSD-1 Hypothesis, Fructose, and Obesity

Local tissue concentrations of corticosterone better predict the promotion and maintenance of obesity than do circulating hormone levels that are not consistently higher in obese rodents compared to lean rodents (Bujalska

TABLE 4.2 Relative Enzyme Message for 11β-HSD-1 and H6PDH in the Liver and Mesenteric Adipose of Rats Given 10 Weeks Access to Either a 16% or 32% Sucrose Solution Compared to Control Rats

	11β-HSD-1 Message		**H6PDH Message**	
Group	**S16**	**S32**	**S16**	**S32**
Liver	54 ± 9[a]	53 ± 10[a]	221 ± 38[a]	159 ± 19
Adipose	2435 ± 978[a]	3294 ± 1108[a]	446 ± 79[a]	181 ± 84[b]

Taken from London, E., Castonguay, T.W., 2011. High fructose diets increase 11beta-hydroxysteroid dehydrogenase type 1 in liver and visceral adipose in rats within 24-h exposure. Obesity (Silver Spring) 19, 925–932.
Values are means± SEM, $n = 8$.
[a]*Different from control, $p < .05$.*
[b]*Different from S16, $p < 0.05$.*

et al., 1997; Walker, 2001). The bidirectional enzyme 11β-HSD-1 interconverts the active hormones cortisol in humans and corticosterone in rats with their inert metabolites cortisone and 11-dehydrocorticosterone, respectively. Highly expressed in adipose tissue, liver, and brain, 11β-HSD-1 acts primarily as an oxoreductase to generate active cortisol or corticosterone. Adipose tissue taken from obese humans has three to four times the 11β-HSD-1 oxoreductase activity compared to adipose taken from lean individuals (Rask et al., 2001). This change in 11β-HSD-1 activity in adipose tissue is likely a commonality of different forms of obesity. We have examined the effect of dietary sucrose on body weight, body composition, and other indices of obesity, including plasma glucose, insulin, and leptin as well as H6PDH and 11β-HSD-1 messaging in mesenteric adipose and liver in rats (London and Castonguay, 2011). Giving rats access to sucrose solutions led to increased 11β-HSD-1 and H6PDH messaging in mesenteric fat while at the same time decreasing 11β-HSD-1 messaging and increasing H6PDH messaging in liver. Refer to Table 4.2. The 11β-HSD-1 activity depends on the activity of H6PDH, which is reliant on the availability of its substrate, primarily glucose-6-phosphate.

The enzyme 11β-HSD-1 is linked to the pentose phosphate pathway and other metabolic pathways via the enzyme hexose-6-phosphate dehydrogenase (London and Castonguay, 2011). Our more recent findings have developed evidence from dietary manipulation experiments that suggests macronutrient composition may elicit changes in 11β-HSD-1 and promote obesity (Table 4.3).

Dietary Sugars and Glucocorticoids: Additional Evidence Linking the Two to Obesity

London and Castonguay (2011) examined the acute effects of ad lib access to 16% solutions of sucrose (S16), fructose (F16), or glucose (G16) and chow and water. Diets high in fructose but not glucose or sucrose increased 11β-HSD1 mRNA within 24h in liver and adipose by greater than two- and threefold, respectively ($p \leq 0.05$). After 1 week, hepatic 11β-HSD1 mRNA and protein were suppressed by >60% in all sugar-fed groups, a phenomenon not previously reported in the absence of obesity. Sucrose- and fructose-fed rats had higher plasma triglycerides than did control or glucose-fed rats at both 24h and 1 week ($p \leq 0.02$), which is consistent with previously reported effects of fructose on lipid metabolism (refer to Fig. 4.2A–F).

Dietary fructose increased 11β-HSD1 mRNA in liver ($p < 0.05$, Fig. 4.2A) and mesenteric adipose ($p = 0.05$, Fig. 4.2B) within the first 24h of exposure when compared to the mean levels of the control, S16, and G16 groups. Continued access to a fructose solution resulted in two outcomes: the suppression of hepatic 11β-HSD1 mRNA ($p < 0.05$, Fig. 4.2A) and an increase in 11β-HSD-1 mRNA in mesenteric adipose 11β-HSD-1 mRNA ($p < 0.05$, Fig. 4.2B). After 1 week of exposure to the experimental diets, 11β-HSD1 mRNA in liver was suppressed by greater than 60% in all of the sugar-fed groups compared to the control ($p < 0.05$, Fig. 4.2B). In mesenteric adipose, the increases in 11β-HSD1 mRNA in the sugar-fed groups at 1 week ranged from two- to sixfold that of the control group, yet mean levels of the S16 and G16 groups did not attain statistical significance.

After 24h or 1 week of exposure to the experimental diets, there were no differences in mean H6PDH mRNA levels in liver or mesenteric adipose in comparison to control levels (Fig. 4.2C and D). All three sugar-fed groups had mean hepatic acetyl-CoA carboxylase (ACC) mRNA levels more than twice that of their respective controls at both 24h and 1 week, although not all of these differences achieved statistical significance (Fig. 4.2F). After 24h, mean hepatic ACC mRNA levels were significantly higher in the F16 and G16 groups ($p < 0.05$; Fig. 4.2F), and

TABLE 4.3 Effect of Overnight Access to Fructose Solution on Message of Appetite Regulating Genes Robust Changes From Control (Minimum 400% Increase or 75% Decrease)

		% Control	
Hypothalamic Region	**Gene**	**Increase**	**Decrease**
FOUND IN THE LATERAL HYPOTHALAMUS			
Glucagon-like peptide 1 receptor	Glp1R		5
Dopamine receptor D1A	Drd1a	1220	
Dopamine receptor D2	Drd2	670	
FOUND IN THE VENTROMEDIAL HYPOTHALAMUS			
Brain-derived neurotrophic factor	Bdnf		2
Glucagon-like peptide 1 receptor	Glp1R		5
Dopamine receptor D1A	Drd1a	1220	
Dopamine receptor D2	Drd2	670	
Agouti-related protein homolog	AGRP		0.4
Attractin	Atrn		0.4
FOUND IN THE ARCUATE NUCLEUS			
Bombesin-like receptor 3	Brs3		5
Agouti-related protein homolog	AGRP		0.4
Insulin receptor	INSR		0.9
Growth hormone 1	Gh1		2
Thyrotropin-releasing hormone receptor	Trhr		3
Attractin	Atrn		0.4
FOUND IN THE PERIVENTRICULAR HYPOTHALAMUS			
Neuromedin B	NMB		3
Insulin receptor	INSR		0.9
Growth hormone 1	Gh1		2
Tumor necrosis factor	TNF		2
Attractin	Atrn		0.4
Thyroid hormone receptor beta	Thrb		4
FOUND IN THE DORSOMEDIAL HYPOTHALAMUS			
Brain-derived neurotrophic factor	Bdnf		2
Thyrotropin-releasing hormone receptor	Trhr		3
FOUND IN THE PERIVENTRICULAR THALAMUS			
Receptor activity modifying protein 3	Ramp3		17

Taken from Colley, D., London, E., Jiang, B., Khural, J., Castonguay, T.W., 2012. in: Collins, B.M.J.a.A.B. (Ed.), Fructose: Synthesis, Functions and Health Implications. Nova Science Publishers Hauppauge, NY, pp. 129–143.

after 1 week the mean hepatic ACC mRNA level was increased in the G16 group compared to controls ($p < 0.05$; Fig. 4.2F). No changes in ACC mRNA levels were observed in mesenteric adipose.

Fructose increased 11β-HSD1 protein expression in liver after 24h ($p < 0.05$, Fig. 4.2E), which was the same trend observed in 11β-HSD1 mRNA in the fructose-fed group. After 1 week, mean hepatic 11β-HSD1 protein levels were

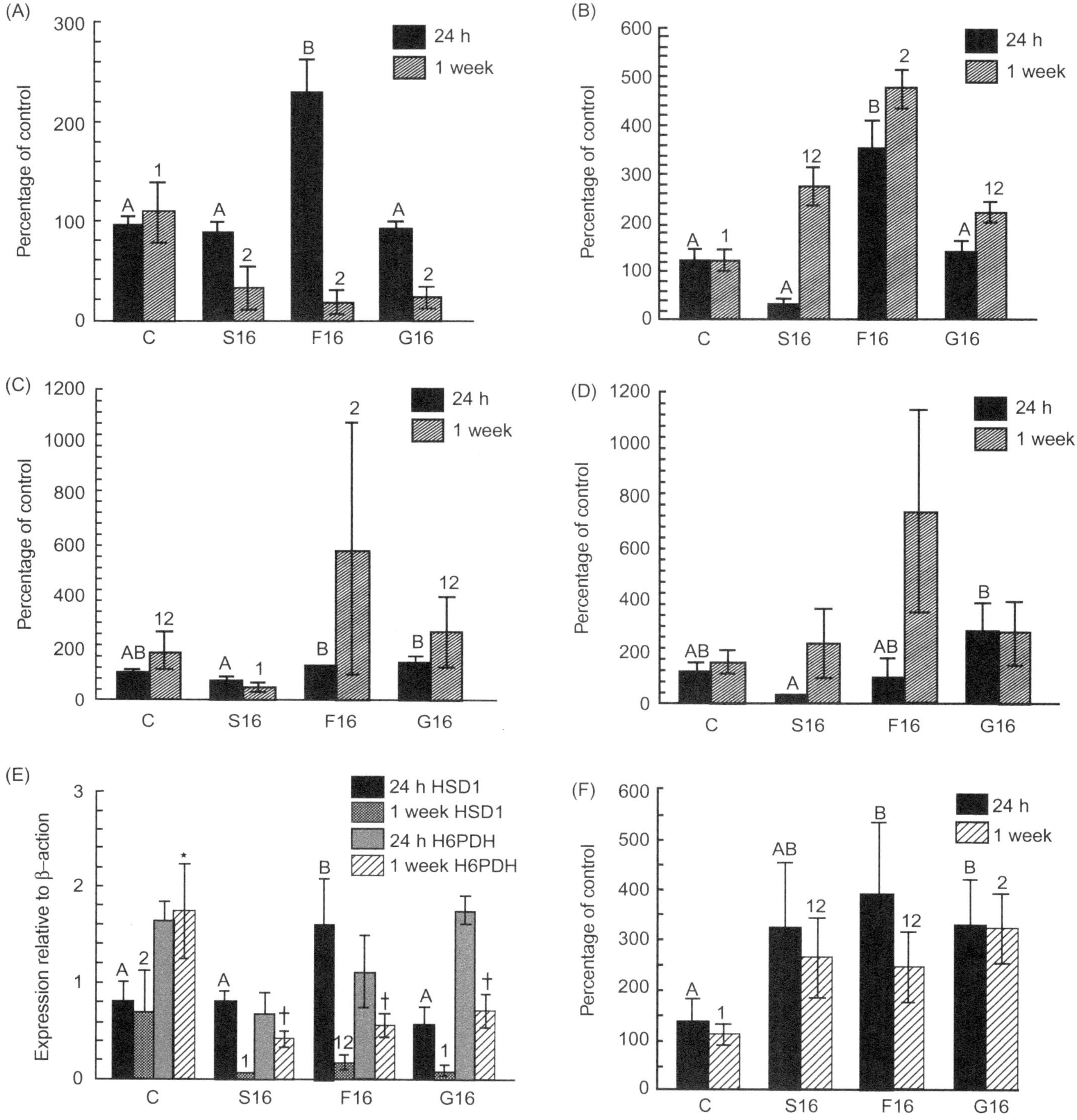

FIGURE 4.2 Effect of different sugar solutions on mRNA and protein expression in liver and mesenteric adipose of 10-week-old male Sprague-Dawley rats. The messenger RNA (mRNA) levels were determined by qRT-PCR and expressed as levels relative to β-actin. (A) Hepatic 11β-HSD-1 mRNA at 24 h and 1 week. (B) Mesenteric adipose 11β-HSD-1 mRNA at 24 h and 1 week. (C) Hepatic H6PDH mRNA at 24 h and 1 week. (D) Mesenteric adipose H6PDH mRNA at 24 h and 1 week. (E) Hepatic 11β-HSD-1 and H6PDH protein expression at 24 h and 1 week as quantified by Western blot. (F) Hepatic acetyl-CoA carboxylase (ACC) mRNA at 24 h and 1 week. The values were expressed as mean± SEM. Means comparisons were limited to within time groupings (24 h or 1 week). Means not sharing a common letter are significantly different from one another, $p \leq 0.05$. *Source: Taken from London, E., Castonguay, T.W., 2011. High-fructose diets increase 11beta-hydroxysteroid dehydrogenase type 1 in liver and visceral adipose in rats within 24-h exposure. Obesity (Silver Spring) 19, 925–932.*

suppressed in the S16 and G16 groups ($p < 0.05$, Fig. 4.2E). Mean hepatic 11β- HSD1 protein of the F16 group was ~25% that of the control and approached being statistically significance versus the control ($p = 0.06$, Fig. 4.2E). There were no changes in hepatic H6PDH protein levels after 24 h of exposure to the experimental diets. After 1 week, the mean hepatic H6PDH protein levels were lower in all sugar-fed groups when compared to the mean level of the control group ($p < 0.05$, Fig. 4.2E).

One of the most important observations of the present work was that fructose, but not glucose, promoted increased 11β-HSD-1 message within 24 h of initial access. We can only speculate that the transient increases in mesenteric adipose and liver followed by suppression in hepatic message that was observed 1 week later was due to the fact that fructose, unlike glucose, bypasses the key regulatory step in glycolysis that otherwise limits flux through the cycle. Mechanistic studies aimed at a better understanding of how unregulated glycolytic activity can affect the expression or activity (or both) of 11β-HSD-1 and H6PDH are clearly warranted. One likely explanation is that the accumulation of glycolytic products triggers an acute inflammatory response and that increased local cytokine production in these key metabolic tissues impacts the transcriptional regulation of these genes.

Clearly, the postingestive effects of fructose change some of the fundamental controls of intracellular glucocorticoid regulation in both liver and adipose. Before this work, changes in 11β-HSD1 had been observed in several models of human and animal obesity, but it remained a question whether high-sugar diets can initiate changes in 11β-HSD1 or whether changes in 11β-HSD1 were the effect of increased adiposity caused by a high-sugar diet. The diet-induced obesity paradigm, as opposed to the use of a genetic obesity model, has enabled us to separate cause and effect to address this question. Fructose causes a disruption in the controls of intracellular glucocorticoid concentrations such as increased adipose 11β-HSD1 mRNA and protein. Similar disruptions have been repeatedly associated with the development of obesity.

SUGAR SOLUTIONS AND THE HYPOTHALAMUS

Despite the extensive behavioral examinations of the rat's avidity for sugar solutions, relatively little work has been focused on the impact of sugar intake on the central mechanisms controlling intake. For example, fructose can upregulate fatty acid amide hydrolase, an enzyme involved in the degradation of hypothalamic endocannabinoids, as well as other enzymes involved in the synthesis of endocannabinoids (Erlanson-Albertsson and Lindqvist, 2010). In addition, sugar solutions can have an effect on the release of dopamine in the nucleus accumbens, the brain's so-called reward center (Avena et al., 2008). In addition to dopamine release, sugar consumption can alter receptor gene expression in reward areas of the brain. Rats with intermittent sugar and chow access also have decreases in dopamine receptor D2 mRNA in the nucleus accumbens compared with ad libitum chow controls (Spangler et al., 2004). Sucrose intake can influence D2R density specifically in subregions of the striatum (Bello et al., 2002) Given the dearth of work relating sugar to changes in the central nervous system as well as our observations on how brief access to fructose can double circulating triglycerides and liver and adipose 11βHSD-1 expression, we next turned our attention to the neural controls of food intake using the same experimental design where rats are given access to a dilute sugar solution overnight and compared with rats that had free access to food and water but no sugar solution.

The availability of a number of new gene-screening tools has given us the opportunity to monitor a large number of genes simultaneously. One such tool is a qPCR array developed by SABioscience (Gaithersburg, MD). In our first uses of this technology, we chose to screen the RNA extracted from the hypothalami of rats fed water, chow diet, and a 16% fructose solution. Controls were fed water and chow diet only. The rats were maintained on their respective diets overnight and then killed. At the time of sacrifice, brains were dissected and flash frozen at −80°C for subsequent analyses. Frozen brains were sectioned using an IEC Minot Custom Microtome (Damon/IEC Division) and 10 consecutive 20-μ-thick tissue hypothalamic region slices were sectioned. See Colley et al. (2012) for more details.

Dopamine receptors 1a and 2 and neuropeptide Y (NPY) were upregulated in the hypothalami taken from the fructose-fed group compared to control. Galanin, Brs3, agouti-related protein (AGRP), INSR, Gh1, Trhr, Atrn, NMB, tumor necrosis factor (TNF), and Thrb were downregulated in the fructose-fed group. Presented in Table 4.4 are the results of comparisons between fructose-fed and control-fed groups that were particularly pronounced. The PCR Array analyses revealed a number of genes that were either dramatically upregulated or silenced by overnight access to fructose. The data reported here include the observation that fructose can upregulate genes in the hypothalamus associated with the dopaminergic pathways. Smith and his group reported similar conclusions: hypothalamic dopamine plays an integral role in the control of sucrose intake (Simansky et al., 1985; Smith et al., 1987; Weatherford et al., 1990). In our preliminary array scan, we observed that overnight access to fructose led to

TABLE 4.4 Fasting Metabolites Are Predictive of Hypothalamic Response

Metabolite Correlations		Fasting Metabolite	Correlation Coefficient	*p*-value
Volume	12 oz.	Triglyceride	0.567	0.003
		Insulin	0.518	0.007
		Glucose	−0.160	0.435
	6 oz.	Triglyceride	0.575	0.002
		Insulin	0.445	0.023
		Glucose	−0.039	0.851
Treatment	Cola	Triglyceride	0.577	0.002
		Insulin	0.468	0.014
		Glucose	−0.133	0.507
	Water	Triglyceride	0.555	0.004
		Insulin	0.503	0.010
		Glucose	−0.079	0.710

Taken from Hudgins, S.M., Schlappal, A., Castonguay, T.W., 2014. Chapter 28, Appetite and Reward Signals in the Brain: Sugar Intake Effects on Brain Activity as Measured by Functional Magnetic Resonance Imaging in: Watson, R.R. (Ed.), Nutrition in the Prevention and Treatment of Abdominal Obesity. Academic Press, San Diego, pp. 307–314.

This table shows the correlation between overall average hypothalamic signal intensity and each of the three fasting metabolites, triglycerides, insulin, and glucose. These data are separated by volume and treatment.

significant upregulation in mRNA for both dopamine 1 and 2 receptors, consistent with their conclusions using microdialysis or dopamine antagonists.

The significance of this observation is that both fructose and sucrose have an effect on this dopaminergic system despite their separate metabolic fates. It is tempting to conclude that sensory properties associated with the intake of both sugars are determining this component of the response to the sugars. By contrast, the suppression of genes in the hypothalamus that are related to insulin (GLP1r, INSR, AGRP, and MCRh1 to name a few) suggests that other processes are involved. Presumably some of these endpoints are also part of the regulatory system involved in promoting increased intake, while others may be more involved in adjusting chow intake subsequent to the influx of calories from fructose. Only a more in-depth side-by-side comparison of the effects of different sugars will permit attribution to which of the changes reported here are specific to fructose and which are common to sugars.

In a follow-up study male, Sprague-Dawley rats were given access to food, water, and one of five different sugar solutions for 24h, after which blood and tissues were collected. Access to the fructose solution (as opposed to other sugars that were tested) resulted in a doubling of circulating triglycerides. Glucose consumption resulted in upregulation of seven satiety-related hypothalamic peptides whereas changes in gene expression were mixed for remaining sugars. Also, following multiple verification assays, six satiety-related peptides were verified as being affected by sugar intake. These data provide evidence that not all sugars are equally effective in affecting the control of intake.

As encouraging as these results were, we were left with several questions that needed to be answered before going further. In particular, although we measured changes in whole hypothalamus, we still had no insight into which hypothalamic pathways were affected. As a consequence, we have subsequently replicated our earlier findings that overnight access to sugar solutions can affect hypothalamic gene expression but that some of these changes were specific to particular regions of the hypothalamus (Zhao et al., 2015a; Zhao and Castonguay, 2016; Zhao et al., 2015b).

Different hypothalamic structures and regions influence hunger and satiety. More than 60 years ago, Stellar proposed that the ventromedial nucleus of the hypothalamus and the lateral hypothalamic (LH) area acted together to control food intake. The dual-center hypothesis was one of the most studied theses in 20th-century neuroscience (Stellar, 1954). The paraventricular nucleus (PVN) was added to this mix later, noting that there were differences in metabolic and behavioral controls of hunger (Weingarten et al., 1985). Many neuropeptides synthesized in these hypothalamic regions play critical roles in energy maintenance. Accordingly, Zhao et al. examined how these neuropeptides were affected by different sugars in three hypothalamic regions: the paraventricular hypothalamic nuclei, the ventromedial hypothalamus (VMH), and the lateral hypothalamus (Zhao et al., 2015a).

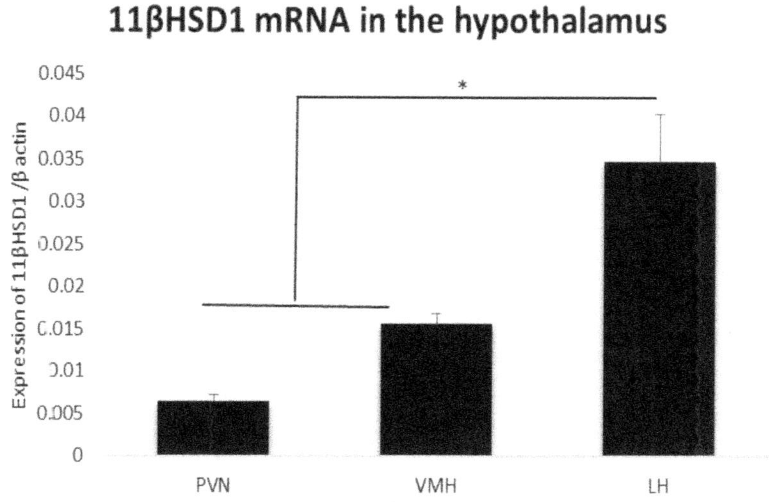

FIGURE 4.3 Expression of 11β-HSD1 mRNA in three regions of the hypothalamus. *Source: Taken from Zhao, C., Tschiffely, A.E., Castonguay, T.W., 2015. Effect of sugars on mRNA expression of 11β-HSD1 in the hypothalamus of rats after 24 hour exposure. Journal of Agriculture and Life Sciences 2, 1–6.*

Sprague-Dawley rats were provided with 24-h access to 15% solutions of glucose, fructose, sucrose, or HFCS and then killed. Portions of the PVN, VMH, and LH were then dissected. Expression of several neuropeptides in these tissues, all of which were previously shown to be influenced by free access to sugar solutions using PCR array, was subsequently measured. Of the four sugar solutions tested, only fructose decreased expression of cholecystokinin significantly and only in the PVN. Other differences between sugar-fed groups included the observation that glucose- and sucrose-fed rats significantly increased the expression of TNF-α only in the PVN and fructose and sucrose fed rats had decreased growth hormone in the VMH.

Zhao et al. went on to quantify the effects of access to different sugar solutions on the expression of hypothalamic 11b HSD-1 (Zhao et al., 2015b), finding that 11β-HSD1 was abundantly expressed in the hypothalamus. Specifically, 11β-HSD1 was mostly expressed in the LH. The remaining two hypothalamic regions (PVN and VMH) also produced 11β-HSD1 (see Fig. 4.3).

None of the sugars used had a significant effect on 11β-HSD1 expression in the PVN, VMH, or LH when compared to controls that were fed chow only. Interestingly, HFCS promoted an increase in 11β-HSD1 expression when compared with glucose- and sucrose-fed groups in both the PVN and VMH.

SUGARS AND THE HYPOTHALAMUS: EVIDENCE FROM HUMANS

Recently, we have begun using functional magnetic resonance imaging to gather further details about how sugars can and do affect the hypothalamus. Smeets et al. (2005b) has reported that oral consumption of a 25-g or 75-g glucose solution elicited a 1–2.5% signal decrease in the hypothalamus shortly after consumption. Furthermore, the 75-g dose induced a greater reduction in hypothalamic activity compared to the 25-g dose. Smeets et al. (2005a) also demonstrated that glucose infusion does not decrease hypothalamic activity to the same magnitude as oral glucose, thus the change in hypothalamic activity is only partially attributed to blood glucose concentration. When Page et al. (2013) compared glucose to fructose, hypothalamic response to both solutions was quite different. Fructose increased hypothalamic activity, while glucose decreased hypothalamic activity by the same magnitude from the baseline. Fructose is rapidly and efficiently taken up by the liver after digestion, leaving little available to reach the brain. As a consequence, the effects of fructose are most likely a secondary response to fructose metabolism.

We set out to identify the effects of HFCS on hypothalamic activity via cola. HFCS comes in many glucose-to-fructose ratios. The most common is 45:55 glucose to fructose. Given the opposing effects of glucose and fructose, hypothalamic activity could remain unchanged when administered simultaneously. However, glucose acts directly on the brain in conjunction with insulin, whereas fructose does not. As a result, we predicted hypothalamic response would reflect the effects of the glucose.

Correlational analyses were used to analyze the relationship between hypothalamic response and circulating metabolites. Hypothalamic response as measured by average hypothalamic signal intensity was positively correlated with fasting triglycerides as well as fasting insulin but not fasting glucose. Refer to Table 4.4. Higher-fasting triglycerides and insulin were associated with higher hypothalamic signal intensity, thus the hypothalamus was less responsive to treatment. High-fasting triglycerides and insulin are indicators of metabolic dysfunction, thus the hypothalamic response is partially inhibited by errors of metabolism.

Our results suggest that circulating triglycerides and circulating insulin influence hypothalamic responses. Insulin binds to many neurons within the hypothalamus as a modulator of intake, including NPY and AGRP neurons. Triglycerides are digested into free fatty acids that might indirectly modulate hypothalamic activity by regulating leptin activity. Glucose acts on the glucose-sensing neurons of the hypothalamus. However, the exact function of these neurons has not been determined. The locations of these neurons are most dense in the lateral hypothalamus. Unfortunately, the lateral hypothalamus may be poorly represented due to scanning limitations.

Body mass index (BMI) does not correlate with hypothalamic signal intensity. This result may be due to BMI's inability to reliably measure metabolic dysfunction. While a BMI greater than 30 is the definition of obesity, BMI is a ratio of height to weight but does not reliably measure body composition or unhealthy fat deposits such as abdominal obesity that are better indicators of metabolic dysfunction.

CONCLUSIONS AND SUMMARY

The body of literature that has been presented in this review is only a fraction of the work that surrounds the question "Does fructose induce obesity?" Our answer to this question is "Fructose can." Here we have presented three different approaches to answering the question, and all three sets of experiments provide evidence that fructose consumption is "not simply sugar," but rather that fructose can promote physiological changes in brain, adipose tissue, and liver that are all conducive to the increased deposition of body fat. Fructose intake changes circulating lipids, promotes an increase in intracellular glucocorticoid concentrations in liver and adipose, and causes changes in genes that control hunger and appetite. One question that has been resolved by some of this work has to do with answering the question of whether or not it was the obesity induced by fructose access that was responsible for the changes in gene expression and intracellular steroids. Our overnight access paradigm has offered a resolution to this question: it is the sugar that is inducing these changes, long before excessive adiposity takes place.

Finally, we would like to echo the comment made by London several years ago (London and Castonguay, 2011). We advocate that mechanistic studies be conducted that are aimed at a better understanding of how unregulated glycolytic activity can affect the expression or activity of 11β-HSD-1 and H6PDH. Future research should be conducted that provides an explanation of how the accumulation of glycolytic products triggers an acute inflammatory response and that increased local cytokine production in these key metabolic tissues impacts the transcriptional regulation of these genes.

References

Avena, N., Rada, P., Hoebel, B.G., 2008. Underweight rats have enhanced dopamine release and blunted acetylcholine response in the nucleus accumbens while bingeing on sucrose. Neuroscience 156, 865–871.

Bar-On, H., Stein, Y., 1968. Effect of Glucose and Fructose Administration on Lipid Metabolism in the Rat. J. Nutr. 94, 95–105.

Bello, N., Lucas, L., Hajnal, A., 2002. Repeated sucrose access influences dopamine D2 receptor density in the striatum. Neuroreport 13, 1575–1578.

Bocarsly, M.E., Powell, E.S., Avena, N.M., Hoebel, B.G., 2010. High-fructose corn syrup causes characteristics of obesity in rats: increased body weight, body fat and triglyceride levels. Pharmacol. Biochem. Behav. 97, 101–106.

Bray, G.A., 2010. Soft drink consumption and obesity: it is all about fructose. Curr. Opin. Lipidol. 21, 51–57.

Bujalska, I., Kumar, S., Stewart, P.M., 1997. Does central obesity reflect "Cushing's disease of the omentum"? Lancet 349, 1210–1213.

Castonguay, T.W., Campbell, E.S., 2014. Fructose intake and circulating triglycerides: an examination of the role of APOC 3. J. Diabetes Obesity 1, 1–7.

Castro, G., Cardoso, J., Vannucchi, H., Zucoloto, S., Jordao, A., 2011. Fructose and NAFLD: metabolic implications and models of induction in rats. Acta Cir. Bras. 26, 45–50.

Castro, G., Massa, M., Schinella, G., Gagliardino, J., Francini, F., 2013. Lipoic acid prevents liver metabolic changes induced by administration of a fructose-rich diet. Biochim. Biophys. Acta 1830, 2226–2232.

Colley, D., London, E., Jiang, B., Khural, J., Castonguay, T.W., 2012. In: Johnston, B.M., Collins, A.B. (Eds.), Fructose: Synthesis, Functions and Health Implications. Nova Science Publishers Hauppauge, New York, pp. 129–143.

Erlanson-Albertsson, C., Lindqvist, A., 2010. Fructose affects enzymes involved in the synthesis and degradation of hypothalamic endocannabinoids. Regulat. Peptid. 161, 87–91.

Hudgins, S.M., Schlappal, A., Castonguay, T.W., 2014. Chapter 28—appetite and reward signals in the brain: sugar intake effects on brain activity as measured by functional magnetic resonance imaging. In: Watson, R.R. (Ed.), Nutrition in the Prevention and Treatment of Abdominal Obesity. Academic Press, San Diego, CA, pp. 307–314.

Jong, M.C., Hofker, M.H., Havekes, L.M., 1999. Role of ApoCs in lipoprotein metabolism: functional differences between ApoC1, ApoC2, and ApoC3. Arterioscl. Thrombos. Vasc. Biol. 19, 472–484.

London, E., Castonguay, T.W., 2011. High fructose diets increase 11beta-hydroxysteroid dehydrogenase type 1 in liver and visceral adipose in rats within 24-h exposure. Obesity (Silver Spring) 19, 925–932.

London, E., Lala, G., Berger, R., Panzenbeck, A., Kohli, A.A., Renner, M., et al., 2007. Sucrose access differentially modifies 11beta-hydroxysteroid dehydrogenase-1 and hexose-6-phosphate dehydrogenase message in liver and adipose tissue in rats. J. Nutr. 137, 2616–2621.

Ogden, C L., Carroll, M.D., Kit, B.K., Flegal, K.M., 2014. Prevalence of childhood and adult obesity in the United States, 2011-2012. JAMA 311, 806–814.

Page, K.A., Chan, O., Arora, J., Belfort-Deaguiar, R., Dzuira, J., Roehmholdt, B., et al., 2013. Effects of fructose vs glucose on regional cerebral blood flow in brain regions involved with appetite and reward pathways fructose consumption and weight gain. JAMA 309, 63–70.

Rask, E., Olsson, T., Soderberg, S., Andrew, R., Livingstone, D., Johnson, O., et al., 2001. Tissue-specific dysregulation of cortisol metabolism in human obesity. J. Clin. Endocrinol. Metab. 86, 1418–1421.

Simansky, K., Bourbonais, K., Smith, G., 1985. Food-related stimuli increase the ratio of 3,4-dihydroxyphenylacetic acid to dopamine in the hypothalamus. Pharm. Biochem. Behav. 23, 253–258.

Smeets, P., de Graaf, C., Stafleu, A., van Osch, M., van der Grond, J., 2005a. Functional magnetic resonance imaging of human hypothalamic responses to sweet taste and calories. Am. J. Clin. Nutr. 82, 1011–1016.

Smeets, P., de Graaf, C., Stafleu, A., van Osch, M., van der Grond, J., 2005b. Functional MRI of human hypothalamic responses following glucose ingestion. Neuroimage 24, 363–368.

Smith, G., Bourbonais, K., Jerome, C., Simansky, K., 1987. Sham feeding of sucrose increases the ratio of 3,4-dihydroxyphenylacetic acid to dopamine in the hypothalamus. Pharm. Biochem. Behav. 26, 585–591.

Spangler, R., Wittkowski, K., Goddard, N., Avena, N., Hoebel, B., Leibowitz, S., 2004. Opiate-like effects of sugar on gene expression in reward areas of the rat brain. Brain Res. Mol. Brain Res. 124, 134–142.

Stanhope, K.L., Griffen, S.C., Bair, B.R., Swarbrick, M.M., Keim, N.L., Havel, P.J., 2008. Twenty-four-hour endocrine and metabolic profiles following consumption of high-fructose corn syrup-, sucrose-, fructose-, and glucose-sweetened beverages with meals. Am. J. Clin. Nutr. 87, 1194–1203.

Stellar, E., 1954. The physiology of motivation. Psychol. Rev. 61, 5–22.

Teff, K.L., Elliott, S.S., Tschop, M., Kieffer, T.J., Rader, D., Heiman, M., et al., 2004. Dietary fructose reduces circulating insulin and leptin, attenuates postprandial suppression of ghrelin, and increases triglycerides in women. J. Clin. Endocrinol. Metab. 89, 2963–2972.

Teff, K.L., Grudziak, J., Townsend, R.R., Dunn, T.N., Grant, R.W., Adams, S.H., et al., 2009. Endocrine and metabolic effects of consuming fructose- and glucose-sweetened beverages with meals in obese men and women: influence of insulin resistance on plasma triglyceride responses. J. Clin. Endocrinol. Metab. 94, 1562–1569.

Walker, B., 2001. Activation of the hypothalamic-pituitary-adrenal axis in obesity: cause or consequence? Growth Horm. IGF Res. 11, S91–95.

Weatherford, S., Greenberg, D., Gibbs, J., Smith, G., 1990. The potency of D-1 and D-2 receptor antagonists is inversely related to the reward value of sham-fed corn oil and sucrose in rats. Pharm. Biochem. Behav. 37, 317–323.

Weingarten, H., Chang, P.K., McDonald, T.J., 1985. Comparison of the metabolic and behavioral disturbances following paraventricularo- and ventromedial-hypothalamic lesions. Brain Res. Bull. 14, 551–559.

Zhao, C., Castonguay, T.W., 2016. Effects of free access to sugar solutions on the control of energy intake. Food Rev. Inter. null-null.

Zhao, C., Campbell, E.S., Tschiffely, A.E., Castonguay, T.W., 2015a. Overnight access to sugar solutions affects mRNA expression of several neuropeptides in different hypothalamic regions in rats. J. Food Nutr. Res. 3, 69–76.

Zhao, C., Tschiffely, A.E., Castonguay, T.W., 2015b. Effect of sugars on mRNA expression of 11β-HSD1 in the hypothalamus of rats after 24 hour exposure. J. Agr. Life Sci. 2, 1–6.

CHAPTER

5

Appetite Regulation in Healthy Aging

Stijn Soenen and Ian Chapman
Royal Adelaide Hospital, Adelaide, SA, Australia

INTRODUCTION

Aging is associated with various physiological changes in appetite and body weight, and many older people are obese or undernourished. Compared with younger adults, older adults have reduced hunger and energy intake; in some cases, suppression of energy intake comes with the ingestion of nutrient preloads (Wurtman et al., 1988; Rolls et al., 1995; Clarkston et al., 1997; MacIntosh et al., 2001a,b; Sturm et al., 2003, 2004; Soenen and Chapman, 2013; Soenen et al., 2014, 2015, 2016; Giezenaar et al., 2016). Malnutrition is a common condition in elderly residents in long-term care (85%) as well as in hospitalized (23–62%) and community dwelling elderly (15%) (Wysokinski et al., 2015). Both low body weight and weight loss are strong predictors of poor outcomes (Newman et al., 2001; Somes et al., 2002), including the development of pathological undernutrition and sarcopenia and reduced functional capacity and frailty (Rolland et al., 2011). The increased prevalence of obesity among older people results largely from the increasing proportion of people entering old age already obese; body weight increases on average to peak at about age 55–60 years before stabilizing and then slowly decreasing thereafter (Ng et al., 2014). The effects of obesity are modified by age. The body weight and body mass index (BMI) associated with maximum life expectancy increase with age; the BMI associated with greatest life expectancy in people older than 65 is in the range of 27–30 kg/m^2 compared to 20–25 kg/m^2 in younger adults (Thinggaard et al., 2010). Both over- and undernutrition in the elderly—a BMI of less than 22 or more than 30 kg/m^2—are associated with substantial reductions in functional independence and quality of life, as well as increases in morbidity, mortality, and health-care utilization (Chapman, 2006; De Hollander et al., 2012; Soenen and Chapman, 2013). More recently, dynamic weight change (i.e., weight change per year)—both increases and decreases in body weight—is increasingly recognized as a critical factor that directly affects health and both all-cause as well as cause-specific mortality risk (i.e., cardiovascular disease and cancer) in older people (French et al., 1997; Somes et al., 2002; Korkeila et al., 2009).

REDUCED APPETITE AND ENERGY INTAKE DURING AGING

On average, healthy older people are less hungry and more full and consume less food and energy compared to healthy younger adults. This physiological process has been termed the *physiological anorexia of aging* (Morley and Silver, 1988; Soenen and Chapman, 2013). Compared with younger adults, some older adults also have diminished energy intake from ingesting nutrient preloads (Fig. 5.1) (Rolls et al., 1995; Soenen and Chapman, 2013; Soenen et al., 2014, 2015, 2016; Giezenaar et al., 2016).

A recent meta-analysis indicated that energy intake decreases by approximately 0.5% per year of increasing age, and this progressive reduction is likely to contribute to weight loss in older people and the development of pathological undernutrition (Giezenaar et al., 2016). This meta-analysis examined the effect of healthy aging on appetite and energy intake in adults, including data from >7500 subjects on energy intake and >500 subjects on appetite derived from 59 studies. Energy intake was less in healthy older (~70 years) than younger (~26 years) adults. The calculated reduction

Nutrition and Functional Foods for Healthy Aging.
DOI: http://dx.doi.org/10.1016/B978-0-12-805376-8.00005-8

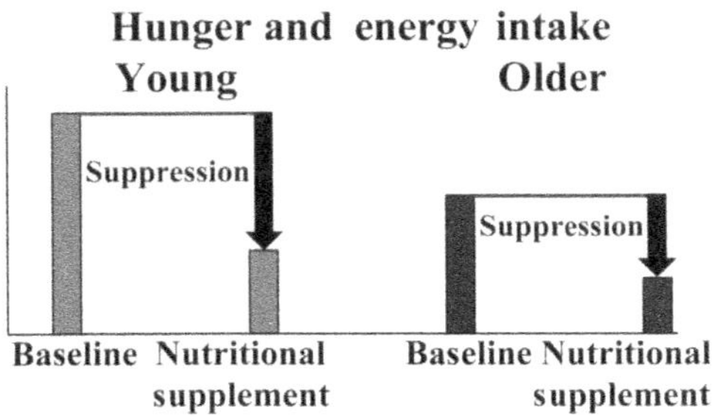

FIGURE 5.1 Scheme of the concept of the physiological anorexia of aging. While hunger and energy intake are lower at baseline (in a fasted state) in healthy older adults compared to younger adults, the suppressive effects of nutritional supplements on hunger and subsequent energy intake are also less in older adults.

fell into quite a narrow range at 16–20%, despite studies of the fasting and fed states and energy intake being calculated by a variety of methods, including intake at an acute study meal, during prolonged periods at home or using weighed food records, 24-h food intake recalls, and food frequency questionnaires—i.e., a robust finding regardless of the method of intake evaluation. Earlier studies indicated a reduced energy intake of ~30% between ages 20 and 80 (Wurtman et al., 1988; Briefel et al., 1995). A 7-year New Mexico longitudinal study of 156 persons aged 64–91 years reported a decrease of 19 kcal/day/year in women and 25 kcal/day/year in men (Koehler, 1994), while a Swedish longitudinal study of 98 people found an even greater decline of energy intake of 610 kcal/day in men and 440 kcal/day in women between ages 70 and 76 (Sjogren et al., 1994). A population-based study indicated that older people ages 60–74 years consume ~500–700 kcal/day less than their younger counterparts ages 20–39 (Briefel et al., 1995).

Perceptions of hunger are predictive of energy intake in both healthy younger and older subjects (Parker et al., 2004). The results of the meta-analysis by Giezenaar et al. show that older people (~73 years) feel less hungry than younger adults (~26 years), both fasting (25%) and after they have consumed food (39%), and they also feel more full in the fasting state (37%)—i.e., changes of about 0.5% per year for hunger and about 0.7% per year for fullness, respectively (Giezenaar et al., 2016).

LESS SUPPRESSION OF APPETITE AND ENERGY INTAKE IN OLDER PEOPLE

The regulation of appetite and energy intake may be impaired in the elderly. For example, the acute suppression of energy intake by dietary protein, whether ingested orally or infused directly into the small intestine (i.e., bypassing *orosensory* and *intragastric* factors), is less in healthy older than younger adults, and in the elderly it may even increase overall energy intake (Soenen et al., 2014; Giezenaar et al., 2015). In the meta-analysis by Giezenaar et al., energy intake was measured in 203 subjects during a single ad libitum buffet-style meal at the research facility both after overnight fasting and in the postprandial state, energy intake decreases on average 11% less in the older than younger adults (Giezenaar et al., 2016). Older people do not show the same ability to regulate food intake after prolonged over- or underfeeding as young individuals (Roberts et al., 1994; Rolls et al., 1995; Moriguti et al., 2000; Parker and Chapman, 2004). For example, younger and older men were underfed for 21 days, during which the younger and older groups lost comparable amounts of weight. After the underfeeding period, the men were allowed to again eat ad libitum. The younger men were shown to eat more than at baseline (before underfeeding) and promptly returned to normal weight, whereas the older men failed to compensate and returned only to their baseline intake and not above it, so they did not regain the weight they had lost (Roberts et al., 1994). This strongly supports the concept that after an anorectic insult (such as major surgery), older adults usually take longer than younger adults to regain the weight, particularly muscle lost, and are at increased risk of vitamin and other dietary deficiencies as well as being more susceptible to superimposed illnesses, often infections.

GASTROINTESTINAL REGULATION OF APPETITE AND ENERGY INTAKE

Appetite and energy intake are dependent on the precise coordination of interrelated *intragastric* and *small intestinal* mechanisms triggered by the interaction with the nutrients ingested. Gastric emptying reflects the coordinated motor activity of the proximal stomach, distal stomach (antrum and pylorus), and duodenum, which is controlled primarily by feedback from neural and humoral signals generated by the interaction of nutrients with the small intestine. Ghrelin is secreted by the stomach and stimulates appetite and energy intake, whereas cholecystokinin (CCK), peptide tyrosine tyrosine (PYY), and glucagon-like polypeptide-1 (GLP-1), among others, are secreted by the small intestine in response to food intake and suppress food intake. The gastric and small intestinal motor and humoral mechanisms underlying normal gastric emptying in humans are complex and highly variable: ingested food must be stored, mixed with digestive enzymes, ground into small particles, and delivered in a liquefied form into the duodenum at a rate that allows efficient digestion and absorption.

Intragastric mechanisms that reduce energy intake include a slowed rate of gastric emptying—i.e., nutrients empty from the stomach at an overall rate of 1–4 kcal/min irrespective of volume in young adults (Meyer et al., 1981; Brener et al., 1983; Horowitz et al., 1994; Gentilcore et al., 2006), increased antral distension (Sturm et al., 2004; Gentilcore et al., 2006), and inhibition of plasma ghrelin concentrations (Sturm et al., 2003; Bowen et al., 2006; Pilichiewicz et al., 2007a). Energy intake is inversely related to antral area and directly to plasma ghrelin concentrations (Jones et al., 1997; Sturm et al., 2004; Bowen et al., 2006).

Small intestinal mechanisms are highly sensitive to the nutrients ingested, and small amounts of nutrients delivered directly into the small intestine have the capacity to reduce appetite and energy intake associated with the suppression of antral motility and increased pyloric motility (Brennan et al., 2008), which results in slowing of gastric emptying and stimulation of gut hormone secretion (i.e., CCK, GLP-1, PYY, and gastric inhibitory peptide, or GIP) (Jones et al., 1997; Pilichiewicz et al., 2007a,b) and the suppression of ghrelin (Pilichiewicz et al., 2007a,b). Appetite and energy intake have been shown to be related inversely to plasma CCK (Bowen et al., 2006) and GLP-1 (Lejeune et al., 2006) as well as the number of isolated pyloric pressure waves (Brennan et al., 2008).

APPETITE REGULATION IN HEALTHY OLDER SUBJECTS

The senses of smell and taste deteriorate with age (Doty et al., 1984), leading to a reduced capacity to enjoy food and develop sensory-specific satiety (Rolls and McDermott, 1991). This normal decline in the pleasantness of a particular food's taste after it has been consumed leads to a decrease in its consumption and a tendency to shift consumption to other food choices during a meal. Age-related reduction in sensory-specific satiety favors a less varied, more monotonous diet and the development of micronutrient deficiencies.

The gastrointestinal mechanisms underlying appetite and energy intake are affected by healthy aging as well; motor function is generally well preserved, whereas deficits in sensory function are more apparent. Healthy aging is associated with the modest slowing of gastric emptying of both solids and liquids (Evans et al., 1981; Moore et al., 1983; Horowitz et al., 1984; Wegener et al., 1988; Clarkston et al., 1997; O'Donovan et al., 2005; Giezenaar et al., 2015, 2016; Soenen et al., 2016), but the rate of emptying generally remains within the range for healthy young subjects (i.e., 1–4 kcal/min) (Soenen et al., 2015). We have recently shown that aging appears especially to affect the initial phase of gastric emptying of protein drinks (Giezenaar et al., 2015), although the dose-dependent slowing of gastric emptying with ingestion of increasing loads of protein was of comparable magnitude in both healthy young and older men. The slightly slower gastric emptying in older subjects is indicative of changes in intragastric mechanisms.

Healthy aging is accompanied by loss of enteric neurons and interstitial cells of Cajal throughout the gut; motor function is generally well preserved, whereas deficits in sensory function are more apparent. Perception of gastric distension is diminished in the healthy elderly (Rayner et al., 2000), indicating a reduction in visceral sensitivity. As a group, older adults have greater antral area (Sturm et al., 2004) and lower plasma ghrelin concentrations (Rigamonti et al., 2002; Sturm et al., 2003) than younger adults. There is evidence that the higher prevalence of *Helicobacter pylori* infection and atrophic gastritis in the elderly compared with the young is associated with a decline in levels of the orexigenic peptide ghrelin (Sturm et al., 2003; Salles, 2007).

In addition to mechanical stimuli, perception of chemical stimuli such as acid and humoral responses to duodenal nutrient exposure decrease with age. There is evidence for altered responses to the presence of nutrients in the small intestine in older people when compared to younger people, including greater stimulation of phasic pyloric pressure waves by intraduodenal lipid infusion (Cook et al., 1997), a greater satiating effect of intraduodenal glucose infusion (MacIntosh et al., 2001a,b), and higher fasting and postprandial CCK and GLP-1 concentrations, which may contribute to slowing of gastric emptying (Berthelemy et al., 1992; Gutzwiller et al., 1999; MacIntosh et al., 2001a,b; Sturm et al., 2003, 2004). It is uncertain whether these changes are due to aging per se or reflect changes in nutrient intake. Healthy older people seem to retain their sensitivity to the satiating effects of exogenous GLP-1 (Gutzwiller et al., 1999), and they may have increased sensitivity to the satiating effects of CCK (MacIntosh et al., 2001a,b). Aging is associated with increased postprandial circulating insulin concentrations (Fraze et al., 1987), mainly due to insulin resistance and associated impaired glucose tolerance (Scheen, 2005), which may reflect increased adiposity and changes in the secretion of incretins GLP-1 and GIP (Trahair et al., 2012). Plasma concentrations of the anorectic hormone leptin may increase with aging. In women, this may be largely attributable to the increased fat mass that also accompanies aging (Baumgartner et al., 1999) and in men, the age-related decrease in circulating testosterone concentrations, which is potentiated by obesity (Hislop et al., 1999).

APPETITE REGULATION IN MALNOURISHED OLDER SUBJECTS

In young adults, there is evidence to support the concept of BMI-related differences in responses to energy intake. Young obese individuals exhibit a less precise compensatory response to ingested energy than lean individuals (Rolls et al., 1994; Ebbeling et al., 2004). For example, suppression of energy intake at a buffet-style meal 30 min after oral mixed macronutrient yogurt ingestion of 161 kcal compared to control (no yogurt) was less in 12 obese than in 12 lean young women ($p < .05$) (Rolls et al., 1994).

Although only a limited number of studies have examined the effects of undernutrition on the regulation of appetite and food intake in older individuals, there is persuasive evidence of substantial differences between undernourished and well-nourished older people. These differences may be the outcome of undernutrition and contribute to the undernourished state (Sturm et al., 2003; Serra-Prat et al., 2009, 2013). Undernourished older adults had significantly reduced hunger in the fasted state and in the postprandial state and significant greater fullness in the fasted state when compared to healthy older (Serra-Prat et al., 2013) and young adults (Sturm et al., 2003; Serra-Prat et al., 2013). In undernourished older women, energy intake was not suppressed by a mixed nutrient preload unlike well-nourished older and young women. The undernourished were also characterized by higher fasting and postpreload ghrelin concentrations, irrespective of a reduction in hunger ratings (Sturm et al., 2003). Hence, it is likely that increased plasma ghrelin concentrations represent a compensatory response to undernutrition at any age, particularly as there is a rise in fasting ghrelin concentrations in normal weight individuals before meals (Cummings et al., 2001), with diet-induced weight loss in the obese (Cummings et al., 2002), and in association with anorexia nervosain young adults (Otto et al., 2001). In another study of undernourished older subjects, plasma concentrations of CCK were shown to be higher than in well-nourished older subjects (Berthelemy et al., 1992), further suggesting that increased CCK activity may be a cause of undernutrition in older people and may act to perpetuate it.

LOSS OF BODY WEIGHT DURING AGING

When compared to younger adults, older adults are more likely to lose than gain weight (Evans and Campbell, 1993). Even apparently healthy, illness-free people exhibit a tendency to lose weight as they age (Wurtman et al., 1988). In some cases, weight loss is due to an illness, which is primarily responsible for the poor outcome. Weight loss in older people occurs because there is a decrease in daily energy intake that is greater than the decrease in energy expenditure. Reduced energy expenditures in the elderly are due to reduced physical exercise, loss of energy-demanding lean tissue, and decreased metabolic cost of metabolizing the smaller amount of consumed food (Fukagawa et al., 1990; Vaughan et al., 1991; Roberts et al., 1995). Various physiological and nonphysiological factors have been identified as being associated with and probably contributing to weight loss in older people (Morley and Kraenzle, 1994; Chapman, 2011; Soenen and Chapman, 2013). These factors include dementia, depression, reduced functional status, medical conditions and medications, poor dentition, social isolation, and poverty (Kerstetter et al., 1992; Gilmore et al., 1995; Chapman, 2007).

It is well documented in population-based, cross-sectional, and longitudinal studies that weight loss is more common than weight gain in adults aged 65 years and older (Wright, 1993; Morley and Kraenzle, 1994; Blaum et al., 1995; Newman et al., 2001; Somes et al., 2002). For example, in the prospective US Cardiovascular Health Study, weight loss over 3 years of ≥5%, was more common than weight gain of ≥5% (17% compared with 13%) and associated with a 70% increase in mortality; weight stability and weight gain were not associated with increased mortality (Newman et al., 2001). Similarly, in the Systolic Hypertension in the Elderly Program, weight loss of 1.6 kg/year in people aged 60 and older was associated with an approximately five times greater death rate than those without significant weight change (i.e., −0.7 to +0.5 kg/year) (Somes et al., 2002).

Longitudinal studies have shown that body weight decreases in older people at approximately 0.5% per year (Wallace et al., 1995; Newman et al., 2001; Arnold et al., 2010), and the rate of weight loss in nursing home residents is slightly higher than in their community-dwelling peers (Blaum et al., 1995; Pizzato et al., 2015; Wirth et al., 2015).

Weight loss of >4–5%, probably irrespective of starting weight (Newman et al., 2001), is associated with increased mortality in older people, both those in the community (Wallace et al., 1995; Reynolds et al., 1999; Newman et al., 2001; Murphy et al., 2014) and those in nursing homes (Ryan et al., 1995; Sullivan et al., 2004; Wirth et al., 2015). Low body weight is also associated with adverse outcomes in older people (Murden and Ainslie,1994; Ryan et al., 1995; Wallace et al., 1995; Flacker and Kiely, 1998; Reynolds et al., 1999; Sullivan et al., 2004; Murphy et al., 2014; Wirth et al., 2015). The body weight and BMI associated with maximum life expectancy increases with increasing age (Decaria et al., 2012), as does the BMI value below which there is an increase in associated mortality. Studies in older people indicate that a BMI less than approximately 23 kg/m^2 is associated with increased mortality (Soenen and Chapman, 2013).

LOSS OF MUSCLE MASS DURING AGING

Weight loss in older people has been associated consistently with adverse outcomes, including increased mortality. This is particularly so in people who lose weight involuntarily and who are already of low body weight (Thinggaard et al., 2010). Adverse effects of weight loss in older people are likely to result, at least in part, from decreases in already reduced skeletal muscle mass. Skeletal muscle mass decreases after ages 20–30, with a decrease of lean mass, mainly muscle, of approximately 3 kg per decade after age 50 (Evans and Campbell, 1993). The loss of muscle mass in the elderly is associated with reduced physical performance, loss of function, increased rates of falls, and increased prevalence of chronic metabolic diseases such as type 2 diabetes (Mathus-Vliegen and Obesity Management Task Force of the European Association for the Study of 2012). When muscle loss is excessive, it results in sarcopenia, which is characterized by generalized loss of muscle mass and strength, and it is associated with increased rates of functional limitation and disability and the need to move to nursing home care (Pajecki et al., 2014). Sarcopenia is usually defined as the combination of very low skeletal muscle mass (e.g., more than two standard deviations below the young adult mean as measured by dual-energy X-ray absorptiometry (Rolland et al., 2009)), and functional impairments such as reduced grip strength or decreased gait speed (Malafarina et al., 2013). The prevalence of sarcopenia in older people varies according to the population studied and diagnostic criteria used, but it is in the range of 6–15% in people 65 and older (Maleki et al., 2000) and up to four times higher in those over 85 than in those 70–75 years of age (Castillo et al., 2003).

In contrast to the loss of lean tissue with age, fat tissue, particularly visceral tissue, increases with age. As a result of these contrasting changes, the percentage of body fat is as much as twice as high in the elderly as in young adults of the same weight (Prentice and Jebb, 2001). With increasing age, fat is increasingly deposited in the skeletal muscle and liver, which is associated with increasing insulin resistance and the development of glucose intolerance (Dominguez and Barbagallo, 2007). Both aging and obesity are characterized by increased inflammation, with reduced immune function, and increased circulating concentrations of tumor necrosis factor alpha (TNF-α), interleukin 6 (IL-6), and C-reactive protein. TNF-α and IL-6 have catabolic effects on muscle mass and further predispose the older person to the development of sarcopenia and frailty. Perhaps it is not surprising, therefore, that obesity in older people is associated with high rates of sarcopenia, a combination referred to as *sarcopenic obesity*. Sarcopenic obesity is associated with two to three times higher rates of disability than either obesity or sarcopenia alone (Dominguez and Barbagallo, 2007). Increased cytokine levels, which may reflect the "stress" of aging per se or the amplified stressful effects of other pathologies, could partly account for the decline in appetite and body weight that occurs in most older people (Yeh and Schuster, 1999). Circulating levels of the cytokines IL-1 and IL-6 appear to decrease energy intake and reduce body weight via a number of central and peripheral pathways. IL-1 and IL-6 levels are elevated in older people with cachexia, while plasma IL-6 concentrations increase as a function of normal aging and correlate inversely with functional ability in older people (Yeh and Schuster, 1999).

CONCLUSION

Healthy older people are less hungry, more full, and consume less food and energy compared to healthy younger adults. They also have a diminished suppression of energy intake by ingestion of a nutrient preload. The gastrointestinal tract has important actions in regulating appetite and food intake that are modified by healthy aging. The reduction in energy intake equates to approximately 0.5% per year of increasing age, and this is likely to contribute to loss of weight in older people and the development of pathological undernutrition in predisposed older people.

Potential competing interests: None of the authors have any conflicts of interest to declare.
Sources of support: SS was supported by Royal Adelaide Hospital Florey Fellowship.

References

Arnold, A.M., Newman, A.B., Cushman, M., Ding, J., Kritchevsky, S., 2010. Body weight dynamics and their association with physical function and mortality in older adults: the Cardiovascular Health Study. J. Gerontol. A Biol. Sci. Med. Sci. 65 (1), 63–70.

Baumgartner, R.N., Waters, D.L., Morley, J.E., Patrick, P., Montoya, G.D., Garry, P.J., 1999. Age-related changes in sex hormones affect the sex difference in serum leptin independently of changes in body fat. Metabolism 48 (3), 378–384.

Berthelemy, P., Bouisson, M., Vellas, B., Moreau, J., Nicole, V., Albarede, J.L., et al., 1992. Postprandial cholecystokinin secretion in elderly with protein-energy undernutrition. J. Am. Geriatr. Soc. 40 (4), 365–369.

Blaum, C.S., Fries, B.E., Fiatarone, M.A., 1995. Factors associated with low body mass index and weight loss in nursing home residents. J. Gerontol. A Biol. Sci. Med. Sci. 50 (3), M162–M168.

Bowen, J., Noakes, M., Clifton, P.M., 2006. Appetite regulatory hormone responses to various dietary proteins differ by body mass index status despite similar reductions in ad libitum energy intake. J. Clin. Endocrinol. Metab. 91 (8), 2913–2919.

Brener, W., Hendrix, T.R., McHugh, P.R., 1983. Regulation of the gastric emptying of glucose. Gastroenterology 85 (1), 76–82.

Brennan, I.M., Little, T.J., Feltrin, K.L., Smout, A.J., Wishart, J.M., Horowitz, M., et al., 2008. Dose-dependent effects of cholecystokinin-8 on antropyloroduodenal motility, gastrointestinal hormones, appetite, and energy intake in healthy men. Am. J. Physiol. Endocrinol. Metab. 295 (6), E1487–E1494.

Briefel, R.R., McDowell, M.A., Alaimo, K., Caughman, C.R., Bischof, A.L., Carroll, M.D., et al., 1995. Total energy intake of the US population: the third National Health and Nutrition Examination Survey, 1988–1991. Am. J. Clin. Nutr. 62 (Suppl. 5), 1072S–1080S.

Castillo, E.M., Goodman-Gruen, D., Kritz-Silverstein, D., Morton, D.J., Wingard, D.L., Barrett-Connor, E., 2003. Sarcopenia in elderly men and women: the Rancho Bernardo study. Am. J. Prev. Med. 25 (3), 226–231.

Chapman, I.M., 2006. Nutritional disorders in the elderly. Med. Clin. North Am. 90 (5), 887–907.

Chapman, I.M., 2007. The anorexia of aging. Clin. Geriatr. Med. 23 (4), 735–756.

Chapman, I.M., 2011. Weight loss in older persons. Med. Clin. North Am. 95 (3), 579–593. xi.

Clarkston, W.K., Pantano, M.M., Morley, J.E., Horowitz, M., Littlefield, J.M., Burton, F.R., 1997. Evidence for the anorexia of aging: gastrointestinal transit and hunger in healthy elderly vs. young adults. Am. J. Physiol. Regul. Integr. Comp. Physiol. 272 (1), R243–R248.

Cook, C.G., Andrews, J.M., Jones, K.L., Wittert, G.A., Chapman, I.M., Morley, J.E., et al., 1997. Effects of small intestinal nutrient infusion on appetite and pyloric motility are modified by age. Am. J. Physiol. 273 (2 Pt 2), R755–R761.

Cummings, D.E., Purnell, J.Q., Frayo, R.S., Schmidova, K., Wisse, B.E., Weigle, D.S., 2001. A preprandial rise in plasma ghrelin levels suggests a role in meal initiation in humans. Diabetes 50 (8), 1714–1719.

Cummings, D.E., Weigle, D.S., Frayo, R.S., Breen, P.A., Ma, M.K., Dellinger, E.P., et al., 2002. Plasma ghrelin levels after diet-induced weight loss or gastric bypass surgery. N. Engl. J. Med. 346 (21), 1623–1630.

De Hollander, E.L., Van Zutphen, M., Bogers, R.P., Bemelmans, W.J., De Groot, L.C., 2012. The impact of body mass index in old age on cause-specific mortality. J. Nutr. Health Aging 16 (1), 100–106.

Decaria, J.E., Sharp, C., Petrella, R.J., 2012. Scoping review report: obesity in older adults. Int. J. Obes. 36 (9), 1141–1150.

Dominguez, L.J., Barbagallo, M., 2007. The cardiometabolic syndrome and sarcopenic obesity in older persons. J. Cardiometab. Syndr. 2 (3), 183–189.

Doty, R.L., Shaman, P., Applebaum, S.L., Giberson, R., Siksorski, L., Rosenberg, L., 1984. Smell identification ability: changes with age. Science 226 (4681), 1441–1443.

Ebbeling, C.B., Sinclair, K.B., Pereira, M.A., Garcia-Lago, E., Feldman, H.A., Ludwig, D.S., 2004. Compensation for energy intake from fast food among overweight and lean adolescents. JAMA 291 (23), 2828–2833.

Evans, M.A., Triggs, E.J., Cheung, M., Broe, G.A., Creasey, H., 1981. Gastric emptying rate in the elderly: implications for drug therapy. J. Am. Geriatr. Soc. 29 (5), 201–205.

Evans, W.J., Campbell, W.W., 1993. Sarcopenia and age-related changes in body composition and functional capacity. J. Nutr. 123 (2S), 465–468.

Flacker, J.M., Kiely, D.K., 1998. A practical approach to identifying mortality-related factors in established long-term care residents. J. Am. Geriatr. Soc. 46 (8), 1012–1015.

Fraze, E., Chiou, Y.A., Chen, Y.D., Reaven, G.M., 1987. Age-related changes in postprandial plasma glucose, insulin, and free fatty acid concentrations in nondiabetic individuals. J. Am. Geriatr. Soc. 35 (3), 224–228.

French, S.A., Folsom, A.R., Jeffery, R.W., Zheng, W., Mink, P.J., Baxter, J.E., 1997. Weight variability and incident disease in older women: the Iowa Women's Health Study. Int. J. Obes. Relat. Metab. Disord. 21 (3), 217–223.

Fukagawa, N.K., Bandini, L.G., Young, J.B., 1990. Effect of age on body composition and resting metabolic rate. Am. J. Physiol. 259 (2 Pt 1), E233–E238.

Gentilcore, D., Hausken, T., Horowitz, M., Jones, K.L., 2006. Measurements of gastric emptying of low- and high-nutrient liquids using 3D ultrasonography and scintigraphy. Neurogastroenterol. Motil. 18 (12), 1062–1068.

Giezenaar, C., Trahair, L.G., Rigda, R., Hutchison, A.T., Feinle-Bisset, C., Luscombe-Marsh, N.D., et al., 2015. Lesser suppression of energy intake by orally ingested whey protein in healthy older men compared with young controls. Am. J. Physiol. Regul. Integr. Comp. Physiol. 309 (8), R845–R854. ajpregu 00213 02015.

Giezenaar, C., Chapman, I., Luscombe-Marsh, N., Feinle-Bisset, C., Horowitz, M., Soenen, S., 2016. Ageing is associated with decreases in appetite and energy intake-a meta-analysis in healthy adults. Nutrients 309 (8), R845–R854.

Gilmore, S.A., Robinson, G., Posthauer, M.E., Raymond, J., 1995. Clinical indicators associated with unintentional weight loss and pressure ulcers in elderly residents of nursing facilities. J. Am. Diet. Assoc. 95 (9), 984–992.

Gutzwiller, J.P., Goke, B., Drewe, J., Hildebrand, P., Ketterer, S., Handschin, D., et al., 1999. Glucagon-like peptide-1: a potent regulator of food intake in humans. Gut 44 (1), 81–86.

Hislop, M.S., Ratanjee, B.D., Soule, S.G., Marais, A.D., 1999. Effects of anabolic-androgenic steroid use or gonadal testosterone suppression on serum leptin concentration in men. Eur. J. Endocrinol. 141 (1), 40–46.

Horowitz, M., Dent, J., Fraser, R., Sun, W., Hebbard, G., 1994. Role and integration of mechanisms controlling gastric emptying. Dig. Dis. Sci. 39 (Suppl. 12), 7S–13S.

Horowitz, M., Maddern, G.J., Chatterton, B.E., Collins, P.J., Harding, P.E., Shearman, D.J., 1984. Changes in gastric emptying rates with age. Clin. Sci. (Lond) 67 (2), 213–218.

Jones, K.L., Doran, S.M., Hveem, K., Bartholomeusz, F.D., Morley, J.E., Sun, W.M., et al., 1997. Relation between postprandial satiation and antral area in normal subjects. Am. J. Clin. Nutr. 66 (1), 127–132.

Kerstetter, J.E., Holthausen, B.A., Fitz, P.A., 1992. Malnutrition in the institutionalized older adult. J. Am. Diet. Assoc. 92 (9), 1109–1116.

Koehler, K.M., 1994. The New Mexico aging process study. Nutr. Rev. 52 (8 Pt 2), S34–S37.

Korkeila, M., Rissanen, A., Sorensen, T.I., Kaprio, J., 2009. BMI, weight stability and mortality among adults without clinical co-morbidities: a 22-year mortality follow-up in the Finnish twin cohort. Obes. Facts 2 (6), 344–351.

Lejeune, M.P., Westerterp, K.R., Adam, T.C., Luscombe-Marsh, N.D., Westerterp-Plantenga, M.S., 2006. Ghrelin and glucagon-like peptide 1 concentrations, 24-h satiety, and energy and substrate metabolism during a high-protein diet and measured in a respiration chamber. Am. J. Clin. Nutr. 83 (1), 89–94.

MacIntosh, C.G., Horowitz, M., Verhagen, M.A., Smout, A.J., Wishart, J., Morris, H., et al., 2001a. Effect of small intestinal nutrient infusion on appetite, gastrointestinal hormone release, and gastric myoelectrical activity in young and older men. Am. J. Gastroenterol. 96 (4), 997–1007.

MacIntosh, C.G., Morley, J.E., Wishart, J., Morris, H., Jansen, J.B., Horowitz, M., et al., 2001b. Effect of exogenous cholecystokinin (CCK)-8 on food intake and plasma CCK, leptin, and insulin concentrations in older and young adults: evidence for increased CCK activity as a cause of the anorexia of aging. J. Clin. Endocrinol. Metab. 86 (12), 5830–5837.

Malafarina, V., Uriz-Otano, F., Iniesta, R., Gil-Guerrero, L., 2013. Effectiveness of nutritional supplementation on muscle mass in treatment of sarcopenia in old age: a systematic review. J. Am. Med. Dir. Assoc. 14 (1), 10–17.

Maleki, D., Locke 3rd, G.R., Camilleri, M., Zinsmeister, A.R., Yawn, B.P., Leibson, C., et al., 2000. Gastrointestinal tract symptoms among persons with diabetes mellitus in the community. Arch. Intern. Med. 160 (18), 2808–2816.

Mathus-Vliegen, E.M., O.Obesity Management Task Force of the European Association for the Study of, 2012. Prevalence, pathophysiology, health consequences and treatment options of obesity in the elderly: a guideline. Obes. Facts 5 (3), 460–483.

Meyer, J.H., Ohashi, H., Jehn, D., Thomson, J.B., 1981. Size of liver particles emptied from the human stomach. Gastroenterology 80 (6), 1489–1496.

Moore, J.G., Tweedy, C., Christian, P.E., Datz, F.L., 1983. Effect of age on gastric emptying of liquid--solid meals in man. Dig. Dis. Sci. 28 (4), 340–344.

Moriguti, J.C., Das, S.K., Saltzman, E., Corrales, A., McCrory, M.A., Greenberg, A.S., et al., 2000. Effects of a 6-week hypocaloric diet on changes in body composition, hunger, and subsequent weight regain in healthy young and older adults. J. Gerontol. A Biol. Sci. Med. Sci. 55 (12), B580–B587.

Morley, J.E., Kraenzle, D., 1994. Causes of weight loss in a community nursing home. J. Am. Geriatr. Soc. 42 (6), 583–585.

Morley, J.E., Silver, A.J., 1988. Anorexia in the elderly. Neurobiol. Aging 9 (1), 9–16.

Murden, R.A., Ainslie, N.K., 1994. Recent weight loss is related to short-term mortality in nursing homes. J. Gen. Intern. Med. 9 (11), 648–650.

Murphy, R.A., Patel, K.V., Kritchevsky, S.B., Houston, D.K., Newman, A.B., Koster, A., et al., 2014. Weight change, body composition, and risk of mobility disability and mortality in older adults: a population-based cohort study. J. Am. Geriatr. Soc. 62 (8), 1476–1483.

Newman, A.B., Yanez, D., Harris, T., Duxbury, A., Enright, P.L., Fried, L.P., G. Cardiovascular Study Research, 2001. Weight change in old age and its association with mortality. J. Am. Geriatr. Soc. 49 (10), 1309–1318.

Ng, M., Fleming, T., Robinson, M., Thomson, B., Graetz, N., Margono, C., et al., 2014. Global, regional, and national prevalence of overweight and obesity in children and adults during 1980-2013: a systematic analysis for the Global Burden of Disease Study 2013. Lancet 384 (9945), 766–781.

O'Donovan, D., Hausken, T., Lei, Y., Russo, A., Keogh, J., Horowitz, M., et al., 2005. Effect of aging on transpyloric flow, gastric emptying, and intragastric distribution in healthy humans—impact on glycemia. Dig. Dis. Sci. 50 (4), 671–676.

Otto, B., Cuntz, U., Fruehauf, E., Wawarta, R., Folwaczny, C., Riepl, R.L., et al., 2001. Weight gain decreases elevated plasma ghrelin concentrations of patients with anorexia nervosa. Eur. J. Endocrinol. 145 (5), 669–673.

Pajecki, D., Santo, M.A., Kanagi, A.L., Riccioppo, D., de Cleva, R., Cecconello, I., 2014. Functional assessment of older obese patients candidates for bariatric surgery. Arq. Gastroenterol. 51 (1), 25–28.

Parker, B.A., Chapman, I.M., 2004. Food intake and ageing—the role of the gut. Mech. Ageing Dev. 125 (12), 859–866.

Parker, B.A., Sturm, K., MacIntosh, C.G., Feinle, C., Horowitz, M., Chapman, I.M., 2004. Relation between food intake and visual analogue scale ratings of appetite and other sensations in healthy older and young subjects. Eur. J. Clin. Nutr. 58 (2), 212–218.

Pilichiewicz, A.N., Chaikomin, R., Brennan, I.M., Wishart, J.M., Rayner, C.K., Jones, K.L., et al., 2007a. Load-dependent effects of duodenal glucose on glycemia, gastrointestinal hormones, antropyloroduodenal motility, and energy intake in healthy men. Am. J. Physiol. Endocrinol. Metab. 293 (3), E743–E753.

Pilichiewicz, A.N., Papadopoulos, P., Brennan, I.M., Little, T.J., Meyer, J.H., Wishart, J.M., et al., 2007b. Load-dependent effects of duodenal lipid on antropyloroduodenal motility, plasma CCK and PYY, and energy intake in healthy men. Am. J. Physiol. Regul. Integr. Comp. Physiol. 293 (6), R2170–R2178.

Pizzato, S., Sergi, G., Bolzetta, F., De Rui, M., De Ronch, I., Carraro, S., et al., 2015. Effect of weight loss on mortality in overweight and obese nursing home residents during a 5-year follow-up. Eur. J. Clin. Nutr. 69 (10), 1113–1118.

Prentice, A.M., Jebb, S.A., 2001. Beyond body mass index. Obes. Rev. 2 (3), 141–147.

Rayner, C.K., MacIntosh, C.G., Chapman, I.M., Morley, J.E., Horowitz, M., 2000. Effects of age on proximal gastric motor and sensory function. Scand. J. Gastroenterol. 35 (10), 1041–1047.

Reynolds, M.W., Fredman, L., Langenberg, P., Magaziner, J., 1999. Weight, weight change, mortality in a random sample of older community-dwelling women. J. Am. Geriatr. Soc. 47 (12), 1409–1414.

Rigamonti, A.E., Pincelli, A.I., Corra, B., Viarengo, R., Bonomo, S.M., Galimberti, D., et al., 2002. Plasma ghrelin concentrations in elderly subjects: comparison with anorexic and obese patients. J. Endocrinol. 175 (1), R1–R5.

Roberts, S.B., Fuss, P., Heyman, M.B., Evans, W.J., Tsay, R., Rasmussen, H., et al., 1994. Control of food intake in older men. JAMA 272 (20), 1601–1606.

Roberts, S.B., Fuss, P., Heyman, M.B., Young, V.R., 1995. Influence of age on energy requirements. Am. J. Clin. Nutr. 62 (Suppl. 5), 1053S–1058S.

Rolland, Y., Abellan van Kan, G., Gillette-Guyonnet, S., Vellas, B., 2011. Cachexia versus sarcopenia. Curr. Opin. Clin. Nutr. Metab. Care 14 (1), 15–21.

Rolland, Y., Lauwers-Cances, V., Cristini, C., Abellan van Kan, G., Janssen, I., Morley, J.E., et al., 2009. Difficulties with physical function associated with obesity, sarcopenia, and sarcopenic-obesity in community-dwelling elderly women: the EPIDOS (EPIDemiologie de l'OSteoporose) Study. Am. J. Clin. Nutr. 89 (6), 1895–1900.

Rolls, B.J., Dimeo, K.A., Shide, D.J., 1995. Age-related impairments in the regulation of food intake. Am. J. Clin. Nutr. 62 (5), 923–931.

Rolls, B.J., Kim-Harris, S., Fischman, M.W., Foltin, R.W., Moran, T.H., Stoner, S.A., 1994. Satiety after preloads with different amounts of fat and carbohydrate: implications for obesity. Am. J. Clin. Nutr. 60 (4), 476–487.

Rolls, B.J., McDermott, T.M., 1991. Effects of age on sensory-specific satiety. Am. J. Clin. Nutr. 54 (6), 988–996.

Ryan, C., Bryant, E., Eleazer, P., Rhodes, A., Guest, K., 1995. Unintentional weight loss in long-term care: predictor of mortality in the elderly. South Med. J. 88 (7), 721–724.

Salles, N., 2007. Basic mechanisms of the aging gastrointestinal tract. Dig. Dis. 25 (2), 112–117.

Scheen, A.J., 2005. Diabetes mellitus in the elderly: insulin resistance and/or impaired insulin secretion? Diab. Metab. 31 (2) 5S27-25S34.

Serra-Prat, M., Mans, E., Palomera, E., Clave, P., 2013. Gastrointestinal peptides, gastrointestinal motility, and anorexia of aging in frail elderly persons. Neurogastroenterol. Motil. 25 (4) 291-e245.

Serra-Prat, M., Palomera, E., Clave, P., Puig-Domingo, M., 2009. Effect of age and frailty on ghrelin and cholecystokinin responses to a meal test. Am. J. Clin. Nutr. 89 (5), 1410–1417.

Sjogren, A., Osterberg, T., Steen, B., 1994. Intake of energy, nutrients and food items in a ten-year cohort comparison and in a six-year longitudinal perspective: a population study of 70- and 76-year-old Swedish people. Age Ageing 23 (2), 108–112.

Soenen, S., Chapman, I.M., 2013. Body weight, anorexia, and undernutrition in older people. J. Am. Med. Dir. Assoc. 14 (9), 642–648.

Soenen, S., Giezenaar, C., Hutchison, A.T., Horowitz, M., Chapman, I., Luscombe-Marsh, N.D., 2014. Effects of intraduodenal protein on appetite, energy intake, and antropyloroduodenal motility in healthy older compared with young men in a randomized trial. Am. J. Clin. Nutr. 100 (4), 1108–1115.

Soenen, S., Rayner, C.K., Horowitz, M., Jones, K.L., 2015. Gastric emptying in the elderly. Clin. Geriat. Med. http://dx.doi.org/10.1016/j.cger.2015.04.003.

Soenen, S., Rayner, C.K., Jones, K.L., Horowitz, M., 2016. The ageing gastrointestinal tract. Curr. Opin. Clin. Nutr. Metab. Care 19 (1), 12–18.

Somes, G.W., Kritchevsky, S.B., Shorr, R.I., Pahor, M., Applegate, W.B., 2002. Body mass index, weight change, and death in older adults: the systolic hypertension in the elderly program. Am. J. Epidemiol. 156 (2), 132–138.

Sturm, K., MacIntosh, C.G., Parker, B.A., Wishart, J., Horowitz, M., Chapman, I.M., 2003. Appetite, food intake, and plasma concentrations of cholecystokinin, ghrelin, and other gastrointestinal hormones in undernourished older women and well-nourished young and older women. J. Clin. Endocrinol. Metab. 88 (8), 3747–3755.

Sturm, K., Parker, B., Wishart, J., Feinle-Bisset, C., Jones, K.L., Chapman, I., et al., 2004. Energy intake and appetite are related to antral area in healthy young and older subjects. Am. J. Clin. Nutr. 80 (3), 656–667.

Sullivan, D.H., Johnson, L.E., Bopp, M.M., Roberson, P.K., 2004. Prognostic significance of monthly weight fluctuations among older nursing home residents. J. Gerontol. A Biol. Sci. Med. Sci. 59 (6), M633–M639.

Thinggaard, M., Jacobsen, R., Jeune, B., Martinussen, T., Christensen, K., 2010. Is the relationship between BMI and mortality increasingly U-shaped with advancing age? A 10-year follow-up of persons aged 70–95 years. J. Gerontol. A Biol. Sci. Med. Sci. 65 (5), 526–531.

Trahair, L.G., Horowitz, M., Rayner, C.K., Gentilcore, D., Lange, K., Wishart, J.M., et al., 2012. Comparative effects of variations in duodenal glucose load on glycemic, insulinemic, and incretin responses in healthy young and older subjects. J. Clin. Endocrinol. Metab. 97 (3), 844–851.

Vaughan, L., Zurlo, F., Ravussin, E., 1991. Aging and energy expenditure. Am. J. Clin. Nutr. 53 (4), 821–825.

Wallace, J.I., Schwartz, R.S., LaCroix, A.Z., Uhlmann, R.F., Pearlman, R.A., 1995. Involuntary weight loss in older outpatients: incidence and clinical significance. J. Am. Geriatr. Soc. 43 (4), 329–337.

Wegener, M., Borsch, G., Schaffstein, J., Luth, I., Rickels, R., Ricken, D., 1988. Effect of ageing on the gastro-intestinal transit of a lactulose-supplemented mixed solid-liquid meal in humans. Digestion 39 (1), 40–46.

Wirth, R., Streicher, M., Smoliner, C., Kolb, C., Hiesmayr, M., Thiem, U., et al., 2015. The impact of weight loss and low BMI on mortality of nursing home residents-Results from the nutrition day in nursing homes. Clin. Nutr. 34 (6), 1274.

Wright, B.A., 1993. Weight loss and weight gain in a nursing home: a prospective study. Geriatr. Nurs. 14 (3), 156–159.

Wurtman, J.J., Lieberman, H., Tsay, R., Nader, T., Chew, B., 1988. Calorie and nutrient intakes of elderly and young subjects measured under identical conditions. J. Gerontol. 43 (6), B174–B180.

Wysokinski, A., Sobow, T., Kloszewska, I., Kostka, T., 2015. Mechanisms of the anorexia of aging-a review. Age (Dordr) 37 (4), 9821.

Yeh, S.S., Schuster, M.W., 1999. Geriatric cachexia: the role of cytokines. Am. J. Clin. Nutr. 70 (2), 183–197.

CHAPTER

6

Human Microbiome and Aging

Seema Joshi and Melissa Navinskey

Dwight D. Eisenhower Veterans Affairs Medical Center, Leavenworth, KS, United States

INTRODUCTION

The role of microorganisms in disease causation has been well established, and the scientific emphasis until recently has been on the prevention and cure of diseases caused by microbes. A dramatic improvement in mortality and morbidity has been seen through improved hygiene, immunization, and antibiotic therapy. However, most interactions between humans and microorganisms do not result in disease. Humans and their microbiome have coevolved over the millennia and live intimately to their mutual benefit (Steves et al., 2016). Recent advances in molecular biology have changed the pathogen-dominated view of human-associated microorganisms, and there has been an increasing interest in the role of the microbiome in human health. Approaches based on gene sequencing have recently allowed complex microbial communities to be characterized more comprehensively and have removed the constraint of being able to identify only microorganisms that can be cultured, greatly increasing knowledge about commensal microorganisms and the mutualistic microorganisms of humans (Dethlefsen et al., 2007).

Joshua Lederberg coined the term *human microbiome* to describe the ecological community of symbiotic and pathogenic microorganisms that inhabit the human body (Lederberg and McCray, 2001). The human intestinal tract is a nutrient-rich environment packed with as many as 100 trillion microbes, whose collective genome is termed the *microbiome* (Ley et al., 2006). Collectively, gut microorganisms encode 150-fold more unique genes than the human genome. The gut microbiome may be conceptualized as an additional organ undertaking a vast amount of metabolic reactions that influence the normal physiology and host metabolism (Steves et al., 2016).

HUMAN MICROBIOME

Advances in bacterial deoxyribonucleic acid sequencing have allowed for characterization of the human commensal bacterial community (microbiota) and its corresponding genome (microbiome). Surveys of healthy adults reveal that a signature composite of bacteria characterizes each unique body habitat (e.g., gut, skin, oral cavity, and vagina) (Zapata and Quagliarello, 2015). Although host-associated microbes are presumably acquired from the environment, the composition of the mammalian microbiota, especially in the gut, is surprisingly different from free-living microbial communities. In the human gut and across human-associated habitats, bacteria comprise the bulk of the biomass and diversity, although archaea, eukaryotes, and viruses are also present in smaller numbers and cannot be neglected (Ursell et al., 2012).

Estimates of the human gene catalog and the diversity of the human genome pale in comparison to estimates of the diversity of the microbiome. The MetaHIT consortium reported a gene catalog of 3.3 million nonredundant genes in the human gut microbiome alone as compared to the 22,000 genes present in the entire human genome (Qin et al., 2010; Consortium IHGS, 2004). Similarly, the diversity among the microbiome of individuals is immense compared to genomic variation: individual humans are about 99.9% identical to one another in terms of their host genome but can be 80–90% different from one another in terms of the microbiome of their hand or gut (Ursell et al., 2012).

Nutrition and Functional Foods for Healthy Aging.
DOI: http://dx.doi.org/10.1016/B978-0-12-805376-8.00006-X

The Human Microbiome Project (HMP), a multidisciplinary international effort, was launched in 2007 to characterize the microbial community within the human body. In 2012, the consortium reported a large study that recruited 242 healthy US adults of both sexes aged 18–40 years to further characterize the microbiota and microbiome. Subjects underwent sampling from various body sites, including the skin, nose, mouth, throat, vagina, and feces. The study confirmed previous findings that each body habitat had a distinct microbial community with a signature composite of taxa. Most metabolic pathways were uniformly distributed across individuals and body habitats, indicating a redundancy in bacterial metabolism. The oral cavity and the stool had the most diverse bacterial communities (the most alpha diversity). Conversely, the vaginal microbial community showed the lowest alpha diversity, with domination by *Lactobacillus* species. The oral cavity had the lowest diversity between subjects (beta diversity), whereas the skin had the highest beta diversity. In the gut, microbiota showed an inverse relationship between the phyla Bacteroidetes and Firmicutes; subjects dominant in Bacteroidetes had a minority of Firmicutes (Zapata and Quagliarello, 2015; Human Microbiome Project Consortium, 2012).

MICROBIOME THROUGH THE HUMAN LIFE CYCLE

The establishment of a stable microbial population involves complex processes such as bacterial succession and host microbe interactions (Lakshminarayanan et al., 2014). Newborns have bacterial communities that reflect the mode of delivery. Vaginally delivered newborns have bacterial communities dominated by vaginal flora such as *Lactobacillus* species. Conversely, newborns delivered by cesarean section have microbiota dominant in skin flora, such as *Staphylococcus* species. The microbiota of the infant gut become more diverse over time with dietary changes. Ingestion of solid food results in an increase in gut Bacteroidetes. By age three, composition of the gut microbiota in children approximates that seen in adults (Dominguez-Bello et al., 2010; Koenig et al., 2011; Yatsunenko et al., 2012).

It has been noted that species diversity of the intestinal microbiota changes with age. *Bifidobacterium* species are decreased while *Bacteroides* increase in the elderly when compared to younger adults (Hopkins et al., 2002). Factors such as clinical changes associated with aging and exposure to multiple medications, including antibiotics, may contribute to changes in the microbiota. A study that analyzed stool samples from more than 35,000 adults reported that colony-forming units remained stable and showed no age- or sex-related changes. However, individual bacterial species such as *Escherichia coli* and *Enterococcus* species constantly and significantly increased with age; *Bacteroides* spp. decreased with increasing age, while *Lactobacilli* and *Bifidobacteria* remained stable through the lifespan. The colonic microbiota demonstrated the most profound changes during the last decades of life (age >60 years). It remains to be shown whether these changes reflect direct changes of the gut microbiota, the mucosal innate immunity, or indirect consequences of age-related altered nutrition (Enck et al., 2009).

The study reported by the HMP consortium in 2012 suggested that the bacterial communities from various human habitats were relatively stable from baseline to repeat sampling within the same subject, but there was large variation between subjects. The stability of the microbiome within an individual therefore suggests a mutually beneficial stable coexistence between the microbiota and the human host. This may imply that any disturbance in the microbiota may be predictive of disease (Human Microbiome Project Consortium, 2004; Zapata and Quagliarello, 2015).

MICROBIOME AND THE IMMUNE RESPONSE

The study by Biagi et al. to explore the age-related differences in both the inflammatory status and the gut ecosystem composition of not only young adults (20–40 years old) and elderly (60–80 years old) but also centenarians revealed that centenarians harbor a less diverse microbiota. Bacteroidetes and Firmicutes still constitute the dominant phyla with enrichment of potentially pathogenic Proteobacteria. The microbiota show a marked decrease in *Faecalibacterium prausnitzii* and relative symbiotic species with reported antiinflammatory properties (Biagi et al., 2010). A subsequent functional microbiome profiling of selected, well-characterized samples from this cohort indicated increased abundance of genes involved in aromatic amino acid metabolism, decreased abundance of those involved in short-chain (≤6) fatty acid production and an enrichment of *pathobionts*, low-abundance microbiota that promote and sustain proinflammatory conditions (Rampelli et al., 2013).

The aging process thus deeply affects the structure of the human gut microbiota as well as their homeostasis with the host's immune system. The presence of a compromised microbiota is associated with an increased inflammatory status, which is also known as *inflammaging*. This is reflected by an increase in proinflammatory cytokines

(IL-6 and IL-8) in the peripheral blood and correlates with changes in the gut microbiota profile of centenarians (Biagi et al., 2010).

This study by Biagi et al. revealed a rearrangement in the population of butyrate-producing bacteria in centenarians. Butyrate is a short-chain fatty acid mainly produced in the gut by Firmicutes of the *Clostridium* clusters IV and XIVa, which is receiving a growing interest in the gut ecology because it represents a major energy source for the enterocytes and has been implicated in the protection against inflammatory bowel diseases. Several butyrate producers were found in lower amounts in centenarians than in other age groups (Biagi et al., 2010).

The microbiota play a crucial role in the host physiology and health status, thus age-related differences in the gut microbiota composition may contribute to inflammaging or itself be affected by the systemic inflammatory status. It may also be related to the progression of diseases and frailty in the elderly population (Biagi et al., 2010).

IMPACT OF DIET ON MICROBIOTA

Several factors—including age, genetics, and diet—may influence the microbiome composition. Of these, diet is the easiest to modify and presents the simplest route for therapeutic intervention. A high fat–low fiber Western diet contributes to a *Bacteroides*-dominant gut microbiome, whereas a low fat–high fiber diet is associated with a Firmicutes-dominant microbiome. There appears to be a strong correlation between long-term diet and enterotypes (gut microbial variants) (Wu et al., 2011).

A study by David et al. examined the impact of dietary interventions on gut microbial communities and revealed that an animal-based diet increased the abundance of bile-tolerant microorganisms (*Alistipes*, *Bilophila*, and *Bacteroides*) and decreased the levels of Firmicutes (*Roseburia*, *Eubacterium rectale*, and *Ruminococcus bromii*) that metabolize dietary plant polysaccharides. Microbial activity mirrored differences between herbivorous and carnivorous mammals, reflecting trade-offs between carbohydrate and protein fermentation (David et al., 2014).

By promoting changes in host bile acid composition, dietary fats can dramatically alter conditions for gut microbial assemblage, resulting in dysbiosis that can perturb immune homeostasis. Increases in the abundance and activity of *Bilophila wadsworthia* on an animal-based diet support a link between dietary fat, bile acids, and the outgrowth of microorganisms capable of triggering inflammatory bowel disease. Current data provide a plausible mechanistic basis by which Western-type diets high in certain saturated fats might increase the prevalence of complex immune-mediated diseases such as inflammatory bowel diseases in genetically susceptible hosts (Devkota et al., 2012). Ultimately, the impact of diet on the human gut microbiota may be an important environmental factor involved in the pathogenesis of disease states that are rapidly growing in industrialized nations (Bushman et al., 2013).

THERAPEUTIC INTERVENTIONS FOR MICROBIAL MANIPULATION

Functional Foods: Prebiotics and Probiotics

Prebiotics are nondigestible food ingredients that beneficially affect the host by selectively stimulating the growth or activity of one or a limited number of bacterial species already resident in the colon and thus attempt to improve host health. Gibson et al. defined three criteria for classifying a food ingredient as a prebiotic. These include (1) resistance to gastric acidity, hydrolysis by mammalian enzymes, and gastrointestinal absorption; (2) fermentation by intestinal microflora; and (3) selective stimulation of the growth or activity of intestinal bacteria associated with health and well-being (Gibson and Roberfroid, 1995; Gibson et al., 2004). Currently, the prebiotics that fulfill these three criteria are fructooligosaccharides, galactooligosaccharides (GOS), lactulose, and nondigestible carbohydrates (inulin, resistant starches, cellulose, hemicellulose, pectins, and gums) (Yoo and Kim, 2016).

Aging is associated with various changes to the human colonic microbiota. Most relevant is a reduction in *Bifidobacteria*, which is a health-positive genus. Prebiotics such as GOS are dietary ingredients that selectively fortify beneficial gut microbial groups. Therefore, they have the potential to reverse the age-related decline in *Bifidobacteria* and modulate associated health parameters. Vulevic et al. assessed the effect of a Bimuno and GOS (B-GOS) on gut microbiota, markers of immune function, and metabolites in 40 older (age 65–80 years) volunteers in a randomized, double-blind, placebo-controlled, crossover study. The intervention periods consisted of 10 weeks with daily doses of 5.5 g/day with a 4-week washout period in between. Blood and fecal samples were collected for the analyses of fecal bacterial populations and immune and metabolic biomarkers. B-GOS consumption led to significant increases in *Bacteroides* and *Bifidobacteria*, the latter correlating with increased lactic acid in fecal waters. Higher IL-10, IL-8, natural killer cell activity, and C-reactive protein and lower IL-1β were also observed. The authors suggested that administration of B-GOS to elderly volunteers may be useful in positively affecting the microbiota and some markers of immune function associated with aging (Vulevic et al., 2015).

The term *probiotic* originates from the Greek and means "for life." Probiotics have been defined as live microbial feed supplements that beneficially affect the host animal by improving its intestinal balance (Fuller, 1989). At the beginning of the 20th century, Metchnikoff associated healthy aging with a specific type of gut microbiota. He observed that populations with a high yogurt consumption also showed increased longevity. He proposed that the consumption of yogurt containing *Lactobacillus* would result in a decrease in toxin-producing bacteria in the gut and increase in host longevity (Mackowiak, 2013). Subsequent studies noted a reduction in serum cholesterol following consumption of copious amounts of milk fermented with *Lactobacillus* or *Bifidobacterium* or both (Sharp et al., 2008; Mann, 1977). A randomized, double-blind, placebo-controlled, 4-week crossover study using a *synbiotic* (synergistic combinations of a probiotic and prebiotic) was done on healthy volunteers ages 65–90 years. The synbiotic comprised the probiotic *Bifidobacterium longum* and an inulin-based prebiotic. Treatment group was noted to have increased numbers of Bifidobacteria, Actinobacteria, and Firmicutes ($p < .0001$) and a reduction in Proteobacteria ($p < .0001$). Synbiotic feeding was associated with increased butyrate production and significantly reduced proinflammatory cytokine TNF-α in the peripheral blood at 2 and 4 weeks postsynbiotic consumption. The study suggested that short-term synbiotic use may be effective in improving the composition and metabolic activities of colonic bacterial communities and immune parameters in older people (Macfarlane et al., 2013).

Bacteriotherapy

Fecal microbial transplantation (FMT) to restore the normal microbiome of the colon is performed for recurrent and severe *Clostridium difficile* infection (CDI). A meta-analysis that included two randomized controlled trials and multiple case series covering 516 patients found an 85% success rate with FMT compared with only 20% success for vancomycin for the treatment of CDI (Drekonja et al., 2015). A recent randomized trial was stopped early because of the overwhelming superiority of FMT: 90% success rate compared with 26% for vancomycin (Cammarota et al., 2015).

FMT or bacteriotherapy is now routinely offered in 500 centers across the United States. It is possible that donor or engineered microbial transplantation could also be used to treat other microbe-associated diseases. However, there is a need for firm evidence supporting its efficacy, along with a better understanding of the mechanism of action and safety in other disease processes. Intervention studies targeting the gut microbiome in age-related diseases might provide an insight and help determine whether there is a clinical window for microbiome manipulations to reduce severity of diseases in the elderly (Spector and Knight, 2015; Petrof and Khoruts, 2014).

IMPLICATIONS FOR HEALTH AND DISEASE

The role of host-associated microbiota, especially the gut microbiome, has received tremendous interest for their potential association with health. Age-associated changes in the colonic microbiota are profound, especially in the last decades of life. An important concern exists regarding the biological significance of alterations in the microbiota and their impact on disease causation.

The gut microbiota have a large impact on the immune system and deal with a large number of bacterial antigenic substances on a daily basis. In fact, there is no larger immune organ in the body than the gut. Thus the gut–microbe interaction is critical for the establishment of a healthy immune system. It is possible that the gut microbiota have a role in stimulating production of the inflammatory molecules that are a hallmark of persistent inflammation in the elderly and lead to chronic health conditions and modulation of the aging process (Lynch et al., 2015; Zapata and Quagliarello, 2015).

Currently, definitive evidence for disease causation by the microbiota is lacking. However, there seems to be an alteration of the microbiota with age and disease processes. The following is a review of some disease states and possible associations with the microbiome.

Frailty

The medical community has not agreed on one specific definition of frailty, but the general consensus is that *frailty* is a term used to describe multisystem physiological changes (cognition, energy, health, and physical ability) that can render an individual vulnerable (Rockwood Mitnitski, 2007; Rockwood et al., 2005). Jackson et al. describes frailty as a useful indicator of overall health deficit, describing a physiological loss of reserve capacity and reduced resistance to stressors (Jackson et al., 2016). An assessment of an individual's frailty is thought to predict unfavorable outcomes such as mortality and hospitalization better than chronological age (Jackson et al., 2016; Mitnitski et al., 2001).

A study of 23 elderly individuals reviewed the composition of the fecal microbiota and the link between the composition and an individual's frailty score. This study revealed that the anaerobic microorganisms *Lactobacilli, Bacteroides,* and *Faecalibacterium prausnitzii* were significantly reduced in the individuals with high frailty scores (Van Tongeren et al., 2005). The same study also concluded that members of the Enterobacteriaceae family were present in higher amounts in individuals with high frailty scores (Van Tongeren et al., 2005). *Lactobacilli, Bacteroides,* and *Faecalibacterium* species are known producers of butyrate, a beneficial short-chain fatty acid required for a healthy colon (Meehan et al., 2015; Hague et al., 1997). The decrease of these species in elderly individuals may have an inverse effect on the health of the gut and could have implications for an individual's frailty score (Claesson et al., 2012). The potential link between frailty and an individual's microbiota is evident from past research, but other factors associated with aging may also contribute to frailty such as diet, changes in living conditions, permanent moves to long-term care facilities, and more frequent visits to hospitals (Claesson et al., 2012). When assessing frailty in an individual, one cannot rule out the importance the microbiome may play on an individual's overall health and wellness. Further studies are needed to determine if altering an elderly individual's microbiome with the addition of probiotics and diet positively impact the frailty index and improve perceived health.

Sarcopenia

Sarcopenia is the loss of muscle mass in an older person. The scientific definition is a measure of muscle mass loss that is two standard deviations less than the mean for young persons (Morley, 2008; Morley, 2012). Disability is regularly associated with sarcopenia, and it occurs in approximately one in every 20 persons ages 65 years and can occur in 50% of those greater than 80 years of age (Morley, 2012). The associated disability related to sarcopenia can lead to increased risk of falls, loss of independence, impaired ability to perform activities of daily living, and increased risk of death (Steves et al., 2016). A proposed link between the gut microbiome and muscle wasting was studied by Bindles and colleagues. This study conducted research on the gut microbiota in mouse models with leukemia, which in later stages can display muscle atrophy, anorexia, inflammation, and loss of fat mass. The study revealed an imbalance and a selective modulation in *Lactobacillus* species in the mice inoculated with leukemia when compared with the control group. The leukemia group was then orally supplemented with *Lactobacillus* species (*L. reuteri* and *L. gasseri*) and doing so produced reduced expression of atrophy markers (Bindels et al., 2012). While human studies are needed to further explore the link between the human gut microbiome and its relationship to sarcopenia, the study by Bindels and colleagues does suggest that a potential link exists.

Clostridium Difficile Infection

Clostridium difficile is a gram-positive, spore-forming, anaerobic bacillus, first discovered in 1978 as the leading bacterial cause of pseudomembranous colitis and antibiotic-associated diarrhea (AAD) (Mylonakis et al., 2001; Bartlett et al., 1978; De Pestel and Aronoff, 2013). *Clostridium difficile* is the most commonly recognized cause of infections diarrhea in health-care settings and accounts for 20–30% of cases of AAD (Cohen et al., 2010). Incidence rates of *C. difficile* infection are highest among those 65 and older compared to other age groups. Hospitalization rates for CDI are highest for those 85 and older (1089 per 100,000 population) (Lucado et al., 2012). *Clostridium difficile* does not cause major disease unless there is a disruption of the intestinal flora, which can happen with antibiotic use. Associated proliferation of *C. difficile* can lead to inflammation and damage to the lining of the intestine with resulting life-threatening illness (Bien et al., 2013; Wilson, 1993). Research was conducted by Rea and colleagues on *C. difficile* carriage in elderly subjects and associated changes in the intestinal microbiota. Their findings revealed large variabilities in the composition of the microbiota among subjects in the *C. difficile* negative and positive groups (Rea et al., 2012). Research related to the manipulation of the gut microbiota and the potential link between the prevention of *C. difficile*–associated diarrhea has revealed varied results with regard to probiotic therapy. A pilot study of 150 subjects by Plummer and colleagues researched the effect of probiotic supplementation on the incidence of *C. difficile* diarrhea during antibiotic treatment in the elderly. In the subjects who developed diarrhea, *C. difficile*–associated toxin was found to be less in the probiotic group compared to the placebo group. Also samples from the probiotic group had less occurrence of being toxinpositive when compared to the placebo group (Plummer et al., 2004).

Recently, the PLACIDE trial conducted by Allen and colleagues studied 2981 subjects and the effect of administering *Lactobacilli* and *Bifidobacteria* in the prevention of AAD and *C. difficile* diarrhea (CDD) in older inpatients. The trial found no significant difference in prevention of AAD or CDD between the microbial preparation group and the placebo group (Allen et al., 2013). FMT, another manipulation strategy of the gut microbiota, has been studied in patients suffering from recurrent CDI. Preliminary results related to FMT for the treatment of CDI have been promising with reported cure rates of more than 80% (Youngster et al., 2014; Van Nood et al., 2013). A meta-analysis of two randomized controlled trials and multiple case series found an 85% success rate with FMT as opposed to a 20% success rate with vancomycin for CDI. Another randomized trial was stopped early because of the overwhelming superiority of FMT when compared with to vancomycin for the treatment of CDI (Drekonja et al., 2015; Cammarota et al., 2015).

Larger, randomized controlled trials are needed to determine if FMT can be generalized across different patient subtypes or if this option provides long-term cure rate for those suffering from recurrent CDI.

Irritable Bowel Syndrome

Irritable bowel syndrome (IBS) is a functional bowel disorder characterized by symptoms of abdominal pain or discomfort that is associated with disturbed defecation (Drossman et al., 2002). Patients with IBS typically present in the third or fourth decade of life; IBS is characteristically more prevalent in females (Saito et al., 2002; Bennett and Talley, 2002; Ruigomez et al., 1999). A systematic review of IBS in North America revealed that the prevalence of IBS did not change significantly with age and occurs in approximately one in 10 individuals across all ages. However, research conducted by Ruigomez and colleagues concluded that newly diagnosed cases of IBS occur less frequently in people greater than 60 years old when compared to other age groups (Bennett and Talley, 2002; Ruigomez et al., 1999). Evidence suggests there is a reduction in IBS prevalence in the elderly due to reduced pain perception with age (Lagier et al., 1999). Also bear in mind that the geriatric population has a higher prevalence of other diseases such as colon cancer and mesenteric ischemia, which can be displayed as intermittent IBS symptoms on presentation (Bennett and Talley, 2002). Research conducted by Tana and colleagues studied the correlation between gastrointestinal microbiota and their contribution to IBS symptoms through increased levels of organic acids. Twenty-six IBS patients were matched with 26 age- and sex-matched controls. The results of the study revealed IBS patients showed significantly higher counts of *Veillonella* and *Lactobacillus* when compared to controls. Study participants with IBS also had higher levels of acetic acid and propionic acid than did the controls. Acetic acid and propionic acid are known by-products of *Veillonella* and *Lactobacillus*, and high levels of these acids may be associated with abdominal symptoms, impaired quality of life, and negative emotions in those who suffer from IBS (Tana et al., 2010).

Based on current research, there appears to be a preliminary link between a disruption in intestinal microbiota and development of IBS. However, one must also consider the complex pathophysiology of IBS and other factors such as dietary indiscretions, lifestyle changes, and psychological stress that may also trigger symptoms (Drossman et al., 2002). Pharmacologic modalities are available to treat IBS, but cure and complete resolution of symptoms are perplexing due to the poorly defined pathophysiology related to IBS (Distrutti et al., 2016). Distrutti and colleagues discussed several systematic reviews that have been conducted related to the use of probiotics and have reported improvement in IBS symptoms. They concluded the evidence related to the manipulation of gut microbiota as an effective cure for IBS is increasing, and probiotic supplementation is a promising strategy for treatment. However, adequate randomized controlled trials of proper length are still needed to definitively determine whether addition of probiotics would be a primary treatment strategy for patients with IBS (Distrutti et al., 2016).

Anxiety and Depression

The US Centers for Disease Control and Prevention estimate that the rate of occurrence of major depression in older adults ranges from less than 1% to 5% for those living in the community, 11.5% in older hospitalized patients, and 13.5% among those who require home healthcare. In 2014, older adults were at an increased risk of depression and associated morbidity with a suicide risk as high as 16.6% among individuals 65 years and older (Drapeu and McIntosh, 2015).

Historically, research related to depression and anxiety has largely focused on neurotransmitters in the brain, and researchers have concentrated on the central nervous system (CNS) and how it controls exhibited behaviors and moods. Recently, a change in this approach and new research has illuminated the distinctive role of gut microbes and their effect on emotional and stress responses (Friedrich, 2015; Foster and McVey Neufeld, 2013). Research on the gut microbes and their effect on mood has been conducted in animals such as mice. A review by Carabotti et al. looked at the research related to the gut–brain axis and the bidirectional communication between the central and enteric nervous system. This review suggests that the gut microbiome plays an important role in the two-way interaction between the CNS and the gut. The gut microbiome interacts with CNS by regulating brain chemistry and influencing neuroendocrine systems associated with stress response, anxiety, and memory function (Carabotti et al., 2015).

Bravo and colleagues tested the manipulation of the gut microbiome on mouse models with the ingestion of *Lactobacillus* and the effect it had on emotional behavior and central gamma-aminobutyric acid receptor expression. The findings resulted in reduced stress-induced corticosterone and anxiety- and depression-related behavior in the group that ingested *Lactobacillus*. Moreover, the neurochemical and behavioral effects were not found in vagotomized mice, identifying the vagus as a major modulatory constitutive communication pathway between the bacteria exposed to the gut and the brain (Bravo et al., 2011).

Most studies related to the microbiome–gut–brain axis have been conducted on mice. Validation of the role of the gut–brain axis on modulation of human behavior is still needed. Current studies offer intriguing opportunities to develop microbially based strategies such as pre- or probiotics for the treatment of stress-related behavioral disorders.

CONCLUSION

Interest in the role of the human microbiome in health has been increasing over the years. Recent advances in molecular biology have shifted our pathogen-dominated view of microorganisms to their role in human health. There has been a dramatic increase in knowledge related to the mutually beneficial stable coexistence between microbiota and the human host. Aging affects the structure of the human gut microbiota, as well as their homeostasis with the host's immune system. Presence of a compromised microbiota has been associated with an increased inflammatory status, which is known as *inflammaging*. The implications of this knowledge are intriguing and suggest that a disturbance in the microbiota may be predictive of disease.

There also appears to be a strong correlation between long-term diet and microbial variants in the gut. Thus, diet may impact the human microbiota by making them an important environmental factor in the pathogenesis of diseases that are rapidly increasing in incidence in industrialized nations.

The impact of fecal transplants in *C. difficile* infections has highlighted the possible role of microbiome manipulation in treatment and prevention of disease. Although more human trials will be needed, there appears to be a tremendous potential for developing microbially based strategies for the treatment and prevention of diseases in the elderly.

Acknowledgment

This material is the result of work supported with resources and the use of facilities at the Dwight D. Eisenhower Veterans Affairs Medical Center, Leavenworth, KS, USA.

References

Allen, S.J., Wareham, K., Wang, D., Bradley, C., Hutchings, H., Harris, W., et al., 2013. Lactobacilli and bifidobacteria in the prevention of antibiotic-associated diarrhea and Clostridium difficile diarrhea in older patients (PLACIDE): a randomized, double-blind, placebo-controlled, multicenter trial. Lancet 382, 1249–1257.

Bartlett, J.G., Chang, T.W., Gurwith, M., Gorbach, S.L., Onderdonk, A.B., 1978. Antibiotic-associated pseudomembranous colitis due to toxin-producing clostridia. N. Engl. J. Med. 298, 531–534.

Bennett, G., Talley, N.J., 2002. Irritable bowel syndrome in the elderly. Clin. Gastroenterol. 16 (1), 63–76.

Biagi, E., Nylund, L., Candela, M., Ostan, R., Bucci, L., Pini, E., et al., 2010. Through ageing, and beyond: gut microbiota and inflammatory status in seniors and centenarians. PLoS One 5 (5), e10667.

Bien, J., Palagani, V., Bozko, P., 2013. The intestinal microbiota dysbiosis and clostridium difficile infection: is there a relationship with inflammatory bowel disease? Ther. Adv. Gastroenterol. 6 (1), 53–68.

Bindels, L.B., Beck, R., Schakman, O., Martin, J.C., De Backer, F., Sohet, F.M., et al., 2012. Restoring specific lactobacilli levels decreases inflammation and muscle atrophy markers in an acute leukemia mouse model. PLoS One 7 (6), e37971.

Bravo, J.A., Forsythe, P., Chew, M.V., Escaravage, E., Savignac, H.M., Dinan, T.G., et al., 2011. Ingestion of *Lactobacillus* strain regulates emotional behavior and central GABA receptor expression in a mouse via the vagus nerve. PNAS 108 (38), 16050–16055.

Bushman, F.D., Lewis, J.D., Wu, G.D., 2013. Diet, gut enterotypes and health: is there a link? Nestle Nutr. Inst. Workshop Ser. 77, 65–73.

Cammarota, G., Masucci, L., Ianiro, G., Ianiro, G., Bibbo, S., Dinoi, G., et al., 2015. Randomised clinical trial: faecal microbiota transplantation by colonoscopy vs vancomycin for the treatment of recurrent Clostridium difficile infection. Aliment Pharm. Ther. 41, 835–843.

Carabotti, M., Scirocco, M.M.A., Severi, M., 2015. The gut-brain axis: interactions between enteric microbiota, centeral and enteric nervous systems. Ann. Gastroenterol. 28, 203–209.

Claesson, M.J., Jeffery, I.B., Conde, S., Power, S.E., O'Conner, E.M., Cusack, S., et al., 2012. Gut microbiota composition correlates with diet and health in the elderly. Nature 488, 178–185.

Cohen, S.H., Gerding, D.N., Johnson, S., Kelly, C.P., Loo, V.G., McDonald, C., et al., 2010. Clinical practice guidelines for *Clostridium difficile* infection in adults: 2010 update by the Society of Healthcare Epidemiology of America (SHEA) and the Infectious Diseases Society of America (IDSA). Infect. Control. Hosp. Epidemiol. 31 (5), 431–455.

Consortium IHGS, 2004. Finishing the euchromatic sequence of the human genome. Nature 431, 931–945.

David, L.A., Maurice, C.F., Carmody, R.N., Gootenberg, D.B., et al., 2014. Diet rapidly and reproducibly alters the human gut microbiome. Nature 505 (7484), 559–563.

DePestel, D.D., Aronoff, D.M., 2013. Epidemiology of *Clostridium difficile* infection. J. Pharm. Pract. 26 (5), 464–475.

Dethlefsen, L., McFall-Ngai, M., Relman, D.A., 2007. An ecological and evolutionary perspective on human–microbe mutualism and disease. Nature 449, 811–818.

Devkota, S., et al., 2012. Dietary-fat-induced taurocholic acid promotes pathobiont expansion and colitis in Il10−/− mice. Nature 487, 104–108.

Distrutti, E., Monaldi, L., Ricci, P., Fiorucci, S., 2016. Gut microbiota role in irritable bowel syndrome: new therapeutic strategies. World J. Gastroenterol. 22 (7), 2219–2241.

Dominguez-Bello, M.G., Costello, E.K., Contreras, M., et al., 2010. Delivery mode shapes the acquisition and structure of the initial microbiota across multiple body habitats in newborns. Proc. Natl. Acad. Sci. U S A 107, 11971–11975.

Drapeu, C.W., McIntosh, J.L., 2015. U.S.A. suicide 2014: Official final data. Washington, DC: American Association of Suicidology, dated December 22, 2015, downloaded from http://www.suicidology.org. Accessed March 15, 2016.

Drekonja, D., Reich, J., Gezahegn, S., Greer, N., Shauka, A., MacDonald, R., et al., 2015. Fecal microbiota transplantation for *Clostridium difficile* infection: a systematic review. Ann. Intern. Med. 162, 630–638.

Drossman, D.A., Camilleri, M., Mayer, E.A., Whitehead, W.E., 2002. AGA technical review on irritable bowel syndrome. Gastroenterology 123, 2108–2131.

Enck, P., Zimmermann, K., Rusch, K., et al., 2009. The effects of ageing on the colonic bacterial microflora in adults. Z. Gastroenterol. 47, 653–658.

Foster, J.A., McVey Neufeld, K.A., 2013. Gut-brain axis: how the microbiome influences anxiety and depression. Trends Neurosci. 36 (5), 305–312.

Friedrich, M.J., 2015. Unraveling the influence of gut microbes on the mind. JAMA 313 (17), 1699–1701.

Fuller, R., 1989. Probiotics in man and animals. J. Appl. Bacteriol. 66, 365–378.

Gibson, G.R., Probert, H.M., Loo, J.V., Rastall, R.A., Roberfroid, M.B., 2004. Dietary modulation of the human colonic microbiota: updating the concept of prebiotics. Nutr. Res. Rev. 17, 259–275.

Gibson, G.R., Roberfroid, M.B., 1995. Dietary modulation of the human colonic microbiota: introducing the concept of prebiotics. J. Nutr. 1995 (125), 1401–1412.

Hague, A., Singh, B., Paraskeva, C., 1997. Butyrate acts as a survival factor for colonic epithelial cells: further fuel for the in vivo in vitro debate. Gastroenterology 112 (3), 1036–1040.

Hopkins, M.J., Sharp, R., Macfarlane, G.T., 2002. Variation in human intestinal microbiota with age. Dig. Liver Dis. 34 (Suppl. 2), S12–S18.

Human Microbiome Project Consortium, 2012. Structure, function and diversity of the healthy human microbiome. Nature 486, 207–214.

Jackson, M., Jeffery, I.B., Beaumont, M., Bell, J.T., Clark, A.G., Ley, R.E., et al., 2016. Signatures of frailty in the gut microbiota. Genome Med. 8 (8), 1–11.

Koenig, J.E., Spor, A., Scalfone, N., et al., 2011. Succession of microbial consortia in the developing infant gut microbiome. Proc. Natl. Acad. Sci. USA 108 (Suppl. 1), 4578–4585.

Lagier, E., Delvaux, M., Vellas, B., Fioramonti, J., Bueno, L., Albarede, J.L., et al., 1999. Influence of age on rectal tone and sensitivity to distension in healthy subjects. Neurogastroenterol. Mot. 11, 101–107.

Lakshminarayanan, B., Stanton, C., O'Toole, P.W., Ross, R.P., 2014. Compositional dynamics of the human intestinal microbiota with aging: implications for health. J. Nutr. Health Aging 18 (9), 773–786.

Lederberg, J., Mccray, A., 2001. Ome Sweet'Omics—a genealogical treasurey of words. Scientist. 15(8). http://lhncbc.mlm.nih.gov/publication/lhncbc-2001-047.

Ley, R.E., Peteresen, D.A., Gordon, J.L., 2006. Ecological and evolutionary forces shaping microbial diversity in the human intestine. Cell 124 (4), 837–848.

Lucado, J., Gould, C., Elixhauser, A., 2012. *Clostridium difficile* Infections (CDI) in Hospital Stays, 2009. HCUP Statistical Brief #124. Agency for Healthcare Research and Quality, Rockville, MD. http://www.hcup-us.ahrg.gove/reports/statbriefs/sb124.pdf. Accessed April 16, 2016.

Lynch, D.B., Jeffery, I.B., O'Toole, P.W., 2015. The role of the microbiota in ageing: current state and perspectives. WIREs Syst. Biol. Med. 7, 131–138.

Macfarlane, S., Cleary, S., Bahrami, B., Reynolds, N., Macfarlane, G.T., 2013. Synbiotic consumption changes the metabolism and composition of the gut microbiota in older people and modifies inflammatory processes: a randomised, double-blind, placebo-controlled crossover study. Aliment Pharm. Ther. 38, 804–816.

Mackowiak, P.A., 2013. Recycling Metchnikoff: probiotics, the intestinal microbiome and the quest for long life. Front Public Health 1, 52.

Mann, G.V., 1977. A factor in yogurt which lowers cholesteremia in man. Atherosclerosis 26, 335–340.

Meehan, C.J., Langille, M.G.I., Beiko, R.G., 2015. Frailty and the microbiome. Interdiscipl. Top. Gerontol. Geriatr. 41, 54–65.

Mitnitski, A.B., Mogilner, A.J., Rockwood, K., 2001. Accumulation of deficits as a proxy measure of aging. Sci. World J. 1, 323–336.

Morley, J.E., 2008. Sarcopenia: diagnosis and treatment. J. Nutr. Health Aging 12 (7), 452–456.

Morley, J.E., 2012. Sarcopenia in the elderly. Family Pract. 29, i44–i48.

Mylonakis, E., Ryan, E.T., Calderwood, S.B., 2001. *Clostridium difficle*-associated diarrhea: a review. Arch. Intern. Med. 161, 525–533.

Petrof, E.O., Khoruts, A., 2014. From stool transplants to next-generation microbiota therapeutics. Gastroenterology 146 (6), 1573–1582.

Plummer, S., Weaver, M.A., Harris, J.C., Dee, P., Hunter, J., 2004. Clostridium difficile pilot study: effects of probiotic supplementation on the incidence of *C. difficlie* diarrhea. Intern. Microbiol. 7, 59–62.

Qin, J., Li, R., Raes, J., Arumugam, M., Burgdorf, K.S., Manichanh, C., et al., 2010. A human gut microbial gene catalogue established by metagenomic sequencing. Nature 464, 59–465.

Rampelli, S., Candela, M., Turroni, S., Biagi, E., Collino, S., Franceschi, C., et al., 2013. Functional metagenomic profiling of intestinal microbiome in extreme ageing. Aging 5, 902–912.

Rea, M.C., O'Sullivan, I., Shanahan, F., O'Toole, P.W., Stanton, C., Ross, R.P., et al., 2012. *Clostridium difficile* carriage in elderly subjects and associated changes in the intestinaal microbiota. J. Microbiol. 50 (3), 867–875.

Rockwood, K., Mitnitski, A., 2007. Frailty in relation to the accumulation of deficits. J. Gerontol. 62A (7), 722–727.

Rockwood, K., Xiaowei, S., MacKnight, C., Bergman, H., Hogan, D.B., McDowell, I., et al., 2005. A global clinical measure of fitness and frailty in elderly people. CMAJ 173 (5), 489–495.

Ruigomez, A., Wallander, M.A., Johansson, S., Rodriguez, A.G., 1999. One-year follow up of newly diagnosed irritable bowel syndrome patients. Aliment Pharm. Ther. 13, 1097–1102.

Saito, Y.A., Schoenfeld, P., Locke, G.R., 2002. The epidemiology of irritable bowel syndrome in North America: a systematic review. Am. J. Gastroenterol. 97 (8), 1910–1915.

Sharp, M.D., McMahon, D.J., Broadbent, J.R., 2008. Comparative evaluation of yogurt and low-fat cheddar cheese as delivery media for probiotic lactobacillus casei. J. Food Sci. 73, M375–M377.

Spector, T., Knight, R., 2015. Faecal transplants. BMJ 351, h5149.

Steves, C.J., Bird, S., Williams, F.M.K., Spector, T.D., 2016. The microbiome and the musculoskeletal conditions of aging: a review of evidence for impact and potential therapeutics. J. Bone Miner. Res. 2, 261–269.

Tana, C., Umesaki, Y., Imaoka, A., Imaoka, A., Handra, T., Kanazawa, M., et al., 2010. Altered profiles of intestinal microbiota and organic acids may be the origin of symptoms in irritable bowel syndrome. Neurogastroenterol. Mot. 22, 512-e115.

Ursell, K.L., Metcalf, J.L., Wegener Parfrey, L., Knight, R., 2012. Defining the human microbiome. Nutr Rev 70 (Suppl. 1), S38–S44.

Van Nood, E., Vrieze, A., Nieuwdrop, M., Fuentes, S., Zoefendal, E.G., de Vos, W.M., et al., 2013. Duodenal infusion of donor feces for recurrent *Clostridium difficile*. N. Engl. J. Med. 368 (5), 407–415.

Van Tongeren, S.P., Slaets, J.P.J., Harmsen, H.J.M., Welling, G.W., 2005. Fecal microbiota composition and frailty. Appl. Environ. Microbiol. 71 (10), 6438–6442.

Vulevic, J., Juric, A., Walton, G.E., et al., 2015. Influence of galacto-oligosaccharide mixture (B-GOS) on gut microbiota, immune parameters and metabonomics in elderly persons. Br. J. Nutr. 114 (4), 586–595.

Wilson, K.H., 1993. The microecology of *Clostridium difficile*. Clin. Infect. Dis. 16, 214–218.

Wu, G.D., Chen, J., Hoffmann, C., Bittinger, K., Chen, Y.-Y., Keilbaugh, S.A., et al., 2011. Linking long-term dietary patterns with gut microbial enterotypes. Science 334, 105–108.

Yatsunenko, T., Rey, F.E., Manary, M.J., et al., 2012. Human gut microbiome viewed across age and geography. Nature 486, 222–227.

Yoo, J.Y., Kim, S.S., 2016. Probiotics and prebiotics: present status and future perspectives on metabolic disorders. Nutrients 8, 173.

Youngster, I., Sauk, J., Pindar, C., Wilson, R.G., Kaplan, J.L., Smith, M.B., et al., 2014. Fecal microbiota transplant for relapsing clostridium difficile infection using a frozen inoculum from unrelated donors: a randomized, open-label, controlled pilot study. Clin. Infect. Dis. 58 (11), 1515–1522.

Zapata, H.J., Quagliarello, V.J., 2015. The microbiota and microbiome in aging: potential implications in health and age-related diseases. J. Am. Geriatr. Soc. 63 (4), 776–781.

CHAPTER

7

Fibromyalgia Syndrome: Role of Obesity and Nutrients

Manisha J. Oza[1,2], *Mayuresh S. Garud*[1], *Anil Bhanudas Gaikwad*[3] and *Yogesh A. Kulkarni*[1]

[1]Shobhaben Pratapbhai Patel School of Pharmacy & Technology Management, SVKM's NMIMS, Mumbai, Maharashtra, India [2]SVKM's Dr. Bhanuben Nanavati College of Pharmacy, Mumbai, Maharashtra, India [3]Birla Institute of Technology and Science, Pilani, Rajasthan, India

INTRODUCTION

Fibromyalgia syndrome (FMS) is an idiopathic form of rheumatism characterized by diffuse nonarticular musculoskeletal pain along with generalized tender body areas such as muscles, tendons, and joints. The chronic pain in fibromyalgia is widespread and mainly affects the neck, shoulders, upper back, arms, and chest. According to American College of Rheumatology criteria, the duration of widespread pain is at least 3 months, and pain on pressure should be 11–18 specific tender points at minimum (White and Harth, 2001; Neumann and Buskila, 2003; Marcus and Deodhar, 2011; Wolfe et al., 1990). FMS is always associated with other complications, especially sleep disturbances, morning stiffness, fatigue after mild physical exertion, paresthesias, cognitive disturbances (especially memory loss), anxiety, tension headaches, irritable bowel syndrome, mitral valve prolapse, primary dysmenorrhea, depression, and psychological disturbance (Branco et al., 2010; Arnold et al., 2006). It is frequently connected with severe functional damage and work inability, and its effects are comparable to those reported for osteoarthritis and other rheumatic disorders (Walker et al., 1997; Hawley and Wolfe, 1991). Approximately 2–2.7% of the world's population suffers from FMS, and the rate of incidence is higher in younger and middle-aged women, obese people, and aged patients (Queiroz, 2013; Fitzcharles et al., 2013). The prevalence rate of FMS in the United States is 6–15%, with a five times higher incidence among women than men (Jahan et al., 2012). From 40% to 70% of the fibromyalgia patients are suffering from obesity, and increased body mass index (BMI) is correlated with higher levels of fatigue and pain in fibromyalgia (Bennett et al., 2007; Neumann et al., 2008). The level of oxidative stress, type of diet, and nutritional status are also associated factors that increase the risk of FMS (Li and Micheletti, 2011; Arranz et al., 2010; Percival et al., 1997) (Fig. 7.1).

PATHOPHYSIOLOGY OF FIBROMYALGIA

The pathophysiology of FMS includes multiple abnormalities and altered mechanisms. The aberrations of the autonomic and central nervous systems, genetic factors, environmental factors, psychological factors, the hypothalamic–pituitary–adrenal (HPA) axis hormones, and oxidative stress are all involved in the pathogenesis of FMS. Abnormalities in several neuroendocrine transmitters—in particular, nerve growth hormone (GH), 5-hydroxytryptamine, cortisol, norepinephrine, and substance P—are reported in FMS (Bradley, 2009; Ozgocmen et al., 2006).

Nutrition and Functional Foods for Healthy Aging.
DOI: http://dx.doi.org/10.1016/B978-0-12-805376-8.00007-1

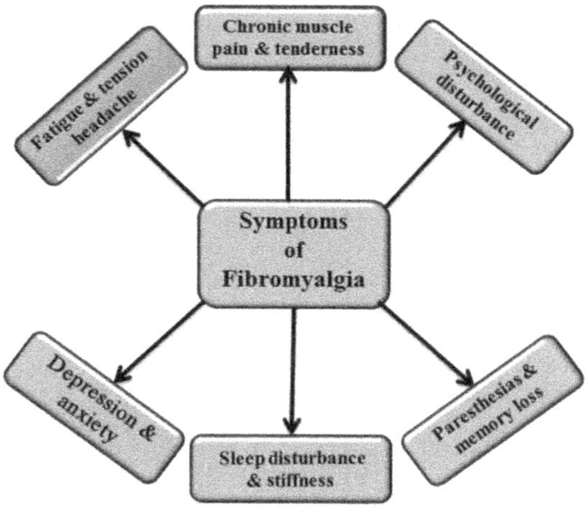

FIGURE 7.1 Associated factors that increase the risk of FMS.

Chronic pain in FMS is a result of central sensitization, abnormal descending inhibitory pain pathways, and altered level of neurotransmitters. Central sensitization is considered the major mechanism involved in chronic pain. It is a result of spontaneous nerve action, enlarged receptive fields, and augmented response to the stimuli conveyed by the primary afferent nerve (Bellato et al., 2012; Ozgocmen et al., 2006). In FMS, central sensitization causes abnormal windup processes, which results in neuronal hyperexcitability in the spinal cord. It is mediated by *N*-methyl-D-aspartate receptors via nitric oxide (NO) and peroxynitrite pathways and plays a vital role in pain processing (Woolf, 2011; Staud et al., 2001; Staud et al., 2004; Latremoliere and Woolf, 2009). Glial cell activation through various stimuli also plays a significant role in pain processes. The activation of glial cell increases the release of NO, reactive oxygen species, and proinflammatory cytokines and ultimately prolongs neuronal hyperexcitability (Watkins et al., 2001). Several neurotransmitters and modulators are involved in the central sensitization and chronic pain. For example, serotonin and noradrenalin levels in the central nervous system appear to be reduced in FMS and lead to dysfunctional descending pathways, while substance P and glutamate levels are increased in cerebrospinal fluid, which increases pain sensitivity. Alteration of these neurotransmitters also affects sleep and mood in FMS patients (Becker et al., 2011; McCarley, 2007; Raison, 2009). The HPA axis functions abnormally in FMS because of chronic pain-induced stress (Crofford, 2002; Demitrack and Crofford, 1998). Furthermore, hyposecretion of corticotropin-releasing hormone in FMS patients elevates the level of adrenocorticotropic hormone and cortisol in response to stress (Neeck and Crofford, 2000; Riedel et al., 1998; Neeck and Crofford, 2002). The secretion of GH and insulin-like growth factor (IGF-1) is also decreased. Inadequate secretion of GH and IGF-1 are significant factors of sleep disturbance in FMS patients (Prinz et al., 1995; Van Cauter et al., 1998). Genetic modifications such as nucleotide polymorphism in various genes such as the serotonin transporter (5-HTT) gene, the catechol-*O*-methyltransferase gene, and dopamine D4 receptor gene are also reported in FMS. Environmental factors such as infections caused by various viruses such as the human immunodeficiency virus, parvoviruses, the hepatitis C virus, and some bacteria also play important roles in pathogenesis by activating glial cells and releasing cytokines (Rivera et al., 1997; Leventhal et al., 1991; Buskila et al., 1990; Nicolson et al., 1999; Furr and Marriott, 2012).

FIBROMYALGIA AND OBESITY

Obesity is defined as a complex disease with immoderate deposition of fat in adipose tissue (Ravussin and Swinburn, 1992; Ursini et al., 2011). It can be considered a major risk factor for the development of several medical problems such as hypertension, respiratory diseases, type 2 diabetes, gout, strokes, osteoarthritis, and musculoskeletal disorders, including fibromyalgia (Must and Strauss, 1999). BMI is considered worldwide as an important measure of obesity and is divided into three classes: a BMI $<25\,kg/m^2$ is considered as normal weight status, a BMI of $25–30\,kg/m^2$ is categorized as overweight, and a BMI >30 is considered obese (Gremese et al., 2014). Physical dysfunction and musculoskeletal pain have been more commonly observed in obese individuals. Several clinical reports also revealed relationships between fibromyalgia and obesity (Peltonen et al., 2003; Hooper et al., 2007; De Sá Pinto et al., 2006). Yunus and coworkers examined a connection between fibromyalgia and obesity in 211 female patients and demonstrated significant correlation between BMI and fibromyalgia (Yunus et al., 2002). Neumann and coworkers evaluated the link between fibromyalgia symptoms (physical activity, muscle tenderness, and quality of life) and obesity in 100 FMS female patients. The result showed negative correlation between quality of life, tenderness threshold, and BMI and positive correlation between obesity and physical dysfunction. In the same study, pain sensitivity was found to be high in obese FMS patients (Neumann et al., 2008). Similar outcomes were obtained by Kim et al. and Timmerman et al. in their study conducted on 888 patients and 179 women suffering from FMS, respectively (Kim et al., 2012; Timmerman et al., 2013). Findings from a few more studies showed that low levels of physical exercise in overweight and obese patients increases the risk of FMS development (Mork et al., 2010; Vincent et al., 2014). Furthermore, FMS was found to be more common in obese and overweight twins than nonobese twins (Wright et al., 2010). All of these reported studies indicate a strong correlation between fibromyalgia and obesity.

SYMPTOMS OF FMS AND OBESITY

Obesity deleteriously affects the musculoskeletal system. Mechanical loading, inflammation, and psychological status are three major mechanisms involved in obesity-related musculoskeletal pain (Vincent et al., 2013; Messier et al., 2005; Kaur, 2014; Marcus, 2004). Mechanical loading is responsible for anabolic stimulus to the bone and improves bone strength, size, and shape by improving tissue density (Turner and Robling, 2004). Obesity induces joint pain by increasing mechanical loading on the musculoskeletal system. It subsequently reduces strength to control loading on cartilaginous areas of the joint and affects alignment of the joints. Furthermore, loading may increase toward a small cross-sectional area of the joint and cause tissue damage (Andriacchi et al., 2004). Axial joints are also victim of central obesity and cause back pain (Menegoni et al., 2009). Tissues such as tendons, cartilages, and fascia are also affected by obesity (Wearing et al., 2006). Recent evidence suggests that in obese person adipocytes enlarge and cause alteration in systemic metabolism (Greenberg and Obin, 2006). Furthermore increases in BMI and fat volume also cause adiposopathy and increased tissue pain because more macrophages are able to enter adipose tissue (Seaman, 2013). The release of several inflammatory markers such as C-reactive proteins, cytokines, and interleukins (specifically IL-6) is higher in obese individuals suffering from chronic musculoskeletal pain compared to lean individuals (Deere et al., 2012; Briggs et al., 2013). Cytokines are known to play a role in diverse clinical processes and phenomena such as fatigue, fever, sleep, pain, stress, and aching (Wallace, 2006). Increases in the release of these inflammatory markers also increases pain severity (Bas et al., 2014). Obesity also alters functions of the HPA axis and increases cortisol levels (Okifuji et al., 2009). Psychological factors also play a major role in severity of pain in obese patients, who have more fear of movement and thus are more inactive and lethargic, which ultimately increases multisite pain (Vincent et al., 2010; Seaman, 2013). Obesity is also associated with insomnia, sleep disturbances, and excessive daytime sleepiness, creating a major risk for sleep apnea. It has also been reported that sleep duration is inversely propositional to BMI while daytime sleepiness in directly proportional to BMI. Obesity reduces sleep duration and quality of sleep in fibromyalgia patients (Hargens et al., 2013; Dixon et al., 2001; Watenpaugh, 2009; St-Onge et al., 2009; Algul et al., 2009; De Araújo et al., 2015). Okifuji and coworkers observed similar outcomes in their study conducted on 215 patients suffering from fibromyalgia. The pain sensitivity was high in obese patients along with poor sleep quality and reduced physical strength (Okifuji et al., 2010). Aparicio and coworkers found that weight status affected fibromyalgia symptoms in 175 and 177 women suffering from fibromyalgia, which showed increased levels of anxiety, fatigue, stiffness, morning tiredness, and depression in overweight and obese patients compared to nonobese patients. Furthermore, the quality of life, motor agility, cardiorespiratory fitness, and upper-body flexibility was damaged more in obese patients (Aparicio et al., 2011; Aparicio et al., 2013; Aparicio et al., 2014).

Based on the fact that obesity is playing an important role in pathophysiology of fibromyalgia, many studies have been carried out by various groups of researchers that showed positive improvement in the symptoms of fibromyalgia after weight reduction. In 2005, Shapiro and coworkers investigated the relationship between BMI and FMSs in 42 obese women to determine the effect of behavioral weight-loss treatment in these patients. The outcome of the 20-week treatment showed significant reduction in FMS and pain interference and improved the patients' quality of life (Shapiro et al., 2005). Evidence showed that weight loss through bariatric surgery in obese subjects reduced FMS up to 92% and also improved musculoskeletal health in obese people (Hooper et al., 2007; Saber et al., 2008).

A randomized controlled trial was also carried out using 86 obese fibromyalgia patients to study the effect of weight loss in improving the FMS. After a 6-month dietary weight loss program, significant improvement was observed in terms of quality of life, improved sleep quality, reduced depression, and reduced tender-point count. The C-reactive protein and interleukin-6 level were also reduced after weight-loss treatment (Senna et al., 2012). There is

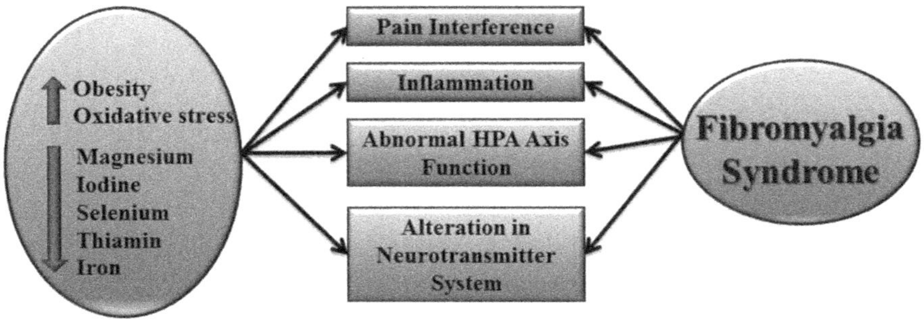

FIGURE 7.2 Factors that increase and decrease the risk of fatigue in FMS patients.

evidence for the beneficial role of exercise in obese fibromyalgia patients to reduce fatigue because exercise leads to increased resistin and IGF-1 levels in serum that are inversely proportional to fatigue (Bjersing et al., 2013) (Fig. 7.2).

ROLE OF DIET AND MICRONUTRIENTS IN FIBROMYALGIA

The eating habits, type of food, and nutritional level of the diet play significant role in the improvement of fibromyalgia symptoms along with pharmacological therapies (Batista et al., 2015; Arranz et al., 2012). It has been reported that nutritional factors are associated with immune and inflammatory processes and can modify the symptoms of FMS (Henderson and Panush, 1999). According to the Brazilian Rheumatology Society, nutrients play a potential role in FMS. Increased consumption of salt, sugar, fat, and alcohol worsens the symptoms of FMS while increased intake of fruits, vegetables, fluids, and fibers have beneficial effects for FMS patients. In addition, nutritional supplementation of micronutrients such as magnesium, iodine, calcium, manganese, iron, thiamine, vitamin D, melatonin, malic acid, thiamine, and sources of tryptophan are important in improving fibromyalgia symptoms (Batista et al. 2015; Arranz et al., 2010).

Diet

Vegetarian diets rich in antioxidants, beta carotene, minerals, and fibers have been reported to improve some of the fibromyalgia symptoms. These diets mainly reduce inflammation in the body by regulating the level of antioxidants, essential fatty acids and arachidonic acid (Smedslund et al., 2010). According to the Donaldson's observational study, fibromyalgia symptoms such as chronic pain in the shoulder and neck, quality of life, and psychosocial behavior in the patients can be improved by dietary intervention of pure vegetarian diet (Donaldson et al., 2001). A study by Kaartinen showed that vegan diets rich in lactobateria improve joint stiffness, quality of sleep, and visual analog scale. It also improved BMI, serum cholesterol and peroxide levels, apolipoproteins, and plasma fibrinogen levels in fibromyalgia patients (Kaartinen et al., 2000; Hostmark et al., 1993). Another study found that a vegan diet rich in antioxidants that mainly contains carotenoids, vitamin C, and vitamin E reduces pain and self-reported morning joint stiffness in rheumatic disorders (Hänninen et al., 2000). Brain tryptophan level is important in the synthesis of serotonin, which is an important neurotransmitter in pain pathway. Increased intake of large neutral amino acids present in animal proteins decreases brain tryptophan levels in fibromyalgia patients and affects the pain pathway (Juhl, 1998). Azad and coworkers conducted an open, controlled, and randomized trial on 78 fibromyalgia patients to investigate the effects of a vegetarian diet (free of animal proteins) in reducing pain and morbidity. The study outcome showed a significant reduction in pain score (Azad et al., 2000). The reports showed that food additives containing aspartate and glutamate, monosodium glutamate, aspartame, autolyzed yeast extract, and branched-chain amino acids present in food act as excitatory neurotransmitters and play a potential role in pain via central sensitization. In addition, food coloring, cow's milk, chocolate, caffeine, and shellfish also trigger fibromyalgia symptoms (Holton et al., 2009; Li and Micheletti, 2011). According to a community-based study, immune reactants such as monosodium glutamate, food colors, chocolate, caffeine, dairy products, and aspartame alter the neuroimmune hormonal feedback control system in fibromyalgia patients. In the same study, replacement of foods containing these substances with dietary supplements that included antioxidants and minerals consumed by patients for 6 months brought improved fibromyalgia symptoms, including reductions in pain, depression, morning stiffness, and fatigue (Deuster and Jaffe, 1998).

Micronutrients

Micronutrients are vital constituents of biological structures. A diet's nutritional status is an important aspect to be considered in fibromyalgia patients because nutritional deficiencies are possible with FMS. Arranz and coworkers have reported the role of nutritional deficiency of magnesium, iodine, iron, selenium, and other micronutrients in the pathogenesis of fibromyalgia (Arranz et al., 2010). The following discusses important nutrients that have a role in FMS.

Magnesium

Magnesium is an important micronutrient required for the production of energy through adenosine triphosphate (ATP) synthesis in the presence of oxygen, substrates, adenosine diphosphate, and phosphate. High levels of cytosolic calcium and aluminum reduces ATP production by inhibiting glycolysis and oxidative phosphorylation. An adequate amount of magnesium is required to maintain low levels of cytosolic calcium and reduce aluminum toxicity (Siesjö et al., 1988; Allen, 1987). Intracellular magnesium and calcium concentrations play a vital role in muscle contraction. The results obtained from a study conducted by Magaldi et al. also showed the potential role of magnesium and calcium in FMS patients for muscular hypertonus (Magaldi et al., 1999). It has been reported that the level of magnesium is below normal range in fibromyalgia patients. A deficiency of magnesium affects the Krebs cycle and reduces lung capacity which ultimately leads to the development of such symptoms as fatigue, headache, muscle pain, irritable bowel syndrome, and depression in FMS patients (Abraham and Flechas, 1992; Romano and John, 1994). A sufficient concentration of magnesium is required to reduce relative hypoxia condition in FMS patients by reducing blood lactate levels and oxygen consumption (Schmidt et al., 1989). A magnesium deficiency also causes mitochondrial swelling and reduces the number of mitochondria per cell (Heaton and Rayssiguier, 1987). Yunus and coworkers also observed similar mitochondrial changes in tender-point muscle biopsies of FM patients (Yunus et al., 1988) and has been associated with muscle pain. Based on this association, Eisinger and coworkers examined magnesium levels in 22 patients suffering from muscle pain in fibromyalgia. The outcome of the study showed increased leukocyte level of magnesium while erythrocyte levels of magnesium decreased in the patients (Eisinger et al., 1994a,b). In one study, the correlation between clinical symptoms of fibromyalgia, especially fatigue and serum magnesium levels, were evaluated in 32 fibromyalgia patients. The results of the study showed significant reduction in serum magnesium levels, and significant correlation has been found between fatigue and serum magnesium levels in patients (Sendur et al., 2008).

Since magnesium concentration in serum plays an important role in fibromyalgia symptoms, magnesium supplementation may improve the symptomatic condition in FMS. In one study conducted in an open clinical setting, the effect of magnesium supplementation at a dosage of 300–600 mg along with malic acid (1200–2400 mg) was evaluated for 4–8 weeks in 15 FMS patients. The outcome of the study showed improvements in the pain condition and significant reductions in the tender-point index after magnesium supplementation (Abraham and Flechas, 1992). Similar finding were obtained in another randomized, double-blind, crossover study carried out by Russell et al. in 24 fibromyalgia patients. In this study, dose escalation of magnesium for 6 months showed significant reduction in pain and tenderness (Russell et al., 1995). A group of researcher evaluated the effect of magnesium citrate and magnesium citrate in combination with amitriptyline in the clinical symptoms of FMS such as pain threshold, number of tender points, pain intensity, tender-point index, Beck Anxiety Scale score and depression in 60 premenopausal women. The outcome of the study showed reduction in tender points, the tender-point index, and the Beck Depression Scale after magnesium citrate treatment and magnesium citrate in combination of amitriptyline showed significant improvement in all fibromyalgia symptoms (Bagis et al., 2013).

Iodine

Iodine is an essential micronutrient required for a healthy life (Prashanth et al., 2015). Approximately 70 μg/day of iodine is used by the thyroid gland to synthesis required amounts of thyroxine (T4) and triiodothyronine (T3) to regulate metabolism, normal growth, and development (Miller, 2006). It acts as an antioxidant by scavenging free hydroxyl radicals and increasing antioxidant levels in human serum (Winkler et al., 2000). An iodine deficiency causes thyroid dysfunction, and this leads to clinical symptoms like those found in fibromyalgia such as chronic aches, abnormal tenderness, sleep disturbances, fatigue, lethargy, and reduced physical and mental functions (Navia, 1970). Evidence showed a link between hypothyroidism, thyroid autoimmunity, and FMS (Friedman, 2013). In one clinical study conducted on 92 fibromyalgia patients, 52 patients were found to have either primary or central hypothyroidism (Lowe et al., 1998). The rate of occurrence of thyroid antibody mainly thyroglobulin and thyroid peroxidase in fibromyalgia patients is double compared to healthy humans (Bazzichi et al., 2007; Pamuk and Çakir, 2007). In addition, the characteristic pain, pressure pain threshold, and pain distribution observed in fibromyalgia patients may be positively associated with increased levels of thyroid antibodies in muscle proteins, low concentration of intracellular T3, and hypothyroidism (Bazzichi et al., 2007; Ruchala et al., 2007; Lowe et al., 2006). Reduced T3 levels in fibromyalgia patients cause increases in the synthesis and secretion of substance P, a neuropeptide that is responsible for pain signaling (Savard et al., 1984). Moreover, mitochondrial dysfunction, one of the factors responsible for impaired thyroid transport, has also been present in fibromyalgia patients (Friedman, 2013). This indicates that thyroid functions become disturbed in FMS. Because iodine deficiency is a major factor associated with thyroid dysfunctions, iodine supplementation may improve thyroid functions and symptoms in FMS patients.

Manganese

Manganese is an important micronutrient with its highest concentration found in grains, nuts, and cereals (Burch et al., 1975). It is an important component of metalloenzymes and plays a significant role in oxidative phosphorylation and metabolism as an enzyme activator (Rehnberg et al., 1982). It is an essential component of antioxidant defense in mitochondria in the form of manganese superoxide dismutase. Since the antioxidant defense has been altered in fibromyalgia patients, a manganese deficiency might be considered in the syndrome's pathophysiology (Kim et al., 2011). Fatigue is one prominent symptom of FMS that can be linked with manganese-dependent neuroendocrine changes because they directly affect the metabolic rate via manganese's participation in the hypothalamic–pituitary–thyroid axis (Ferraccioli et al., 1990).

Selenium

Selenium is a vital element of selenoprotein enzymes and acts as a redox center for these enzymatic functions (O'Dell and Sunde, 1997). Selenium-dependent glutathione peroxidase reduces hydrogen peroxide, organic hydroperoxidases, and main membrane integrity and reduces oxidative damage to biomolecules (Diplock, 1994). A selenium nutritional deficiency is one causative factor in the musculoskeletal noninflammatory disorder known as Kashin–Beck Disease (KBD). KBD symptoms such as morning stiffness in the joint and joint pain are comparable with the symptoms of FMS (Allander, 1994; Rayman, 2000). Low levels of selenium are also observed in rheumatoid arthritis and psoriatic arthritis (Tarp, 1994; Michaelsson et al., 1988). A selenium deficiency, along with an iodine deficiency, aggravates hypothyroidism (Vanderpas et al., 1990). A selenium insufficiency leads to depressed mood, anxiety, fatigue, and depression, which are also observed in fibromyalgia patients (Hawkes and Hornbostel, 1996; Benton and Cook, 1990). The above facts revealed a link between selenium deficiency and the symptoms of fibromyalgia. Based on these facts, a study was conducted by Reinhard and coworkers of 68 fibromyalgia patients to check their serum concentrations of selenium. The outcome of the study showed significant differences in serum selenium levels between FM patients and healthy blood donors, with the fibromyalgia patients showing lower serum selenium levels (Reinhard et al., 1998). The reports showed that dietary supplements of selenium significantly improved mood, anxiety, depression, and tiredness in a US study and double-blind crossover study conducted in the United Kingdom in FMS patients (Finley and Penland, 1998; Benton and Cook, 1990).

Thiamine

Thiamine or vitamin B_1 is important to the respiratory chain. It acts as a coenzyme (magnesium-coordinated thiamin pyrophosphate) in metabolizing carbohydrates and amino acids. A thiamine deficiency leads to reduced carbohydrate and branched-chain amino acid metabolism, which subsequently affect the formation of acetylcholine, which is required for normal neuronal functions (Vorhees et al., 1977; Mann and Quastel, 1940). Moreover, a thiamine deficiency alters the brain's turnover rate of serotonin, which plays a significant role in FMS (Plaitakis et al., 1982). The symptoms of thiamine deficiency mainly include anorexia, weakness, apathy, muscle tenderness, fatigue, burning sensations in feet and hands, confusion, sleep disturbance, low blood pressure, reduced metabolism, and depression (Prinzo, 1999). The majority of symptoms observed for a thiamine deficiency are also found in FMS patients. An important study published by Monroe revealed a metabolism abnormality of thiamine in fibromyalgia mainly due to a reduction in the activation of thiamine to thiamine pyrophosphate (Monroe et al., 1998). This abnormality causes impaired glycolysis, and decreased NO and glutathione and causes serotonin depletion in FM, which is responsible for symptoms such as muscle soreness, fatigue, and abnormal muscle relaxation (Eisinger et al.,

1994a,b; Eisinger et al., 1997; Eisinger and Ayavou, 1990). In their study results, Costantini et al. commented that the classical symptoms of fibromyalgia such as depression, anxiety, fatigue, and insomnia are the result of thiamine deficiency and can be overcome by high-dose thiamine therapy in fibromyalgia patients (Costantini and Pala, 2013).

Iron

Iron is an essential element used by cytochrome oxidase enzyme to generate energy. It is required for the synthesis of neurotransmitter such as serotonin, norepinephrine, and dopamine, which are involved in the pathophysiology of fibromyalgia. An iron deficiency results in chronic tiredness, myalgia, unusual fatigue, poor endurance, and sleep disturbances (Beard et al., 1993; Gerwin, 2005). An iron deficiency also reduces the pain threshold and increases pain sensation (Dowling et al., 2009). This indicates that iron might play a significant role in the pathophysiology of fibromyalgia. Ortancil and coworkers suggested from their study carried out on 46 fibromyalgia patients that iron deficiency may have a role in etiology of some fibromyalgia symptoms because it act as a cofactor in serotonin and dopamine synthesis (Ortancil et al., 2010). The clinical study carried out on 205 patients with iron deficiency anemia (IDA) patients, 40 patients with thalassemia minor (TM), and 100 healthy volunteers detected a higher frequency of fibromyalgia in IDA patients and TM patients compare to the healthy volunteers (Pamuk et al., 2008).

SUMMARY

FMS is a rheumatic disease that affects the quality of life of people around the world. Its etiology is unknown, but various scientific and nonscientific reports show the strong involvement of obesity and lowered nutritional levels of antioxidants and essential micronutrients in its pathophysiology. Furthermore, current therapies used to treat fibromyalgia symptoms include not only pharmacological agents but also physical activities and other alternative regimens (i.e., weight-loss programs, diet modifications, and the use of antioxidant and micronutrient supplements).

The assessed clinical data showed that obesity plays a major role in FMS. The severity of symptoms in obese people is more than in nonobese fibromyalgia patients. Various clinical studies demonstrated improvement in the FMS after the use of weight-loss programs and nutritional intervention of vegetarian and vegan diets rich in antioxidants. Nevertheless, more complete and detailed studies are required to confirm the positive effects of these diets on FMS. Some nutritional deficiencies have been suggested to be involved in FMS, although detailed clinical reports on these are lacking. Few studies have been carried out that point to nutritional deficiencies of magnesium, iodine, selenium, iron, thiamine, and manganese as linked with FMS or related conditions such as chronic pain syndrome and hypothyroidism. The importance of some micronutrients in FMS has been evaluated in some studies with positive outcome. This suggests that more detailed and specific investigations are required in FMS patients to understand the beneficial effect of the cited nutrients. In conclusion, current dietary advice is necessary for FMS patients so they can maintain normal weight and enjoy the nutritional benefits of micronutrients that will reduce the severity of their symptoms.

References

Abraham, G.E., Flechas, J.D., 1992. Management of fibromyalgia: rationale for the use of magnesium and malic acid. J. Nutr. Med. 3 (1), 49–59.

Algul, A., Ates, M.A., Semiz, U.B., Basoglu, C., Ebrinc, S., Gecici, O., et al., 2009. Evaluation of general psychopathology, subjective sleep quality, and health-related quality of life in patients with obesity. Int. J. Psychiatry Med. 39 (3), 297–312.

Allander, E., 1994. Kashin-Beck disease. An analysis of research and public health activities based on a bibliography 1849–1992. Scand. J. Rheumatol. 23 (suppl. 99), 1–36.

Allen, V.G., 1987. Influence of aluminum on magnesium metabolism. In: Altura, B.M., Durlach, J., Seelig, M.S., Mildred, S. (Eds.), Magnesium in Cellular Processes and Medicine. Karger Publishers, Basel, pp. 50–66.

Andriacchi, T.P., Mündermann, A., Smith, R.L., Alexander, E.J., Dyrby, C.O., Koo, S., 2004. A framework for the in vivo pathomechanics of osteoarthritis at the knee. Ann. Biomed. Eng. 32 (3), 447–457.

Aparicio, V.A., Ortega, F.B., Carbonell-Baeza, A., Camiletti, D., Ruiz, J.R., Delgado-Fernández, M., 2011. Relationship of weight status with mental and physical health in female fibromyalgia patients. Obes. Facts 4 (6), 443–448.

Aparicio, V.A., Ortega, F.B., Carbonell-Baeza, A., Gatto-Cardia, C., Sjöström, M., Ruiz, J.R., et al., 2013. Fibromyalgia's key symptoms in normal-weight, overweight, and obese female patients. Pain Manage. Nurs. 14 (4), 268–276.

Aparicio, V.A., Segura-Jiménez, V., Alvarez-Gallardo, I.C., Estévez-López, F., Camiletti-Moirón, D., Latorre, P.A., et al., 2014. Are there differences in quality of life, symptomatology and functional capacity among different obesity classes in women with fibromyalgia? The al-Ándalus project. Rheumatol. Inter. 34 (6), 811–821.

Arnold, L.M., Hudson, J.I., Keck, P.E., Auchenbach, M.B., Javaras, K.N., Hess, E.V., 2006. Comorbidity of fibromyalgia and psychiatric disorders. J. Clin. Psychiatry 67 (8), 1–478.

Arranz, L.I., Canela, M.Á., Rafecas, M., 2010. Fibromyalgia and nutrition, what do we know? Rheumatol. Inter. 30 (11), 1417–1427.

Arranz, L.I., Canela, M.Á., Rafecas, M., 2012. Dietary aspects in fibromyalgia patients: results of a survey on food awareness, allergies, and nutritional supplementation. Rheumatol. Inter. 32 (9), 2615–2621.

Azad, K.A., Alam, M.N., Haq, S.A., Nahar, S., Chowdhury, M.A., Ali, S.M., et al., 2000. Vegetarian diet in the treatment of fibromyalgia. Bangladesh Med. Res. Counc. Bull. 26 (2), 41–47.

Bagis, S., Karabiber, M., As, I., Tamer, L., Erdogan, C., Atalay, A., 2013. Is magnesium citrate treatment effective on pain, clinical parameters and functional status in patients with fibromyalgia? Rheumatol. Int. 33 (1), 167–172.

Bas, S., Finckh, A., Puskas, G.J., Suva, D., Hoffmeyer, P., Gabay, C., et al., 2014. Adipokines correlate with pain in lower limb osteoarthritis: different associations in hip and knee. Inter. Orthopaed. 38 (12), 2577–2583.

Batista, E.D., Andretta, A., de Miranda, R.C., Nehring, J., dos Santos Paiva, E., Schieferdecker, M.E.M., 2015. Food intake assessment and quality of life in women with fibromyalgia. Revista Brasileira de Reumatologia (English Edition).

Bazzichi, L., Rossi, A., Giuliano, T., De Feo, F., Giacomelli, C., Consensi, A., et al., 2007. Association between thyroid autoimmunity and fibromyalgic disease severity. Clin. Rheumatol. 26 (12), 2115–2120.

Beard, J.L., Connor, J.R., Jones, B.C., 1993. Iron in the brain. Nutr. Rev. 51 (6), 157–170.

Becker, S., Schweinhardt, P., 2011. Dysfunctional neurotransmitter systems in fibromyalgia, their role in central stress circuitry and pharmacological actions on these systems. Pain Res. Treat. 2012, 741–746.

Bellato, E., Marini, E., Castoldi, F., Barbasetti, N., Mattei, L., Bonasia, D.E., et al., 2012. Fibromyalgia syndrome: etiology, pathogenesis, diagnosis, and treatment. Pain Res. Treat. 2012, 426130.

Bennett, R.M., Jones, J., Turk, D.C., Russell, I., Matallana, L., 2007. An internet survey of 2,596 people with fibromyalgia. BMC Musculoskelet. Dis. 8 (1), 1.

Benton, D., Cook, R., 1990. Selenium supplementation improves mood in a double-blind crossover trial. Psychopharmacology 102 (4), 549–550.

Bjersing, J.L., Erlandsson, M., Bokarewa, M.I., Mannerkorpi, K., 2013. Exercise and obesity in fibromyalgia: beneficial roles of IGF-1 and resistin? Arthritis. Res. Ther. 15, R34.

Bradley, L.A., 2009. Pathophysiology of fibromyalgia. Am. J. Med. 122 (12), S22–S30.

Branco, J.C., Bannwarth, B., Failde, I., Carbonell, J.A., Blotman, F., Spaeth, M., et al., 2010. Prevalence of fibromyalgia: a survey in five European countries. Seminars in Arthritis and Rheumatism 39 (6), 448–453. WB Saunders.

Briggs, M.S., Givens, D.L., Schmitt, L.C., Taylor, C.A., 2013. Relations of C-reactive protein and obesity to the prevalence and the odds of reporting low back pain. Arch. Phys. Med. Rehabil. 94 (4), 745–752.

Burch, R.E., Hahn, H.K., Sullivan, J.F., 1975. Newer aspects of the roles of zinc, manganese, and copper in human nutrition. Clin. Chem. 21 (4), 501–520.

Buskila, D., Gladman, D.D., Langevitz, P., Urowitz, S., Smythe, H.A., 1990. Fibromyalgia in human immunodeficiency virus infection. J. Rheumatol. 17 (9), 1202–1206.

Costantini, A., Pala, M.I., 2013. Thiamine and fatigue in inflammatory bowel diseases: an open-label pilot study. J. Altern. Complement. Med. 19 (8), 704–708.

Crofford, L.J., 2002. The hypothalamic–pituitary–adrenal axis in the pathogenesis of rheumatic diseases. Endocrinol. Netab. Clin. North Am. 31 (1), 1–13.

De Araújo, T.A., Mota, M.C., Crispim, C.A., 2015. Obesity and sleepiness in women with fibromyalgia. Rheumatol. Inter. 35 (2), 281–287.

De Sá Pinto, A.L., De Barros Holanda, P.M., Radu, A.S., Villares, S.M., Lima, F.R., 2006. Musculoskeletal findings in obese children. J. Paediatr. Child Health 42 (6), 341–344.

Deere, K.C., Clinch, J., Holliday, K., McBeth, J., Crawley, E.M., Sayers, A., et al., 2012. Obesity is a risk factor for musculoskeletal pain in adolescents: findings from a population-based cohort. PAIN 153 (9), 1932–1938.

Demitrack, M.A., Crofford, L.J., 1998. Evidence for and pathophysiologic implications of hypothalamic-pituitary-adrenal axis dysregulation in fibromyalgia and chronic fatigue syndrome. Ann. NY Acad. Sci. 840 (1), 684–697.

Deuster, P.A., Jaffe, R.M., 1998. A novel treatment for fibromyalgia improves clinical outcomes in a community-based study. J. Musculoskelet. Pain 6 (2), 133–149.

Diplock, A.T., 1994. Antioxidants and disease prevention. Mol. Aspects Med. 15 (4), 293–376.

Dixon, J.B., Schachter, L.M., O'Brien, P.E., 2001. Sleep disturbance and obesity: changes following surgically induced weight loss. Arch. Internal med. 161 (1), 102–106.

Donaldson, M.S., Speight, N., Loomis, S., 2001. Fibromyalgia syndrome improved using a mostly raw vegetarian diet: an observational study. BMC Complemen. Alternat. Med. 1 (1), 1.

Dowling, P., Klinker, F., Amaya, F., Paulus, W., Liebetanz, D., 2009. Iron-deficiency sensitizes mice to acute pain stimuli and formalin-induced nociception. J. Nutr. 139 (11), 2087–2092.

Eisinger, J., Ayavou, T., 1990. Transketolase stimulation in fibromyalgia. J. Am. Coll. Nutr. 9 (1), 56–57.

Eisinger, J., Gandolfo, C., Zakarian, H., Ayavou, T., 1997. Reactive oxygen species, antioxidant status and fibromyalgia. J. Musculoskelet. Pain 5 (4), 5–15.

Eisinger, J., Plantamura, A., Ayavou, T., 1994a. Glycolysis abnormalities in fibromyalgia. J. Am. Coll. Nutr. 13 (2), 144–148.

Eisinger, J., Plantamura, A., Marie, P.A., Ayavou, T., 1994b. Selenium and magnesium status in fibromyalgia. Magnes. Res. 7 (3–4), 285–288.

Ferraccioli, G., Cavalieri, F., Salaffi, F., Fontana, S., Scita, F., Nolli, M., et al., 1990. Neuroendocrinologic findings in primary fibromyalgia (soft tissue chronic pain syndrome) and in other chronic rheumatic conditions (rheumatoid arthritis, low back pain). J. Rheumatol. 17 (7), 869.

Finley, J.W., Penland, J.G., 1998. Adequacy or deprivation of dietary selenium in healthy men: clinical and psychological findings. J. Trace Elem. Exp. Med. 11 (1), 11–27.

Fitzcharles, M.A., Shir, Y., Ablin, J.N., Buskila, D., Amital, H., Henningsen, P., et al., 2013. Classification and clinical diagnosis of fibromyalgia syndrome: recommendations of recent evidence-based interdisciplinary guidelines. Evid. Based Complemen. Alternat. Med. 2013, 528952.

Friedman, M., 2013. Fibromyalgia, thyroid dysfunction and treatment modalities. J. Restorat. Med. 2 (1), 60–69.

Furr, S.R., Marriott, I., 2012. Viral CNS infections: role of glial pattern recognition receptors in neuroinflammation. Front. Microbiol. 3, 201.

Gerwin, R.D., 2005. A review of myofascial pain and fibromyalgia–factors that promote their persistence. Acupunct. Med. 23 (3), 121–134.

Greenberg, A.S., Obin, M.S., 2006. Obesity and the role of adipose tissue in inflammation and metabolism. Am. J. Clin. Nutr. 83 (2), 461S–465S.

Gremese, E., Tolusso, B., Gigante, M.R., Ferraccioli, G., 2014. Obesity as a risk and severity factor in rheumatic diseases (autoimmune chronic inflammatory diseases). Front. Immunol. 5, 576.

Hänninen, O., Kaartinen, K., Rauma, A.L., Nenonen, M., Törrönen, R., Häkkinen, S., et al., 2000. Antioxidants in vegan diet and rheumatic disorders. Toxicology 155 (1), 45–53.

Hargens, T.A., Kaleth, A.S., Edwards, E.S., Butner, K.L., 2013. Association between sleep disorders, obesity, and exercise: a review. Nat. Sci. Sleep 5, 27–35.

Hawkes, W.C., Hornbostel, L., 1996. Effects of dietary selenium on mood in healthy men living in a metabolic research unit. Biol. Psychiatry 39 (2), 121–128.

Hawley, D.J., Wolfe, F., 1991. Pain, disability, and pain/disability relationships in seven rheumatic disorders: a study of 1,522 patients. J. Rheumatol. 18 (10), 1552–1557.

Heaton, F.W., Rayssiguier, Y., 1987. Magnesium deficiency and membrane properties, 121–130.

Henderson, C.J., Panush, R.S., 1999. Diets, dietary supplements, and nutritional therapies in rheumatic diseases. Rheum. Dis. Clin. North Am. 25 (4), 937–968.

Holton, K.F., Kindler, L.L., Jones, K.D., 2009. Potential dietary links to central sensitization in fibromyalgia: past reports and future directions. Rheum. Dis. Clin. North Am. 35 (2), 409–420.

Hooper, M.M., Stellato, T.A., Hallowell, P.T., Seitz, B.A., Moskowitz, R.W., 2007. Musculoskeletal findings in obese subjects before and after weight loss following bariatric surgery. Inter. J. Obes. 31 (1), 114–120.

Hostmark, A.T., Lystad, E., Vellar, O.D., Hovi, K., Berg, J.E., 1993. Reduced plasma fibrinogen, serum peroxides, lipids, and apolipoproteins after a 3-week vegetarian diet. Plant Foods Human Nutr. 43 (1), 55–61.

Jahan, F., Nanji, K., Qidwai, W., Qasim, R., 2012. Fibromyalgia syndrome: an overview of pathophysiology, diagnosis and management. Oman Med. J. 27 (3), 192–195.

Juhl, J.H., 1998. Fibromyalgia and the serotonin pathway. Alternat. Med. Rev. 3, 367–375.

Kaartinen, K., Lammi, K., Hypen, M., Nenonen, M., Hänninen, O., Rauma, A.L., 2000. Vegan diet alleviates fibromyalgia symptoms. Scand. J. Rheumatol. 29 (5), 308–313.

Kaur, J., 2014. A comprehensive review on metabolic syndrome. Cardiol. Res. Pract. 2014, 943162.

Kim, C.H., Luedtke, C.A., Vincent, A., Thompson, J.M., Oh, T.H., 2012. Association of body mass index with symptom severity and quality of life in patients with fibromyalgia. Arthrit. Care Res. 64 (2), 222–228.

Kim, Y.S., Kim, K.M., Lee, D.J., Kim, B.T., Park, S.B., Cho, D.Y., et al., 2011. Women with fibromyalgia have lower levels of calcium, magnesium, iron and manganese in hair mineral analysis. J. Korean Med. Sci. 26 (10), 1253–1257.

Latremoliere, A., Woolf, C.J., 2009. Central sensitization: a generator of pain hypersensitivity by central neural plasticity. J. Pain 10 (9), 895–926.

Leventhal, L.J., Naides, S.J., Freundlich, B., 1991. Fibromyalgia and parvovirus infection. Arthrit. Rheum. 34 (10), 1319–1324.

Li, S., Micheletti, R., 2011. Role of diet in rheumatic disease. Rheum. Dis. Clin. North Am. 37 (1), 119–133.

Lowe, J.C., Reichman, A.J., Honeyman, G.S., Yellin, J., 1998. Thyroid status of fibromyalgia patients. Clin. Bull. Myofas. Ther. 3 (1), 69–70.

Lowe, J.C., Yellin, J., Honeyman-Lowe, G., 2006. Female fibromyalgia patients: lower resting metabolic rates than matched healthy controls. Med. Sci. Monitor Basic Res. 12 (7), CR282–CR289.

Magaldi, M., Moltoni, L., Biasi, G., Marcolongo, R., 1999. Changes in intracellular calcium and magnesium ions in the physiopathology of the fybromyalgia syndrome. Minerva Medica 91 (7-8), 137–140.

Mann, P.J.G., Quastel, J.H., 1940. Vitamin B1 and acetylcholine formation in isolated brain. Nature 145 (856), 59.

Marcus, D.A., 2004. Obesity and the impact of chronic pain. Clin. J. Pain 20 (3), 186–191.

Marcus, D.A., Deodhar, A., 2011. Fibromyalgia Definition and Epidemiology Fibromyalgia. Springer, New York.

McCarley, R.W., 2007. Neurobiology of REM and NREM sleep. Sleep Med. 8 (4), 302–330.

Menegoni, F., Galli, M., Tacchini, E., Vismara, L., Cavigioli, M., Capodaglio, P., 2009. Gender-specific effect of obesity on balance. Obesity 17 (10), 1951–1956.

Messier, S.P., Gutekunst, D.J., Davis, C., DeVita, P., 2005. Weight loss reduces knee-joint loads in overweight and obese older adults with knee osteoarthritis. Arthrit. Rheum. 52 (7), 2026–2032.

Michaelsson, G., Berne, B., Carlmark, B., Strand, A., 1988. Selenium in whole blood and plasma is decreased in patients with moderate and severe psoriasis. Acta Dermato-Venereologica 69 (1), 29–34.

Miller, D.W., 2006. Extrathyroidal benefits of iodine. J. Am. Phys. Surg. 11 (4), 106.

Monroe, B.A., 1998. Fibromyalgia--a hidden link? J. Am. Coll. Nutr. 17 (3), 300.

Mork, P.J., Vasseljen, O., Nilsen, T.I., 2010. Association between physical exercise, body mass index, and risk of fibromyalgia: longitudinal data from the Norwegian Nord-Trøndelag Health Study. Arthrit. Care Res. 62 (5), 611–617.

Must, A., Strauss, R.S., 1999. Risks and consequences of childhood and adolescent obesity. Inter. J. Obes. Related Metab. Dis 23, S2–S11.

Navia, J.M., 1970. Effect of minerals on dental caries Dietary Chemicals vs Dental Caries. American Chemical Society, Washington, DC.

Neeck, G., 2002. Pathogenic mechanisms of fibromyalgia. Ageing Res. Rev. 1 (2), 243–255.

Neeck, G., Crofford, L.J., 2002. Neuroendocrine perturbations in fibromyalgia and chronic fatigue syndrome. Rheum. Dis. Clin. North Am. 26 (4), 989–1002.

Neumann, L., Buskila, D., 2003. Epidemiology of fibromyalgia. Curr. Pain Headache Rep. 7 (5), 362–368.

Neumann, L., Lerner, E., Glazer, Y., Bolotin, A., Shefer, A., Buskila, D., 2008. A cross-sectional study of the relationship between body mass index and clinical characteristics, tenderness measures, quality of life, and physical functioning in fibromyalgia patients. Clin. Rheumatol. 27 (12), 1543–1547.

Nicolson, G.L., Nasralla, M., Haier, J., Erwin, R., Nicolson, N.L., Ngwenya, R., 1999. Mycoplasmal infections in chronic illnesses: fibromyalgia and chronic fatigue syndromes, Gulf War illness, HIV-AIDS and rheumatoid arthritis. Med. Sentinel. 4, 172–176.

O'Dell, B.L., Sunde, R.A. (Eds.), 1997. Handbook of Nutritionally Essential Mineral Elements. CRC Press, Boca Raton, FL.

Okifuji, A., Bradshaw, D.H., Olson, C., 2009. Evaluating obesity in fibromyalgia: neuroendocrine biomarkers, symptoms, and functions. Clin. Rheumatol. 28 (4), 475–478.

Okifuji, A., Donaldson, G.W., Barck, L., Fine, P.G., 2010. Relationship between fibromyalgia and obesity in pain, function, mood, and sleep. J. Pain 11 (12), 1329–1337.

Ortancil, O., Sanli, A., Eryuksel, R., Basaran, A., Ankarali, H., 2010. Association between serum ferritin level and fibromyalgia syndrome. Eur. J. Clin. Nutr. 64 (3), 308–312.

Ozgocmen, S., Ozyurt, H., Sogut, S., Akyol, O., 2006. Current concepts in the pathophysiology of fibromyalgia: the potential role of oxidative stress and nitric oxide. Rheumatol. Int. 26 (7), 585–597.

Pamuk, Ö.N., Çakir, N., 2007. The frequency of thyroid antibodies in fibromyalgia patients and their relationship with symptoms. Clin. Rheumatol. 26 (1), 55–59.

Pamuk, G.E., Pamuk, Ö.N., Set, T., Harmandar, O., Yeşil, N., 2008. An increased prevalence of fibromyalgia in iron deficiency anemia and thalassemia minor and associated factors. Clin. Rheumatol. 27 (9), 1103–1108.

Peltonen, M., Lindroos, A.K., Torgerson, J.S., 2003. Musculoskeletal pain in the obese: a comparison with a general population and long-term changes after conventional and surgical obesity treatment. Pain 104 (3), 549–557.

Percival, M., 1997. Fibromyalgia nutritional support. Clin. Nutr. Insights 3.

Plaitakis, A., Hwang, E.C., Woert, M.H., Szilagyi, P.I., Berl, S., 1982. Effect of thiamin deficiency on brain neurotransmitter systems. Ann. NY Acad. Sci. 378 (1), 367–381.

Prashanth, L., Kattapagari, K.K., Chitturi, R.T., Baddam, V.R.R., Prasad, L.K., 2015. A review on role of essential trace elements in health and disease. J. Dr. NTR University Health Sci. 4 (2), 75.

Prinz, P.N., Moe, K.E., Dulberg, E.M., Larsen, L.H., Vitiello, M.V., Toivola, B., et al., 1995. Higher plasma IGF-1 levels are associated with increased delta sleep in healthy older men. J. Gerontol. Series A Biol. Sci. Med. Sci. 50 (4), M222–M226.

Prinzo, Z.W., 1999. Thiamine deficiency and its prevention and control in major emergencies. In Micronutrient Series. World Health Organization (WHO). Department of Nutrition for Health and Development; Office of the United Nations High Commissioner for Refugees (UNHCR).

Queiroz, L.P., 2013. Worldwide epidemiology of fibromyalgia. Curr. Pain Headache Rep. 17 (8), 1–6.

Raison, V.M.C.L., 2009. Neurobiology of depression, fibromyalgia and neuropathic pain. Front. Biosci. 14, 5291–5338.

Ravussin, E., Swinburn, B.A., 1992. Pathophysiology of obesity. Lancet 340 (8816), 404–408.

Rayman, M.P., 2000. The importance of selenium to human health. Lancet 356 (9225), 233–241.

Rehnberg, G.L., Hem, J.F., Carter, S.D., Linko, R.S., Laskey, J.W., 1982. Chronic ingestion of Mn3O4 by rats: tissue accumulation and distribution of manganese in two generations. J. Toxicol. Environ. Health, Part A Curr. Issues 9 (2), 175–188.

Reinhard, P., Schweinsberg, F., Wernet, D., Kötter, I., 1998. Selenium status in fibromyalgia. Toxicol. Lett. 96, 177–180.

Riedel, W., Layka, H., Neeck, G., 1998. Secretory pattern of GH, TSH, thyroid hormones, ACTH, cortisol, FSH, and LH in patients with fibromyalgia syndrome following systemic injection of the relevant hypothalamic-releasing hormones. Zeitschrift für Rheumatologie 57 (2), S81–S87.

Rivera, J., De Diego, A., Trinchet, M., Monforte, A.G., 1997. Fibromyalgia-associated hepatitis C virus infection. Rheumatology 36 (9), 981–985.

Romano, T.J., John, W.S., 1994. Magnesium deficiency in fibromyalgia syndrome. J. Nutr. Med. 4 (2), 165–167.

Ruchala, M., Kosowicz, J., Baumann-Antczak, A., Skiba, A., Zamyslowska, H., Sowinski, J., 2007. The prevalence of autoantibodies to: myosin, troponin, tropomyosin and myoglobin in patients with circulating triiodothyronine and thyroxine autoantibodies (THAA). Neur. Endocrinol. Lett. 28 (3), 259–266.

Russell, I.J., Michalek, J.E., Flechas, J.D., Abraham, G.E., 1995. Treatment of fibromyalgia syndrome with Super Malic: a randomized, double blind, placebo controlled, crossover pilot study. J. Rheumatol. 22 (5), 953–958.

Saber, A.A., Boros, M.J., Mancl, T., Elgamal, M.H., Song, S., Wisadrattanapong, T., 2008. The effect of laparoscopic Roux-en-Y gastric bypass on fibromyalgia. Obes. Surg. 18 (6), 652–655.

Savard, P., Blanchard, L.M., Mérand, Y., Bédard, P., Dussault, J.H., Dupont, A., 1984. Influences of both thyroid and bovine growth hormones on substance P, thyrotropin-releasing hormone, serotonin and 5-hydroxyindoleacetic acid contents in the lumbar spinal cord of developing rats. Develop. Brain Res. 13 (1), 105–110.

Schmidt, M., Pohlmann, U., Golf, S., Temme, H., Graef, V., Roka, L., et al., 1989. The effects of a magnesium supplementation on the energy metabolism in competitive swimmers. Magnes. Res. 2, 281–283.

Seaman, D.R., 2013. Body mass index and musculoskeletal pain: is there a connection? Chirop. Manual Ther. 21 (1), 1.

Sendur, O.F., Tastaban, E., Turan, Y., Ulman, C., 2008. The relationship between serum trace element levels and clinical parameters in patients with fibromyalgia. Rheumatol. Inter. 28 (11), 1117–1121.

Senna, M.K., Sallam, R.A.E.R., Ashour, H.S., Elarman, M., 2012. Effect of weight reduction on the quality of life in obese patients with fibromyalgia syndrome: a randomized controlled trial. Clin. Rheumatol. 31 (11), 1591–1597.

Shapiro, J.R., Anderson, D.A., Danoff-Burg, S., 2005. A pilot study of the effects of behavioral weight loss treatment on fibromyalgia symptoms. J. Psychosom. Res. 59 (5), 275–282.

Siesjö, B.K., 1988. Calcium and cell death. Magnesium 8 (5–6), 223–237.

Smedslund, G., Byfuglien, M.G., Olsen, S.U., Hagen, K.B., 2010. Effectiveness and safety of dietary interventions for rheumatoid arthritis: a systematic review of randomized controlled trials. J. Am. Diet. Assoc. 110 (5), 727–735.

Staud, R., Price, D.D., Robinson, M.E., Mauderli, A.P., Vierck, C.J., 2004. Maintenance of windup of second pain requires less frequent stimulation in fibromyalgia patients compared to normal controls. Pain 110 (3), 689–696.

Staud, R., Vierck, C.J., Cannon, R.L., Mauderli, A.P., Price, D.D., 2001. Abnormal sensitization and temporal summation of second pain (wind-up) in patients with fibromyalgia syndrome. Pain 91 (1), 165–175.

St-Onge, M.P., Perumean-Chaney, S., Desmond, R., Lewis, C.E., Yan, L.L., Person, S.D., et al., 2009. Gender differences in the association between sleep duration and body composition: the Cardia Study. Int. J. Endocrinol. 2010, 726071.

Tarp, U., 1994. Selenium and the selenium-dependent glutathione peroxidase in rheumatoid arthritis. Danish Med. Bull. 41 (3), 264–274.
Timmerman, G.M., Calfa, N.A., Stuifbergen, A.K., 2013. Correlates of body mass index in women with fibromyalgia. Orthopaed. Nurs. Natl. Assoc. Orthopaed. Nurs. 32 (2), 113.
Turner, C.H., Robling, A.G., 2004. Mechanical loading and bone formation. BoneKEy-Osteov. 1 (9), 15–23.
Ursini, F., Naty, S., Grembiale, R.D., 2011. Fibromyalgia and obesity: the hidden link. Rheumatol. Inter. 31 (11), 1403–1408.
Van Cauter, E., Plat, L., Copinschi, G., 1998. Interrelations between sleep and the somatotropic axis. Sleep 21 (6), 553–566.
Vanderpas, J.B., Contempre, B., Duale, N.L., Goossens, W., Bebe, N.G.O., Thorpe, R., et al., 1990. Iodine and selenium deficiency associated with cretinism in northern Zaire. Am. J. Clin. Nutr. 52 (6), 1087–1093.
Vincent, H.K., Adams, M.C., Vincent, K.R., Hurley, R.W., 2013. Musculoskeletal pain, fear avoidance behaviors, and functional decline in obesity: potential interventions to manage pain and maintain function. Reg. Anesthes. Pain Med. 38 (6), 481–491.
Vincent, A., Clauw, D., Oh, T.H., Whipple, M.O., Toussaint, L.L., 2014. Decreased physical activity attributable to higher body mass index influences fibromyalgia symptoms. PM&R 6 (9), 802–807.
Vincent, H.K., Lamb, K.M., Day, T.I., Tillman, S.M., Vincent, K.R., George, S.Z., 2010. Morbid obesity is associated with fear of movement and lower quality of life in patients with knee pain-related diagnoses. PM&R 2 (8), 713–722.
Vorhees, C.V., Schmidt, D.E., Barrett, R.J., Schenker, S., 1977. Effects of thiamin deficiency on acetylcholine levels and utilization in vivo in rat brain. J. Nutr. 107 (10), 1902–1908.
Walker, E.A., Keegan, D., Gardner, G., Sullivan, M., Katon, W.J., Bernstein, D., 1997. Psychosocial factors in fibromyalgia compared with rheumatoid arthritis: I. Psychiatric diagnoses and functional disability. Psychosom. Med. 59 (6), 565–571.
Wallace, D.J., 2006. Is there a role for cytokine based therapies in fibromyalgia. Curr. Pharm. Des. 12 (1), 17–22.
Watenpaugh, D.E., 2009. The role of sleep dysfunction in physical inactivity and its relationship to obesity. Curr. Sports Med. Rep. 8 (6), 331–338.
Watkins, L.R., Milligan, E.D., Maier, S.F., 2001. Spinal cord glia: new players in pain. Pain 93 (3), 201–205.
Wearing, S.C., Hennig, E.M., Byrne, N.M., Steele, J.R., Hills, A.P., 2006. Musculoskeletal disorders associated with obesity: a biomechanical perspective. Obes. Rev. 7 (3), 239–250.
White, K.P., Harth, M., 2001. Classification, epidemiology, and natural history of fibromyalgia. Curr. Pain Headache Rep. 5 (4), 320–329.
Winkler, R., Griebenow, S., Wonisch, W., 2000. Effect of iodide on total antioxidant status of human serum. Cell Biochem. Funct. 18 (2), 143–146.
Wolfe, F., Smythe, H.A., Yunus, M.B., Bennett, R.M., Bombardier, C., Goldenberg, D.L., et al., 1990. The American College of Rheumatology 1990 criteria for the classification of fibromyalgia. Arthrit. Rheum. 33 (2), 160–172.
Woolf, C.J., 2011. Central sensitization: implications for the diagnosis and treatment of pain. Pain 152 (3), S2–S15.
Wright, L.J., Schur, E., Noonan, C., Ahumada, S., Buchwald, D., Afari, N., 2010. Chronic pain, overweight, and obesity: findings from a community-based twin registry. J. Pain 11 (7), 628–635.
Yunus, M.B., Arslan, S., Aldag, J.C., 2002. Relationship between body mass index and fibromyalgia features. Scand. J. Rheumatol. 31 (1), 27–31.
Yunus, M.B., Kalyan-Raman, U.P., Kalyan-Raman, K., 1988. Primary fibromyalgia syndrome and myofascial pain syndrome: clinical features and muscle pathology. Arch. Phys. Med. Rehabil. 69 (6), 451–454.

CHAPTER

8

Aging and Gait

Kunal Singhal[1] *and Jeffrey B. Casebolt*[2]

[1]University of Tennessee Health Science Center, Memphis, TN, United States [2]West Texas A&M University, Canyon, TX, United States

INTRODUCTION

Human locomotion and gait occur as a result of complex interplays of multiple muscle contractions across multiple joints as affected by different environmental conditions (internal and external) in which these contractions occur. For successful locomotion, we must consider not only that a person has traversed a distance from one point to another but also factors such as pain, fatigue, balance, safety, and quality of movement. Age-associated declines in body functions can affect most of these factors in unison or in various combinations. Failure to maintain an effective gait could be a result of any of these factors or their underlying causes, which might disrupt activities of daily living and result in increased fall risk, especially in older adults.

Successfully completing daily living activities and maintaining independence are closely associated with quality of life, and a healthy gait is essential for both. In this regard, gait analysis and interpreting gait adaptations in older adults as a function of health status and falls has been of prime importance for more than 20 years for physical therapists, biomechanists, and physicians. In this chapter, we will focus on age-induced changes in gait on level surfaces along with changes in the neuromuscular system that may result in alterations that predispose older adults to increased risk of falls.

The chapter is divided into two broad sections: (1) mechanics of gait changes and (2) changes in physiological functions. In the first section, changes in gait in older adults will be approached from two primary directions: changes in mobility and changes in stability. Changes in mobility will address biomechanical parameters of forward progression. Changes in stability will explain factors that affect older adults' gait stability using conventional biomechanical variables of stability during gait. The second section will incorporate changes in balance and how various systems integral to maintaining balance change with age. This will be followed by changes in functioning of the core gait apparatus: the human neuromuscular system.

MECHANICS OF CHANGES IN GAIT

Changes in Mobility

Gait is a function of the entire body and is directly and indirectly affected by almost everybody system. Here we will be talking strictly about aging-induced changes in the neuromuscular system and their effects on gait. These neuromuscular processes involve changes at muscle level, motor neurons, and the central nervous system (CNS). Changes in gait with aging can be attributed to pathology or healthy aging or both, so it is important while reviewing literature that demographic characteristics of population tested are well described and understood. One primary reason for such elucidation is that healthy older adults living an active lifestyle maintain gait changes that are similar to young adults well into old age (Bloem et al., 1992; Verghese et al., 2006). Some of the changes in gait such as slowness, increased step width, and stooped posture can be attributed to subclinical pathologies that may

Nutrition and Functional Foods for Healthy Aging.
DOI: http://dx.doi.org/10.1016/B978-0-12-805376-8.00008-3

affect overall quality of life and independence in older adults. Regardless, certain changes in gait do occur with increasing old age. Some of these changes are irreversible but others can be arrested and their damages minimized through exercises and physical therapy.

As people age, the speed they prefer to walk without restriction significantly declines. Reasons for the decline in this *preferred gait velocity* include reduction in lower-body muscle strength (Bassey et al., 1992), aerobic capacity (Mian et al., 2006), cognitive function status (Buchner et al., 1996), and physical health (Cesari et al., 2006). Mechanically, reduced gait speed is associated with reduced step length, an increase in the double-stance phase, and gait stability ratio.

Murray and coauthors studied gait parameters for 64 men ranging in age from 20 to 87 years of age and reported that the oldest three age groups—67–73, 74–80, and 81–87 years of age—produced the slowest preferred gait speed of 1.18, 1.23, and 1.18 m/s and fast walking speeds of 1.63, 1.67, and 1.60 m/s, respectively (Murray et al., 1969), when compared to the other age groups. The younger groups averaged 1.52 and 2.15 m/s for preferred and fast walking speeds (Murray et al., 1969). Stride length was significantly reduced for the oldest three walking groups during both preferred and fast walking speeds at 1.36, 1.41, and 1.26 m and 1.60, 1.59, and 1.40 m, respectively. Therefore, males younger than 65 years of age averaged stride lengths that were approximately 89% of their height; for those 67 and older, the percentage drops to 79% of height for preferred walking speed. At fast gait speeds, the percentages climbed to 107% and 90% for the younger groups in comparison to the three older groups (Murray et al., 1969).

Elble and colleagues compared gait parameters for 20 young (30.0 ± 6.1 years) and 20 older adults (74.7 ± 6.6 years) who walked a 10-m walkway four times at their preferred and fast walking speeds (Elble et al., 1991). The preferred and fast gait speeds were 1.18 and 1.67 m/s and 0.94 and 1.39 m/s, respectively for young and older adults, which equated to a 20% and 17% decline for the older adults in comparison to the young adults. The older adults had 1.08 and 1.26-m stride lengths for preferred and fast walking speed in comparison to young adults at 1.32 and 1.58 m. However, these changes were not due to cadence because cadence was reported to be similar at 107 and 104 steps/min and 126 and 128 steps/min for young and older adults at preferred and fast walking speeds (Elble et al., 1991). These results indicate that healthy older adults take shorter steps at a similar frequency resulting in a decrease in gait velocity for both preferred and fast gait speeds. In addition, the shorter steps taken by the older adults increase the amount of time spent in stance and the double-support phase (Elble et al., 1991).

Nigg and Skleryk (1988) determined that older adults reduced their preferred walking speed either as a result of increased joint stiffness or because of a need to increase safety and balance (Nigg and Skleryk, 1988). This study alludes to an important aspect of age-associated adaptation: whether the changes in gait are a result of a pathology or a need to increase safety. In either situation, the physiological or pathological changes in the human body need to be understood before any judgment can be passed on gait in older adults. This idea has been well explained in an excellent review by McGibbon (2003). As correctly pointed out in that paper, the clarity between adaptations to a primary pathology and changes related to aging itself needs to be explained further. The article argues that most of the changes in gait due to age are a manifestation of a primary pathology.

One prominent change has been a shift to a hip-dominant strategy from an ankle-dominant strategy for forward propulsion (DeVita and Hortobagyi, 2000; Franz and Kram, 2014; Kerrigan et al., 1998). Once again, the shift in strategy is related to the gait speed, and one of the key differences while reviewing various studies arises from whether walking speed was self-selected or not. Judge and colleagues (1996) tested young and older adults at self-selected walking speeds and found a significant reduction in ankle plantar flexor power that was replaced by increased hip flexor power during late stance in older adults. They reported that the primary age-limiting factor in reduction of gait velocity comes from reduction of the ankle plantar flexor push-off. This has been contradicted by other studies that have found that older adults can increase their hip contribution to match young adults at a faster gait velocity but the limitation is in the hip extension range of motion (Kerrigan et al., 1998; Riley et al., 2001; Riley et al., 2001). Riley et al. (2001) analyzed age-associated gait differences and the contribution of lower-extremity joint moment to gait velocity and forward progression. When the elderly were asked to walk at higher velocity, they were able to increase the contribution of ankle plantar flexor power at higher velocity but could not increase their hip contribution, which suggests a limitation in hip extension moments during gait.

DeVita and Hortobagyi (2000) stated that overall support moment is similar between older and young adults, although the moments are redistributed between lower-extremity joints with the hip increasing its role and the ankle decreasing its contribution (DeVita and Hortobagyi, 2000). Increased hip concentric power during early stance and reduced ankle push-off during late stance in old adults suggests this altered gait strategy. Similar results have been reported by other authors comparing various combination of speed (preferred, slow, and fast). The verdict is clear that old adults reduce their ankle plantar flexor push-off and increase the hip concentric and eccentric load in order to continue forward progression. Also, that limitation in an old adult's ability to generate power through hip joint affects gait velocity more than reduction in ankle moments. However, this last assertion has to be questioned. First, redistribution of support moments occurs as a result of ankles producing lower push-off, therefore changes in hip moments are an adaptation themselves. Second, ankle push-off reduces first, which increases the demand on hip muscles. Third, plantar flexors can still increase their effort if need arises but hip muscles cannot. What needs to be understood is whether the changes in gait strategy is a function of greater or faster rate of strength loss in ankle plantar flexors or is an alteration in joint proprioception and balance. Since the muscle strength was not measured in these studies, it cannot be conclusively said whether these changes are adaptations for weak ankle plantar flexors or are a part of normal aging. Nevertheless, plenty of evidence for reduction in plantar flexor strength in older adults along with other concomitant changes in neuromotor processes is available. Also, changes in hip extensors with aging is also well documented (Dean et al., 2004). Therefore, the loss of strength in hip and ankle muscles cannot by itself explain the change in gait strategy.

On the other hand, the knee joint moments are essential components of support moment required to maintain a dynamic vertical posture during gait, therefore the role of the quadriceps' muscle strength should be considered a potential mechanism of falling. Quadriceps strength reduces with age similar to other muscles of the lower extremities, but the weakness is associated with failure to maintain upright stance, difficulty in moving from sitting to standing, and instability while going up and down stairs. An indirect link between reduced quadriceps strength and falls can be inferred from the results of a study that found that participants who were obese and had limited knee extensor strength showed a fast decline in their gait velocity, thus predisposing them to increased risk of fall and mortality (White et al., 2013). Quadriceps strength has been considered a significant predictor of falls over a 3-year period in community-dwelling healthy older women (Scott et al., 2014). Quadriceps strength was also a better predictor of first incidence of falls compared to gait velocity. Since ankle and hip muscle strength were not measured, the results cannot be used to compare the relative importance of strength loss in different muscle groups across lower-extremity joints. However, if all the evidence presented here is considered, we need to ask the following questions. Ankle plantar flexors (during high gait speed) and hip extensors can compensate for one weakness in another, but is there a mechanism for compensating for quadriceps strength loss? Mechanically increased activity of hip extensors and ankle plantar flexors can passively extend the knee and provide a rigid lever in the lower extremity. Does that mean the functional loss of quadriceps strength increases the burden on other muscles and is the primary mechanism that predisposes healthy older adults to a fall risk? Research thus far does not provide a clear answer to that question.

Changes in Stability

Stability and *balance* are related terms in motor control and biomechanical literature that carry multiple definitions. Clinically, falls occur as a result of loss of balance, whereas stability can be loosely defined as the ability to resist perturbations or forces that result in loss of balance. An analysis of stability during gait can be undertaken using multiple methods, and each method defines stability accordingly. We are going to limit the discussion on stability by utilizing a conventional linear variable called *gait stability ratio*; kinematic variables such as *toe clearance*, *foot inclination*, *lateral trunk sway*, and *heel velocity*; and a kinetic variable such as *angular momentum*. The list is in not all-encompassing because the analysis strategies have differed over the decades and left us an accumulation of variables that can be used to show differences in gait stability among age groups.

Gait Stability Ratio

Gait stability ratio was first introduced to account for a decrease in preferred walking speed as the ratio of cadence (steps/s) to gait velocity (m/s) and is reported as steps per meter (Cromwell et al., 2001). An increase in the number of steps per unit of distance coupled with a decrease in preferred walking speed is an indication of walking stability, which equates to an increase in the amount of time spent in the double-stance phase (Cromwell and Newton, 2004). An increase in the amount of time spent in the double-stance phase reduces the dynamic component of walking while increasing gait stability (Maki, 1997).

The gait stability ratio for older adults significantly increased when compared to young adults, 1.48 ± 0.19 to 1.36 ± 0.17 steps/m, respectively (Cromwell and Newton, 2004). The increase in gait stability ratio indicates that older adults take more steps per unit of distance, thereby increasing stability while walking at their preferred speed. An increase in stability while walking allows them to compensate for reductions in balance thus maximizing walking stability, creating resistance to perturbations, and reducing fall potential.

The older adults reduce gait velocity, decrease step length, and increase gait stability ratio, which increases time spent in the double-support phase. Age-related adaptations during gait are considered to be mechanisms that increase stability at the cost of reducing mobility (Cromwell and Newton, 2004); however, this results in individuals becoming less efficient by reducing the forward progression within each gait cycle. The reduced gait velocity brings about a mechanical reduction in the amount of forward progression in a given amount of time and lowering the momentum of the body. This loss of momentum is sometimes considered critical in preventing falls. Conversely, gait patterns among young adults are distinguished by phases of instability, which produces a much more efficient forward progression and therefore a preferred walking speed that is quicker.

Kinematic Variables

The primary focus of fall risk kinematics in the older adults has been tripping, slipping, and lateral movement of the trunk while walking. Tripping and loss of balance remain significant reasons why older adults fall while walking. Tripping accounts for approximately 53% of falls among older adults (Blake et al., 1988) and is separated into two classifications: stubbing the toe and catching the bottom of the foot during the swing phase. A decrease in ankle dorsiflexion during the swing phase, as suggested by Oberg et al. (1994), increases the chances of stubbing the toe along with a greater probability of catching the bottom of the foot. The initial mechanism can be understood by analyzing toe clearance, while the latter can be investigated using the foot's inclination angle.

Tripping is associated with stubbing the toes on a walking surface or on an obstacle at approximately the midpoint during the swing phase of the gait cycle when the toe velocity is greatest and toes are at their minimal height above the ground (Schulz, 2011; Winter, 1992). The tripping mechanism occurs without an apparent obstacle causing the stumble due to a foot catch at the lowest point of the swing phase or immediately prior to heel strike (Chen et al., 1994). Older adults demonstrate less toe clearance at a point during the swing phase when the velocity of the distal end of the foot is the greatest (Barrett et al., 2010), which increases the chances of catching the toe on an obstacle or the floor. Maximal foot clearance is the minimum vertical clearance between the lowest point of the foot of the swing leg and the walking surface (Barrett et al., 2010), and it is associated with reduced foot inclination during the swing phase of the gait cycle (Chiba et al., 2005).

An increase in lateral sway among older adults while walking is indicated to be a fall variable (Chiba et al., 2005), especially as preferred gait velocity decreases. Lateral sway ratio is the relationship between the center of mass (COM) of the body and the base of support created by the foot placement in the frontal plane (van den Kroonenberg et al., 1996). The displacement of the COM close to or outside the base of support will increase the instability and can potentially result in a fall. Lateral gait unsteadiness has been considered a determining factor in lateral fall risk assessment (Helbostad and Moe-Nilssen, 2003) because the COM displacement in the frontal plane is a source of greater concern because it might result in people falling on their sides. This can potentially cause more debilitating injuries to the pelvis and hip complex and affect long-term outcomes in older adults, including the quality of life.

Chiba and associates compared the differences between fallers and nonfallers among community-dwelling individuals using minimum toe clearance, maximum foot inclination, and the trunk's lateral sway ratio. Fifty-six older adults were separated into two groups: 25 fallers (76.0 ± 6.6 years) and 31 age- and gender-matched nonfallers (74.9 ± 7.2 years) who walked a 6-m walkway at their preferred walking speed (Chiba et al., 2005). When compared with the nonfallers, the fallers produced less toe clearance (12.0 ± 0.7 mm and 15.2 ± 1.0 mm, respectively), lower maximal sole inclination angle (7.4 ± 0.8 degrees and 14.3 ± 0.9 degrees, respectively), and larger lateral trunk sway (0.23 ± 0.01 and 0.18 ± 0.01, respectively). This indicates altered ankle–foot dynamics in fallers, which increases the risk of trips while walking on a level smooth terrain. The increase in lateral sway ratio for fallers in comparison to nonfallers indicated a problem with the whole body during the gait, which may be a result of increased lower-extremity variability, reduced muscle strength, and altered reflexes (Chiba et al., 2005). However, none of this was tested and therefore can only be treated as speculation. Variability in trunk movement patterns in older adults demonstrate a different motor control strategy in the mediolateral direction compared to other anteroposterior and vertical directions (Moe-Buksseb and Helbostad, 2005). Therefore, it is essential to test gait stability in both the anteroposterior and mediolateral directions.

Slips are another important cause of falls (Lloyd and Stevenson, 1992). Just like trips, slips can be analyzed using a multitude of variables. The one we are explaining in detail is heel velocity and how it indicates increased risk of falls in older adults, especially as the foot approaches heel contact. The heel velocity immediately prior to heel strike is an indication of foot trajectory during the swing phase and the end-point control (Winter, 1992), so higher heel velocity indicates an increased risk for slipping (Winter et al., 1990). When compared to young adults, the older adults produced significantly higher heel velocity (1.15 and 0.87 m/s, respectively) immediately prior to heel strike

(Winter et al., 1990; Winter, 1992), thus indicating greater risk for slipping in older adults even though their preferred walking speed was significantly less (1.29 ± m/s compared to 1.43 ± m/s) than young adults (Winter et al., 1990).

Kinetic Variables

Since gait is a combination of angular movements occurring at the lower extremity and the upper-extremity joint, their combined movement generates angular momentum. Failure to control the angular momentum of the body can result in instability and therefore predispose an individual to an increased risk of falls. Whole-body angular momentum is considered to be a highly controlled variable (Bennett et al., 2010; Neptune and McGowan, 2011) during different human tasks. It may be important in maintaining balance and stability from sitting to standing (Riley et al., 1997) and in trip events (Pijnappels et al., 2004). It has been suggested that angular momentum while walking is controlled by the CNS and the control synergies emanating from it. Thus, the altered regulation of the angular momentum may be a sign of an increased risk of fall (Popovic et al., 2004). Altered patterns of angular momentum regulation has been reported between older men and women while negotiating stairs (Singhal et al., 2015), which highlights the increased risk of falls in older women. However, more studies need to be undertaken to understand age-associated differences in the regulation of angular momentum.

CHANGES IN BODY STRUCTURE AND PHYSIOLOGICAL FUNCTIONS

Changes in Balance

Analysis of balance in itself is a complicated task because of the multiple body systems involved: visual, vestibular, and proprioceptive. Obvious changes in vision due to glaucoma, macular degeneration, diabetic retinopathy, and bifocal lenses can lead to a loss of balance and are relatively easier to comprehend. However, subtle changes in depth perception, ground overlay, three-dimensional forms, and slant characteristics are much more difficult to discern but have been found to be reduced in older adults. All these changes would affect older adults' ability to navigate natural environment and would either increase their risk of falls or cause adaptations in gait that would allow them to be more unstable while walking. Vestibular causes of imbalance can range from specific pathologies such as benign paroxysmal positional vertigo and Méniére's disease to idiopathic changes in vestibular apparatus. An age-associated decrease in functional vestibular connectivity and an increase in its variability have been reported in the vestibular cortical network (Cyran et al., 2016). The authors have suggested reduced cortico–cortical inhibition as a potential mechanism for this impairment, which may increase the risk of falls.

Proprioception is a neural correlate of balance and comprises inputs through mechanoreceptors located in the joints and muscles to the CNS. The two components of proprioception—the joint position sense and the sense of limb movement—are both essential for coordinated movement patterns, motor control during posture, and gait and motor learning (Ghez et al., 1995; Ghez and Sainburg, 1995; Hiemstra et al., 2001; Pickard et al., 2003; Tsang and Hui-Chan, 2003). People of all age groups are more dependent on proprioception to maintain balance than vision and vestibular sensation (Colledge et al., 1994). The occurrence of proprioceptive decline with age and its effects on balance and motor control have long been identified (Barrack et al., 1984; Bullock-Saxton et al., 2001; Horak et al., 1989; Kaplan et al., 1985; Lord and Ward, 1994; Manchester et al., 1989; Pai et al., 1997; Petrella et al., 1997; Skinner et al., 1984; Woollacott et al., 1986), as has its role in increasing the incidence of falls (Lord et al., 1999; Overstall et al., 1977; Sorock and Labiner, 1992; Tinetti et al., 1988). The underlying theme is that the loss of proprioception is prevalent with old age in the ankle, knee, and upper-extremity joints. The mechanism through which these changes occur are both central and peripheral. Central mechanisms involve feedback loops between sensory and motor areas (McCloskey, 1978), whereas the peripheral mechanism includes alterations in cutaneous, articular, and Golgi tendon organ receptors. Each of these mechanisms have been investigated in various papers (Aydog et al., 2006; Iwasaki et al., 2003; Morisawa, 1998; Ribeiro and Oliveira, 2007).

Muscle Structure and Function

Aging-induced reductions in muscle strength and function begin in the second decade. The changes in gait with aging have largely been attributed to muscle weakness. Muscle weakness in turn can be due to alterations in the muscle structure and motor unit complex within one or more muscle groups. The studies in this domain can be grouped into three broad categories depending on their focus: muscle strength, muscle structure physiology, and neuromuscular physiology.

Changes in gluteal muscles strength have been observed in healthy women, with hip extensors showing a decrease from the fourth decade onward and hip abductors showing a decrease from the fifth decade onward (Akbari and Mousavikhatir, 2012). Hip flexor and extensor maximal isometric strength has been reported to be reduced to about 22% and 31% in older women as compared to young women (Dean et al., 2004). The changes in maximal isometric voluntary contractions, especially at the ankle, have been shown to be affected more by changes in muscle fibers and motor unit physiology (Vandervoort and McComas, 1986). Although this provides some insight into strength changes, these results cannot be directly applied to incidences of falls when older adults are undergoing dynamic transformations in posture. In addition, gait does not require lower-extremity muscles to produce forces at their maximal capacity. While climbing stairs, the ankle joint power exerted by both young and old adults was found to be similar. However, when ankle power was normalized to the maximal isokinetic power at the closest ankle angular velocity of a stair gait, it was found that older adults were operating close to their maximal capacity. Therefore, any additional stress occurring as a result of perturbation or loss of balance will increase the risk of falls because muscles may not be able to provide extra power to resist the loss of balance. This provides a direct clinical evidence that there is a loss of functional strength in older adults and that absolute measure of strength does not necessarily provide a complete picture of an individual's performance or susceptibility to adverse events.

The preceding findings are supported by evidence of slower contractile properties and slower action potential discharge rates in the muscles of older adults. Muscles of older adults have slower contractile properties, which has been demonstrated by smaller rates of maximal torque development and decay within the tibialis anterior muscle of older adults as compared to young (Baudry et al., 2005). This occurs in conjunction with lower rates of action potential discharge and smaller torque generation in ankle dorsiflexors during rapid submaximal contractions in older adults (Klass et al., 2005, 2007, 2008). Two situations arise out of this evidence: (1) if this phenomenon can be extrapolated to other muscle groups critical in maintaining the gait velocity and balance and (2) if this is restricted to ankle dorsiflexors alone or affects ankle dorsiflexors more than any other muscle group associated with continuance of the gait. The first scenario clearly provides an explanation for an increased risk of fall both as a result of failure to carry the movement (because of velocity) and to maintain balance. The second scenario provides a potential reason for a shift in balance strategy in older adults from ankle dominant to hip dominant, especially when encountering a challenging environment or condition such as a ramp (Casebolt and Singhal, in preparation).

Muscle structural changes can occur because of sarcopenia or atrophy. Sarcopenia—or loss of muscle mass and its contractility occurring as a result of old age—results from changes in tissue matrix and cellular structure, which are distinct from the changes that occur due to chronic lack of use, which leads to atrophy. These changes are beyond the scope of this chapter, but both sarcopenia and muscle atrophy cause reduced muscle strength and increased susceptibility to muscle injury. Contraction-induced damage and subsequent regenerative capacity of type II muscle has been reported to be most affected in old adults (Faulkner et al., 1995; Schultz and Lipton, 1982; Singh et al., 1999). It has also been shown that the internal environment of the muscle rather than the myofibrils themselves have an effect on muscle regeneration (Carlson and Faulkner, 1989; Conboy et al., 2005) such that new myofibrils are thinner and more fragile, which may result in increased susceptibility to contraction-induced injury (Renault et al., 2000). Another study has observed that there is a greater amount of atrophy in type II fibers and not a loss of number of fibers with old age (Klein et al., 2003). This does not mean that type I fibers do not undergo changes because cross-sectional areas for both type I and type II vastus lateralis fibers have been found to be decreased in older women (Hunter et al., 1999). These studies highlight not only that the capacity to generate quick and high forces is reduced in older adults but also that their susceptibility to and recovery from an injury increases in cases of sudden perturbations.

The role of strength training in improving muscle strength has been well documented. The guidelines for dosage published by the American College of Sports Medicine can be used to provide a starting point, but an older adult needs to be properly evaluated in order to rule out any other underlying pathology that may require alterations to any rehabilitation plan. Besides an obvious increase in muscle strength, high to moderate resistance training has been associated with increases in antiinflammatory IL-1ra in males and the reversal in pretraining expression of 179 genes (Forti et al., 2016; Melov et al., 2007). These gene expression changes were similar to characteristics of a younger population, implying that resistance training not only reduces inflammatory markers but also reverses certain aspects of aging. A systematic review compared functions in older adults after strength training or power training and found that power training results in better functional outcomes, but the review could not come to any conclusion regarding the safety of any of the methods (Tschopp et al., 2011).

Changes in muscle structure are accompanied by changes in motor unit physiology. A motor unit comprises a motor neuron and the muscle fibers it innervates. All muscle fibers in a motor unit are of one type, and all show contractions at the same time once there is a stimulus. During old age, the changes in motor unit occur in the number of motor neurons available (Campbell et al., 1973), which will consequentially result in some muscle denervation.

Some of these denervated fibers undergo degeneration, but there is evidence that motor units are redistributed, with some of these fibers being reinnervated by other motor neurons (Payne et al., 2006). Thus, there is an overall loss in the number of motor units and an increase in twitch force production from the redistributed motor units. However, these changes affect fine motor activity in hand muscles more than the larger muscle groups utilized in gait. On the lower-extremity front, plantarflexor force production abilities have been shown to be associated with walking velocity (Clark et al., 2013). The rate of force production and electromyography (EMG) muscle activation during rapid maximal heel raise is associated with the fastest walking velocities in older adults. The adults who had a lower fastest velocity showed much lower rate of force and EMG activation in medial gastrocnemius. The muscle cross-section area in medial gastrocnemius was similar in both the groups. Although the study was able to show independent associations between walking velocity and ankle plantarflexors force generation capabilities, these are not similar to dynamic walking tasks and one has to be cautious while inferring that limited plantarflexor neuromuscular activation and force generation limits walking speed.

Changes in the Central Nervous System

Age-associated changes have been observed in the soleus H-reflex (the EMG equivalent of the stretch reflex) in different standing positions and reduced modulation in reciprocal inhibition of muscles (between agonist and antagonists) during low-force contractions (Kido et al., 2004; Tsuruike et al., 2003). However, changes in the H-reflex were not seen during walking or in complex standing tasks (Chalmers and Knutzen, 2002; Kido et al., 2004; Mynark and Koceja, 2002). These findings again reinforce that the human gait is intrinsically a very different process than standing or any other postural task. Therefore, findings obtained during other activities should be cautiously applied when drawing similarities with gait. Discussion on the presence of spinal circuitry that may aid in controlling locomotion (also referred to as the central pattern generator) is beyond the scope of this chapter.

Imaging studies have shown increased activation in older adults' cortical and subcortical areas while doing simple upper-extremity motor tasks. Similar cortical adaptations may be associated with observed changes in voluntary activation of the quadriceps femoris during isometric contractions (Klass et al., 2007, 2008). Here again we need to be careful in interpreting the relationships to actual walking tasks. As far as walking or stepping is concerned, evidence suggests the presence of coactivation of agonist and antagonist, which may reduce the overall strength of contraction (Hortobagyi and DeVita, 2000). This coactivation is controlled by descending motor pathways independently of agonist activation (Hortobagyi and Devita, 2006; Levenez et al., 2005), which suggests an adaptation in higher cortical control. The presence of coactivation of muscles works to reduce the net force of contraction acting at the joint, which provides an additional mechanism of strength loss. In addition, coactivation of muscles at a joint is an important mechanism for increasing joint stability, so it may be correlated with changes in proprioception. However, more research is required to establish direct correlation in CNS activity and gait changes.

CONCLUSION

In conclusion, the underlying physiological changes occurring among the elderly begin as early as the fourth decade but do not become recognizable until much later in life. As a result, the elderly are more likely to slow their gait velocity to accommodate changes in muscle strength, aerobic capacity, cognitive function, and overall physical health. Gait adaptations in old age can be due to age or any other underlying pathology. It is extremely difficult but important to differentiate the cause of these changes clinically in order to ensure an older individual's proper rehabilitation. A decrease in gait speed increases the chances of a fall. As a person ages, there seems to be a transition from an ankle strategy to one that places increased emphasis on the hip, which is primarily responsible for carrying the upper body during ambulation; therefore, utilizing a hip strategy to produce forward progression while balancing the upper body may prove too demanding if a perturbation should occur. These changes in gait occur due to the conjunction of altered physiology and body structure. Altered sensations affect balance, deteriorating neuromuscular processes affect muscle strength characteristics, and changes in CNS affect overall control and execution. Numerous studies have been conducted to elucidate these effects, but care should be taken to infer whether these can be applied to walking tasks. The studies correlating changes in CNS and locomotion are limited both in number and scope due to the difficulty of measuring CNS activity while a person is ambulating. Technological advances, especially in ambulatory electroencephalography and near-infrared spectroscopy, have made this a possibility, and significant research in this arena can be expected in the near future.

References

Akbari, M., Mousavikhatir, R., 2012. Changes in the muscle strength and functional performance of healthy women with aging. Med. J. Islam Repub. Iran 26 (3), 125–131. Retrieved from <http://www.ncbi.nlm.nih.gov/pubmed/23482911>.

Aydog, S.T., Korkusuz, P., Doral, M.N., Tetik, O., Demirel, H.A., 2006. Decrease in the numbers of mechanoreceptors in rabbit ACL: the effects of ageing. Knee Surg. Sports Traumatol. Arthrosc. 14 (4), 325–329. http://dx.doi.org/10.1007/s00167-005-0673-2.

Barrack, R.L., Skinner, H.B., Cook, S.D., 1984. Proprioception of the knee joint. Paradoxical effect of training. Am. J. Phys. Med. 63 (4), 175–181. Retrieved from <http://www.ncbi.nlm.nih.gov/pubmed/6465302>.

Barrett, R.S., Mills, P.M., Begg, R.K., 2010. A systematic review of the effect of ageing and falls history on minimum foot clearance characteristics during level walking. Gait Posture 32 (4), 429–435. http://dx.doi.org/10.1016/j.gaitpost.2010.07.010.

Bassey, E.J., Fiatarone, M.A., O'Neill, E.F., Kelly, M., Evans, W.J., Lipsitz, L.A., 1992. Leg extensor power and functional performance in very old men and women. Clin. Sci. (Lond) 82 (3), 321–327. Retrieved from <http://www.ncbi.nlm.nih.gov/pubmed/1312417>.

Baudry, S., Klass, M., Duchateau, J., 2005. Postactivation potentiation influences differently the nonlinear summation of contractions in young and elderly adults. J. Appl. Physiol. (1985) 98 (4), 1243–1250. http://dx.doi.org/10.1152/japplphysiol.00735.2004.

Bennett, B.C., Russell, S.D., Sheth, P., Abel, M.F., 2010. Angular momentum of walking at different speeds. Hum. Mov. Sci. 29 (1), 114–124. http://dx.doi.org/10.1016/j.humov.2009.07.011.

Blake, A.J., Morgan, K., Bendall, M.J., Dallosso, H., Ebrahim, S.B., Arie, T.H., et al., 1988. Falls by elderly people at home: prevalence and associated factors. Age Ageing 17 (6), 365–372. Retrieved from <http://www.ncbi.nlm.nih.gov/pubmed/3266440>.

Bloem, B.R., Haan, J., Lagaay, A.M., van Beek, W., Wintzen, A.R., Roos, R.A., 1992. Investigation of gait in elderly subjects over 88 years of age. J. Geriatr. Psychiatry Neurol. 5 (2), 78–84. Retrieved from <http://www.ncbi.nlm.nih.gov/pubmed/1590914>.

Buchner, D.M., Cress, M.E., Esselman, P.C., Margherita, A.J., deLateur, B.J., Campbell, A.J., et al., 1996. Factors associated with changes in gait speed in older adults. J. Gerontol. Series a-Biol. Sci. Med. Sci. 51 (6), M297–M302. Retrieved from < Go to ISI> ://WOS:A1996WD35200018.

Bullock-Saxton, J.E., Wong, W.J., Hogan, N., 2001. The influence of age on weight-bearing joint reposition sense of the knee. Exp. Brain Res. 136 (3), 400–406. Retrieved from <http://www.ncbi.nlm.nih.gov/pubmed/11243482>.

Campbell, M.J., McComas, A.J., Petito, F., 1973. Physiological changes in ageing muscles. J. Neurol. Neurosurg. Psychiatry 36 (2), 174–182. Retrieved from <http://www.ncbi.nlm.nih.gov/pubmed/4708452>.

Carlson, B.M., Faulkner, J.A., 1989. Muscle transplantation between young and old rats: age of host determines recovery. Am. J. Physiol. 256 (6 Pt 1), C1262–1266. Retrieved from <http://www.ncbi.nlm.nih.gov/pubmed/2735398>.

Cesari, M., Onder, G., Russo, A., Zamboni, V., Barillaro, C., Ferrucci, L., et al., 2006. Comorbidity and physical function: Results from the aging and longevity study in the Sirente geographic area (ilSIRENTE study). Gerontology 52 (1), 24–32. http://dx.doi.org/10.1159/000089822.

Chalmers, G.R., Knutzen, K.M., 2002. Soleus H-reflex gain in healthy elderly and young adults when lying, standing, and balancing. J. Gerontol. A Biol. Sci. Med. Sci. 57 (8), B321–329. Retrieved from <http://www.ncbi.nlm.nih.gov/pubmed/12145358>.

Chen, H.C., Ashtonmiller, J.A., Alexander, N.B., Schultz, A.B., 1994. Age effects on strategies used to avoid obstacles. Gait Posture 2 (3), 139–146. doi:10.1016/0966-6362(94)90001-9.

Chiba, H., Ebihara, S., Tomita, N., Sasaki, H., Butler, J., 2005. Differential gait kinematics between fallers and non-fallers in community-dwelling elderly people. Geriatr. Gerontol. Int. 5, 127–134.

Clark, D.J., Manini, T.M., Fielding, R.A., Patten, C., 2013. Neuromuscular determinants of maximum walking speed in well-functioning older adults. Exp. Gerontol. 48 (3), 358–363. http://dx.doi.org/10.1016/j.exger.2013.01.010.

Colledge, N.R., Cantley, P., Peaston, I., Brash, H., Lewis, S., Wilson, J.A., 1994. Ageing and balance: the measurement of spontaneous sway by posturography. Gerontology 40 (5), 273–278. Retrieved from <http://www.ncbi.nlm.nih.gov/pubmed/7959084>.

Conboy, I.M., Conboy, M.J., Wagers, A.J., Girma, E.R., Weissman, I.L., Rando, T.A., 2005. Rejuvenation of aged progenitor cells by exposure to a young systemic environment. Nature 433 (7027), 760–764. http://dx.doi.org/10.1038/nature03260.

Cromwell, R.L., Newton, R.A., 2004. Relationship between balance and gait stability in healthy older adults. J. Aging Phys. Act. 12 (1), 90–100. Retrieved from <https://www.ncbi.nlm.nih.gov/pubmed/15211023>.

Cromwell, R.L., Newton, R.A., Forrest, G., 2001. Head stability in older adults during walking with and without visual input. J. Vestib. Res. Equilibrium Orientat. 11 (2), 105–114. Retrieved from < Go to ISI> ://WOS:000174334000005.

Cyran, C.A., Boegle, R., Stephan, T., Dietrich, M., Glasauer, S., 2016. Age-relateddecline in functional connectivity of the vestibular cortical network. Brain Struct. Funct. 221 (3), 1443–1463. Retrieved from <https://www.ncbi.nlm.nih.gov/pubmed/25567421>.

Dean, J.C., Kuo, A.D., Alexander, N.B., 2004. Age-related changes in maximal hip strength and movement speed. J. Gerontol. A Biol. Sci. Med. Sci. 59 (3), 286–292. Retrieved from <http://www.ncbi.nlm.nih.gov/pubmed/15031315>.

DeVita, P., Hortobagyi, T., 2000. Age causes a redistribution of joint torques and powers during gait. J. Appl. Physiol. (1985) 88 (5), 1804–1811. Retrieved from <http://www.ncbi.nlm.nih.gov/pubmed/10797145>.

Elble, R.J., Thomas, S.S., Higgins, C., Colliver, J., 1991. Stride-dependent changes in gait of older people. J. Neurol. 238 (1), 1–5. Retrieved from <http://www.ncbi.nlm.nih.gov/pubmed/2030366> .

Faulkner, J.A., Brooks, S.V., Zerba, E., 1995. Muscle atrophy and weakness with aging: contraction-induced injury as an underlying mechanism. J. Gerontol. A Biol. Sci. Med. Sci. 50 (Spec No), 124–129. Retrieved from <http://www.ncbi.nlm.nih.gov/pubmed/7493205>.

Forti, L.N., Van Roie, E., Njemini, R., Coudyzer, W., Beyer, I., Delecluse, C., et al., 2016. Load-specific inflammation mediating effects of resistance training in older persons. J. Am. Med. Dir. Assoc. http://dx.doi.org/10.1016/j.jamda.2016.02.010.

Franz, J.R., Kram, R., 2014. Advanced age and the mechanics of uphill walking: a joint-level, inverse dynamic analysis. Gait Posture 39 (1), 135–140. http://dx.doi.org/10.1016/j.gaitpost.2013.06.012.

Ghez, C., Gordon, J., Ghilardi, M.F., 1995. Impairments of reaching movements in patients without proprioception. II. Effects of visual information on accuracy. J. Neurophysiol. 73 (1), 361–372. Retrieved from <http://www.ncbi.nlm.nih.gov/pubmed/7714578>.

Ghez, C., Sainburg, R., 1995. Proprioceptive control of interjoint coordination. Can. J. Physiol. Pharmacol. 73 (2), 273–284. Retrieved from <http://www.ncbi.nlm.nih.gov/pubmed/7621366>.

Helbostad, J.L., Moe-Nilssen, R., 2003. The effect of gait speed on lateral balance control during walking in healthy elderly. Gait Posture 18 (2), 27–36. doi:10.1016/S0966-6362(02)00197-2.

Hiemstra, L.A., Lo, I.K., Fowler, P.J., 2001. Effect of fatigue on knee proprioception: implications for dynamic stabilization. J. Orthop. Sports Phys. Ther. 31 (10), 598–605. http://dx.doi.org/10.2519/jospt.2001.31.10.598.

Horak, F.B., Shupert, C.L., Mirka, A., 1989. Components of postural dyscontrol in the elderly: a review. Neurobiol. Aging 10 (6), 727–738. Retrieved from <http://www.ncbi.nlm.nih.gov/pubmed/2697808>.

Hortobagyi, T., DeVita, P., 2000. Muscle pre- and coactivity during downward stepping are associated with leg stiffness in aging. J. Electromyogr. Kinesiol. 10 (2), 117–126. Retrieved from <http://www.ncbi.nlm.nih.gov/pubmed/10699559>.

Hortobagyi, T., Devita, P., 2006. Mechanisms responsible for the age-associated increase in coactivation of antagonist muscles. Exerc. Sport. Sci. Rev. 34 (1), 29–35. Retrieved from <http://www.ncbi.nlm.nih.gov/pubmed/16394812>.

Hunter, S.K., Thompson, M.W., Ruell, P.A., Harmer, A.R., Thom, J.M., Gwinn, T.H., et al., 1999. Human skeletal sarcoplasmic reticulum Ca2+ uptake and muscle function with aging and strength training. J. Appl. Physiol. (1985) 86 (6), 1858–1865. Retrieved from <http://www.ncbi.nlm.nih.gov/pubmed/10368350>.

Iwasaki, T., Goto, N., Goto, J., Ezure, H., Moriyama, H., 2003. The aging of human Meissner's corpuscles as evidenced by parallel sectioning. Okajimas Folia Anat Jpn 79 (6), 185–189. Retrieved from <http://www.ncbi.nlm.nih.gov/pubmed/12776944>.

Judge, J.O., Davis 3rd, R.B., Ounpuu, S., 1996. Step length reductions in advanced age: the role of ankle and hip kinetics. J. Gerontol. A Biol. Sci. Med. Sci. 51 (6), M303–312. Retrieved from <http://www.ncbi.nlm.nih.gov/pubmed/8914503>.

Kaplan, F.S., Nixon, J.E., Reitz, M., Rindfleish, L., Tucker, J., 1985. Age-related changes in proprioception and sensation of joint position. Acta Orthop. Scand. 56 (1), 72–74. Retrieved from <http://www.ncbi.nlm.nih.gov/pubmed/3984706>.

Kerrigan, D.C., Todd, M.K., Della Croce, U., Lipsitz, L.A., Collins, J.J., 1998. Biomechanical gait alterations independent of speed in the healthy elderly: evidence for specific limiting impairments. Arch. Phys. Med. Rehabil. 79 (3), 317–322. Retrieved from <http://www.ncbi.nlm.nih.gov/pubmed/9523785>.

Kido, A., Tanaka, N., Stein, R.B., 2004. Spinal excitation and inhibition decrease as humans age. Can. J. Physiol. Pharmacol. 82 (4), 238–248. http://dx.doi.org/10.1139/y04-017.

Klass, M., Baudry, S., Duchateau, J., 2005. Aging does not affect voluntary activation of the ankle dorsiflexors during isometric, concentric, and eccentric contractions. J. Appl. Physiol. (1985) 99 (1), 31–38. http://dx.doi.org/10.1152/japplphysiol.01426.2004.

Klass, M., Baudry, S., Duchateau, J., 2007. Voluntary activation during maximal contraction with advancing age: a brief review. Eur. J. Appl. Physiol. 103 (5), 543–551. http://dx.doi.org/10.1007/s00421-006-0205-x.

Klass, M., Baudry, S., Duchateau, J., 2008. Age-related decline in rate of torque development is accompanied by lower maximal motor unit discharge frequency during fast contractions. J. Appl. Physiol. (1985) 104 (3), 739–746. http://dx.doi.org/10.1152/japplphysiol.00550.2007.

Klein, C.S., Marsh, G.D., Petrella, R.J., Rice, C.L., 2003. Muscle fiber number in the biceps brachii muscle of young and old men. Muscle Nerve 28 (1), 62–68. http://dx.doi.org/10.1002/mus.10386.

Levenez, M., Kotzamanidis, C., Carpentier, A., Duchateau, J., 2005. Spinal reflexes and coactivation of ankle muscles during a submaximal fatiguing contraction. J. Appl. Physiol. (1985) 99 (3), 1182–1188. http://dx.doi.org/10.1152/japplphysiol.00284.2005.

Lloyd, D.G., Stevenson, M.G., 1992. An Investigation of Floor Surface Profile Characteristics That Will Reduce the Incidence of Slips and Falls. ME17, No. 2, September. Mechanical Engineering Transactions-Institute of Engineers, Australia.99–105

Lord, S.R., Ward, J.A., 1994. Age-associated differences in sensori-motor function and balance in community dwelling women. Age Ageing 23 (6), 452–460. Retrieved from <http://www.ncbi.nlm.nih.gov/pubmed/9231937>.

Lord, S.R., Rogers, M.W., Howland, A., Fitzpatrick, R., 1999. Lateral stability, sensorimotor function and falls in older people. J. Am. Geriatr. Soc. 47 (9), 1077–1081. Retrieved from <http://www.ncbi.nlm.nih.gov/pubmed/10484249>.

Maki, B.E., 1997. Gait changes in older adults: predictors of falls or indicator of fear? J. Am. Geriatri. Soc. 45, 313–320.

Manchester, D., Woollacott, M., Zederbauer-Hylton, N., Marin, O., 1989. Visual, vestibular and somatosensory contributions to balance control in the older adult. J. Gerontol. 44 (4), M118–127. Retrieved from <http://www.ncbi.nlm.nih.gov/pubmed/2786896>.

McCloskey, D.I., 1978. Kinesthetic sensibility. Physiol. Rev. 58 (4), 763–820. Retrieved from <http://www.ncbi.nlm.nih.gov/pubmed/360251>.

McGibbon, C.A., 2003. Toward a better understanding of gait changes with age and disablement: neuromuscular adaptation. Exp. Sport Sci. Rev. 31 (2), 102–108.

Melov, S., Tarnopolsky, M.A., Beckman, K., Felkey, K., Hubbard, A., 2007. Resistance exercise reverses aging in human skeletal muscle. PLoS One 2 (5), e465. http://dx.doi.org/10.1371/journal.pone.0000465.

Mian, O.S., Thom, J.M., Ardigo, L.P., Narici, M.V., Minetti, A.E., 2006. Metabolic cost, mechanical work, and efficiency during walking in young and older men. Acta Physiol. (Oxf) 186 (2), 127–139. http://dx.doi.org/10.1111/j.1748-1716.2006.01522.x.

Moe-Buksseb, R., Helbostad, J.L., 2005. Interstride trunk acceleration variability but not step width variability can differentiate between fit and frail older adults. Gait Posture 21 (2), 164–70. Retrieved from <https://www.ncbi.nlm.nih.gov/pubmed/15639395>.

Morisawa, Y., 1998. Morphological study of mechanoreceptors on the coracoacromial ligament. J. Orthop. Sci. 3 (2), 102–110. Retrieved from <http://www.ncbi.nlm.nih.gov/pubmed/9654563>.

Murray, M.P., Kory, R.C., Clarkson, B.H., 1969. Walking patterns in healthy old men. J. Gerontol. 24 (2), 169–178. Retrieved from <http://www.ncbi.nlm.nih.gov/pubmed/5789252>.

Mynark, R.G., Koceja, D.M., 2002. Down training of the elderly soleus H reflex with the use of a spinally induced balance perturbation. J. Appl. Physiol. (1985) 93 (1), 127–133. http://dx.doi.org/10.1152/japplphysiol.00007.2001.

Neptune, R.R., McGowan, C.P., 2011. Muscle contributions to whole-body sagittal plane angular momentum during walking. J. Biomech. 44 (1), 6–12. http://dx.doi.org/10.1016/j.jbiomech.2010.08.015.

Nigg, B.M., Skleryk, B.N., 1988. Gait characteristics of the elderly. Clin. Biomech. (Bristol, Avon) 3 (2), 79–87. http://dx.doi.org/10.1016/0268-0033(88)90049-6.

Oberg, T., Karsznia, A., Oberg, K., 1994. Joint angle parameters in gait: reference data for normal subjects, 10-79 years of age. J. Rehab. Res. Dev. 31 (3), 199–213.

Overstall, P.W., Exton-Smith, A.N., Imms, F.J., Johnson, A.L., 1977. Falls in the elderly related to postural imbalance. Br. Med. J. 1 (6056), 261–264. Retrieved from <http://www.ncbi.nlm.nih.gov/pubmed/837061>.

Pai, Y.C., Rymer, W.Z., Chang, R.W., Sharma, L., 1997. Effect of age and osteoarthritis on knee proprioception. Arthritis Rheum. 40 (12), 2260–2265. doi:10.1002/1529-0131(199712)40:12<2260::AID-ART22>3.0.CO;2-S.

Payne, A.M., Zheng, Z., Messi, M.L., Milligan, C.E., Gonzalez, E., Delbono, O., 2006. Motor neurone targeting of IGF-1 prevents specific force decline in ageing mouse muscle. J. Physiol. 570 (Pt 2), 283–294. http://dx.doi.org/10.1113/jphysiol.2005.100032.

Petrella, R.J., Lattanzio, P.J., Nelson, M.G., 1997. Effect of age and activity on knee joint proprioception. Am. J. Phys. Med. Rehabil. 76 (3), 235–241. Retrieved from <http://www.ncbi.nlm.nih.gov/pubmed/9207711>.

Pickard, C.M., Sullivan, P.E., Allison, G.T., Singer, K.P., 2003. Is there a difference in hip joint position sense between young and older groups? J. Gerontol. A Biol. Sci. Med. Sci. 58 (7), 631–635. Retrieved from <http://www.ncbi.nlm.nih.gov/pubmed/12865479>.

Pijnappels, M., Bobbert, M.F., van Dieen, J.H., 2004. Contribution of the support limb in control of angular momentum after tripping. J. Biomechan. 37, 1811–1818.

Popovic, M, Hofmann, A, & Herr, H (2004). *Angular momentum regulation during human walking: Biomechanics and control.* Paper presented at the IEEE International Conference on Robotics & Automation, New Orleans, LA.

Renault, V., Piron-Hamelin, G., Forestier, C., DiDonna, S., Decary, S., Hentati, F., et al., 2000. Skeletal muscle regeneration and the mitotic clock. Exp. Gerontol. 35 (6-7), 711–719. Retrieved from <http://www.ncbi.nlm.nih.gov/pubmed/11053661>.

Ribeiro, F., Oliveira, J., 2007. Aging effects on joint proprioception: the role of physical activity in proprioception preservation. Eur. Rev. Aging Phys. Activity 4 (2), 71–76. http://dx.doi.org/10.1007/s11556-007-0026-x.

Riley, P.O., Della Croce, U., Kerrigan, D.C., 2001. Propulsive adaptation to changing gait speed. J. Biomech. 34 (2), 197–202. Retrieved from <http://www.ncbi.nlm.nih.gov/pubmed/11165283>.

Riley, P.O., DellaCroce, U., Kerrigan, D.C., 2001. Effect of age on lower extremity joint moment contributions to gait speed. Gait Posture 14 (3), 264–270. Retrieved from <http://www.ncbi.nlm.nih.gov/pubmed/11600330>.

Riley, P.O., Krebs, D.E., Popat, R., 1997. Biomechanical analysis of failed sit-to-stand. IEEE Translat. Rehabil. Eng. 5, 353–359.

Schultz, E., Lipton, B.H., 1982. Skeletal muscle satellite cells: changes in proliferation potential as a function of age. Mech. Ageing Dev. 20 (4), 377–383. Retrieved from <http://www.ncbi.nlm.nih.gov/pubmed/7166986>.

Schulz, B.W., 2011. Minimum toe clearance adaptations to floor surface irregularity and gait speed. J. Biomech. 44 (7), 1277–1284. http://dx.doi.org/10.1016/j.jbiomech.2011.02.010.

Scott, D., Stuart, A.L., Kay, D., Ebeling, P.R., Nicholson, G., Sanders, K.M., 2014. Investigating the predictive ability of gait speed and quadriceps strength for incident falls in community-dwelling older women at high risk of fracture. Arch. Gerontol. Geriatr. 58 (3), 308–313. http://dx.doi.org/10.1016/j.archger.2013.11.004.

Singh, M.A., Ding, W., Manfredi, T.J., Solares, G.S., O'Neill, E.F., Clements, K.M., et al., 1999. Insulin-like growth factor I in skeletal muscle after weight-lifting exercise in frail elders. Am. J. Physiol. 277 (1 Pt 1), E135–143. Retrieved from <http://www.ncbi.nlm.nih.gov/pubmed/10409137>.

Singhal, K., Kim, J., Casebolt, J., Lee, S., Han, K.H., Kwon, Y.H., 2015. Gender difference in older adult's utilization of gravitational and ground reaction force in regulation of angular momentum during stair descent. Human Movement Sci. 41, 230–239. http://dx.doi.org/10.1016/j.humov.2015.03.004.

Skinner, H.B., Barrack, R.L., Cook, S.D., 1984. Age-related decline in proprioception. Clin. Orthop. Relat. Res. 184, 208–211. Retrieved from <http://www.ncbi.nlm.nih.gov/pubmed/6705349>.

Sorock, G.S., Labiner, D.M., 1992. Peripheral neuromuscular dysfunction and falls in an elderly cohort. Am. J. Epidemiol. 136 (5), 584–591. Retrieved from <http://www.ncbi.nlm.nih.gov/pubmed/1332465>.

Tinetti, M.E., Speechley, M., Ginter, S.F., 1988. Risk factors for falls among elderly persons living in the community. N. Engl. J. Med. 319 (26), 1701–1707. http://dx.doi.org/10.1056/NEJM198812293192604.

Tsang, W.W., Hui-Chan, C.W., 2003. Effects of tai chi on joint proprioception and stability limits in elderly subjects. Med. Sci. Sports Exerc. 35 (12), 1962–1971. http://dx.doi.org/10.1249/01.MSS.0000099110.17311.A2.

Tschopp, M., Sattelmayer, M.K., Hilfiker, R., 2011. Is power training or conventional resistance training better for function in elderly persons? A meta-analysis. Age Ageing 40 (5), 549–556. http://dx.doi.org/10.1093/ageing/afr005.

Tsuruike, M., Koceja, D.M., Yabe, K., Shima, N., 2003. Age comparison of H-reflex modulation with the Jendrassik maneuver and postural complexity. Clin. Neurophysiol. 114 (5), 945–953. Retrieved from <http://www.ncbi.nlm.nih.gov/pubmed/12738442>.

Vandervoort, A.A., McComas, A.J., 1986. Contractile changes in opposing muscles of the human ankle joint with aging. J. Appl. Physiol. (1985) 61 (1), 361–367. Retrieved from <http://www.ncbi.nlm.nih.gov/pubmed/3525504>.

van den Kroonenberg, A., Hayes, W.C., McMahon, T.A., 1996. Hip impact velocities and body configurations for experimental falls form standing height. J. Biomech. 29, 807–811.

Verghese, J., LeValley, A., Hall, C.B., Katz, M.J., Ambrose, A.F., Lipton, R.B., 2006. Epidemiology of gait disorders in community-residing older adults. J. Am. Geriatr. Soc. 54 (2), 255–261. http://dx.doi.org/10.1111/j.1532-5415.2005.00580.x.

White, D.K., Neogi, T., Nevitt, M.C., Peloquin, C.E., Zhu, Y., Boudreau, R.M., et al., 2013. Trajectories of gait speed predict mortality in well-functioning older adults: the Health, Aging and Body Composition study. J. Gerontol. A Biol. Sci. Med. Sci. 68 (4), 456–464. http://dx.doi.org/10.1093/gerona/gls197.

Winter, D.A., 1992. Foot trajectory in human gait—a precise and multifactorial motor control task. Phys. Ther. 72 (1), 45–53. Retrieved from <Go to ISI> ://WOS:A1992GY30700007.

Winter, D.A., Patla, A.E., Frank, J.S., Walt, S.E., 1990. Biomechanical walking pattern changes in the fit and healthy elderly. Phys. Ther. 70 (6), 340–347.

Woollacott, M.H., Shumway-Cook, A., Nashner, L.M., 1986. Aging and posture control: changes in sensory organization and muscular coordination. Int. J. Aging Hum. Dev. 23 (2), 97–114. Retrieved from <http://www.ncbi.nlm.nih.gov/pubmed/3557634>.

CHAPTER

9

Assessment of Nutritional Status in the Elderly

Teresa Kokot[1], *Ewa Malczyk*[2], *Ewa Ziółko*[1], *Małgorzata Muc-Wierzgoń*[1] *and Edyta Fatyga*[1]

[1]Medical University of Silesia in Katowice, Katowice, Poland [2]University of Applied Sciences, Nysa, Poland

INTRODUCTION

Nutritional status is the state of health resulting from the usual food intake, absorption, and utilization of food nutrients and from any pathology influencing these processes. It is determined by many factors, including age, sex, physical activity, comorbidities, used drugs or stimulants, and socioeconomic situation (Charzewska et al., 2010; Donini et al., 2007).

Assessing the nutritional status of the elderly is an integral component of a comprehensive geriatric assessment. It provides information on possible quantitative or qualitative deficiencies of nutrients, helps to identify the risk of protein-energy malnutrition (PEM), overweight, and obesity, and it helps to monitor effectiveness of the nutritional therapy (Ashwell et al., 2012). Assessment of the nutritional status in disabled and bedridden elderly patients presents particular challenges.

Most often, the same indicators and criteria used with adults can assess the nutritional status of the elderly (2006). However, an assessment must consider the physiological and pathophysiological distinctiveness of the aging process (Charzewska et al., 2010; Wojszel, 2011; Green and Watson, 2006; Antczak-Domagała et al., 2013). Proper assessment of the nutritional status in the elderly is carried out by qualified personnel (doctors, nurses, dietitians), and it requires a combination of several methods: medical history, with a particular emphasis on nutritional history; physical examination; anthropometric tests; and determination of biochemical parameters and surveys based on validated questionnaires for assessing nutritional status (Babiarczyk and Turbiarz, 2012).

MEDICAL HISTORY WITH A PARTICULAR EMPHASIS ON THE NUTRITIONAL HISTORY AND PHYSICAL EXAMINATION

Medical History

A medical history interview should be collected from a patient as well as from a family member, especially a caregiver. Additional help can be found in the medical records of the patient (results of specialist consultations, information cards, etc.). Questions about currently occurring acute and chronic disorders, painful conditions, incidents of fainting and falls, acute and chronic stress, recent hospitalizations, and medications and dietary supplements taken are particularly important. The taken pharmacological agents, often polypragmasic, in addition to side effects, also affect the absorption of various nutrients. The interview with the elderly patient should be deepened with questions on mood disorders, with particular emphasis on depression and cognitive impairment. It is also important to learn

Nutrition and Functional Foods for Healthy Aging.
DOI: http://dx.doi.org/10.1016/B978-0-12-805376-8.00009-5

about the degree of a patient's independence, his or her family and social situation (lack of support, discrimination), and present or completed mourning and economic factors.

The interview should also take into account symptoms that are characteristic of the so-called large geriatric problems: dementia, depression, falls and syncope, urinary incontinence, and malnutrition.

Nutritional History

Questions regarding changes in appetite, diet, increases or decreases in body weight in the preceding 3 months, deviations in sense of taste and smell, disorders of the gastrointestinal tract (including dysphagia, odynophagia, diarrhea, and constipation) are important. Analysis primarily includes the amount and quality of meals with regard to food allergies and cultural and economic factors. It is important to check if food meets a person's energy demands and whether it satisfies the requirements for essential nutrients.

Monitoring a patient while eating and noting consumed products in food diaries is used in the prospective assessment. The methodology considers an interview on the food consumption within the preceding 24 h, eating history, a 3-day noting method, and chemical analysis of the recreated daily food rations. The latter is relatively expensive and is not suitable for use with individuals in larger populations.

The 24-h dietary interview is the most commonly used and assesses the average energy value of a daily diet, the content of basic nutrients, and the consumption of selected minerals (calcium, magnesium, phosphorus, sodium). The interview is carried out once with each of the respondents, on any day of the week, and noting the proportions between common days and holidays. Photographs of the products included in a special album of servings and dishes are used during collection of the history.

Physical Examination: Deviations

Physical examination should be carried out in accordance with the accepted medical standards. Particular attention should be paid to the accurate assessment of the skin and subcutaneous tissue atrophy and skin discoloration, enlarged veins, deficient or excess body fat, atrophy of skeletal muscles, impaired wound healing, susceptibility to the development of bedsores, brittle nails, hair loss, exudates from body cavities, and peripheral edema.

The oral cavity should also be subjected to a very accurate assessment, including missing teeth, dental caries, the presence or absence of dentures, inflammation of mucous membranes, and possible ulcerations.

ANTHROPOMETRIC TESTS

Anthropometric tests provide information on body weight, body fat distribution, and body proportions, as well as information on the body's protein-energy reserves. They are noninvasive and easy to make. The measuring sets are highly available and relatively cheap and include a stadiometer (anthropometer) caliper, anthropometric tape, and a scale. An additional advantage is the lack of any contraindications (Antczak-Domagała et al., 2013). Tests include (1) determining body parameters (height and body mass; the circumference of the waist, hip, arm, and calf; and thickness of skin folds) and (2) determination of the body composition.

Body Mass

Body mass is a measure of total body weight, including muscle mass, fat, bone, and water, but generally does not provide information on the relative proportions of each constituent. Body mass is measured in the morning after a person has emptied his or her bladder and without outerwear or footwear on a calibrated scales with an accuracy of at least 0.1 kg (Charzewska et al., 2010; Wronka et al., 2010).

Body mass is a single authoritative indicator of nutritional status and a particular indicator of the risk of PEM in the elderly (Babiarczyk and Turbiarz, 2012). Analysis of body weight changes in time is particularly important in assessing nutritional status (unintentional weight loss) (Charzewska et al., 2010; Blackburn et al., 1977; Charzewska, 2000). Serious weight loss of body mass is defined as >2% weight loss in 1 week, >5% in a month, >7% in 3 months, or >10% in 6 months (Blackburn et al., 1977).

Assessing the nutritional status of the elderly takes into account the percentage of body mass. The optimal body mass can vary within 10% of ideal body weight. A patient is diagnosed as overweight if the optimal body mass is exceeded by 10–20%, while obesity is diagnosed if the optimal body mass is exceeded by more than 20% (Blackburn et al., 1977; Szczygieł et al., 1994).

Body Height

Body height is the distance from the base (the contact point of feet with the ground) to the highest anatomical point of the head (the vertex). The measurement is performed in the morning (due to fluctuations in the body height within a day) using a stadiometer or portable anthropometer with a precision of 0.1 cm. The person being measured should stand freely upright with knees and heels together and toes slightly apart. The result of measurements of the body height is a relatively constant parameter in adults, but with age it may change as a result of involution processes (e.g., osteoporosis). The difference can be as much as 10 cm (Wronka et al., 2010).

Body Mass Index

Measurements of weight and height are the basis for determining body mass index (BMI). The measure is the ratio of body mass in kilograms to the square of height expressed in meters. BMI is widely used as a diagnostic indicator to identify abnormal nutritional status and has been recognized by the World Health Organization (WHO) as a measure of a person's energy and protein nutritional status. A BMI less than 17 kg/m² indicates a risk of malnutrition; 18–24 kg/m² indicates a good nutritional status; 28–29 kg/m² indicates a person is overweight; and more than 30 kg/m² indicates obesity (Charzewska et al., 2010; World Health Organization, 1995, 2010; Kvamme et al., 2012).

Many researchers point to malnutrition among older people with higher values of BMI (Babiarczyk and Turbiarz, 2012; Beck and Ovesen, 1998). BMI values between 24 and 27 kg/m² are associated with reduced risk of mortality and an improved quality of life (Babiarczyk and Turbiarz, 2012; Kvamme et al., 2012).

Older people tend to lose muscle mass (Ness-Abramof and Apovian, 2008) as well as body height (Srikanthan et al., 2009), which can lead to an underestimation of BMI. Therefore, this indicator is a poor predictor of health problems related to body mass in the geriatric population (Kravitz, 2010).

Measuring Body Composition

Assessment of the proportion of body fat to remaining body mass can determine an organism's nutritional status (Charzewska, 2000).

Assessing Fat Content in the Body

Assessing fat content in the body using anthropometric methods is performed by measuring the thickness of skin folds at defined anatomical points on the body: e.g., above the triceps and above the biceps; under the lower angle of the shoulder blades; over the iliac cress; on the belly, chest, and thigh; and above the gastrocnemius muscle (Wronka et al., 2010; Szczygieł et al., 1994).

These measurements (thickness of the skin folds) are carried out using a clipper on the right side of the upright body, with freely lowered upper limbs, at least twice in the same place, calculating an arithmetic mean from the measurements (Harrison et al., 1988).

Points and sites of measurements in the elderly are:

1. above the triceps in a vertical line midway between the acromion and the elbow ulna,
2. above the biceps of the arm in a vertical line midway between the acromion and the elbow ulna, and
3. on the belly in the diagonal, one-quarter of the distance between the navel and the front upper iliac thorn.

Measurement of the triceps skin-fold thickness above the triceps of a person's nondominant arm is the most common way to measure and to determine a person's nutritional status because it helps define the energy reserves of the body (Szczygieł et al., 1994) and calculate body density and the amount of body fat (Jackson and Pollock, 1978, 1985; Jackson et al., 1980; Durnin and Womersley, 1974; Siri, 1961).

The phenomenon of internalizing and centralizing body fat is commonly observed in the elderly, which is why measuring skin-fold thickness is not a diagnostic method (National Institutes of Health, 1998; World Health Organization, 2004).

Indicators of Fat Tissue Distribution

The waist circumference, waist-to-hip ratio (WHR), and waist-to-height ratio (WHtR) are the measurements most often used to evaluate body fat distribution (Ashwell et al., 2012; Bolanowski et al., 2005; Lee et al., 2008).

Waist Circumference

Waist circumference is a diagnostic indicator that reflects abdominal obesity. It is measured by applying a stretch-resistant tape at least twice between the bottom edge of the bottom rib and the top of the iliac crest and perpendicular to the vertical line of the trunk at the end of a gentle exhalation of a person standing with legs together and hands lowered freely (WHO, 2008). In the case of highly obese individuals whose measurements cannot be taken between the edge of the rib and the ridge of the hip, the waist circumference is measured at the navel (Ness-Abramof and Apovian, 2008; Browning et al., 2010; Roszkowski and Chmara-Pawlińska, 2003).

Waist-to-Hip Ratio

When measuring WHR, waist circumference is measured at least twice at the widest part of the buttocks perpendicular to the vertical line of the trunk at the end of a gentle exhalation of a person standing with legs together and hands lowered freely (Welborn and Dhaliwal, 2007). WHR is a measurement of the fat tissue distribution in an organism (Ashwell et al., 2012; Ness-Abramof and Apovian, 2008; Srikanthan et al., 2009; Kravitz, 2010; Browning et al., 2010).

Waist-to-Height Ratio

WHtR is the ratio of waist circumference to body height. In addition to WHR and waist circumference, it is also a measure of fat distribution (Ashwell et al., 2012). Values of WHR higher than 0.50 indicate an increased risk of cardiovascular diseases associated with obesity. WHtR is correlated with the abdominal obesity.

Measuring Lean Body Mass

The elderly are exposed not only to metabolic diseases but also to sarcopenia, protein malnutrition, and vitamin and mineral deficiencies (WHO, 2008; Leischker et al., 2010; Fairweather-Tait et al., 2014). Therefore, measurements of lean body mass, which can be measured by anthropological methods, are also included in any assessment of nutritional status.

Arm Circumference and the Volume Index of the Arm Muscle Area

Measurement of the arm circumference (mid-arm circumference) is performed midway between the anatomical points of the acromion and the olecranon on the nondominant side of the body. A circumference below 21 cm indicates a shortage of muscle tissue and therefore protein malnutrition.

In determining the arm muscle circumference (mid-arm muscle circumference) and arm muscle area (mid-arm muscle area), skin-fold thickness is measured above the nondominant triceps.

Calf Circumference

Calf circumference also provides information about normal muscle mass. It can reflect a decrease in muscle mass with limited physical activity. A result of more than 31 cm is considered normal (Tsai et al., 2008). When measuring the circumference of the arm and calf in the diagnosis of sarcopenia, one should be aware that these measurements may be affected by errors of interpretation due to the presence of edema and possible connective and adipose tissue in place of muscle tissue (Strzelecki et al., 2011). There are no clear standardized criteria in the diagnosis of sarcopenia (Krzymińska-Siemaszko and Wieczorowska-Tobis, 2012).

BIOCHEMICAL TESTS

Laboratory tests are also components of any thorough nutritional status assessment. Based on the results of laboratory tests and patient body mass, one can qualify a person as having normal nutritional status or different degrees of malnutrition. No laboratory test, however, clearly indicates malnutrition in the elderly.

The biochemical tests include the following:

- blood counts—numbers of leukocytes, red blood cells, platelets, hemoglobin concentration, hematocrit, and total lymphocyte counts;
- concentration of albumin, prealbumin, and transferrin in plasma;
- concentration of creatinine, glucose, iron, vitamin B_{12} in serum;
- thyroid-stimulating hormone;
- acute phase protein; and
- lipids.

SURVEY METHODS

Many questionnaires can assess the nutritional status of the elderly, including validated nutritional status questionnaires such as Nutritional Risk Screening (NRS 2002), Mini-Nutritional Assessment (MNA), Subjective Global Assessment (SGA), Seniors in the Community Risk Evaluation for Eating and Nutrition (SCREEN II), Nutritional Risk Index (NRI), and Prognostic Inflammatory and Nutritional Index (PINI) (Phillips et al., 2010; Guigoz and Vellas, 1998; Ożga and Małgorzewicz, 2013; Walsh, 2003; Al-Najjar et al., 2012; Bonnefoy et al., 1998).

Nutritional Risk Screening 2002

The NRS 2002 is a screening method that can assess nutritional status. In hospitalized patients, the scale shows from 39% to 70% sensitivity and from 83% to 93% of specificity. The point survey takes into account inter alia such factors as BMI <20.5 kg/m^2, the percentage of body mass loss (>5% in the last 3 months), changes in food consumption within the preceding week, and the occurrence of severe comorbidity factors (e.g., stroke, liver cirrhosis, chronic obstructive pulmonary disease, and renal failure), the medical treatment (e.g., extensive abdominal surgery, chemotherapy, bone marrow transplantation), and a patient's age. Patients who score three or more points require nutritional therapy. In the case of more than three points, a conservative approach is implemented or the questionnaire is repeated in a week (Ożga and Małgorzewicz, 2013).

Mini-Nutritional Assessment

The MNA is the most widely used questionnaire (developed by Guigoz et al.) for evaluating nutritional status in the elderly (Guigoz and Vellas, 1998). It shows the highest sensitivity (>83%) and specificity (>90%). It consists of a screening part (6 questions) or a patient assessment (12 questions) or both. The survey includes questions on meals, usual body mass, neurological disorders, stress history over the preceding 3 months, BMI measurement, and calf circumference. Rating a patient also means determining frequency of consumption of various food groups and medications, housing quality, and a person's subjective perception of his or her own health and nutritional status. The maximum number of points a patient can get is 30. Scores in the range of 24–30 indicate a normal nutritional status. A range of 17–23 indicates a risk of malnutrition, and below 17 points suggests malnourishment (Ożga and Małgorzewicz, 2013).

Subjective Global Assessment

The SGA is considered a nutritional assessment scale and consists of three parts: history, physical examination, and opinion about the risk of malnutrition.

As part of the interview, a doctor establishes, among other things, whether there has been any recent weight loss (defined as a percentage), whether a patient follows a specific diet or has changed the diet recently, whether there are unwanted gastrointestinal symptoms (nausea, vomiting, anorexia, diarrhea), what the patient's physical capacity is (working, reclining), and whether the main disease increases metabolic demand. During the physical examination, the doctor will assess whether there has been a loss of subcutaneous adipose tissue or muscle (quadriceps, deltoid) and whether the patient has ascites or edema (ankle, above the sacrum). The final SGA conclusion establishes whether the tested person exhibits normal nutritional status, suspected malnutrition or moderate malnutrition, a high risk of malnutrition, or emaciation (Ożga and Małgorzewicz, 2013; Walsh, 2003).

Seniors in the Community: Risk Evaluation for Eating and Nutrition

The SCREEN II questionnaire is particularly useful with older people living in their own homes. Its 17 questions assess the risk of malnutrition based on the amount of food intake, physiological problems with the intake of food, changes in body weight, and social aspects of eating.

NRI and PINI are useful indicators of the risk of malnutrition in hospitalized elderly patients (Ożga and Małgorzewicz, 2013; Al-Najjar et al., 2012).

Nutritional Risk Index

The NRI is calculated from the following formula:

$$(1.5 \times \text{albumin concentration}[\text{g/L}]) + \text{current body mass(kg)/due body mass}$$

A good nutritional status is recognized if the NRI is in the range of 97.5–100. Moderate malnutrition is determined when the NRI ranges from 83.5 to 97.5, and severe malnutrition is determined when the NRI is less than 83.5 (Ożga and Małgorzewicz, 2013).

Prognostic Inflammatory and Nutritional Index

The PINI allows the evaluation of the ratio of acute phase catabolic proteins (alpha 1-acid glycoprotein, CRP) to anabolic proteins (albumin and prealbumin). Life risk is diagnosed when a PINI score is >30; high risk is seen for 21–30, an average risk for 11–20, and a low risk when PINI is in the range of 1–10 (Ożga and Małgorzewicz, 2013; Al-Najjar et al., 2012; Bonnefoy et al., 1998).

CONCLUSION

The biggest nutritional problems with the elderly are malnutrition and severe obesity.

Assessing nutritional status requires only basic medical skills although there is no simple tool for this assessment. Each time the results of a subjective and objective examination and additional tests must be analyzed globally and critically. The nutritional assessment scales are also helpful but do not substitute for a medical conclusion.

There are many methods to assess seniors' nutritional status. Unfortunately, so far we failed to develop a gold standard that will allow us to assess the nutritional status of all elderly patients. Such an evaluation is complex and requires a compilation of many different studies. The results of any nutritional assessment should be documented and completed with proposals on how to proceed, depending on the existing nutritional risk.

References

Al-Najjar, Y., et al., 2012. Prredicting outcome in patients with left ventricular systolic chronic heart failure using a nutritional risk index. Am. J. Cardiol. 109 (9), 1315–1320.

Antczak-Domagała, K., Magierski, R., Wlazło, A., Sobów, T., 2013. Nutritional status and ways of assessment in the elderly and demented patients. Psychiatry Clin. Psychol. 13 (4), 271–277.

Ashwell, M., Gunn, P., Gibson, S., 2012. Waist-to-height ratio is a better screening tool than waist circumference and BMI for adult cardiometabolic risk factors: systematic review and meta-analysis. Obes. Rev. 13 (3), 275–286. http://dx.doi.org/10.1111/j.1467-789X.2011.00952.x. Epub 2011 Nov 23.

Babiarczyk, B., Turbiarz, A., 2012. Body Mass Index in elderly people—do the reference ranges matter. Prog. Health 2 (1), 58–67.

Beck, A.M., Ovesen, L., 1998. At which body mass index and degree of weight loss should hospitalized elderly patients be considered at nutritional risk? Clin. Nutr. 17, 195–198.

Blackburn, G.L., Bistrian, B.R., Maini, B.S., Schlamm, H.T., Smith, M.F., 1977. Nutritional and metabolic assessment of the hospitalized patient. JPEN J. Parenter. Enteral. Nutr. 1 (1), 11–22.

Bolanowski, M., Zadrożna-Śliwka, B., Zatońska, K., 2005. Body composition studies—methods and possible application in hormonal disorders. Nutr. Obes. Metabol. Surg. 1, 20–25.

Bonnefoy, M., Ayzac, L., Ingenbleek, Y., Kostka, T., Boisson, R.C., Bienvenu, J., 1998. Usefulness of the prognostic inflammatory and nutritional index (PINI) in hospitalized elderly patients. Int. J. Vitam. Nutr. Res. 68, 189–195.

Browning, L.M., Hsieh, S.D., Ashwell, M., 2010. A systematic review of waist-to-height ratio as a screening tool for the prediction of cardiovascular disease and diabetes: 0·5 could be a suitable global boundary value. Nutr. Res. Rev. 23 (2), 247–269. http://dx.doi.org/10.1017/S0954422410000144. Epub 2010 Sep 7.

Charzewska, J., 2000. Assessment of nutritional status. In: Gawęcki, J., Hryniewiecki, L. (Eds.), Human Nutrition-Basics of Food Science. PWN, Warsaw, pp. 481–494.

Charzewska, J., Chabros, E., Pachocka, L., 2010. Assesment of nutriotional status. W: Jarosz M. red. IŻŻ, Warsaw, 117–129.
Donini, L.M., Savina, C., Rosano, A., Canella, C., 2007. Systematic review of nutritional status evaluation and screening tools in the elderly. J. Nutr Health Aging 11 (5), 421–432.
Durnin, J V.G.A., Womersley, J., 1974. Body fat assessed from total body density and its estimation from skinfold thickness: measurements on 481 men and women aged from 16 to 72 Years. Br. J. Nutr. 32, 77–97. http://dx.doi.org/10.1079/BJN19740060.
Fairweather-Tait, S.J., Wawer, A.A., Gillings, R., Jennings, A., Myint, P.K., 2014. Iron status in the elderly. Mechan. Ageing . Develop. 136-137, 22.
Green, S.M., Watson, R., 2006. Nutritional screening and assessment tools for older adults: literature review. J. Adv. Nurs. 54, 477–490.
Guigoz, Y., Vellas, B., 1998. Assessing the nutritional status of the elderly:the Mini Nutritional Assessment as part of the geriatic evaluation. Nutr. Rev. 54, 59–65. 33.
Harrison, G.G., Buskirk, E.R., Lindsay Carter, J.E., Johnston, F.E., Lohman, T.G., Pollock, M.L., et al., 1988. Skinfold thickness and measurement technique. In: Lohman, T.G., Roche, A.F., Martorell, R. (Eds.), Anthropometric Standardization Reference Manual. Human Kinetics, Champaign, pp. 55–70.
Jackson, A.S., Pollock, M.L., 1978. Generalized equations for predicting body density of men. Br. J. Nutr. 40, 497–504.
Jackson, A.S., Pollock, M.L., 1985. Practical assessment of body composition. Physician Sport Med. 13, 76–90.
Jackson, A.S., Pollock, M.L., Ward, A., 1980. Generalized equations for predicting body density of women. Med. Sci. Sports Ex. 12, 175–182.
Kravitz, L., 2010. Waist-to-hip ratio, waist circumference and BMI. IDEA Fit. J. 7 (9), 18–21.
Krzymińska-Siemaszko, R., Wieczorowska-Tobis, K., 2012. Sarcopenia—towards standarized criteria. Gerontol 6, 46–49.
Kvamme, J.M., Holmen, J., Wilsgaard, T., Florholmen, J., Midthjell, K., Jacobsen, B.K., 2012. Body mass index and mortality in elderly men and women: the Tromsø and HUNT studies. J. Epidemiol. Community Health 66 (7), 611–617. Published online 2011 Feb 14. http://dx.doi.org/10.1136/jech.2010.123232 PMCID: PMC3368492.
Lee, C.M., Huxley, R.R., Wildman, R P., Woodward, M., 2008. Indices of abdominal obesity are better discriminators of cardiovascular risk factors than BMI. a meta-analysis. J. Clin. Epidemiol. 61, 646–653.
Leischker, A.H., Kolb, G.F., Felschen-Ludwig, S., 2010. Nutritional status, chewing function and vitamin deficiency in geriatric inpatients. Eur. Geriat. Med. 1, 207–212. http://dx.doi.org/10.1016/j.eurger.2010.06.006.
National Institutes of Health, 1998. Clinical Guidelines on the Identification, Evaluation, and Treatment of Overweight and Obesity in Adults. The Evidence Raport. NIH Publication No. 98-4083. Bethesda, MD, U.S. Department of Health and Human Services.
Ness-Abramof, R., Apovian, C.M., 2008. Waist circumference measurement in clinical practice. Nutr. Clin. Pract. 23 (4), 397–404.
Ożga, E., Małgorzewicz, S., 2013. Assesment of nutritional ststus of the elderly. Geriatria 7, 98–103.
Phillips, M.B., Foley, A.L., Barnard, R., Isenring, E.A., Miller, M.D., 2010. Nutritional screening in community-dwelling older adults: a systematic literature review. Asia Pac. J. Clin. Nutr. 19 (3), 440–449.
Roszkowski, W., Chmara-Pawlińska, R., 2003. Somatometria the elderly as an indicator of nutritional status. Yearbook PZH 54 (4), 399–408.
Siri, W.E., 1961. Body composition from fluid space and density. In: Brozek, J., Hanschel, A. (Eds.), Techniques for Measuring Body Composition. National Academy of Science, Washington, DC, pp. 223–244.
Srikanthan, P., Seeman, T.E., Karlamangla, A.S., 2009. Waist-hip-ratio as a predictor of all-cause mortality in high-functioning older adults. Ann. Epidemiol. 19, 724–731.
Strzelecki, A., Ciechanowicz, R., Zdrojewski, Z., 2011. Sarcopenia in the elderly. Gerontol. Pol. 19 (3/4), 134–145.
Szczygieł, B., Pertkiewicz, M., Majewska, K., 1994. Assessment of nutritional status. In: Szczygieł, B., Socha, J. (Eds.), Enteral and Parenteral Nutrition in Surgery. PZWL, Warsaw, pp. 35.
Tsai, A.C., Ku, P.-Y., Tsai, J.-D., 2008. Population specific anthropometric cutoff standards improve the functionality of the Mini Nutritional Assessment without BMI in institutionalized elderly in Taiwan. J. Nutr. Health Aging 12 (10), 696–700.
Walsh, D., 2003. Assessment of nutritional status and prognosis in advanced cancer:interleukin-6, reactive protein, and the prognostic and inflammatory nutritional index. Support Care Cancer 11 (1), 60–62.
Welborn, T.A., Dhaliwal, S.S., 2007. Preferred clinical measures of central obesity for predicting mortality. Eur. J. Clin. Nutr. 61 (12), 1373–1379.
Wojszel, Z.B., 2011. Malnutrition and dilemmas nutritional therapy in geriatrics. Prog. Med. Sci. 8, 649–657.
World Health Organization, 1995. Physical status: the use and interpretation of anthropometry. Report of a WHO Expert Committee WHO Technical Report Series. World Health Organization, Geneva. 854.
World Health Organization, 2004. Obesity: Preventing and Managing the Global Epidemic: Raport of a WHO. Genewa, Switzerland.
World Health Organization, 2008. WHO STEPwise Approach to Surveillance (STEPS). World Health Organization (WHO), Geneva.
World Health Organization, 2010. BMI Classification. http://apps.who.int/bmi/index.jsp?introPage=intro_3.html. (2016.01.28).
Wronka, L., Sińska, B., Wójcik, Z., 2010. Review of methods for assessing nutritional status in adults. Part I. Anthropometric methods. Polish J. Human Nutr. Matabol. 37 (4), 268–280.

CHAPTER

10

Eating Capability Assessments in Elderly Populations

Laura Laguna[1], *Anwesha Sarkar*[1] *and Jianshe Chen*[2]

[1]University of Leeds, Leeds, United Kingdom [2]Zhejiang Gongshang University, Hangzhou, China

INTRODUCTION

Physiologically, with the aging process, there is a decline in the functioning of all organs (Langley-Evans, 2009). There are changes in body composition (Rosenberg and Miller, 1992) such as a decrease in bone density and lean mass and an increase in body fat. Many of these changes translate into declining physical abilities and declining motor performances (Newell et al., 2006) that influence the normal execution of daily activities such as self-feeding. The self-feeding process involves numerous actions to be performed such as opening a food package, heating the meal, manipulating the food by hand or mouth, chewing, masticating, and finally swallowing the food bolus. Opening a package can be a difficult task for many individuals, especially for disabled elderly consumers (Heinö et al., 2008). Other physical impairments also tend to interfere with their abilities such as difficulty in transporting food from the plate to the mouth in the case of Parkinson's disease sufferers, mastication inefficiency in edentulous or denture wearers (Fontijn-Tekamp et al., 2000), or swallowing disorders in dysphagia patients (Scialfa and Geoff, 2006). Elderly individuals who suffer from difficulties performing this entire eating process generally eat less food due to the fatigue and time consumed to perform these actions (McLaren and Dickerson, 2000), and this may result in malnutrition and deterioration of health. In fact, previous studies showed that common barriers among elderly to eat adequately have been related to difficulties in eating as well as the inability to prepare fruit- and vegetable-based meals (Dittus et al., 1995).

To our knowledge, eating difficulties in elderly populations have been studied mostly from the perspective of caregivers using nursing diagnosis through observation and interviews with patients having neurological pathologies (Axelsson, 1988; Jacobsson et al., 1996; Jacobsson, 2000; Norberg et al., 1987; Westergren et al., 2002). Generally in these qualitative studies, different eating actions (e.g., hand movements, oral manipulation, eating time, swallowing) with different levels of aberrancy are monitored. To complement the eating actions, an assessment of an individual's nutritional status is also carried out, which shows a close association between low energy intake and malnutrition. To measure the eating disability in an acute stroke population, McLaren and Dickerson (2000) designed a study measuring eight different categories of eating action inabilities using direct observation. Within each category (arm movement, lip closure, chewing, reflex swallowing, posture, communication, attention and visual field loss, and perceptual loss), numerical values were assigned according to severity and level of impairment ranging from 0 (absence of impairment, disability or dependence) to 1, 2, and 3 (moderate to severe levels of impairment and dependence). As in previous studies, McLaren and Dickerson (2000) found a direct relationship between eating disability and reduced dietary energy intake.

Despite this valuable study, there is a lack of reliable instruments for eating assessments, and the outcomes from such assessments are often not comparable between different studies. Therefore, there is a need to establish easily quantifiable parameters and select methods for objective assessments of eating actions in order to consider elderly group heterogeneity and address appropriate foods for each individual. A new concept called *eating*

Nutrition and Functional Foods for Healthy Aging.
DOI: http://dx.doi.org/10.1016/B978-0-12-805376-8.00010-1

capability (EC) was very recently proposed (Laguna and Chen, 2016) to represent an individual's capability of oral food consumption. Based on the fact that an eating process involves a series of food – body interactions, EC is a combination of one's physical, physiological, and mental coordination capabilities in handling and consuming food. This chapter focuses on the difficulties faced by the elderly during the eating process rather than the digestion of food after oral processing. The main objective of this chapter is to introduce different methodologies that can be used to quantitatively measure the eating process.

EATING CAPABILITY: DEFINITION AND CONSTITUENTS

EC is defined as the physical, physiological, and cognitive capabilities of an individual in handling and consuming food. As shown in Fig. 10.1, the EC comprises different parameters: hand, oral, sensation, and mental and coordination capability. Each parameter of the EC can be characterized separately by measurable parameters. Mental and coordination capability are not discussed in this chapter due to its complexity and the lack of literature information on its implications to eating impairment. Hand, oral, and sensation capability will be discussed in the following sections. The most common devices used to measure these capabilities are shown in Fig. 10.2, which will be referred throughout this section.

Hand Manipulation Capability

Hands are the most versatile parts of the human body and essential tools for handling different situations in our daily lives. Any injury, disability, or distortion of the hand can affect our quality of life (Olandersson et al., 2005). With aging, hands suffer from numerous changes due to normal decline, common metabolic skeletal diseases such as osteoarthritis, rheumatoid arthritis and osteoporosis, hormonal changes, degenerative diseases of the central nervous system (CNS) such as Parkinson's disease (Carmeli et al., 2003), or side effects of malnutrition. These changes result in diminished hand strength (Mathiowetz et al., 1985a) due to decreased muscle mass (Metter et al., 1998), stiffer tendons, and irregular or dense connective tissue (due to biochemical changes), swelling and joint deformation in case of osteoarthritis, fungal infections in nails, and peripheral decrement in tactile sensibility (Carmeli et al., 2003). During the eating process, the capability of hand manipulation is essential both before and during the course of a meal (food preparation and hand cutlery manipulation). This capability can be defined as the ability of an individual to exert an appropriate force in a coordinated manner so as to manipulate food from opening a package to reaching the food to bringing it to the mouth.

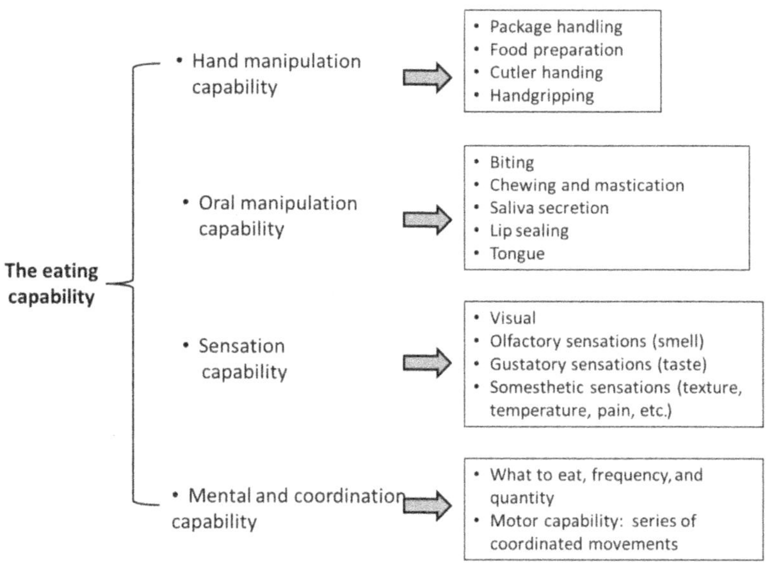

FIGURE 10.1 Components of the eating capability and measurable parameters.

Four types of actions require hand manipulation during the eating process:

1. food package handling and opening,
2. managing food on the plate (e.g., using cutlery or spreading butter),
3. handling and lifting an object (e.g., a glass of water), and
4. transporting food from the plate to the mouth.

When it comes to food packaging, many consumers experience some difficulty in opening certain types of packaging (Heinö et al., 2008). The grip and coordination needed often varies. For instance, a wrist twist is needed to

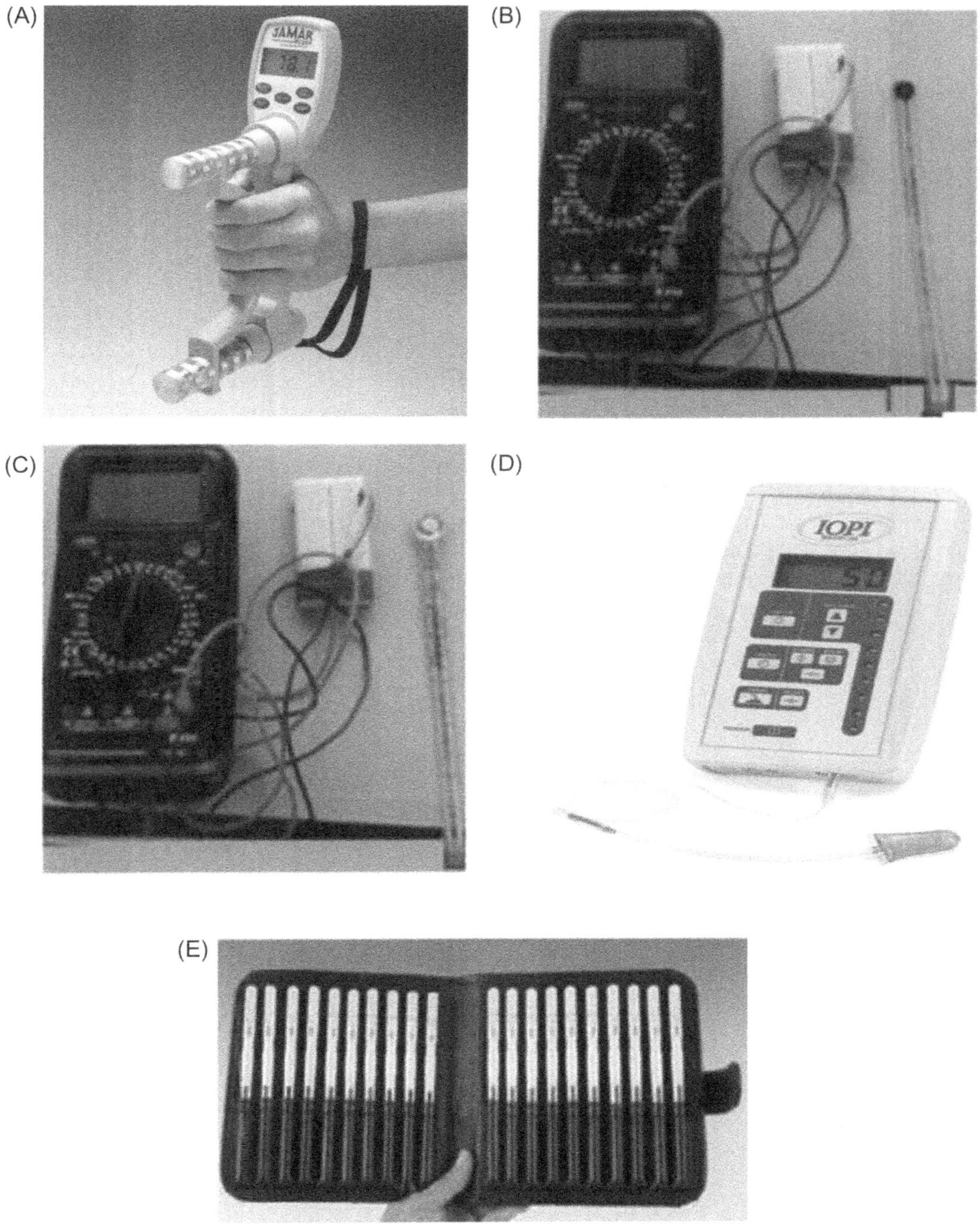

FIGURE 10.2 Devices used to assess eating capability: (A) JAMAR dynamometer for handgripping force, (B) flexisensor with neoprene disk for finger-gripping force, (C) flexisensor with silicone disk for bite force, (D) IOPI for isometric tongue pressure, and (E) Semmi Weinstein monofilaments for touch sensations (Reproduced with permission from Elsevier) (Laguna et al., 2015a).

open big jars, a lateral pick is needed for certain small lids, and a finger grip is required for peelable packaging. Winder et al. (2002) noted that the difficulty in dealing with food package is one of the main barriers for elderly consumers in food consumption and is often a cause of packaging-related accidents, especially when inappropriate tools are used in the opening process (Lewis et al., 2007). Opening peelable induction seal on bottles and glass jars commonly present problems for elderly people, particularly for those who have hand disorders (Duizer et al., 2009). Dittrich and Spanner-Ulmer (2010) found that the main problems were the high forces required to open the packages, tearable openings being too small, and the opening mechanisms being too hard to see.

During the course of the Optimizing Food for the Elderly (OPTIFEL) Project (a European Union FP7 project), European older adults (65 and older) were put into three different categories based on their feeding dependency (Laguna et al., 2016a): (1) living at home and needing help for food purchasing, (2) living at home and needing help for meal preparation or having food delivered, and (3) living in a nursing home or sheltered accommodation and requiring full-time care. Participants were asked about package-related difficulties, and a significantly high percentage of elderly reported experiencing problems, especially when trying to open screw caps. Those elderly who suffered arthritis have great difficulties in opening jars and bottles (Wylie et al., 1999); those who suffer strokes typically have trouble manipulating food on the plate and transporting it to the mouth (Axelsson, 1988; Jacobsson et al., 1996, 2000; Westergren et al., 2001).

The action of grasping and lifting food objects from plate to the mouth is directed by a complex interplay between multiple sensorimotor systems to signal, analyze, and process the mechanical interactions and constraints between body and object (Nowak and Hermsdörfer, 2003). One class of forelimb movement is the reach to eat. In this movement, an individual takes the food up to the mouth (for eating) or to the nose (for smelling). When the hand reaches toward one's face, tactile and proprioceptive (the perception of body position and movements in three-dimensional space) information concerning the location of facial features provides enough sensory information to accurately shape the digits for food grasping. The time to perform an action from visualizing the food to carrying out the required action is longer in the elderly than in younger populations (Coats and Wann, 2011; Seidler-Dobrin and Stelmach, 1998).

To overcome problems of hand manipulation, a range of adaptive eating utensils have been developed. Examples include a nosey cup to avoid bending the neck in the case of dysphagia, cutlery for people with grasping problems, plate guards to avoid spillage for people with low vision, and a weighted mug for those with tremor problems. Even though these tools are helpful, they only deal with a part of the eating difficulties. For example, patients with Parkinson's disease have trembling hands and difficulty in coordinating cutlery on the plate and transporting food to the mouth (Andersson and Sidenvall, 2001), and individuals who suffer from skeletal muscle weakness (due to aging or pathology) have reported problems in handgrip precision and force (Kurillo et al., 2004).

HAND FORCE ASSESSMENTS

The ability to manipulate food packaging and food by hand involves two dimensions: (1) adequate force to perform the movement (e.g., to lift a glass) and (2) a degree of coordination to execute the movement. These two dimensions are related and influence each other. For example, to open a so-called easy-to-open package, one has to have enough hand dexterity (or coordination) to initiate the peel force and then have enough force to tear the plastic apart. So, devices that cover these two dimensions—strength and coordination—will first be considered.

Hand Strength

A *hand dynamometer* is an easy-to-use device for measuring hand strength (Sasaki et al., 2007). The Jamar Grip Strength Dynamometer (Lafayette Instruments, Indiana, USA) is the standard device used by clinicians (American Society of Hand Therapist) (see Fig. 10.2A). For several reasons (validation technique, accessibility to the product, ease of carry, ease of test performance, reproducibility, and price), this device has been used for the hand-strength measurement in assessing EC (Laguna et al., 2015a; Laguna et al., in press b). Previous authors have reported that handgrip strength can be related to lower limb strength (Lauretani et al., 2003) and general muscle strength (Budziareck et al., 2008; Norman et al., 2011). However, elderly patients suffering from different health disorders such as cerebral stroke (Hermsdörfer et al., 2003), peripheral nerve damage (Nowak and Hermsdörfer, 2003) or hand osteoarthritis (de Oliveira et al., 2011) cannot perform grip movements adequately. Other authors such as Kurillo et al. (2004) developed tracking systems to evaluate grip force control with different end objects for different hand positions (nippers, pinch, spherical, lateral, and cylindrical grips). This device is more versatile and capable of providing different types of gripping forces that are used in daily activities. Moreover, this proposed device records the track over time, allowing better understanding of sensory-motor control. Unfortunately, this device has never been replicated or validated.

Finger Force

The B&L pinch gauge (B&L Engineering, California, USA) is a standardized protocol (American Society of Hand Therapists) used in rehabilitation assessment. The Flexisensor (Laguna et al., 2015a) (see Fig. 10.2B) has been used to measure the finger-gripping force with a modified version of the device designed by previous authors (Flanagan et al., 2012). The modified setup consists of a built-in thin flexible force transducer (Tekscan, South Boston, Massachusetts, USA) connected to a multimeter. Two self-adhesive neoprene disks of 1 cm diameter are attached to the sensor to make the assessment comfortable for participants. The multimeter connected to the flexisensor registers resistance in ohms (the larger the force, the lower the resistance). To convert the registered resistance data into force values, a calibration is needed. Forces of magnitude from 5 N to 250 N were applied by a probe attached to the Texture analyzer (Stable Micro Systems, Godalming, UK), and resistance at each applied force was recorded. A standard curve of the applied force (N) and registered resistance can be used to convert the assessment into finger-gripping force. In the study conducted by Laguna et al. (2015a), elderly subjects were asked to squeeze the neoprene adhesive with their thumb and index finger, and the minimum resistance was recorded. Authors found that the finger-gripping assessment had the highest variability among subjects, as this precision assessment picks up even minor variability in subjects suffering from trauma (Palastanga et al., 2012).

Hand Coordination

Technical sensors. Hermsdorfer et al. (2003) developed a method for dynamically holding and transporting different spherical objects to analyze impairments of manipulative grip control in patients with chronic cerebral stroke. Values obtained from such assessments can give an effective indication of the strength and coordination of the hand (as well as finger) muscles and therefore the capability of food handling.

Timing and videorecording actions. Moving different objects at a measured distance depends on bimanual or unimanual movements (Coats and Wann, 2011, 2012). Thus, there is the possibility of using a standardized kit for manual dexterity (Mathiowetz et al., 1985b). This is a performance-based test of unilateral gross manual dexterity. Individuals move as many blocks as they can one at a time from one compartment of a box to another of equal size in 60 s. This kit provides a baseline for motor coordination. The test is quick and simple to administer and suitable for persons with limited motor coordination.

Oral-Processing Capability

Older individuals have altered appetites and slower metabolic absorption of key nutrients, which can affect their nutritional status. This can be worsened by their inability to chew and swallow food (Walls and Steele, 2004) effectively and efficiently. For that, an adequate assessment of oral capability is needed. *Oral capability* is defined as the ability to transform nonswallowable food into a swallowable bolus and to transport it safely from the oral cavity into the stomach. It includes every oral action from the first bite up to swallowing (details are shown in Fig. 10.3). Very often, these oral actions are grouped into two sequential categories: (1) mastication capability and (2) swallowing capability. To perform these two actions, different structures work in a highly coordinated manner under the direction of the CNS: orofacial muscles, lips, cheeks, teeth, tongue, and palate (Koshino et al., 1997).

ACTIONS IN THE ORAL CAVITY: MASTICATION AND SWALLOWING

Mastication

Mastication starts with the first bite of solid or semisolid food and is conducted by the forcible occlusion of the opposing edges of the upper and lower incisors (Okada et al., 2007). Then a succession of chewing cycles occurs (Woda et al., 2006) with the help of saliva or liquid released from the food to form a cohesive bolus (Jalabert-Malbos et al., 2007). The main components of the mastication process and swallowing are shown in Fig. 10.3.

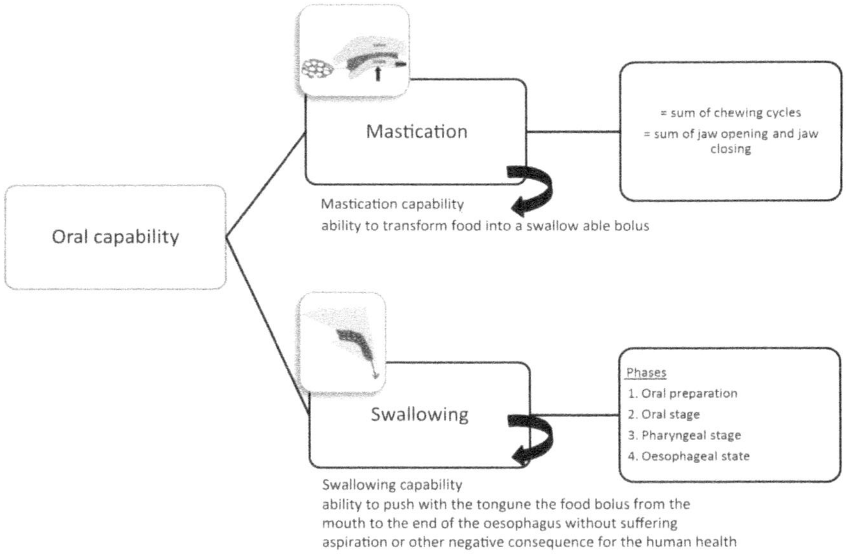

FIGURE 10.3 Schematic illustration of the oral capability.

Mastication takes place inside the oral cavity and has a close interaction with the sensory-motor system, including teeth, orofacial muscles, jaw muscles, labial muscles, the tongue, and the production of salivary secretions. All of these components work in a highly coordinated manner and under close control by the upper CNS, which generates efficient masticatory movements (Koshino et al., 1997). Because of the involvement of different parts, each must function properly. If one part is missing or is dysfunctional, the mastication capability will be diminished. In the elderly, different causes can impair mastication, including the loss of teeth, inadequate secretion of saliva, tongue problems, and loss of muscle mass with consequent decreases in biting force. Also, the pattern and rhythm of mastication is altered with age. For instance, the number of chew cycles increases progressively with age (Feldman et al., 1980; Peyron et al., 2004) to compensate for changes in food hardness, and the time needed for a chewing cycle decreases (Peyron et al., 2004).

The Influence of Dentition in the Mastication Process

The masticatory capability includes the execution of the first bite and the ability to use the teeth to grind or pulverize a chewable food into smaller particles (de Liz Pocztaruk et al., 2011; Hatch et al., 2001). During the first bite, the pressure exertion on teeth causes slight stretching to the periodontal ligaments and thus information is sent to the CNS for texture interpretation. The periodontal ligaments are able to detect extremely small forces (1 N or lower) (Lucas et al., 2004). Masticatory efficiency decreases for subjects who have missing teeth (Fontijn-Tekamp et al., 2000; Miyaura et al., 2000). The contacting area between upper and lower teeth is highly important for food oral breakdown, and fewer teeth means the biting force decreases (Laguna et al., 2015a). Replacing missing teeth with dentures can improve mastication but cannot always fully recover the efficiency of natural teeth (N'Gom and Woda, 2002). People who have lost postcanine teeth and replaced them with removable dentures (Fontijn-Tekamp et al., 2000; Kapur and Soman, 2006; Pocztaruk et al., 2008) have a much reduced masticatory function. Because of this reason, elderly people who usually suffer from tooth loss often have partially depleted mastication capability. Generally speaking, elderly patients with incomplete dentition (which is common in old age) swallow relatively larger food particles even though they may try to compensate for teeth loss by chewing longer (Woda et al., 2006). Bates et al. (1976) observed that loose dentures can even move during eating. In such cases, the tongue has to be used to stabilize and hold dentures within the mouth. This means that there is not only decreased efficiency for food oral breakdown but also the tongue must help position food while trying to retain the dentures. The dentition status can also influence an individual's food choice. When dentition is low (i.e., a patient wears complete dentures), the intake of difficult-to-chew food items (e.g., roots, vegetables, fruits, and meat) becomes less pleasing. It is also possible that they avoid difficult-to-chew foods such as stringy foods like beef, crunchy foods like carrots, and dry foods like crusty bread (Hildebrandt et al., 1997). However, sometimes the desire to eat certain food products overshadows the lack of teeth (Laguna et al., 2015a).

TABLE 10.1 Summary of Problems for Denture Wearers in Comparison With Natural Teeth Bearers

• Less masticatory efficiency
• Difficulty in swallowing large particles and consequent difficulties in digestion
• Diminished food choices leading to less intake of certain vitamins such as A and C and carotenes because fewer fruits and vegetables are consumed
• Extensive food preparation that can lower nutritional quality (e.g., peeling fruit and overcooking vegetables)

When it comes to food preparation, those elderly patients with reduced masticatory efficiency often require extra work to prepare their food. For example, some fruits and vegetables must have their skin removed, and some foods must be overcooked to facilitate mastication (Walls and Steele, 2004). Table 10.1 summarizes the main problems denture wearers suffer in comparison with those who still have their natural teeth.

Mastication and Dentition Assessment

The Bite Force

To measure biting force, different instruments have been used. Their positioning inside the mouth is critical for reliable measurements because different forces can be executed with different teeth and the area of contact is also different. With more teeth involved in the measurement, the assessment of the oral action could be more relevant to reality, even though dental studies commonly assess a single tooth or single tooth position to determine the efficiency of oral tooth implants (Flanagan et al., 2012). Up to now, various types of sensors for biting force quantification have been used. Tortopidis et al. (1998) used three different patterns of stainless steel force transducers to measure the biting force. These transducers used a similar model described earlier by Lyons and Baxendale (1990) in which two stainless steel beams with two strain gauges attached to each side of the beams are used with flexible epoxy resin and wire to form a Wheatstone bridge circuit. Probably the simplest one of these experimental setups is the one with only a single sensor connected to a multimeter (Fernandes et al., 2003; Flanagan et al., 2012; Laguna et al., 2015a; Laguna, 2016c,d; Singh et al., 2011) as shown in Fig. 10.2C. Because the flexisensor is available at an affordable price and reproducible, it has been used most frequently for EC assessments.

The Dental Status

The number of teeth is another important factor. As already noted, fewer teeth results in a decreased bite force. To assess the dental status, researcher can observe and count the number of teeth or directly ask the elderly person if he or she has natural teeth, crowns, is edentulous, is wearing dentures, or a combination of these. Assessment of the impact of tooth loss is available in the Geriatric Oral Health Assessment Index (El Osta et al., 2014), a questionnaire regarding the functional dimension—pain and discomfort—and the psychosocial dimension. This has been used to evaluate problems related to food ingestion.

The Grind-Mastication Capability

Characterization of masticatory capability can be carried out by using a standard (or representative) food material and measuring particle size reduction during mastication to indicate grinding capability. Peanuts, almonds, cocoa, carrots, jelly, hazelnuts, decaffeinated coffee beans, and nuts are the most frequently used food materials for assessing mastication (Gambareli et al., 2007; Schneider and Senger, 2002).

The preferred choices, however, are silicone-based artificial food materials (Pocztaruk et al., 2008). Various artificial test foods have been reported in literature—e.g., OptosilR, Optocal PlusR, and CutterSilR (Fontijn-Tekamp, 2004). The advantages of these materials are that they are inert to water and saliva (they are neither soluble nor enzyme responsive); are of homogeneous size, shape, and toughness; have no seasonal variation; and can be stored easily (Fontijn-Tekamp et al., 2004). Compared to food, artificial gels are much more stable and show little fluctuation in their physical and chemical properties. However, one big limitation is that these gels are not digestible and must not be swallowed (Pocztaruk et al., 2008). Other materials such as chewing gums, gelatin gels, paraffin wax, and a mixture of calcium carbonate have also been used as test foods (Ahmad, 2006).

To study the degree of food fragmentation different methods are often used, such as sieving, colorimetric determination, light scattering, and various image-analysis tools. All these methodologies will require mouth contents to be expectorated (or spitted) before swallowing. A potential problem is that saliva and particles can be swallowed accidentally during chewing. Yamashita et al. (2013) found that during the preparatory phase of swallowing, part of the oral bolus may pass to the pharynx before spontaneous swallowing is initiated. Because of this, caution must be taken when using these methods to assess real food boluses. In contrast to the food breakup method, van der Bilt (2010) developed a method to determine masticatory capability by assessing the mixing and kneading of food inside the mouth. Two chewing gums with different colors were placed in the mouth and chewed. The extent of color mixing was then measured as a function of chewing cycles, and the masticatory efficiency of the individual was assessed.

Recently, to incorporate the mastication assessment in EC assessments, participants were videorecorded (Laguna et al., 2016b). In those videos, participants were asked to eat normally texture-characterized products. By analyzing individual video frames, one can reveal the number of chews and oral-processing time. Other oral-processing aspects, such as expressions of difficulty, could also be taken into account. This technique was reliable for assessing number of chews and time needed to perform the eating process.

Mastication and the Role of Saliva

Saliva is a biological fluid naturally secreted from inside the human mouth. During eating, saliva helps in three processes: chewing, tasting perception, and swallowing. During chewing, saliva helps to form a coherent and smooth bolus by mixing and aggregating food particles (Sarkar et al., 2009). It also contributes to the sensory perception by functioning as a reservoir of food ingredients for a continuous flavor release (Doyennette et al., 2011). In the swallowing process, the mucins present in saliva create a slippery effect so that food bolus can easily slide through the esophagus (Pedersen et al., 2002), which is critically important for safe swallowing (Engelen et al., 2005).

With age, salivary glands can become disturbed and cause a decrease in saliva secretion (Samnieng, 2015). In addition, many pathological conditions linked with old age influence salivary secretion, especially medications that cause diminished salivary secretion. Head and neck irradiation and systemic conditions such as Sjögren's syndrome and type 2 diabetes also can affect saliva production (Anurag Gupta et al., 2006). Elderly patients with xerostomia (i.e., mouth dryness) (Walls and Steele, 2004) not only will have problems of chewing food and swallowing but also problems of tasting and speaking as well as being intolerant of dentures (Narhi et al., 1992).

Salivation Assessment

Saliva quantification is not generally measured in relation to nutrition status but is commonly studied in relation to drug metabolism by different collective methods that can be classified as nonstimulated and stimulated secretion. The latter involves chewing an inert material such as paraffin or being exposed to gustatory stimulation. In both cases, saliva is collected in a container for its biochemical characterization (Crouch, 2005; Topkas et al., 2012). For quantification purposes, Navazesh and Christensen (1982) used four different methods: draining, spitting, suction, and swabbing. Authors concluded that the flow rate did not differ significantly, although the swab technique was the least reproducible method.

Mastication and the Role of the Tongue

The tongue is a mass of mobile muscle tissue inside the oral cavity. Its proper functioning is crucial for both eating and speaking. During oral food processing, the tongue acts as a mechanical device to manipulate and transport the food (Heath, 2002) and the dominant source of energy for initiating bolus flow (Alsanei and Chen, 2014). Chemoreceptors and mechanoreceptors on tongue surface act as the most delicate sensation systems capable of detecting and discriminating the taste and textural properties of food (Hiiemae and Palmer, 1999). The tongue (Hiiemae and Palmer, 1999) also helps to move food distally through the oral cavity, from the anterior to the pharynx (Pereira, 2012). Any dysfunction of the tongue (i.e., lack of coordination or motor disorder) will make eating and swallowing difficult (Ueda et al., 2004). One of the commonly known adverse effects of tongue dysfunction is pneumonia after food aspiration (Steele and Cichero, 2014). Tongue fatigue contributes to an incomplete food clearance, longer time to finish a meal, reduced food intake, and difficulty swallowing. For a young and healthy individual, this effect is not significant, but diminished tongue strength for the elderly often shows a significant decrease after meal consumption (Kays et al., 2010).

TONGUE CAPABILITY ASSESSMENT

The available techniques to study tongue capability can be divided into those that measure the strength of the tongue against the palate and those that record images of tongue movement during oral processing and swallowing. In tongue – palate contact measurements, an indication of the contraction strength of tongue muscles is obtained.

Devices for such assessments normally consist of two parts: a sensor inserted between tongue and palate and a register for data recording using the Iowa Oral Performance Instrument (IOPI), the Handy Probe System, or a multisensory system. Their sensors are the difference between them. IOPI uses a mobile plastic bulb (Ono et al., 2009) (see Fig. 10.2D) just like the Handy Probe System; both, however, are generally uncomfortable due to the presence of a sizable sensor inside the oral cavity. Incorrect bulb placement inside the mouth can cause errors (Butler et al., 2011). Multiple sensing probes are also used where three (or even more) air-filled bulbs are arranged in a sequence. When the tongue presses the hard palate, pressures at different locations can be determined and lead to a tongue-pressure profile rather than the pressure at a single point. However, the main disadvantage of such devices is their inevitable interference with normal tongue movement.

The palatal plate with multisensors consists of a plastic palate with sensors inserted where tongue pressure during both swallowing and mastication can be recorded. However, real applications of palatal plates can be difficult because the prostheses require advanced techniques and are expensive to manufacture. Furthermore, subjects often find them highly uncomfortable and usually need considerable amount of time to get used to the plates. Similar to a palatal plate is a sensor sheet consisting of five measuring points attached directly to the palatal mucosa with a sheet denture adhesive (Hori et al., 2009). The last two multisensors not only can measure the tongue pressing strength but also evaluate the tongue movement during mastication and the initiation of swallowing.

For the study of tongue movement during oral processing and swallowing, imaging techniques such as ultrasound, videofluorography and fiberoptic endoscopy are also available (Hori et al., 2009; Langmore, 2003; Palmer et al., 2000; Yamashita et al., 2013). Although they are useful for studying swallowing and provide a good understanding of the tongue behavior during the entire eating process, these techniques require clinical training, which makes them less accessible for research scientists and community applications. Moreover, they are qualitative techniques, and the time required to complete the test and image analysis is higher than the tongue – palate contact tests. For this reason, IOPI or a Handy Probe could be better choices for quick and reproducible tongue-strength assessments. The sheet sensor developed by Hori et al. (2009) allows accurate assessment of pressure at different points without dramatically interfering with mastication and swallowing. The great advantage of this technique in comparison with multiple sensing and palate sensors is that the superthin sensor sheet can be flexibly adapted to the hard palate without causing too much discomfort to the subject.

The IOPI device shows a decrement of tongue pressure with increases in age (see Fig. 10.4) (Alsanei and Chen, 2014). In the EC assessments carried out in 200 elderly subjects in the United Kingdom and Spain, a similar trend (age–tongue pressure) was found (Laguna et al., 2015a; Laguna et al., 2016b,c,d). The IOPI was chosen as a technique to measure tongue strength in elderly because it is easily available, reproducible, and allows comparison of new results with previously reported results in the literature using the same device in elderly groups.

Bolus Swallowing

Bolus swallowing is a transporting process that moves food from the oral cavity to the stomach via the oral–pharyngeal–esophageal tract. The whole process takes just a few seconds from initiation to completion (Dodds, 1989). A swift switch between breathing and swallowing is vital (Matsuo and Palmer, 2008) and achieved by physical

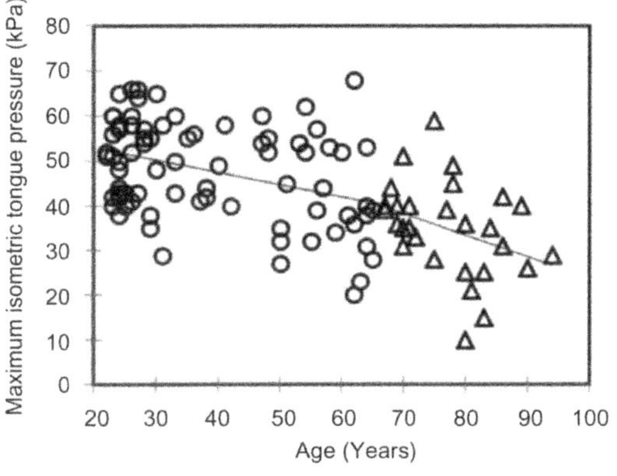

FIGURE 10.4 Maximum tongue pressure and age relation (Reproduced with permission from Wiley) (Alsanei and Chen, 2014).

closure of the airway by elevation of the soft palate (to seal off the nasal cavity) and titling the epiglottis (to seal off the larynx) along with neural suppression of respiration in the brainstem (Nishino and Hiraga, 1991).

A swallowing process is traditionally divided into four stages: (1) oral preparation, (2) the oral propulsive state, (3) the pharyngeal state, and (4) the esophageal state (Logemann, 2007). Disorders affecting the oral preparatory and oral propulsive forces usually result from impaired control of the tongue (Dodds, 1989) or dental problems (Palmer et al., 2000), while disorders in the pharyngeal and esophageal states is usually dictated by abnormality in the motor sequence or obstruction (caused, e.g., by tumors).

Dysphagia is the term often used to refer to swallowing disorders (Hori et al., 2009) in any of the previously described stages. Particularly in elderly population, dysphagia can lead to malnutrition and increase the risk of aspiration and pneumonia, leading to morbidity and mortality (Kaiser et al., 2010; Kikawada et al., 2005). The exact effect of aging on oropharyngeal swallowing is not yet fully understood and will require collaborative efforts from oral physiologists, food scientists, and clinical researchers (Logemann, 2007). The major risks of inappropriate bolus swallowing are aspiration and choking. The former is caused by accidental entering of food residues into the larynx pipe; serious coughing and even infection can follow if oral bacteria enter the larynx. The latter is caused when large food particles block the airway and could lead to fatal consequences such as suffocation. Nonoral feeding may be implemented when the patient cannot achieve adequate nutrition or hydration or if there is risk or aspiration (Leonard et al., 2014). Based on the preceding discussion, we could use the term *swallowing capability* to represent how an individual is capable of transporting the food bolus from the mouth to enter the stomach through the whole oral–pharyngeal–esophagus tract without causing aspiration or some other negative consequence to human health.

SWALLOWING CAPABILITY ASSESSMENT

An objective assessment of swallowing process is not an easy task. The most common diagnosis is the swallowing evaluation in which subjects are asked to swallow a quantity of water and are then assessed for possible coughing or gurgling vocal sounds (Macht et al., 2014). However, this methodology has been criticized for its poor standardization and poor accuracy (McCullough et al., 2001). There are other sets of imaging techniques that can be used to clinically diagnose swallowing disorders such as videofluorography and fiberoptic endoscopy. In a videofluoroscope examination, a food with a certain fluid consistency is mixed with radioactive barium and fed to the patient who sits upright (Langmore, 2003; Palmer et al., 2000). Radiography images are recorded when a subject swallows barium-marked boluses of different consistencies; examiners are then able to determine how capable the patient is in dealing with a bolus (Palmer et al., 2000). Also, with videofluorography recording, the anatomical structure and motion of a food bolus can be monitored (Palmer et al., 2000). The main disadvantage of this technique is that patients are exposed to radiation and an endoscopic view of anatomical abnormalities is not possible.

In a fiber-optic endoscopic evaluation of swallowing, a flexible transnasal laryngoscope is inserted deep into the oropharyngeal region and then used to evaluate the path of bolus entry and coordination during a normal meal (Dua et al., 1997). The advantage of transnasal endoscopy is that it shows real-time swallowing with no oral invasion and therefore no influence on tongue movement. However, the nasal lidocaine that is applied to decrease discomfort during examination can affect the swallowing function (Macht et al., 2014). Despite the advantages of both techniques, their use is largely restricted to clinicians due to the required clinical expertise to use these techniques and therefore is not easily accessible to food scientists or community workers. Koshino et al. (1997) reported the use of ultrasound diagnostic equipment to study bolus movement, the onset and offset of bolus flow, and bolus moving speed. One great advantage of ultrasound assessment is that it is noninvasive. The attachment of ultrasound probes around the neck does not cause any noticeable impediment to bolus movement and actions of the tongue and other swallowing muscles. However, this technique gives qualitative information and frame-by-frame image analysis; unfortunately, the technique is highly time consuming and requires lots of images to be processed to provide statistical relevance.

For EC assessment, the IOPI has been used to measure tongue muscle strength, which is based on the fact that tongue pressing generates the first pushing force in creating bolus flow. However, it must be noted that tongue muscle strength assessment only gives information on oral propulsive capability. It does not provide information about possible abnormalities that occur in the pharyngeal and esophageal areas.

Sensing Capability

Sensing capability is the ability of an individual to evaluate and perceive sensory stimuli of a food through the five human senses (sight, smell, taste, touch, and hearing). The aging process is accompanied by a decreased efficiency

TABLE 10.2 Effects of Sensory Impairment

Sense	Depleted Sensory Effect
Sight	Affects food appetite and intake (by affecting the senses of taste and odor) Difficulty in shopping, food preparation, and cutlery management
Smell	Interferes with hedonic evaluation Less food enjoyment
Taste	Alterations can aggravate anorexic states and contribute to malnutrition Affects food choice: lower preferences for citrus fruits and higher intakes of sweets and fat Less food enjoyment
Touch	Alters perception of pleasantness Alters quality perception in food products (e.g., deterioration of products such as softening due to enzyme activity)
Hearing	Texture appreciation

in sensory perception and aggravated by pathological conditions such as stroke and pathological treatments such as chemotherapy for cancer treatment. The sensing perceptions losses and distortions decrease the perception of a food's hedonic qualities, which decreases the overall enjoyment of eating and thus appetite and overall food intake. Some well-recognized effects of sense impairment on eating process are summarized in Table 10.2.

The consequences of sense impairment lead to decreased food sensory appreciation. Elderly persons with impaired taste sensation typically have decreased food consumption (Stanga, 2009), which contributes to the anorexia of aging. One easy solution is to add flavor enhancers to food (Schiffman and Warwick, 1993). This may help reduce one of the most common complaints by nursing home residents regarding food quality (Stanga, 2009).

ASSESSING SENSING CAPABILITY

To quantitatively assess an individual's sensing capabilities, threshold detection has been found to be most practical. A person's sensing capability can be assessed by three different thresholds (Meilgaard et al., 2006): the absolute or detection threshold, the recognition or identification threshold, and the difference threshold. The absolute or the detection threshold is the lowest intensity of a physical stimulus that is perceivable by human sense of smell, taste, or touch. The recognition or identification threshold is the level at which a stimulus not only can be detected but also recognized or identified. The difference threshold represents the smallest change in stimulation that a person can detect.

Despite their different natures, threshold values can be identified using similar approaches: an incrementing battery of intensities with a forced response of perception. For example, in hearing, the absolute threshold refers to the smallest level of a tone that can be detected by normal hearing when no other interfering sound is present; and in vision, the absolute threshold refers to the lowest level of light that a participant can detect. In relation to food, sensory thresholds to taste and odor are widely used. Various validated methods have been proposed by some organizations such as the American Society for Testing and Materials.

THE EATING CAPABILITY CONCEPT IN USE

In the frame of the OPTIFEL project, several studies have been attempted using the EC concept in both young and elderly populations. With elderly populations, the main objective was to correlate food consistencies (or structure complexity) with individual's EC score (Fig. 10.5). Our hypothesis was that the frailest elderly (with low EC) will find high-consistency or structurally complicated food difficult to eat, while those among EC group will be able to consume food of a wide range of consistencies or complexities. Elderly populations can therefore be grouped into clusters based on their objectively measured eating capabilities. Such clusters can be grouped based on the sum of the different capabilities: hand, oral, swallowing, sensing, and mental.

The EC model is in its early stages and the focus has been on hand, oral, and swallowing capacities. Only non-invasive, reproducible, reliable, and quick assessments have been used.

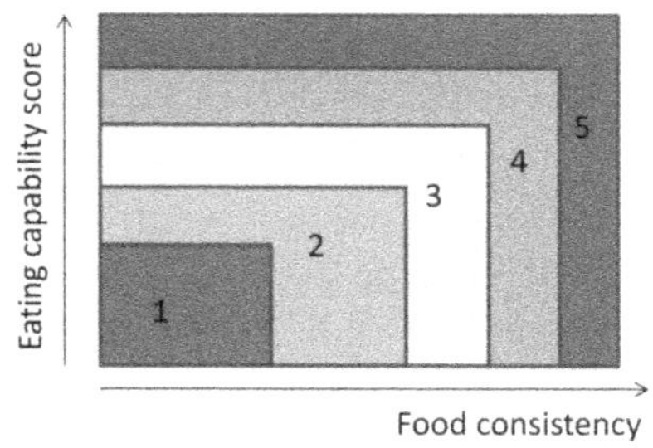

FIGURE 10.5 Hypothesis of a correlation between the eating capability and food consistency (or structural complexity of the food) which is safe to consume by elderly.

First Approach of Eating Capability Assessment

In the first stage (Laguna et al., 2015a,b), overall EC was measured using three key components—hand and oral capabilities and tactile sensitivity—among 203 elderly subjects living in the United Kingdom ($n = 103$ in seven community centers and two sheltered accommodations) and Spain ($n = 100$ in three nursing homes and one community center). Handgripping force was measured with an adjustable handheld dynamometer (JAMAR Dynamometer, Patterson Medical Ltd., Nottinghamshire, UK). Participants were asked to squeeze the hand dynamometer with one hand using maximum effort and maintain that grip for approximately three seconds; the grip on the other hand is then measured (Trampisch et al., 2012). The intensity of handgripping was displayed as the maximum force in the digital panel. Handgripping force was further studied to know if it can be used as a predictor of oral forces (Laguna et al., 2015a).

Finger-gripping force was measured with a modified version of the device designed by previous authors (Flanagan et al., 2012). The chosen technique for touching sensitivity was the Semmes-Weinstein monofilament test (North Coast Medical, Inc., Gilroy, California, USA) (Wiggermann et al., 2012) as shown in Fig. 10.2E. A Touch Sense monofilament was pressed in a perpendicular direction against the skin surface until the filament was bowed—approximately 1.5 s—and then removed. Tests began with the strongest monofilament, which applied a force of 300 g and continued in descending order down to the weakest filament with only 0.008 g force. Subjects were asked to give a signal when they sensed a touch. If no signal was given after filament pressing, this was taken as a failure to detect the touch by the subject. The value of the last monofilament that was detected by the participant was recorded as the touching threshold, which is taken as an indication of tactile sensitivity. Results of those participants who were unable to feel the monofilament of 300 g were eliminated.

For oral capability, denture status was asked and maximum biting force was measured. Participants were asked about their dentures and were classified into six different dental statuses: natural teeth, combination (natural with some crowns and bridges), full dentures, no teeth, just a few natural teeth, and bottom or top denture. For the maximum biting force, the designed device used in the previous study (Flanagan et al., 2012) was used for maximum biting force assessment. Two adhesive silicone disks (1.5 cm diameter, 0.3 cm thickness) were used to sandwich the force sensor. Participants were asked to bite the flexisensor with the incisors and hold the bite for a couple of seconds. The minimum resistance shown by the multimeter was recorded. As a hygienic measure, a new plastic film protector was used for each participant.

Tongue pressure was measured using the IOPI (Medical LLC, Redmond, Washington, USA) (Fig. 10.1E), which recorded tongue-palate pressure (Ono et al., 2009). Participants were asked to place the bulb in the center of the oral cavity between the tongue and the hard palate and press down with their tongues as hard as they could. The maximum pressure was recorded in kPa. Lip-sealing pressure was also measured using the IOPI. Participants were asked to place the bulb between their lips and then to press their lips as hard as they could. The maximum pressure was also recorded in kPa.

As shown in Fig. 10.6, a strong correlation was established between handgripping force and oral forces (tongue pressure, lip pressure, handgripping force, and biting force). The results suggested that the positive correlation between hand and orofacial muscle strengths in the elderly might lead to the possible use of noninvasive methods (hand force) to assess EC. However, this correlation might not be useful for participants who suffer from motor-illness pathologies.

All of the measured parameters (handgripping force, finger-gripping force, biting force, lip-sealing pressure, and tongue pressure) were normalized and converted to a score between 1 and 5, with 1 being the weakest. The collated

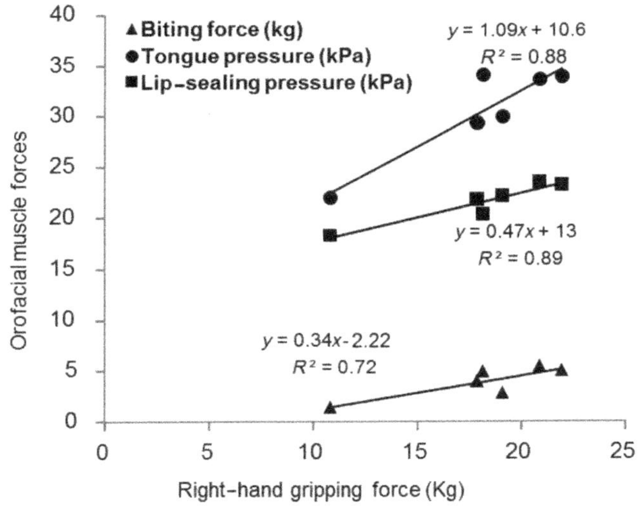

FIGURE 10.6 Relation of right handgripping force with orofacial muscle forces (biting force, maximum tongue pressure, and lip-sealing pressure) in UK elderly participants.

and aggregated measure of *EC* was then used to characterize participants from weakest to strongest in four groups. To test the functional utility of this classification, participants were shown with a series of food pictures and were asked to rate how difficult it was to manage that particular food by hand (manipulating cutlery by performing tasks such as cutting or picking up food) and by mouth (oral processing through chewing, biting, and swallowing). As a conclusion, participants from the lower EC groups perceived fibrous and hard food products as significantly more difficult to consume than did participants with higher EC scores. However, the concept needed to be validated by examining real oral food processing with elderly patients—i.e., by measuring chewing cycles, bolus-swallowing time, and characterization of bolus as a function of EC score.

In a later study (Laguna et al., 2016a,b) food stimuli were given to elderly patients to observe their eating process. The food stimuli consisted of both food products of different textures and flavorless hydrocolloid gels (to avoid psychological and social bias) with different levels of structural heterogeneity. Finger-grip force and touch sensitivity were excluded from EC assessment due to the difficulty perceived by elderly subjects and the relatively low relevance of these assessments to EC assessment. A tool more relevant in terms of grasping and moving objects during the eating process was introduced, and manual dexterity was measured by a standardized kit.

The EC score was quantified this time, using the following equation:

$$EC = \frac{\left(\frac{RH_{Par}}{RH_{Str\ Par}}\right) + \left(\frac{LH_{Par}}{LH_{Str\ Par}}\right)}{2} + \left(\frac{BF_{Par}}{BF_{Str\ Par}}\right) + \left(\frac{TP_{Par}}{TP_{Str\ Par}}\right) + \frac{\left(\frac{RD}{RD_{Str\ Par}}\right) + \left(\frac{LD_{Par}}{LD_{Str\ Par}}\right)}{2}$$

where *RH* is the right handgripping force (kg), *LH* is the left handgripping force (kg), *BF* is the biting force (kg), *TP* is the tongue pressure (KPa), *RD* is the right-hand dexterity count, and *LD* is the left-hand dexterity count (using the manual dexterity kit). Subscripts $_{Par}$ and $_{Str\ Par}$ represent the individual and strongest individual scoring the highest in that particular test, respectively.

The maximum EC score was four points, with each test assessment contributing a maximum of one point. To calculate the value of each force for every individual, a fraction was generated. The denominator was the maximum value obtained for the test by the strongest participant, and the numerator was populated with values for the participant under study. Participants with EC of less than 2 were placed in cluster one (the weakest group); participants with EC between 2 and 3 were placed in cluster two, and participants with eating capabilities of more than 3 were placed in cluster three.

The key conclusion was that bite force differed by EC group, and was significantly different by dental status and influenced both liking, number of chews, and difficulty perceived. Other EC parameters had little influence on the oral processing of real food and gels.

CONCLUSIONS

With ageing, elderly's food and energy intake tend to decrease due to diminished capability for eating, which results in compromised nutritional status for most elderly individuals and an increased incidence of morbidities. These vulnerable consumers may have different problems in food handling, oral manipulation, sensing, and perception as well as swallowing. The causes of these problems are physiological or pathological. One top priority for the food industry and caregiving industry is to provide foods that are safe to consume by these consumers. Objectively measuring an individual's EC may help to correctly assess his or her abilities of food handling, food oral manipulation, sensation, and cognition. This chapter covers different objective assessments of physical and oral capabilities and how such capabilities can be integrated into a unique EC score. Such scoring might help food designers develop foods with textures that are just right for elderly consumers.

References

Ahmad, S., 2006. An insight into the masticatory performance of complete denture wearer. Ann. Dent. 13, 24–33.

Alsanei, W.A., Chen, J., 2014. Studies of the oral capabilities in relation to bolus manipulations and the ease of initiating bolus flow. J. Texture Stud. 45, 1–12.

Andersson, I., Sidenvall, B., 2001. Case studies of food shopping, cooking and eating habits in older women with Parkinson's disease. J. Adv. Nurs. 35, 69–78.

Anurag Gupta, B., Epstein, J.B., Sroussi, H., 2006. Hyposalivation in elderly patients. J. Can. Dent. Assoc. 72, 841–846.

Axelsson, K., 1988. Eating problems and nutritional status after stroke. Umea University Medical Dissertation. New series No 218. Umea, Sweden.

Bates, J., Stafford, G., Harrison, A., 1976. Masticatory function—a review of the literature. J. Oral Rehabil. 3, 57–67.

Budziareck, M.B., Pureza Duarte, R.R., Barbosa-Silva, M.C.G., 2008. Reference values and determinants for handgrip strength in healthy subjects. Clin. Nutr. 27, 357–362.

Butler, S.G., Stuart, A., Leng, X., Wilhelm, E., Rees, C., Williamson, J., et al., 2011. The relationship of aspiration status with tongue and handgrip strength in healthy older adults. J. Gerontol. Series A Biol. Sci. Med. Sci. 66A, 452–458.

Carmeli, E., Patish, H., Coleman, R., 2003. The aging hand. J. Gerontol. Series A Biol. Sci. Med. Sci. 58, M146–M152.

Coats, R.O., Wann, J.P., 2011. The reliance on visual feedback control by older adults is highlighted in tasks requiring precise endpoint placement and precision grip. Experime. Brain Res. 214, 139–150.

Coats, R.O., Wann, J.P., 2012. Reaching a better understanding of the control of bimanual movements in older adults. PloS one. 7, 10. e47222.

Crouch, D.J., 2005. Oral fluid collection: the neglected variable in oral fluid testing. Foren. Sci. Inter. 150, 165–173.

de Liz Pocztaruk, R., Abbink, J.H., de Wijk, R.A., da Fontoura Frasca, L.C., Gavião, M.B.D., van der Bilt, A., 2011. The influence of auditory and visual information on the perception of crispy food. Food Qual. Pref. 22, 404–411.

de Oliveira, D.G., Nunes, P.M., Aruin, A.S., dos Santos, M.J., 2011. Grip force control in individuals with hand osteoarthritis. J. Hand Ther. 24, 345–355.

Dittrich, F., Spanner-Ulmer, B., 2010. Easy opening. DLG-lebensmittel 5, 32–36.

Dittus, K.L., Hillers, V.N., Beerman, K.A., 1995. Benefits and barriers to fruit and vegetable intake: relationship between attitudes and consumption. J. Nutr. Educ. 27, 120–126.

Dodds, W.J., 1989. The physiology of swallowing. Dysphagia 3, 171–178.

Doyennette, M., Deleris, I., Saint-Eve, A., Gasiglia, A., Souchon, I., Trelea, I., 2011. The dynamics of aroma compound transfer properties in cheeses during simulated eating conditions. Food Res. Inter. 44, 3174–3181.

Dua, K.S., Ren, J., Bardan, E., Xie, P., Shaker, R., 1997. Coordination of deglutitive glottal function and pharyngeal bolus transit during normal eating. Gastroenterology 112, 73–83.

Duizer, L., Robertson, T., Han, J., 2009. Requirements for packaging from an ageing consumer's perspective. Packaging Technol. Sci. 22, 187–197.

El Osta, N., Hennequin, M., Tubert-Jeannin, S., Naaman, N.B.A., El Osta, L., Geahchan, N., 2014. The pertinence of oral health indicators in nutritional studies in the elderly. Clin. Nutr. 33, 316–321.

Engelen, L., Fontijn-Tekamp, A., Bilt Avd, 2005. The influence of product and oral characteristics on swallowing. Arch. Oral Biol. 50, 739–746.

Feldman, R.S., Kapur, K.K., Alman, J.E., Chauncey, H.H., 1980. Aging and mastication: changes in performance and in the swallowing threshold with natural dentition†. J. Am. Geriatr. Soc. 28, 97–103.

Fernandes, C.P., Glantz, P.-O.J., Svensson, S.A., Bergmark, A., 2003. A novel sensor for bite force determinations. Dental Mater. 19, 118–126.

Flanagan, D., Ilies, H., O'brien, B., McManus, A., Larrow, B., 2012. Jaw bite force measurement device. J. Oral Implantol. 38, 361–364.

Fontijn-Tekamp, F., Slagter, A., Van Der Bilt, A., Hof, M.V.T., Witter, D., Kalk, W., et al., 2000. Biting and chewing in overdentures, full dentures, and natural dentitions. J. Dental Res. 79, 1519–1524.

Fontijn-Tekamp, F., Van Der Bilt, A., Abbink, J., Bosman, F., 2004. Swallowing threshold and masticatory performance in dentate adults. Physiol. Behav. 83 (3), 431–436.

Gambareli, F.R., Serra, M.D., Pereira, L.J., Gavião, M.B.D., 2007. Influence of measurement technique, test food, teeth and muscle force interactions in the masticatory performance. J. Texture Studies 38 (1), 2–20.

Hatch, J., Shinkai, R., Sakai, S., Rugh, J., Paunovich, E., 2001. Determinants of masticatory performance in dentate adults. Arch. Oral Biol. 46, 641–648.

Heath, M.R., 2002. The oral management of food: the bases of oral success and for understanding the sensations that drive us to eat. Food Qual. Pref. 13, 453–461.

Heinö, R., Åström, A., Antvorskov, H., Mattsson, M., Østergaard, S., 2008. Easy Open Pack–Scientific background for the basis of an international standard for easy-to-open packages. Nordic Cooperation Project (NICe).

Hermsdörfer, J., Hagl, E., Nowak, D.A., Marquardt, C., 2003. Grip force control during object manipulation in cerebral stroke. Clin. Neurophysiol. 114, 915–929.

Hiiemae, K.M., Palmer, J., 1999. Food transport and bolus formation during complete feeding sequences on foods of different initial consistency. Dysphagia 14, 31–42.

Hildebrandt, G.H., Dominguez, B.L., Schork, M.A., Loesche, W.J., 1997. Functional units, chewing, swallowing, and food avoidance among the elderly. J. Prosthet. Dentis. 77, 588–595.

Hori, K., Ono, T., Tamine K-i, Kondo, J., Hamanaka, S., Maeda, Y., et al., 2009. Newly developed sensor sheet for measuring tongue pressure during swallowing. J. Prosthodont. Res. 53, 28–32.

Jacobsson, C., 2000. How people with stroke and healthy older people experience the eating process. J. Clin. Nurs. 9, 255–264.

Jacobsson, C., Axelsson, K., Wenngren, B.I., Norberg, A., 1996. Eating despite severe difficulties: assessment of poststroke eating. J. Clin. Nurs. 5, 23–31.

Jacobsson, C., Axelsson, K., Österlind, P.O., Norberg, A., 2000. How people with stroke and healthy older people experience the eating process. J. Clin. Nurs. 9, 255–264.

Jalabert-Malbos, M.-L., Mishellany-Dutour, A., Woda, A., Peyron, M.-A., 2007. Particle size distribution in the food bolus after mastication of natural foods. Food Qual. Pref. 18, 803–812.

Kaiser, M.J., Bandinelli, S., Lunenfeld, B., 2010. Frailty and the role of nutrition in older people A review of the current literature. Acta Bio Medica Atenei Parmensis 81, 37–45.

Kapur, K.K., Soman, S.D., 2006. Masticatory performance and efficiency in denture wearers. J. Prosthet. Dentis. 95, 407–411.

Kays, S.A., Hind, J.A., Gangnon, R.E., Robbins, J., 2010. Effects of dining on tongue endurance and swallowing-related outcomes. J. Speech Language Hearing Res. 53, 898–907.

Kikawada, M., Iwamoto, T., Takasaki, M., 2005. Aspiration and infection in the elderly. Drugs Aging 22, 115–130.

Koshino, H., Hirai, T., Ishijima, T., Ikeda, Y., 1997. Tongue motor skills and masticatory performance in adult dentates, elderly dentates, and complete denture wearers. J. Prosthet. Dentis. 77, 147–152.

Kurillo, G., Zupan, A., Bajd, T., 2004. Force tracking system for the assessment of grip force control in patients with neuromuscular diseases. Clin. Biomechan. 19, 1014–1021.

Laguna, L., Chen, J., 2016. The eating capability: Constituents and assessments. Food Qual. Pref. 48 (Part B), 345–358.

Laguna, L., Mingioni, M., Maitre, I., Vanwymelbeke, V., Pirttijärvi, T., Artigas, M.G., et al., 2016a. Perception of difficulties encountered in eating process from European elderlies' perspective. J. Texture Stud. 47, 342–352.

Laguna, L., Hetherington, M.M., Chen, J., Artigas, G., Sarkar, A., 2016b. Measuring eating capability, liking and difficulty perception of older adults: a textural consideration. Food Quality Pref. 53, 47–56.

Laguna, L., Aktar, T., Ettelaie, R., Holmes, M., Chen, J., Physiological impact of ageing on eating capabilities J. Texture Stud, 2016c, in press.

Laguna, L.A.T, Ettelaie, R., Holmes, M., Chen, J., 2016d. A comparison between young and elderly adults investigating the manual and oral capabilities during the eating process. J. Texture Stud. 47, 361–372.

Laguna, L., Sarkar, A., Artigas, G., Chen, J., 2015a. A quantitative assessment of the eating capability in the elderly individuals. Physiol. Behav. 147, 274–281.

Laguna, L., Sarkar, A., Chen, J., 2015b. Assessment of eating capability of elderly subjects in UK: a quantitative evaluation. Proc. Nutr. Soc. 74, E167.

Langley-Evans, S.C., 2009. Nutrition: A Lifespan Approach. Wiley-Blackwell, Oxford.

Langmore, S.E., 2003. Evaluation of oropharyngeal dysphagia: which diagnostic tool is superior? Curr. Opin. Otolaryngol. Head Neck Surg. 11, 485–489.

Lauretani, F., Russo, C.R., Bandinelli, S., Bartali, B., Cavazzini, C., Di Iorio, A., et al., 2003. Age-associated changes in skeletal muscles and their effect on mobility: an operational diagnosis of sarcopenia. J. Appl. Physiol. 95, 1851–1860.

Leonard, R.J., White, C., McKenzie, S., Belafsky, P.C., 2014. Effects of bolus rheology on aspiration in patients with Dysphagia. J. Acad. Nutr. Dietet. 114, 590–594.

Lewis, R., Menardi, C., Yoxall, A., Langley, J., 2007. Finger friction: grip and opening packaging. Wear 263, 1124–1132.

Logemann, J.A., 2007. Swallowing disorders. Best Pract. Res. Clin. Gastroenterol. 21, 563–573.

Lucas, P., Prinz, J., Agrawal, K., Bruce, I., 2004. Food texture and its effect on ingestion, mastication and swallowing. J. Texture Stud. 35, 159–170.

Lyons, M., Baxendale, R., 1990. A preliminary electromyographic study of bite force and jaw-closing muscle fatigue in human subjects with advanced tooth wear. J. Oral Rehabil. 17, 311–318.

Macht, M., White, S.D., Moss, M., 2014. Swallowing dysfunction after critical illness. CHEST J. 146, 1681–1689.

Mathiowetz, V., Kashman, N., Volland, G., Weber, K., Dowe, M., Rogers, S., 1985a. Grip and pinch strength: normative data for adults. Arch. Phys. Med. Rehabil. 66, 69–74.

Mathiowetz, V., Volland, G., Kashman, N., Weber, K., 1985b. Adult norms for the Box and Block Test of manual dexterity. Am. J. Occupat. Ther. 39, 386–391.

Matsuo, K., Palmer, J.B., 2008. Anatomy and physiology of feeding and swallowing: normal and abnormal. Phys. Med. Rehabil. Clin. North Am. 19, 691–707.

McCullough, G., Wertz, R., Rosenbek, J., 2001. Sensitivity and specificity of clinical/bedside examination signs for detecting aspiration in adults subsequent to stroke. J. Commun. Dis. 34, 55–72.

McLaren, S., Dickerson, J., 2000. Measurement of eating disability in an acute stroke population. Clin. Effectiv. Nurs. 4, 109–120.

Meilgaard, M.C., Carr, B.T., Civille, G.V., 2006. Sensory Evaluation Techniques. CRC Press, Boca Raton, FL.

Metter, E., Conwit, R., Metter, B., Pacheco, T., Tobin, J., 1998. The relationship of peripheral motor nerve conduction velocity to age-associated loss of grip strength. Aging Clin. Exp. Res. 10, 471–478.

Miyaura, K., Morita, M., Matsuka, Y., Yamashita, A., Watanabe, T., 2000. Rehabilitation of biting abilities in patients with different types of dental prostheses. J. Oral Rehabil. 27, 1073–1076.

Narhi, T., Meurman, J., Ainamo, A., Nevalainen, J., Schmidt-Kaunisaho, K., Siukosaari, P., et al., 1992. Association between salivary flow rate and the use of systemic medication among 76-, 81-, and 86-year-old inhabitants in Helsinki, Finland. J. Dental Res. 71, 1875–1880.

Navazesh, M., Christensen, C., 1982. A comparison of whole mouth resting and stimulated salivary measurement procedures. J. Dental Res. 61, 1158–1162.

Newell, K.M., Vaillancourt, D.E., Sosnoff, J.J., 2006. Aging, complexity, and motor performance. Handbook Psychol. Aging 62, 163–182.

N'Gom, P.I., Woda, A., 2002. Influence of impaired mastication on nutrition. J. Prosthet. Dentis. 87, 667–673.

Nishino, T., Hiraga, K., 1991. Coordination of swallowing and respiration in unconscious subjects. J. Appl. Physiol. 70, 988–993.

Norberg, A., Athlin, E., Winblad, B., 1987. A model for the assessment of eating problems in patients with Parkinson's disease. J. Adv. Nurs. 12, 473–481.

Norman, K., Stobäus, N., Gonzalez, M.C., Schulzke, J.-D., Pirlich, M., 2011. Hand grip strength: outcome predictor and marker of nutritional status. Clin. Nutr. 30, 135–142.

Nowak, D.A., Hermsdörfer, J., 2003. Selective deficits of grip force control during object manipulation in patients with reduced sensibility of the grasping digits. Neurosci. Res. 47, 65–72.

Okada, A., Honma, M., Nomura, S., Yamada, Y., 2007. Oral behavior from food intake until terminal swallow. Physiol. Behav. 90, 172–179.

Olandersson, S, et al., 2005. Finger-force measurement-device for hand rehabilitation. *Rehabilitation Robotics, 2005. ICORR 2005. 9th International Conference on.*

Ono, T., Hori, K., Tamine, K.-i, Maeda, Y., 2009. Evaluation of tongue motor biomechanics during swallowing—from oral feeding models to quantitative sensing methods. Japanese Dental Sci. Rev. 45, 65–74.

Palastanga, N., Field, D., Soames, R., 2012. Anatomy and Human Movement. Structure and Function. Elsevier, Churchill Livingstone, UK.

Palmer, J.B., Drennan, J.C., Baba, M., 2000. Evaluation and treatment of swallowing impairments. Am. Fam. Physician. 61, 2453–2462.

Pedersen, A., Bardow, A., Jensen, S.B., Nauntofte, B., 2002. Saliva and gastrointestinal functions of taste, mastication, swallowing and digestion. Oral Dis. 8, 117–129.

Pereira, L.J., 2012. Oral cavity. Food Oral Processing. Wiley-Blackwell, Oxford (UK).

Peyron, M.-A., Blanc, O., Lund, J.P., Woda, A., 2004. Influence of age on adaptability of human mastication. J. Neurophysiol. 92, 773–779.

Pocztaruk, Rd.L., Frasca, L.Cd.F., Rivaldo, E.G., Fernandes, Ed.L., Gavião, M.B.D., 2008. Protocol for production of a chewable material for masticatory function tests (Optocal-Brazilian version). Brazilian Oral Res. 22, 305–310.

Rosenberg, I.H., Miller, J.W., 1992. Nutritional factors in physical and cognitive functions of elderly people. Am. J. Clin. Nutr. 55, 1237S–1243S.

Samnieng, P., 2015. Association of hyposalivation with oral function, nutrition, and oral health in visual impaired patient. Inter. J. Clin. Prevent. Dentis. 11, 15–20.

Sarkar, A., Goh, K.K.T., Singh, H., 2009. Colloidal stability and interactions of milk-protein-stabilized emulsions in an artificial saliva. Food Hydrocoll. 23, 1270–1278.

Sasaki, H., Kasagi, F., Yamada, M., Fujita, S., 2007. Grip strength predicts cause-specific mortality in middle-aged and elderly persons. Am. J. Med. 120, 337–342.

Schiffman, S.S., Warwick, Z.S., 1993. Effect of flavor enhancement of foods for the elderly on nutritional status: food intake, biochemical indices, and anthropometric measures. Physiol. Behav. 53, 395–402.

Schneider, G., Senger, B., 2002. Clinical relevance of a simple fragmentation model to evaluate human masticatory performance. J. Oral Rehabil. 29 (8), 731–736.

Scialfa, C.T.F., Geoff, R., 2006. Adaptative technology. In: Birren, J.E.S., Warner, K. (Eds.), Handbook of the Psychology of Aging. Elsevier Academic Press, San Diego, pp. 426.

Seidler-Dobrin, R.D., Stelmach, G., 1998. Persistence in visual feedback control by the elderly. Exp. Brain Res. 119, 467–474.

Singh, S., Utreja, A.K., Sandhu, N., Dhaliwal, Y.S., 2011. An innovative miniature bite force recorder. Inter. J. Clin. Pediat. Dentis. 4, 113–118.

Stanga, Z., 2009. Basics in clinical nutrition: nutrition in the elderly. e-SPEN, European e-J. Clin. Nutr. Metabol. 4, e289–e299.

Steele, C.M., Cichero, J.A., 2014. Physiological factors related to aspiration risk: a systematic review. Dysphagia 29 (3), 295–304.

Topkas, E., Keith, P., Dimeski, G., Cooper-White, J., Punyadeera, C., 2012. Evaluation of saliva collection devices for the analysis of proteins. Clin. Chim. Acta 413, 1066–1070.

Tortopidis, D., Lyons, M., Baxendale, R., Gilmour, W., 1998. The variability of bite force measurement between sessions, in different positions within the dental arch. J. Oral Rehabil. 25, 681–686.

Trampisch, U.S., Franke, J., Jedamzik, N., Hinrichs, T., Platen, P., 2012. Optimal Jamar dynamometer handle position to assess maximal isometric hand grip strength in epidemiological studies. J. Hand Surg. 37, 2368–2373.

Ueda, K., Yamada, Y., Toyosato, A., Nomura, S., Saitho, E., 2004. Effects of functional training of dysphagia to prevent pneumonia for patients on tube feeding. Gerodontology 21, 108–111.

Van Der Bilt, A., de Liz Pocztaruk, R., Abbink, J.H., 2010. Skull vibration during chewing of crispy food. J. Texture Studies 41 (6), 774–788.

Walls, A.W.G., Steele, J.G., 2004. The relationship between oral health and nutrition in older people. Mechan. Ageing Develop. 125, 853–857.

Westergren, A., Ohlsson, O., Hallberg, I.R., 2001. Eating difficulties, complications and nursing interventions during a period of three months after a stroke. J. Adv. Nurs. 35, 416–426.

Westergren, A., Unosson, M., Ohlsson, O., Lorefält, B., Hallberg, I.R., 2002. Eating difficulties, assisted eating and nutritional status in elderly (≥ 65 years) patients in hospital rehabilitation. Inter. J. Nurs. Stud. 39, 341–351.

Wiggermann, N.E., Werner, R.A., Keyserling, W.M., 2012. The effect of prolonged standing on touch sensitivity threshold of the foot: a pilot study. PM&R 4, 117–122.

Winder, B., Ridgway, K., Nelson, A., Baldwin, J., 2002. Food and drink packaging: who is complaining and who should be complaining. Appl. Ergon. 33, 433–438.

Woda, A., Foster, K., Mishellany, A., Peyron, M., 2006. Adaptation of healthy mastication to factors pertaining to the individual or to the food. Physiol. Behav. 89, 28–35.

Wylie, C., Copeman, J., Kirk, S., 1999. Health and social factors affecting the food choice and nutritional intake of elderly people with restricted mobility. J. Human Nutr. Dietet. 12, 375–380.

Yamashita, S., Sugita, D., Matsuo, K., 2013. Relationship between stage II transport and number of chewing strokes as mastication progresses. Physiol. Behav. 122, 100–103.

PART II

NUTRIENTS (VITAMINS AND MINERALS) IN HEALTH IN AGING ADULTS

CHAPTER

11

Healthy Food Choice and Dietary Behavior in the Elderly

Christine Brombach[1], Marianne Landmann[2], Katrin Ziesemer[3], Silke Bartsch[4] and Gertrud Winkler[5]

[1]ZHAW, Zurich University of Applied Sciences, Wädenswil, Switzerland [2]Friedrich-Schiller-University Jena, Jena, Germany [3]University of Konstanz, Konstanz, Germany [4]Pädagogische Hochschule Karlsruhe, Karlsruhe, Germany [5]Albstadt-Sigmaringen University, Sigmaringen, Germany

WHY DO WE EAT WHAT WE EAT?

From epidemiological studies we know that well-being and health are related to nutrition (Köster, 2009; Furst et al., 1996; Bisogni et al., 2002; Peel et al., 2005; Conklin et al., 2014; Mozzafarian, 2016). For our biological survival, we need to furnish our body with food. Eating and drinking constitute part of our daily actions to maintain our life. The word *eating* carries a double meaning: the act of nourishing, which refers to our physiological status, and the social act of eating, which is transformed and constituted by norms, values, traditions, and transported *socio-cultural constructs* of what, how, when, and with whom we eat (Furst et al., 1996; Shatenstein et al., 2013; Dickens and Ogden, 2014; Winter Flak et al., 1996; Wansink and Sobal, 2007; Wansink, 2010). Newborns learn that feeding occurs periodically, encompassing specific foods that are (usually) provided by their mothers. A baby´s caretaker resumes her own childhood experiences, thus carrying on the social dissemination of eating habits. Knowing and learning about food, eating, and eating behavior—such as the use of cutlery, the number and typical composition of meals per day, table manners, and taste—are acquired within the primary social group of the family (Methfessel et al., 2016; Edstrom and Devine, 2001; Atkins et al., 2015; Visser et al., 2016; Vabo and Hansen, 2014; Falk et al, 1996).

Studies on eating and eating behavior from the perspective of social sciences provide insights and help answer the question "Why do we eat what we eat?" (Barlösius, 2011; Köster, 2009; Devine et al., 1998; Devine et al., 1999; Wansink and Sobal, 2007; Just and Wansink, 2009). Even so, another paradigm other than a natural scientific approach is required (Table 11.1). Eating behaviors encompass complex actions that are socially shaped and further refined over a person's lifetime (De Castro, 2009; Köhler et al., 2008; Kim, 2016). *Eating behaviors* refers to food-related actions, including growing, shopping, storing, preparing, and eating food, as well as cleaning up afterwards and planning for following eating occasions. It is assumed that eating and nutritional behaviors result from lifelong experiences, so it is important to understand the life course and biographical factors in relation to eating and drinking (Furst et al., 1996; Sobal et al., 1998). Insight into the onset of individual eating behavior requires carrying out studies in which eating behavior is mediated within the frame of everyday life situations (Wansink, 2010). In addition, studying eating behavior in the context of an intergenerational approach might help deepen our understanding of the values passed on through socialization (Jones, 2015). Literature reviews reveal that studies on intergenerational influences on dietary behavior have hardly been examined (Brombach et al., 2014a,b; Stafleu et al., 1994; Vauthier et al., 1996). A study conducted by Ikeda et al. (2006) examined the diets of black American women in the course of three generations. They concluded that the grandmothers influenced the mothers' diets but not those of their granddaughters. In addition, the nutritional quality of the mothers' and daughters' diets was not similar (Ikeda et al., 2006).

Nutrition and Functional Foods for Healthy Aging.
DOI: http://dx.doi.org/10.1016/B978-0-12-805376-8.00011-3

TABLE 11.1 Two Paradigms, Two Sides of Food Behavior in Aging

Natural Science	Social Science
Aging	Getting old
Nutrition	Eating, food behavior
Physiological needs	Sociocultural aspects, eating biography
Nutrients	Food availability, choice, meals, preferences
Aging and food behavior take place in an individual; social and cultural forces shape historical context	

DETERMINANTS OF DIETARY BEHAVIOR

Eating and drinking are daily tasks that furnish our bodies with adequate amounts of nutrients and water and provide energy. On average, each person in a Western society consumes as much as 1.27 metric tons of food per year[1]. In the 1950s, German sociologist Georg Simmel described in an essay the common denominator that all humans share—meals and companionship (Simmel, 1957). Over their lifetimes, humans gather and share food for meals, but the most intimate shared meal is the start of a personal eating biography: when a mother nurses her baby, as anthropologists have assumed for decades (Douglas and Nicod 1974; Goody, 1982; Harnack et al., 1998; Murcott, 1995; Murcott, 1997). How and why do we learn to eat what we do? On which accounts do we make up food choices? We need to understand it first; otherwise we will not be able to support for healthy dietary behavior. In order to understand why people eat what they eat we can learn from elderly since they are experienced in their dietary behavior (Naughton et al., 2012; Ball et al., 2006; Edstrom and Devine, 2001; Wethington, 2005; Dean et al., 2009). On average an 80-year-old person consumed more than 50 metric tons of solid foods and 50 metric tons on liquid foods and consumed around 100,000 meals (own calculation). Despite the fact that eating and drinking are fundamental for our surviving; our daily food intake is by no means just a trivial biological action. Humans have no instincts such as animals do to guide their food intake. Humans have distinct eating behaviors which are culturally shaped and formed according to social rules, norms, and values of a given society (Fischler, 1988; Dean et al., 2009; De Vriendt et al., 2009; Conklin et al., 2014; Köster, 2009; Gatenby, 1997; Gibeny and Wolever, 1997; Blane et al., 2003, Kong et al., 2016). Each society defines which foods are edible or allowed to eat and which are not, which foods are valued and which foods are detested. Such food attribution or connotations differed throughout history of mankind (Goody, 1982; Lévi-Strauss, 1965; Mennell, 1985; Mennell et al., 1992; Barlösius, 2011), and even within individual life course foods considered to be adequate to eat, change. While we eat certain foods solely during infancy such as mushed food or infant food, we consume different foods in adulthood, e.g. wine. At specific times, often distinct foods are eaten and are part of certain festivities such as Christmas cookies or birthday cakes. Foods are valued differently in cultures and religions, while there are some foods forbidden in a culture, the same foods may be highly valued in another (Douglas and Nicod, 1974; Mennell et al., 1992; Goody, 1982). Prominent examples are insects which are not allowed for sales and prohibited on the food markets by most European food laws while insects are treasured foods in e.g. Asian countries or food valued in Europe such as blood sausages are taboo food in other cultures. Values and norms such as religious rules outlaw foods that are culturally accepted in other societies for examples alcoholic beverages or pork. Yet, despite different food habits and food-related norms, all humans share, that foods are eaten in situations we describe as "meals" denoting that there are norms, rituals, times, and routines that accompany food intake. Georg Simmel, a German sociologist described meals as the smallest denominator that all humans share (Simmel, 1957).

Food and eating behavior are inherently connected with many aspects of daily living and are formed and shaped over a lifetime. Eating behavior is guided by numerous practical and social concerns and by traditions, daily routines, and individual rituals (Fischler, 1988; Dean et al., 2009; De Vriendt et al., 2009; Conklin et al., 2014; Köster, 2009; Gatenby, 1997; Gibeny and Wolever, 1997; Blane et al., 2003). Studies of family meals (Brombach, 2001; Mäkela, 1995; Bartsch, 2011) found that the table was the forum for exchanging news and an instrument used by parents to instruct, educate, punish, or reward children in respect to the correct eating behaviors and table manners as well as generally acknowledged correct behaviors and socially shared norms and values (De Almeida Mota Ramalho

[1] On average, we consume 3.5 kg of food, including fluids, per day. This totals 1.27 metric tons annually.

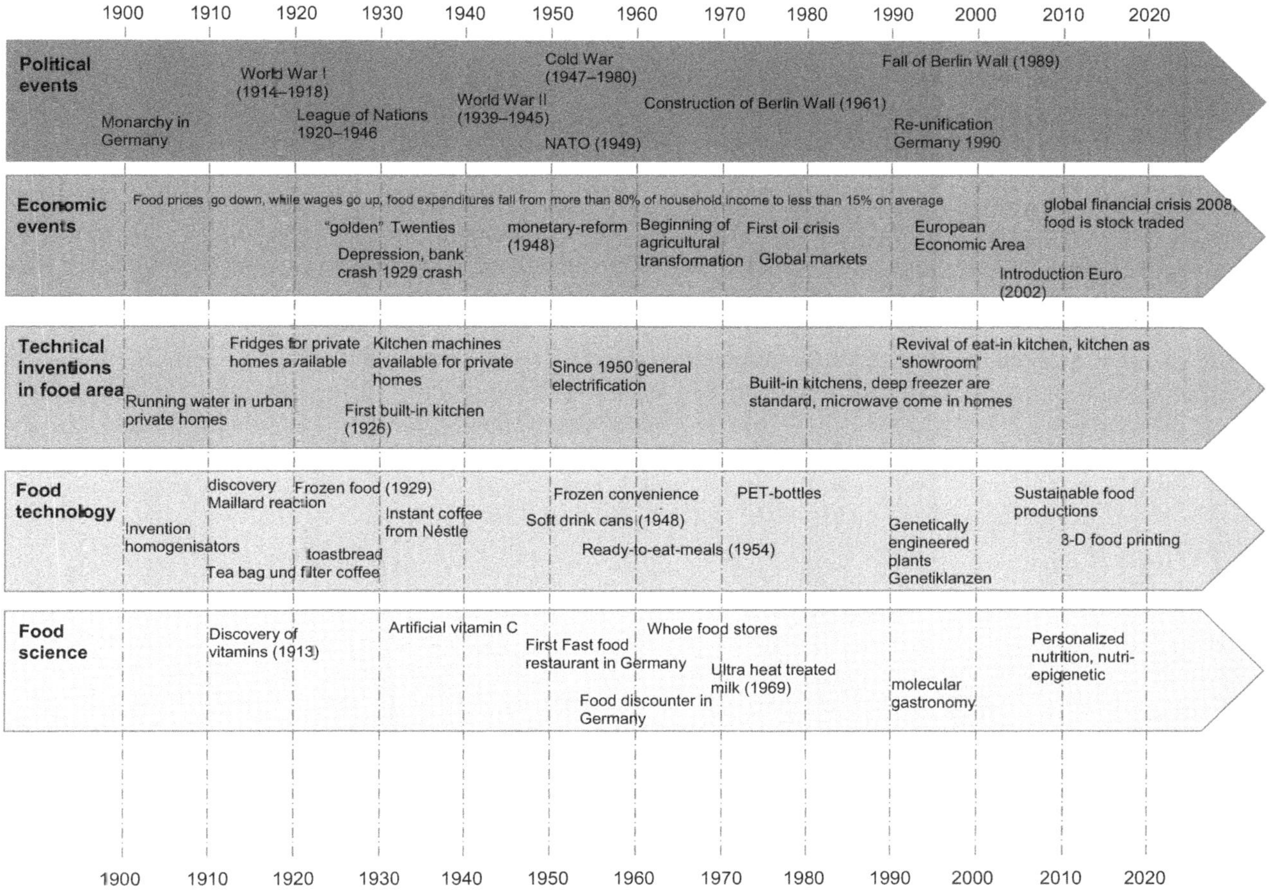

FIGURE 11.1 Contextual influences: sociocultural, technological, food-specific, and political "frames" in Germany, 1900 to the present.

et al., 2016). In his study on distinctions, Bourdieu (1984) found a certain habitus to be a distinctive criterion of class members. Habitus is learned and shaped within the social class an individual is brought up in.

We do not thoroughly understand the complexity of potentially independent and joint influences that shape and model eating behavior over the life course (Hummel and Hoffmann, 2016). Looking from a life course perspective and focusing on healthy elderly people, however, may reveal the trajectory of eating behaviors and their subsequent well-being later in life.

Food choices and life course influences have become a prominent framework in research on food behavior (e.g., Sobal et al., 1998; Sobal and Hanson, 2011; Sobal and Nelson, 2003).

Humans become socialized according to their family upbringings but are also subject to sociocultural factors that help make up any individual's life course. To help our research, we developed an overview of contextual influences in Germany and Switzerland (Fig. 11.1), which we see as an example for the sociocultural, political, and technological influences that shape and model food trajectories and eating behavior throughout the life course. The factors are different in each culture, but we assume the process of contextual shaping and influencing of individuals is general. In our understanding, we assume four main sociocultural "frames" that shape and influence eating behavior during life course. We look at chronologies of events starting in 1900 until 2020, just a few short years away. In our case, we exemplify our idea in four German women: mother, daughter, granddaughter, and great granddaughter. The mother was born in southwest Germany in 1885 and died in 1957. Her daughter was born in 1926 in southwest Germany, is now 90 years old, and still lives independently. The granddaughter was born in 1960 and, like the great granddaughter born in 1988, brought up in southwest Germany.

The mother was raised at the end of the 19th century in a setting that was incredibly different from today in respect to political systems, economic affairs, technological development, and foods available on the market. She was born in a time of monarchy and spent her young adulthood raising her own family during World War I. In her mid-50s, she experienced World War II and saw the founding of the Federal Republic of Germany when she was an old woman. She had 15 children (the oldest born in 1906, the youngest in 1929) who survived into adulthood, while the daughter, child number 14 (born in 1926), had five children (born between 1954 and 1968). The granddaughter (born 1960) had four children, while the great granddaughter, who was born in 1988, has a partner but as of yet no children. Both the mother and her still living 90-year old daughter experienced different political systems, economic crises, food scarcity events, and technological developments. Global foods were not available on the market until the rise of an affluent environment in the late 1950s and early 1960s.

For the mother, cooking and preparing food was hard manual labor. She had to preserve, store, and cook food without the aid of any electrical devices. Her daughter grew up in the 1930s and 1940s with electricity, cars, modern food technology such as refrigerators, pasteurization, and deep freezers in the 1960s. Yet both women share a history of food scarcity after wars and profound "everyday competences" about how to prepare seasonal and locally produced food. They learned to value food but prepared it according to gender roles and habits to which they adhered (e.g., serving husbands first, providing meat for male family members, doing all housework without the assistance of males, training their daughters but not sons to cooking and do kitchen chores). While the daughter knows about microwave ovens and convenience food, she never learned to like or appraise them in the same way as the grand daughter. Both, mother and daughter belong to generations that learned to "make the most" of available food and to avoid food waste. Looking at the third and fourth generations, the grandchildren and great-grandchildren will experience something much different because they were born in the 1960s and late 1980s, respectively, and raised in times of food abundance, food affluence, and even food waste. Still, they are also increasingly aware of food scares and discourses on the sustainability of food production. While sustainability is a current and relevant topic for the great granddaughter, her great grandmother and grandmother also acted with an understanding of sustainability, but for different reasons: food was seen as precious and meat too expensive to waste it or serve it every day. They knew by their own experiences that food was labour intense in preparing and by no means just available. Food was bound in a value system and to waste it was regarded sinful. The experience of hunger after wars was still very present and to have enough food was seen as privilege and by no means self evident. Consuming every part of a slaughtered animal was considered essential and practical. (So-called nose-to-tail consumption of animals was merely considered normal and not worth talking about—and certainly not considered an outstanding skill as we observe today in some food blogs.) Both granddaughter and great granddaughter eat different foods than mother and daughter, eat outside the home far more often, and are familiar with globally processed foods and have integrated scarce and expensive foods more often than their great grandmother and grandmother, who had them only occasionally. Yet even in the fourth generation, some habits and food consumption patterns remain to be passed on, including family recipes and family food events. The values provided to such habits, patterns, and food values lead us to the assumption that some food patterns and behaviors have a specific trajectory within families and might be more persistent and long-lasting than previously imagined and worthy of ongoing study.

DESIGN AND METHODS

To study long-term effects on nutrition behavior, we have to look at individuals' life experience with eating and drinking. Elderly people have had daily experiences of eating and drinking for decades, and perhaps the majority of women also have daily experience with food preparation. We derived the following questions to help guide our research:

- Are biographical methods depicting influencing factors on nutrition behavior?
- Are certain childhood eating patterns also present in adulthood?
- Can we assume an intergenerational approach to better understand eating behavior?

Acquiring insight into eating biographies can follow two strategies that can be classified as quantitative versus qualitative (see Table 11.1). While quantitative methods pursue identification on causes and effects and their mechanisms, qualitative methods focus primarily on the complexity and variety of individuals' everyday life situations (Silvermann, 2013). For this chapter, two qualitative studies will be presented.

The first study is a three-generational explorative study (Brombach et al., 2014a,b) that ran from March to June 2013. Questionnaires with 31 questions on food were distributed to nutrition students at four universities in Germany and Switzerland: Karlsruhe, Jena, and Sigmaringen in Germany and Zurich, Switzerland. Questions addressed intake frequency of selected food groups, meal patterns, cooking skills, food purchasing, food storage, food packaging and handling, and attitudes about nutrition. The students were asked to fill in the questionnaires themselves (F3 generation). Whenever possible, they had to interview at least one parent (F2 generation) and one grandparent (F1 generation). All questions referred to the present and to childhood. The questions referring to current situations and childhood (up to age 14 or so) were identical so we could compare current situations with

TABLE 11.2 Mean Frequency of Intake of Selected Food Groups per Week by Grandparents (F1), Parents (F2). and Children (F3) in Childhood and at Survey Time in 2013 (Intergenerational Differences)

Food Group	Childhood			Differences	Present			Differences
	F1	F2	F3	F1, F2, and F3 Childhood[a]	F1	F2	F3	F1, F2, and F3 Present[a]
Fruits and vegetables	4.0	4.6	5.0	S	5.8	5.6	5.7	NS
Milk and milk products	5.0	5.2	5.5	NS	5.7	5.5	5.7	NS
Wholemeal products	2.1	1.6	2.8	S	3.8	3.3	3.4	S
Fish and seafoods	0.5	0.9	0.9	NS	1.0	1.0	0.8	NS
Alcoholic drinks	0.1	0.0	0.1	NS	1.4	1.9	1.0	S
Meats and sausages	3.0	4.0	4.6	S	4.1	4.2	3.7	NS

Brombach, 2014a, p. 172.
S significant ($\alpha = 0.05$), *NS* not significant.
[a]*$\chi 2$ test.*

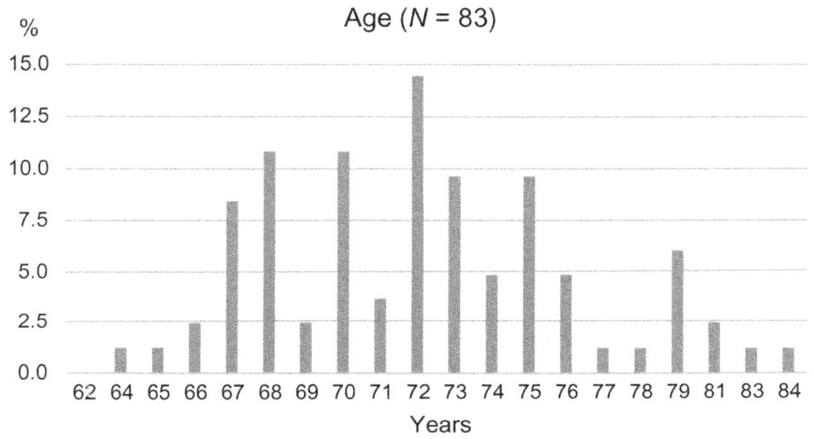

FIGURE 11.2 Age distribution of senpan participants.

childhood situations. In total, 249 persons participated in this study (75.7% women, 24.3% men), including 53 grandparents (F1: 78 ± 6 years), 96 parents (F2: 52 ± 5 years), and 100 children (F3: 23 ± 4 years).

The participants were asked to estimate the frequency of consumption (not the amount) of six food groups in childhood and today. Mean intake frequency was based on a calculation: daily = seven days per week, four to six times = five times per week, one to three times = twice per week, one to three times per month = once per month, less than once a month = 0.5 per month, and never = zero (Table 11.2).

No differences were found in the frequency of intake for milk and milk products, alcoholic drinks, and fish and seafood, between the childhoods of all three generations. When focusing on the F1 generation, we could observe that, with the exemption of milk and milk products, all other food groups changed in their consumption frequency. Other result of this study refer to the cooking and food waste reduction skills (not all results are shown here; see Brombach et al., 2014a,b, for details). In both aspects, the F1 generation performed better than the F2 and F3 generations.

To get a deeper insight and understanding of the elderly, we made a "quasi control group" in a similar age group. For this we used the same questions on the frequency of food group consumptions in childhood and the present in a sample of members of the senior consumer panel—*senpan*—at Zurich University of Applied Sciences in Waedenswil (ZHAW), Switzerland. The consumer panel at ZHAW currently consists of 90 participants over age 62 who live independently but close to ZHAW in private homes. Most of the participants were recruited via a sensory panel or by word of mouth. This panel is not representative because it presents a healthy, well-educated, and mobile segment of Swiss seniors, and almost all senpan participants have access to the Internet. Before participating in the study, all participants had to give their written consent to participate in this survey.

In this survey, which was conducted from March to May 2016, 84 senior consumers over age 62 participated in an online survey. The mean participant age was 72 ± 5 years and consisted of 44 men and 40 women (Fig. 11.2). In

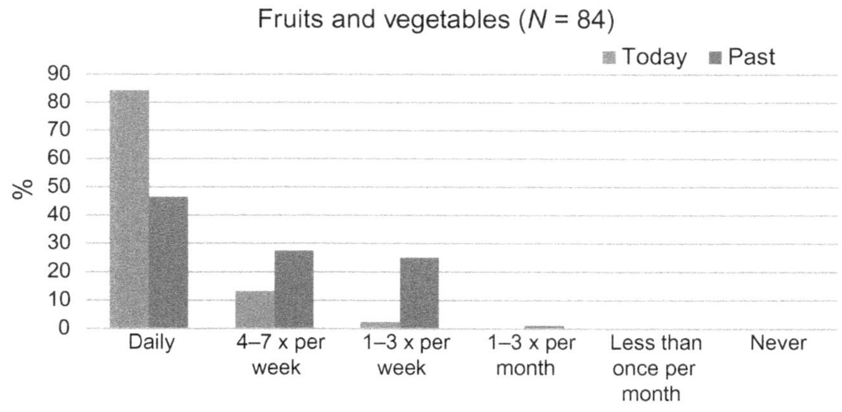

FIGURE 11.3 Frequency of fruits and vegetables consumed today and in childhood.

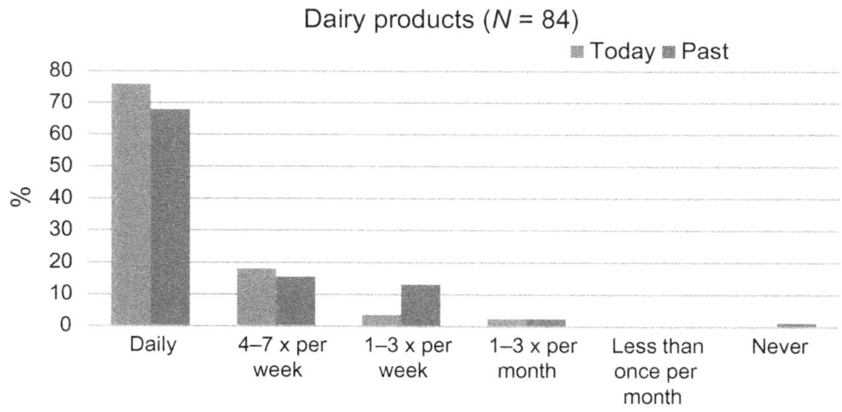

FIGURE 11.4 Frequency of dairy products consumed today and in childhood.

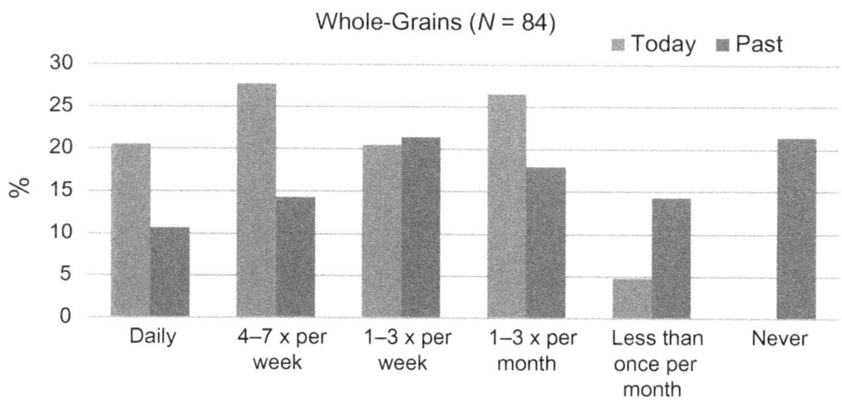

FIGURE 11.5 Frequency of whole grains consumed today and in childhood.

comparison to the three-generation study, results from the senpan showed surprisingly similar results. There are similar changes of frequency in all food groups except for milk and milk products. As can be seen in Figs 11.3–11.8, there are changes in today's and past frequencies in the given food groups.

In the three-generation study, we also addressed criteria used to decide what to cook. As can be seen in Table 11.3, almost the same proportion of senpan participants selected "health" to be a prominent factor in deciding what to cook—almost in the same percentage as in the three-generation study.

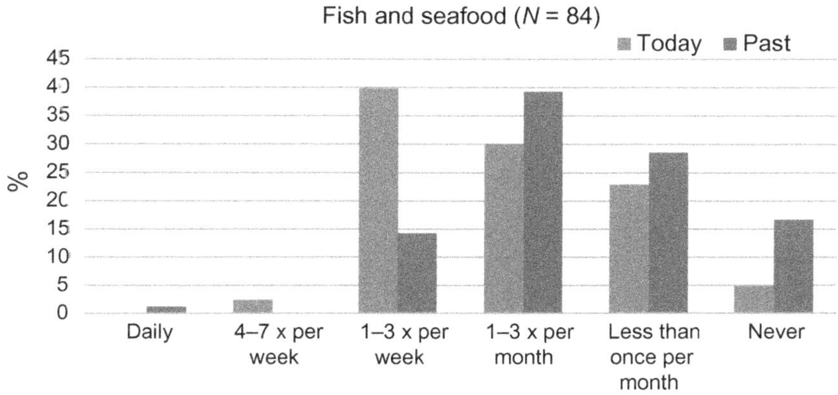

FIGURE 11.6 Frequency of fish and seafood consumed today and in childhood

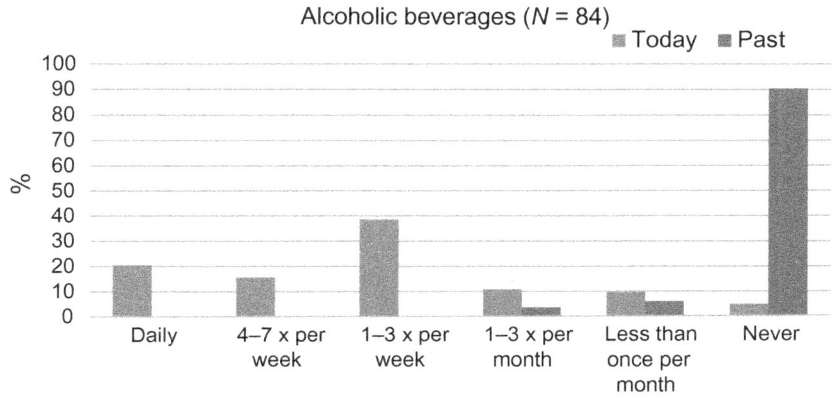

FIGURE 11.7 Frequency of alcoholic beverages consumed today and in childhood.

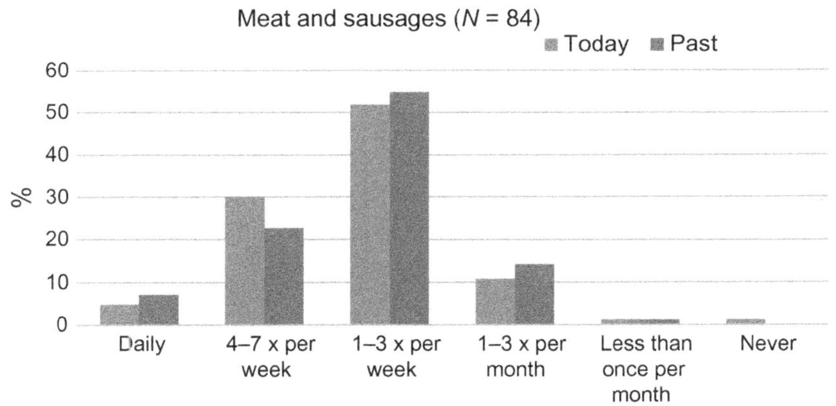

FIGURE 11.8 Frequency of meat and sausages consumed today and in childhood.

DISCUSSION AND APPLICATIONS

From the findings of the two studies, we assume that there are intergenerational effects and biographical factors that can be attributed to a given dietary behavior. We also conclude that cohort effects may lead to similar results in these two pilot studies. Because both studies are explorative, there are limitations and chances for improvement in such studies. In both these studies, there is a low number of participants and an imbalance of distribution. The recruitment

TABLE 11.3 Criteria on What to Cook in the Three-Generation Study and Senpan Participants

Criterion for Deciding Whether to Cook a Dish	Grandparent (F1) (n = 53) (%)	Parent (F2) (n = 96) (%)	Children (F3) (n = 100) (%)	Senpan (n = 84) (%)
Fast preparation	2	23	23	11
Another person cooks and decides	15	9	1	3
It has to be healthy	38	29	21	35
It has to be tasty	55	47	63	45

may cause a bias toward health-conscious participants. Retrospective questions may be inflicted with memory bias, an issue that is hard to control for (Eisinger-Watzl et al., 2015). Results of both studies may not be generalized and should be cautiously interpreted. However, there are striking comparisons with other studies such as the German Nutrition Survey II, which shows that the significance of the health value of food and healthy food behavior increased with age. Generally, cooking skills are more prominent and better in the elderly compared to younger adults, and older Germans in general seem to know better how to handle and reuse leftovers than do younger Germans (Max-Rubner-Institut, 2008; Heuer et al., 2015). Several studies (Visser et al., 2016; Berge, 2009; Brown and Ogden, 2004; Savage et al., 2007) have found that parents influence their children's dietary habits and that there are similarities in the dietary behavior of parents and children. Yet studies over three generations involving grandparents have been rarely examined. Findings of biographical or intergenerational studies might be helpful to understand the onset of dietary behavior. Eating and drinking are integral parts of an upbringing, and it might be helpful to integrate questions on where people were raised to answer what, why, and how they eat. Fritz Stern, a renowned historian, used a biographical approach (Stern, 2006) to interweave historical analysis and understanding with narratives of persons in specific situations.

From the empirical data in the two studies, we can conclude that eating socialization in childhood is a distal factor molding present-day eating behavior. Including biographical aspects of eating behavior in the context of cultural, political, technological, and economic "frames" might help illuminate how, when, in what ways food is eaten today.

References

Atkins, J.L., Ramsay, S.E., Whincup, P.H., Morris, R.W., Lennon, L.T., Wannamethee, S.Goya, 2015. Diet quality in older age: the influence of childhood and adult socio-economic circumstances. Br. J. Nutr. 113, 1441–1452.

Ball, K., Timperio, A.F., Crawford, D.A., 2006. Understanding environmental influences on nutrition and physical activity behaviors: where should we look and what should we count? Int. J. Behav. Nutr. Phys. Activity 3, 33. (2006). http://dx.doi.org/10.1186/1479-5868-3-33.

Barlösius, E., 2011. Soziologie des Essens (2. Aufl.). Juventa Verlag, Weinheim & München.

Bartsch, S., 2011. Familienmahlzeiten aus der Sicht der Jugendlichen. In: Schönberger, G., Methfessel, B. (Eds.), Mahlzeiten. Alte Last oder neue Lust?. VS Verlag, Wiesbaden, pp. 79–94.

Berge, J.M., 2009. A review of familial correlates of child and adolescent obesity: what has the 21 century taught us so far? Int. J. Adolesc. Med. Health 21 (4), 457–483.

Bisogni, C.A., Connors, M., Devine, C.M., Sobal, J., 2002. Who we are and how we eat: a qualitative study of identities in food choice. J. Nutr. Educ. Behav. 34, 128–139.

Blane, D., Abraham, L., Gunnell, D., Maynard, M., Ness, A., 2003. Background influences on dietary choices in early old age. J. R. Soc. Promot. Health 123 (4), 204–209.

Bourdieu, P., 1984. A Social Critique of the Judgement of Taste. Harvard College and Routledge & Kegan Paul Ltd, Massachusetts; USA.

Brombach, C., 2001. Mahlzeit-Familienzeit? Mahlzeiten im heutigen Familienalltag (Mealtime-family time? Meals in todays families). ErnahrungsUmschau 48, 238–242.

Brombach, C., Haefeli, D., Bartsch, S., Clauß, S., Winkler, G., 2014a. What have we kept and what have we changed? A three generation study on nutrition and food handling. ErnahrungsUmschau 61 (11), 171–177. http://dx.doi.org/10.4455/eu.2014.029.

Brombach, C., Haefeli, D., Bartsch, S., Winkler, G., 2014b. Ernährungsmuster im Verlauf von drei Generationen: Gibt es inter- und intraindividuelle Unterschiede? (Dietary patterns in a three-generational approach: are there inter- and intraindividual differences?) IAKE. Mitteilungen 2014, 12–21.

Brown, R., Ogden, J., 2004. Children's eating attitudes and behavior: a study of the modeling and control theories of parental influence. Health Educ. Res. 19, 261–271. http://dx.doi.org/10.1093/her/cyg040.

Charles, N., Kerr, M., 1988. Women, Food and Families. Manchester University Press, Manchester.

Conklin, A.I., Forouhi, N.G., Surtees, P., Khaw, K.-T., Wareham, N.J., Monsivais, P., 2014. Social relationships and healthful dietary behavior: evidence from over-50s in the EPIC cohort, UK. Soc. Sci. Med. 100, 167–175.

Dean, M., Raats, M.M., Grunert, K.G., Lumbers, M., 2009. Factors influencing eating a varied diet in old age. Public Health Nutr. 12 (12), 2421–2427.

De Almeida Mota Ramalho, J., Lachal, J., Ferro Bucher-Maluschke, J.S.N., Moro, M.-R., Revah-Levy, A., 2016. A qualitative study of the role of food in family relationsships: an insight into the families of Brazilian obese adolescents using photo elicitation. Appetite 96, 539–545.

De Castro, J.M., 2009. When, how much and what foods are eaten are related to total daily food intake. Br. J. Nutr. 102 (8), 1228–1237. http://dx.doi.org/10.1017/S0007114509371640.

Devine, C.M., Connors, M., Bisogni, C.A., Sobal, J., 1998. Life course influences on fruit and vegetable trajectories: qualitative analysis of food choices. Soc. Nutr. Educ. 30, 361–370.

Devine, C.M., Wolfe, W.S., Frongillo, E.A., Bisogni, C.A., 1999. Life course events and experiences: association with fruit and vegetable consumption in 3 ethnic groups. J. Am. Diet. Assoc. 99 (3), 309–314.

De Vriendt, T., Matthys, C., Verbeke, W., Pynaert, I., deHenauw, S., 2009. Determinants of nutrition knowledge in young and middle-aged Belgian women and the association with their dietary behavior. Appetite 52, 788–792.

Dickens, E., Ogden, J., 2014. The role of parental control and modeling in predicting a child's diet and relationship with food after they leave home. A prospective study. Appetite 76, 23–29.

Douglas, M., Nicod, M., 1974. Taking the biscuit: the structure of British meals. New Soc. 30 (637), 744–747.

Edstrom, K.M., Devine, C.M., 2001. Consistency in Women's orientations to food and nutrition in midlife and older age: a 10-year qualitative follow-up. J. Nutr. Educ. 33, 215–223.

Eisinger-Watzl, M., Straßburg, A., Ramünke, J., Krems, C., Heuer, T., Hoffmann, I., 2015. Comparison of two dietary assessment methods by food consumption: results of the German National Nutrition Survey II. Eur. J. Nutr. 54, 343–354.

Falk, L.W., Bisogni, C.A., Sobal, J., 1996. Food choice processes of older adults: a qualitative investigation. J. Nutr. Educ. 28, 257–265.

Fischler, C., 1988. Food, self and identity. Soc. Sci. Inform. 27 (2), 275–292.

Furst, T., Connors, M., Bisogni, C.A., Sobal, J., Falk, L.W., 1996. Food choice: a conceptual model of the process. Appetite 26, 247–266.

Gatenby, S.J., 1997. Eating frequency: methodological and dietary aspects. Br. J. Nutr. 77 (Suppl. 1), 7–20.

Gibeny, M.J., Wolever, T.M.S., 1997. Periodicity of eating and human health: present perspective and future directions. Br. J. Nutr. 77 (Suppl. 1), 3–5.

Goody, J., 1982. Cooking, Cuisine, Class. A Study On Comparative Sociology. Cambridge University Press., Cambridge.

Harnack, L., Story, M., Martinson, B., Neumark-Sztainer, D., Stang, J., 1998. Guess who´s cooking? The role of men in meal planning, shopping, and preparation in US families.. J. Am. Diet. Assoc. 98, 995–1000.

Heuer, T., Krems, C., Moon, K., Brombach, C., Hoffmann, I., 2015. Food consumption of adults in Germany: results of the German National Nutrition Survey II based on diet history interviews. Br. J. Nutr. page 1 of 12. http://dx.doi.org/10.1017/s0007114515000744.

Hummel, E., Hoffmann, I., 2016. Complexity of nutritional behavior: capturing and depicting its interrelated factors in a cause-effect model. Ecol. Food Nutr. 55 (3), 241–257.

Ikeda, P.I., Lexion, C.L., Turner, B.J., et al., 2006. Dietary quality is not linked across three generations of black women. Calif. Agric. 60, 154–159.

Jones, A., 2015. Intergenerational educational attainment, family characteristics and child obesity. J. Biosoc. Sci. published online 28 August 2015, http://dx.doi.org/10.1017/S0021932015000280.

Just, D.R., Wansink, B., 2009. Better school meals on a budget: using behavioral economics and food psychology to improve meal selection. Choices 24 (3), 1–6.

Kim, C.-O., 2016. Food choice patterns among frail older adults: the associations between social network, food choice values, and diet quality. Appetite 96 (2016), 116–121.

Kong, K.L., Gillman, M.W., Rifas-Shiman, S.L., Wen, X., 2016. Mid-childhood fruit and vegetable consumption: the roles of early liking, early consumption, and maternal consumption. Appetite (2016), to appear in Appetite, http://dx.doi.org/10.1016/j.appet.2016.05.033.

Köhler, J., Leonhäuser, I.-U., 2008. Changes in food preferences during aging. Ann. Nutr. Metab. 52 (suppl 1), 15–19.

Köster, E.P., 2009. Diversity in the determinants of food choice: a psychological perspective. Food Qual. Preference 20, 70–82. (2009).

Lévi-Strauss, C., 1965. Le triangle culinaire. L'Arc 26, 19–29.

Mäkela, J., 1995. The structure of Finish meals. Ernährungsumschau 42, 112–114.

Max-Rubner-Institut (2008) National Nutrition Survey II, https://www.bmel.de/SharedDocs/Downloads/Ernaehrung/NVS_Ergebnisbericht.pdf?__blob=publicationFile, (retrieved 1.06.2016)

Mennell, S., 1985. All Manners of Food:Eating and Taste in England and France from the Middle Ages to the Present. Basil Blackwell, Oxford.

Mennell, S., Murcott, A., van Otterloo, A.H., 1992. The Sociology of Food: Eating, diet and culture. Sage, London.

Methfessel, B., Höhn, K., Miltner-Jürgensen, B., 2016. Essen und Ernährungsbildung in der KiTa Entwicklung – Versorgung – Bildung. Kohlhammer, Stuttgart.

Mozzafarian, D., 2016. Dietary and policy priorities for cardiovascular disease, diabetes, and obesity. Compreh. Rev. Circul. 133, 187–225. http://dx.doi.org/10.1161/CIRCULATIONAHA.115.018585.

Murcott, A., 1997. Family meals: A thing of the past?. In: Caplan, P. (Ed.), Food Health And Identity. Routledge, London.

Murcott, A., 1995. Raw, cooked and proper meals at home. 219–235 Food Choice and the Consumer

Naughton, S., Crawford, D., Ball, K., Salmon, J., 2012. Understanding determinants of nutrition, physical activity and quality of life among older adults: the Wellbeing, Eating and Exercise for a Long Life (WELL) study. Health Qual. Life Outcomes 10, 109. http://dx.doi.org/10.1186/1477-7525-10-109.

Peel, N.M., McClure, R.J., Bartlett, H.P., 2005. Behavioral determinants of healthy aging. Am. J. Prevent. Med. 28 (3), 298–304. 2005.

Savage, J., Fisher, J.O., Birch, L.L., 2007. Parental influence on eating behavior: conception to adolescence. J. Law Med. Ethics 35 (1), 22–34.

Shatenstein, B., Gauvin, L., Keller, H., Richard, L., Gaudreau, P., Giroux, F., et al., 2013. Baseline determinants of global diet quality in older men and women from the NUAGE cohort. J. Nutr. Health Aging 17 (5), 419–425.

Silvermann, D., 2013. Doing Qualitative Research. SAGE, London.

Simmel, G., (1957): Soziologie der Mahlzeit. In: Susmann, M./LandmannM. (Hrsg.), Brücke und Tor. Essays zur Geschichte, Religion, Kunst und Gesellschaft. Stuttgart: K.F. Koehler.

Sobal, J., Hanson, K., 2011. Marital status, marital history, body weight, and obesity. Marriage Fam. Rev. 47 (7), 474–504.

Sobal, J., Nelson, M.K., 2003. Commensal eating patterns: a community study. Appetite 41, 181–190.

Sobal, J., Khan, L.K., Bisogni, C.A., 1998. A conceptual model of the food and nutrition system. Soc. Sci. Med. 47 (7), 853–863.

Sobal, J., Bisogni, C.A., Devine, C.M., Jastran, M., 2006. A conceptual model of the food choice process over the life course. In: Shepherd, R., Raats, M. (Eds.), The Psychology of Food Choice. CABI Publishing, Cambridge MA, pp. 1–18.

Stafleu, A., van Staveren, W.A., de Graaf, C., et al., 1994. Family resemblance in energy, fat, and cholesterol intake: A study among three generations of women. Prevent. Med. 23, 474–480.

Stern, F., 2006. Five Germanies I Have Known, 2006. Farrar, Straus and Giroux, New York.

Vabo, M., Hansen, H., 2014. The relationship between food preferences and food choice: a theoretical discussion. Int. J. Bus. Soc. Sci. 5 (7), 145–157.

Vauthier, J.M., Luch, A., Lecomte, E., Artur, Y., Herbeth, B., 1996. Family resemblance in energy and macronutrient intakes: the stanislas family study. Int. J. Epidemiol. 25, 1030–1037.

Visser, S.S., Hutter, I., Haisma, H., 2016. Building a framework for theory-based ethnographies for studying intergenerational family food practices. Appetite 97, 49–57.

Wansink, B., 2010. From mindless eating to mindlessly eating better. Physiol. Behav. 100, 454–463.

Wansink, B., Sobal, J., 2007. Mindless eating. Environ. Behav. 39 (1), 106–123.

Wethington, E., 2005. An overview of the life course perspective: implications for health and nutrition. J. Nutr. Educ. Behav. 37 (37), 115–120.

Winter Flak, L., Bisogni, C.A., Sobal, J., 1996. Food choice process of older adults: a qualitative investigation. Soc. Nutr. Educ. 28, 257–265.

CHAPTER

12

Vitamin D and Diabetes in Elderly People

Nicola Veronese[1], *Enzo Manzato*[1,2] *and Giuseppe Sergi*[1]

[1]University of Padova, Padova, Italy [2]National Research Council, Padova, Italy

INTRODUCTION

Diabetes type 2 is one of the most common diseases in older people. More than 40% of all cases of diabetes are diagnosed in people 65 and older, and the number of older people with diabetes is expected to rise exponentially in the next 20 years (Mokdad et al., 2000). Although treatments for diabetes and its complications have improved, the prevention of this condition in the elderly seems to be fundamentally important.

Several factors (e.g., obesity, sedentary lifestyle, hypertension) are known to be potentially modifiable risk factors for diabetes, but their treatment seems to be difficult and produces limited results in the elderly (Pittas et al., 2007b), hence the need to conduct further research in an effort to identify factors that are easier to modify with a view to preventing diabetes.

Low vitamin D levels (hypovitaminosis D) seem to be important in this population. Hypovitaminosis D (usually defined as low circulating serum 25 hydroxyvitamin D (25OHD) levels) is a common condition in older people, with a prevalence ranging from 30% to 60% in populations that include people over 65 (Mosekilde, 2005; Timpini et al., 2011; Veronese et al., 2014a). Hypovitaminosis D is also easily reversible, and its treatment has few side effects even in older individuals. Since diabetes and hypovitaminosis D are both becoming increasingly common among older people, it is hardly surprising that recent research has been trying to find a connection between these two conditions.

In this chapter, we discuss current research on hypovitaminosis D as a potential risk factor for diabetes in the elderly, starting with a brief description of the molecular pathways that may be involved, and outlining the epidemiological research conducted on young and middle-aged people.

POTENTIAL MECHANISMS AND PATHWAYS FOR AN EFFECT OF VITAMIN D IN DIABETES

Experimental research strongly supports a role for vitamin D in the pathogenesis of diabetes. In fact, vitamin D seems to play a part in improving pancreatic beta cell function through both direct mechanisms (transcriptional activation of the human insulin gene by the active form of vitamin D) (Maestro et al., 2002) and indirect mechanisms (normalization of extracellular and intracellular calcium) (Pittas et al., 2007b). Both effects could increase the insulin response to food and glucose stimulation without affecting basal insulin levels (Bourlon et al., 1999; Zeitz et al., 2003).

Another relevant mechanism that has emerged from in vitro and animal research concerns the improvement in insulin resistance: vitamin D stimulates insulin receptor expression in peripheral tissues, thereby improving the action of insulin (Maestro et al., 2000). The modulation of calcium metabolism also could play an important part in improving insulin secretion (Pittas et al., 2007b). Some authors have also hypothesized a role for vitamin D in reducing inflammation (particularly through a downregulation of inflammatory cytokines), although evidence of this effect is less clear (Guadarrama-López et al., 2014). It has to be said, however, that most of the experiments conducted to date involved young or adult animals; to the best of our knowledge, there are no published studies on the role of vitamin D in glucose and insulin metabolism in older animals.

Nutrition and Functional Foods for Healthy Aging.
DOI: http://dx.doi.org/10.1016/B978-0-12-805376-8.00012-5

EPIDEMIOLOGICAL EVIDENCE OF HYPOVITAMINOSIS D AS A RISK FACTOR FOR DIABETES

Case-Control and Cross-Sectional Studies

In case-control studies, diabetic people usually have significantly lower serum 25OHD levels than those who are age- and sex-matched healthy controls, and this association seems to be scarcely affected by potential confounders such as obesity (Christiansen et al., 1982; Cigolini et al., 2006; Hyppönen and Power, 2006). As Pittas et al. concluded in their systematic review (Pittas et al., 2007b), however, the cohorts considered in case-control studies were generally younger than 65 years or included more young adults than older participants.

Examining pooling data from 12 large cross-sectional studies, Pittas et al. found that participants with higher serum 25OHD levels had an approximately 46% lower prevalence of diabetes, but this finding was not statistically significant and was characterized by a high degree of heterogeneity (Pittas et al., 2007b).

Some cross-sectional studies produced data on hypovitaminosis D and diabetes in the elderly. For instance, in a cohort of 142 older diabetic people (with a mean age of 76), Baynes et al. (1997) found no significant association between 25OHD and fasting plasma glucose or 2-h oral glucose tolerance test results. Another study confirmed the lack of association between hypovitaminosis D and diabetes in 1235 participants with a mean age of 75: after adjusting for potential confounders, those with hypovitaminosis D were not more likely to have diabetes (Snijder et al., 2006). More recently, two other large studies seem to support the conviction that there is no association between hypovitaminosis D and diabetes or altered glucose parameters, particularly after accounting for adiposity (Dalgård et al., 2011; Hirani et al., 2014).

Prospective Studies

A large meta-analysis involving 21 prospective studies and 76,220 participants at the baseline found that having higher serum 25OHD levels protected against the onset of diabetes. Every 10nmol/L increase in vitamin D levels corresponded to a 4% reduction in the chances of developing diabetes in the future (Song et al., 2013). Among the 21 studies considered, however, only three concerned people over 65 or a sample with a mean age above this cutoff (Bolland et al., 2010; Pilz et al., 2012; Robinson et al., 2011), and all three studies reported no significant association between baseline serum 25OHD status and incident diabetes.

After this meta-analysis published in 2013, other longitudinal studies investigated the potential association between poor vitamin D status and diabetes in the elderly. In a subgroup analysis on 1583 participants in the German ESTHER study over 65 years old, no significant association emerged between baseline 25OHD and the onset of diabetes during an 8-year follow-up (Schöttker et al., 2013). Schafer et al. further confirmed this lack of association in 5463 older women followed up for about 9 years (Schafer et al., 2014): they found a significant association between poor vitamin D status and diabetes, but it disappeared after adjusting for body mass index (BMI) (Schafer et al., 2014). Finally, we also found no association between baseline serum 25OHD levels and incident diabetes in a cohort of 2227 older men and women participating in the Progetto Veneto Anziani study (Veronese et al., 2014b).

Randomized Controlled Trials on Vitamin D Supplementation in Diabetes

In a meta-analysis of 43 randomized controlled trials (RCTs) and 43,407 participants, oral supplementation with vitamin D did not seem to improve insulin resistance, insulin secretion, or glycosylated hemoglobin levels compared with placebo or no intervention (Seida et al., 2014). Vitamin D supplementation was also unable to prevent progression to diabetes in four large trials (Seida et al., 2014).

Five RCTs only considered individuals over 65 given vitamin D supplementation, always comparing them with a control group taking a placebo (Avenell et al., 2009; Breslavsky et al., 2013; Pittas et al., 2007a; Witham et al., 2010; Yiu et al., 2013). They basically reported that oral vitamin D supplementation had no effect on glucose parameters, neither in participants with diabetes (Breslavsky et al., 2013; Witham et al., 2010; Yiu et al., 2013) nor in participants at high risk of diabetes (Avenell et al., 2009; Pittas et al., 2007a). On the whole, the quality of these studies seems to be adequate, the doses of cholecalciferol used were 700 international units per day or more, and the follow-up was long enough for any significant changes to emerge in the metabolic parameters investigated (Seida et al., 2014).

VITAMIN D AND DIABETES IN THE ELDERLY

The current literature suggests that a poor vitamin D status (represented by low serum 25OHD levels) is not associated with diabetes in the elderly, in contrast with the results obtained for middle age participants when hypovitaminosis D does seem to be significantly associated with diabetes. The possible reasons for these differences are outlined in the following and in Fig. 12.1.

Epidemiological and Demographic Reasons

The depletion of the susceptible effect might play an important part in the association between vitamin D and diabetes (Tournier et al., 2008). People with low 25OHD levels who reach old age may be less prone to the health hazards relating to hypovitaminosis D than those with low 25OHD levels who developed diabetes when they were younger (Schöttker et al., 2013). This effect is somewhat similar to the effect of a high BMI in older subjects (Veronese et al., 2015). Unlike the case of obesity in which a sizable body of literature has shown a protective factor for mortality in the elderly (Cereda et al., 2011; Sergi et al., 2005; Veronese et al., 2015), serum 25OHD levels are not associated with the onset of diabetes, suggesting that other characteristics of older people with hypovitaminosis D must have an important influence. It may be that hypovitaminosis D is a stronger predictor of mortality than diabetes in older people, as shown by some papers on this issue (Johansson et al., 2012; Samefors et al., 2014), and subjects with low serum 25OHD would therefore die before developing diabetes.

The Role of Obesity

Conditions associated with both hypovitaminosis D and diabetes might feasibly play a more important part in older adults than in the middle-aged. Several other conditions are commonly found in association with hypovitaminosis D or diabetes (or both)—including multiple comorbidities, disability, and frailty—but adiposity seems to be the most important in explaining why low 25OHD levels are not associated with diabetes in older people (Hirani et al., 2014). This hypothesis is supported by some of the previously mentioned studies, which found that the significant association identified between poor vitamin D status and diabetes disappeared after controlling for BMI and other adiposity measures (Dalgård et al., 2011; Hirani et al., 2014; Pilz et al., 2012; Schafer et al., 2014).

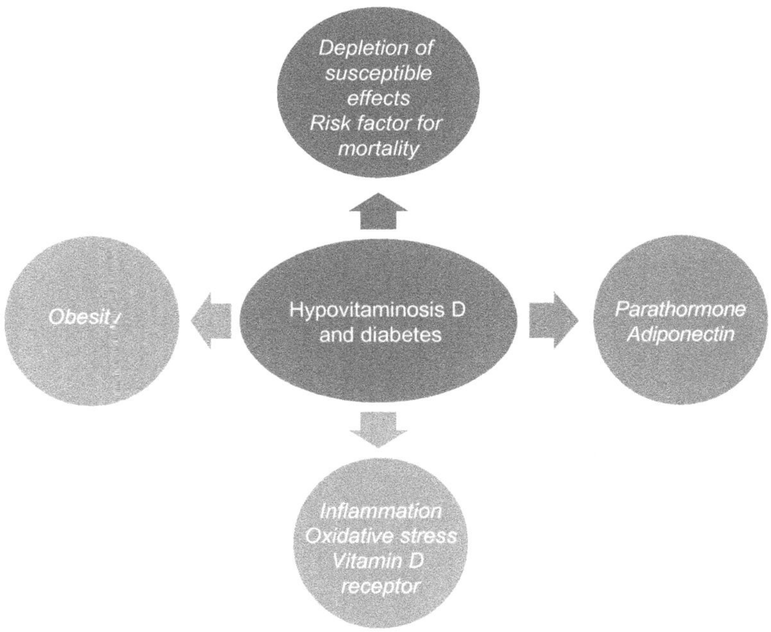

FIGURE 12.1 Possible explanations for the lack of association between hypovitaminosis D and diabetes in older people.

Fat mass is well known to strongly influence 25OHD levels, especially in older people (Pereira-Santos et al., 2015; Seo et al., 2012), so obesity, which has a role also in the onset of diabetes, could help to explain why hypovitaminosis D is not associated with a poor glycemic control in older people. Taken together, these findings suggest that low vitamin D levels are more a marker than a causal factor for diabetes in the elderly as recently claimed in various reports (Ye et al., 2014).

Metabolic and Molecular Pathways

The molecular pathways involved in the association between hypovitaminosis D and diabetes have unfortunately been little explored in the elderly. The animal research that sustained the influence of vitamin D on glucose parameters was conducted on young animals, which probably differ from older animals in terms of their body composition and metabolic pathways.

In human beings, older people have higher inflammatory and oxidative stress parameters and lower sex hormone levels (Rizza et al., 2014). More specifically, as regards blood glucose parameters, aging coincides with an increase in both insulin and glucose levels, predisposing the elderly to a higher risk of diabetes (Rizza et al., 2014).

The role of a vitamin D receptor (VDR) seems to be relevant in explaining the lack of association between hypovitaminosis D and diabetes in the elderly. VDR occurs largely in the skeletal muscle, which is the most important regulator of insulin sensitivity. Since muscle mass decreases linearly with age, it may be that VDR concentrations drop and that higher 25OHD concentrations are consequently needed to achieve the same effect on glucose metabolism as in younger adults (Gallagher, 2013).

Additional Regulators of Insulin Resistance

Parathyroid hormone (PTH) and 25OHD are closely related. An increasing body of research is showing an independent effect of high PTH levels on glucose metabolism. In a meta-analysis of 17 studies, e.g., individuals with primary hyperthyroidism had higher levels of adiposity and glucose than did healthy controls (Bolland et al., 2005). These findings also seem partially applicable to older people, in whom this condition is associated with a higher rate of obesity and consequently insulin resistance (Conroy et al., 2003). Increased PTH levels could therefore play a part in the onset of diabetes by causing an increase in fat mass.

When it comes to the possible role of hyperparathyroidism secondary to low 25OHD levels in predicting diabetes in older people, however, there is only one study available, and it found no significant association between high serum PTH levels and diabetes (Veronese et al., 2014b). Further epidemiological studies are therefore needed to better elucidate the role of PTH in glucose metabolism.

Similar findings are available for adiponectin. This hormone is significantly related to a better control over glucose metabolism, and its levels are lower in the obese than in people of normal weight. Several studies have reported a significant association between 25OHD and adiponectin, albeit mediated by the quantity of fat mass (Bidulescu et al., 2014; Cekmez et al., 2012). No studies focusing specifically on the association between 25OHD and adiponectin in the elderly are yet available, however.

Vitamin D Supplementation and Diabetes in the Elderly

The evidence emerging from RCTs on the effect of vitamin D supplementation on glucose parameters in the elderly is not comforting. Even when it is delivered in adequate doses and for an appropriate period of time, vitamin D supplementation seems unable to improve several metabolic parameters in people with diabetes or at high risk of diabetes, reinforcing the conviction that the association between poor vitamin D status and diabetes is unlikely to be causal (Ye et al., 2014). It seems more likely that hypovitaminosis D in older people is a marker of other conditions that are associated with a high risk of diabetes (obesity, limited physical activity, and limited exposure to the sun). Based on this hypothesis, 25OHD levels could be measured to identify older people at higher risk of diabetes and propose timely appropriate interventions (such as weight loss and physical exercise) to prevent diabetes in this population.

CONCLUSIONS

Diabetes and hypovitaminosis D are two common conditions in the elderly, and both are increasing exponentially in this age group, but current research does not support an etiological role for hypovitaminosis D in the onset of diabetes. Since various studies on this population have reported that the statistical association between hypovitaminosis D and diabetes disappears after adjusting for potential confounders, we recommend measuring 25OHD levels as a possible marker of diabetes and metabolic diseases in the elderly. Further investigations are nonetheless needed to shed light on whether supplementation with oral vitamin D could have any influence in preventing or delaying diabetes in the elderly.

References

Avenell, A., Cook, J.A., MacLennan, G.S., McPherson, G.C., 2009. Vitamin D supplementation and type 2 diabetes: a substudy of a randomised placebo-controlled trial in older people (RECORD trial, ISRCTN 51647438). Age Ageing 38, 606–609. http://dx.doi.org/10.1093/ageing/afp109.

Baynes, K.C., Boucher, B.J., Feskens, E.J., Kromhout, D., 1997. Vitamin D, glucose tolerance and insulinaemia in elderly men. Diabetologia 40, 344–347. http://dx.doi.org/10.1007/s001250050685.

Bidulescu, A., Morris, A.A., Stoyanova, N., Meng, Y.-X., Vaccarino, V., Quyyumi, A.A., et al., 2014. Association between vitamin D and adiponectin and its relationship with body mass index: the META-health study. Front. Public Health 2, 193. http://dx.doi.org/10.3389/fpubh.2014.00193.

Bolland, M.J., Bacon, C.J., Horne, A.M., Mason, B.H., Ames, R.W., Wang, T.K., et al., 2010. Vitamin D insufficiency and health outcomes over 5 y in older women. Am. J. Clin. Nutr. 91, 82–89. http://dx.doi.org/10.3945/ajcn.2009.28424.

Bolland, M.J., Grey, A.B., Gamble, G.D., Reid, I.R., 2005. Association between primary hyperparathyroidism and increased body weight: a meta-analysis. J. Clin. Endocrinol. Metab. 90, 1525–1530. http://dx.doi.org/10.1210/jc.2004-1891.

Bourlon, P.M., Billaudel, B., Faure-Dussert, A., 1999. Influence of vitamin D3 deficiency and 1,25 dihydroxyvitamin D3 on de novo insulin biosynthesis in the islets of the rat endocrine pancreas. J. Endocrinol. 160, 87–95.

Breslavsky, A., Frand, J., Matas, Z., Boaz, M., Barnea, Z., Shargorodsky, M., 2013. Effect of high doses of vitamin D on arterial properties, adiponectin, leptin and glucose homeostasis in type 2 diabetic patients. Clin. Nutr. 32, 970–975. http://dx.doi.org/10.1016/j.clnu.2013.01.020.

Cekmez, F., Aydemir, G., Aydinoz, S., Pirgon, O., Genc, F.A., Tunc, T., et al., 2012. Low 25-hydroxyvitamin D level and adiponectin is associated with insulin sensitivity in large gestational age infants. Cytokine 59, 156–158. http://dx.doi.org/10.1016/j.cyto.2012.04.031.

Cereda, E., Pedrolli, C., Zagami, A., Vanotti, A., Piffer, S., Opizzi, A., et al., 2011. Body mass index and mortality in institutionalized elderly. J. Am. Med. Dir. Assoc. 12, 174–178. http://dx.doi.org/10.1016/j.jamda.2010.11.013.

Christiansen, C., Christensen, M.S., McNair, P., Nielsen, B., Madsbad, S., 1982. Vitamin D metabolites in diabetic patients: decreased serum concentration of 24,25-dihydroxyvitamin D. Scand. J. Clin. Lab. Invest. 42, 487–491.

Cigolini, M., Iagulli, M.P., Miconi, V., Galiotto, M., Lombardi, S., Targher, G., 2006. Serum 25-hydroxyvitamin D3 concentrations and prevalence of cardiovascular disease among type 2 diabetic patients. Diabetes Care 29, 722–724.

Conroy, S., Moulias, S., Wassif, W.S., 2003. Primary hyperparathyroidism in the older person. Age Ageing 32, 571–578.

Dalgård, C., Petersen, M.S., Weihe, P., Grandjean, P., 2011. Vitamin D status in relation to glucose metabolism and type 2 diabetes in septuagenarians. Diabetes Care 34, 1284–1288. http://dx.doi.org/10.2337/dc10-2084.

Gallagher, J.C., 2013. Vitamin D and aging. Endocrinol. Metab. Clin. North Am. 42, 319–332. http://dx.doi.org/10.1016/j.ecl.2013.02.004.

Guadarrama-López, A.L., Valdés-Ramos, R., Martínez-Carrillo, B.E., 2014. Type 2 diabetes, PUFAs, and vitamin D: their relation to inflammation. J. Immunol. Res. 2014, 860703. http://dx.doi.org/10.1155/2014/860703.

Hirani, V., Cumming, R.G., Le Couteur, D.G., Naganathan, V., Blyth, F., Handelsman, D.J., et al., 2014. Low levels of 25-hydroxy vitamin D and active 1,25-dihydroxyvitamin D Independently associated with type 2 diabetes mellitus in older Australian men: the concord health and ageing in men project. J. Am. Geriatr. Soc., 1741–1747. http://dx.doi.org/10.1111/jgs.12975.

Hyppönen, E., Power, C., 2006. Vitamin D status and glucose homeostasis in the 1958 British birth cohort: the role of obesity. Diabetes Care 29, 2244–2246. http://dx.doi.org/10.2337/dc06-0946.

Johansson, H., Odén, A., Kanis, J., McCloskey, E., Lorentzon, M., Ljunggren, Ö., et al., 2012. Low serum vitamin D is associated with increased mortality in elderly men: MrOS Sweden. Osteoporos. Int. 23, 991–999. http://dx.doi.org/10.1007/s00198-011-1809-5.

Maestro, B., Campión, J., Dávila, N., Calle, C., 2000. Stimulation by 1,25-dihydroxyvitamin D3 of insulin receptor expression and insulin responsiveness for glucose transport in U-937 human promonocytic cells. Endocr. J. 47, 383–391.

Maestro, B., Molero, S., Bajo, S., Dávila, N., Calle, C., 2002. Transcriptional activation of the human insulin receptor gene by 1,25-dihydroxyvitamin D(3). Cell Biochem. Funct. 20, 227–232. http://dx.doi.org/10.1002/cbf.951.

Mokdad, A.H., Ford, E.S., Bowman, B.A., Nelson, D.E., Engelgau, M.M., Vinicor, F., et al., 2000. Diabetes trends in the U.S.: 1990–1998. Diabetes Care 23, 1278–1283.

Mosekilde, L., 2005. Vitamin D and the elderly. Clin. Endocrinol. (Oxf) 62, 265–281. http://dx.doi.org/10.1111/j.1365-2265.2005.02226.x.

Pereira-Santos, M., Costa, P.R.F., Assis, A.M.O., Santos, C.A.S.T., Santos, D.B., 2015. Obesity and vitamin D deficiency: a systematic review and meta-analysis. Obes. Rev. 16, 341–349. http://dx.doi.org/10.1111/obr.12239.

Pilz, S., van den Hurk, K., Nijpels, G., Stehouwer, C.D.A.D.A., Van't Riet, E., Kienreich, K., et al., 2012. Vitamin D status, incident diabetes and prospective changes in glucose metabolism in older subjects: The Hoorn study. Nutr. Metab. Cardiovasc. Dis. 22, 883–889. http://dx.doi.org/10.1016/j.numecd.2012.03.008.

Pittas, A.G., Harris, S.S., Stark, P.C., Dawson-Hughes, B., 2007a. The effects of calcium and vitamin D supplementation on blood glucose and markers of inflammation in nondiabetic adults. Diabetes Care 30, 980–986. http://dx.doi.org/10.2337/dc06-1994.

Pittas, A.G., Lau, J., Hu, F.B., Dawson-hughes, B., 2007b. REVIEW: the role of vitamin D and calcium in type 2 diabetes. A systematic review and meta-analysis. J. Clin. Endocrinol. Metab. 92, 2017–2029. http://dx.doi.org/10.1210/jc.2007-0298.

Rizza, W., Veronese, N., Fontana, L., 2014. What are the roles of calorie restriction and diet quality in promoting healthy longevity? Ageing Res. Rev. 13, 38–45. http://dx.doi.org/10.1016/j.arr.2013.11.002.

Robinson, J.G., Manson, J.E., Larson, J., Liu, S., Song, Y., Howard, B.V., et al., 2011. Lack of association between 25(OH)D levels and incident type 2 diabetes in older women. Diabetes Care 34, 628–634. http://dx.doi.org/10.2337/dc10-1632.

Samefors, M., Östgren, C.J., Mölstad, S., Lannering, C., Midlöv, P., Tengblad, A., 2014. Vitamin D deficiency in elderly people in Swedish nursing homes is associated with increased mortality. Eur. J. Endocrinol. 170, 667–675. http://dx.doi.org/10.1530/EJE-13-0855.

Schafer, A.L., Napoli, N., Lui, L., Schwartz, A.V., Black, D.M., 2014. Serum 25-hydroxyvitamin D concentration does not independently predict incident diabetes in older women. Diabet. Med. 31, 564–569. http://dx.doi.org/10.1111/dme.12368.

Schöttker, B., Herder, C., Rothenbacher, D., Perna, L., Müller, H., Brenner, H., 2013. Serum 25-hydroxyvitamin D levels and incident diabetes mellitus type 2: a competing risk analysis in a large population-based cohort of older adults. Eur. J. Epidemiol. 28, 267–275. http://dx.doi.org/10.1007/s10654-013-9769-z.

Seida, J.C., Mitri, J., Colmers, I.N., Majumdar, S.R., Davidson, M.B., Edwards, A.L., et al., 2014. Effect of vitamin D_3 supplementation on improving glucose homeostasis and preventing diabetes: a systematic review and meta-analysis. J. Clin. Endocrinol. Metab. 99, 3551–3560. http://dx.doi.org/10.1210/jc.2014-2136.

Seo, J.A., Cho, H., Eun, C.R., Yoo, H.J., Kim, S.G., Choi, K.M., et al., 2012. Association between visceral obesity and sarcopenia and vitamin D deficiency in older Koreans: the Ansan Geriatric Study. J. Am. Geriatr. Soc. 60, 700–706. http://dx.doi.org/10.1111/j.1532-5415.2012.03887.x.

Sergi, G., Perissinotto, E., Pisent, C., Buja, A., Maggi, S., Coin, A., et al., 2005. An adequate threshold for body mass index to detect underweight condition in elderly persons: the Italian Longitudinal Study on Aging (ILSA). J. Gerontol. A. Biol. Sci. Med. Sci. 60, 866–871.

Snijder, M., van Dam, R., Visser, M., Deeg, D., Seidell, J., Lips, P., 2006. To: Mathieu C, Gysemans C, Giulietti A, Bouillon R (2005) Vitamin D and diabetes. Diabetologia 48:1247–1257. Diabetologia 49, 217–8. doi:10.1007/s00125-005-0047-9.

Song, Y., Wang, L., Pittas, A.G., Del Gobbo, L.C., Zhang, C., Manson, J.E., et al., 2013. Blood 25-hydroxy vitamin D levels and incident type 2 diabetes: a meta-analysis of prospective studies. Diabetes Care 36, 1422–1428. http://dx.doi.org/10.2337/dc12-0962.

Timpini, A., Pini, L., Tantucci, C., Cossi, S., Grassi, V., 2011. Vitamin D and health status in elderly. Intern. Emerg. Med. 6, 11–21. http://dx.doi.org/10.1007/s11739-010-0407-4.

Tournier, M., Moride, Y., Lesk, M., Ducruet, T., Rochon, S., 2008. The depletion of susceptibles effect in the assessment of burden-of-illness: the example of age-related macular degeneration in the community-dwelling elderly population of Quebec. Can. J. Clin. Pharmacol. 15, e22–e35.

Veronese, N., Bolzetta, F., De Rui, M., Zambon, S., Corti, M.C.M.-C., Musacchio, E., et al., 2014a. Serum 25-hydroxyvitamin D and orthostatic hypotension in old people: the Pro.V.A. study. Hypertension 64, 481–486. http://dx.doi.org/10.1161/HYPERTENSIONAHA.114.03143.

Veronese, N., Cereda, E., Solmi, M., Fowler, S.A., Manzato, E., Maggi, S., et al., 2015. Inverse relationship between body mass index and mortality in older nursing home residents: a meta-analysis of 19,538 elderly subjects. Obes. Rev. http://dx.doi.org/10.1111/obr.12309.

Veronese, N., Sergi, G., De Rui, M., Bolzetta, F., Toffanello, E.D., Zambon, S., et al., 2014b. Serum 25-Hydroxyvitamin D and Incidence of Diabetes in Elderly People: the Pro.V.a Study. J. Clin. Endocrinol. Metab. 99, jc20133883. http://dx.doi.org/10.1210/jc.2013-3883.

Witham, M.D., Dove, F.J., Dryburgh, M., Sugden, J.A., Morris, A.D., Struthers, A.D., 2010. The effect of different doses of vitamin D(3) on markers of vascular health in patients with type 2 diabetes: a randomised controlled trial. Diabetologia 53, 2112–2119. http://dx.doi.org/10.1007/s00125-010-1838-1.

Ye, Z., Sharp, S.J., Burgess, S., Scott, R.A., Imamura, F., Langenberg, C., et al., 2014. Association between circulating 25-hydroxyvitamin D and incident type 2 diabetes: a Mendelian randomisation study. Lancet. Diabetes Endocrinol. 3, 35–42. doi:10.1016/S2213-8587(14)70184-6.

Yiu, Y.-F., Yiu, K.-H., Siu, C.-W., Chan, Y.-H., Li, S.-W., Wong, L.-Y., et al., 2013. Randomized controlled trial of vitamin D supplement on endothelial function in patients with type 2 diabetes. Atherosclerosis 227, 140–146. http://dx.doi.org/10.1016/j.atherosclerosis.2012.12.013.

Zeitz, U., Weber, K., Soegiarto, D.W., Wolf, E., Balling, R., Erben, R.G., 2003. Impaired insulin secretory capacity in mice lacking a functional vitamin D receptor. FASEB J. 17, 509–511. http://dx.doi.org/10.1096/fj.02-0424fje.

CHAPTER

13

Vitamin D and the Elderly Orthopedic Patient

Gerrit Steffen Maier[1], *Andreas Alois Kurth*[3], *Konstantin Horas*[2], *Kristina Kolbow*[1], *Jörn Bengt Seeger*[4], *Klaus Edgar Roth*[5], *Djordje Lazovic*[1] and *Uwe Maus*[1]

[1]Carl-von-Ossietzky-University, Oldenburg, Germany [2]Julius-Maxilians-University, Würzburg, Germany [3]Themistocles Gluck Hospital, Ratingen, Germany [4]Justus-Liebig-University, Giessen, Germany [5]Johannes-Gutenberg-University, Mainz, Germany

INTRODUCTION

Vitamin D is a key player in calcium homeostasis and bone health. Beyond these well-known effects, new data suggest that vitamin D deficiency potentiates a variety of chronic disease states, including diabetes, cancer, and depression. Extremely low vitamin D levels have been associated with osteomalacia and impaired muscle function, both core elements in the field of orthopedic surgery. Good muscle function and healthy bones are essential for fast rehabilitation and positive outcome after orthopedic surgery as well, especially in elderly patients seeking a return to good physical functioning. Physical function is important for the preservation of independence in daily life and for the prevention of falls, which are associated with fractures and high mortality. This review focuses on the role of vitamin D deficiency in elderly orthopedic patients.

VITAMIN D

Vitamin D is a fat-soluble, secosteroid hormone required for proper regulation of many body systems and normal human growth and development (Hoffmann et al., 2015). Two common forms exist: vitamins D_2 (ergocalciferol) and D_3 (cholecalciferol). Vitamin D uptake or acquisition is regulated both through nutritional means (10–20%) and by the intradermal synthesis under the action of sunlight (80–90%). The main circulation form is 25-hydroxyvitamin D ($25(OH)_2D$), the result of hydroxylation in the liver of vitamin D_2 or D_3. It is yielded into the biologically active form of vitamin D, calcitriol, or $1,25(OH)_2D$, through hydroxylation in the kidney. The active $1,25(OH)_2D$ acts through specific vitamin D receptors to regulate calcium metabolism, differentiation, and division of various cell types (Holick and DeLuca, 1974).

The major source of vitamin D for most people is casual exposure of the skin to sunlight (Godar et al., 2011). When the precursor, 7-dehydrocholesterol, is exposed to ultraviolet light, it converts to previtamin D_3 (Baggerly et al., 2015). Previtamin D_3 undergoes nonenzymatic thermal transformation, which results in the production of vitamin D_3 (Hoffmann et al., 2015). Due to the necessity of sun exposure and ultraviolet light, the endogenous synthesis can be affected by many different factors. Decreased synthesis of vitamin D can be attributed to high latitude, darker skin pigmentation, advanced age, and the use of sunblock and protective clothing (Adams et al., 1982; Clemens et al., 1982; Dowdy et al., 2010).

Nutrition and Functional Foods for Healthy Aging.
DOI: http://dx.doi.org/10.1016/B978-0-12-805376-8.00013-7

A limited number of foods naturally contain vitamin D, including fish, egg yolk, and offal such as liver. Because dietary intake of such foods is generally low in many countries, the use of supplements is important and should be recommended for groups prone to develop vitamin D deficiency such as infants and inactive elderly (Lips, 2007).

Vitamin D Status Assessment

Circulating 1,25-(OH)-D concentrations are under homeostatic control, limiting the value of 1,25-(OH)-D as a nutritional marker of vitamin D status (Hill et al., 2013). Serum concentrations closely reflect the amount of vitamin D synthesized in the skin and ingested in the diet. For this reason, 25-OH-D is widely accepted as a good biomarker of vitamin D status (Hill et al., 2013). During winter months in countries with a geographies above 40 degrees northern or southern latitude, the skin is not capable of synthesizing vitamin D for as long as 4–5 months (Webb et al., 1988). Therefore, it is assumed that during winter the circulating 25-OH-D levels are related to late-summer concentrations, oral intake, and body stores (Hill et al., 2013).

Vitamin D Deficiency

Vitamin D status has been studied on all continents and in most countries of the world (van Schoor and Lips, 2011). The best determinant of the serum vitamin D status is the serum concentration of 25-hydroxyvitamin D (25-OH-D) (Lips, 2001). As yet, there is no consensus on what constitutes normal vitamin D levels (Perez-Lopez et al., 2011). Many studies suggest 30 ng/mL as an optimal level, whereas others suggest 40 ng/mL, especially under particular conditions such as cancer involvement (Grant et al., 2009). The Institute of Medicine of the US National Academies has recommended an increase in minimal daily requirements for vitamin D and also raised its recommendation of an upper limit on a safe dose of vitamin D to 4000 international units (IUs) per day (Perez-Lopez et al., 2011). The US Endocrine Society guideline defines vitamin D deficiency as a serum 25-OH-D level less than 20 ng/mL (50 nmol/L) and vitamin D insufficiency as 25-OH-D values between 21 and 29 ng/mL (Pramyothin and Holick, 2012).

Hypovitaminosis D has been described in several studies in numerous segments of the global population. It is estimated to affect more than 1 billion people of all races, age groups, and ethnic backgrounds (Mithal et al., 2009). High rates of vitamin D deficiency in particular have been described among the elderly. One British study revealed a lower vitamin D level in people 65 and older than in the general public (Glowacki et al., 2003; Hirani and Primatesta, 2005). In postmenopausal American women taking antiosteoporotic medicine, more than 50% showed inadequate low vitamin D levels (Glowacki et al., 2003). Even young and healthy cohorts are at risk of developing hypovitaminosis D. In an American study from 2004, 52% of Boston-based adolescents of Hispanic and African American origin were suffering from hypovitaminosis D (Gordon et al., 2004).

Data on vitamin D status among the German population frequently reveals low vitamin D levels. In 14,000 individuals between one and 79 years of age, 62% of adolescent boys, 64% of adolescent girls, 57% of men, and 58% of women demonstrated vitamin D levels below 20 ng/mL (Hintzpeter et al., 2008). A study of 1578 elderly care rehabilitation facility patients in Germany published in 2012 showed severe vitamin D deficiencies with values below 10 ng/mL in 68% of patients. Only 4% of the patients had levels in the target range of 30–60 ng/mL (Schilling, 2012).

Among inpatients of geriatric acute care units, lower vitamin D serum levels have been associated with a greater severity of chronic diseases, increased risks of acute decompensation, and a higher risk of in-hospital mortality (Annweiler et al., 2010; Beauchet et al., 2012; Sutra Del Galy et al., 2009). In line with this, hypovitaminosis D doubled the risk of hospitalization for more than 14 days in a geriatric acute care unit (Beauchet et al., 2013).

Although several studies reported a widespread rate of vitamin D deficiency, epidemic data on elderly orthopedic patients is scarce. Data revealing the prevalence of vitamin D insufficiency and deficiency in elderly patients may be of value for treating orthopedic surgeons and geriatricians to prevent potential negative consequences in the operative and postoperative settings to maintain good physical function and to preserve independence in daily life. We reported in 2013 on an association between hypovitaminosis D and elderly orthopedic patients in general and found a high prevalence of vitamin D deficiency and insufficiency in such patients in an orthopedic department in central Germany (Maier et al., 2015a; Sutra Del Galy et al., 2009). We were able to show not only that orthopedic patients with hip or vertebral fractures have low vitamin D levels but also that elderly orthopedic patients in general had such low levels. A novelty in this study was that mainly nonhospitalized elderly patients were tested. Extremely low vitamin D levels have been associated with osteomalacia and impaired muscle function, both core elements in the field of orthopedic surgery. Good muscle function and healthy bones are essential for fast rehabilitation and positive outcome after orthopedic surgery as well as good physical function, especially in elderly patients (LeBoff et al., 2008; Maier et al., 2013a).

Physical function is important for the preservation of independence in daily life and for the prevention of falls, which are associated with fractures and high mortality (Annweiler et al., 2010; Bischoff-Ferrari et al., 2005; Bruyere et al., 2007). Vitamin D depletion has been linked with impaired cognition and specific damage to executive functions and speed of information processing, which can directly impact the selection of postural control strategies and reaction to falls (Annweiler and Beauchet, 2015; Annweiler et al., 2010). Low vitamin D levels negatively affect muscle strength, which may impact fall patterns, their severity, and reaction to them (Hamilton, 2010). Furthermore, several studies showed that lower 25-OH-D serum levels are a risk factor for orthostatic hypotension, which was reported to deteriorate the functional autonomy of older patients and to have a close relation with mortality and morbidity in the elderly (McCarroll et al., 2012; Soysal et al., 2014). In a study of 546 elderly patients aged 65 and older, vitamin D deficiency was shown to be a factor in the development of orthostatic hypotension. The authors concluded that during the evaluation of orthostatic hypotension serum, 25-OH-D levels should be checked and detected deficiencies should be treated (Soysal et al., 2014).

Vitamin D and Fracture Prevention

Vitamin D plays a pivotal role in bone mineralization. Vitamin D deficiency results in decreased bone mineralization as well as secondary hyperparathyroidism and increased cortical bone loss. In certain cases, severe vitamin D deficiencies can lead to osteomalacia. An autopsy study of deceased with clinically healthy bones found histopathological signs of osteomalacia with vitamin D levels below 30 ng/mL in 25% of all bone samples taken. Of note, samples with correlating vitamin D levels above 30 ng/mL did not show any signs of bone pathology (Priemel et al., 2010).

The relationship between vitamin D status and osteoporosis is of growing interest. Vitamin D levels below 20 ng/mL lead to malabsorption of intestinal calcium, and osteomalacia in the elderly as well as rickets in children (Holick, 2007; Lips, 2001). Several studies revealed that vitamin D status influences various outcomes of osteoporosis (Dawson-Hughes et al., 2005; Nakamura et al., 2011). One serious outcome of osteoporosis is fracture. Hip fractures are one of the most common fractures of the elderly (Maier et al., 2013b). Recent studies suggest that measurement of vitamin D serum concentrations might serve as a biomarker for hip-fracture risks among elderly patients (LeBoff et al., 1999; Lopes et al., 2009; Nuti et al., 2004). Current studies have shown a widespread rate of vitamin D deficiency in women with hip fractures (Dhanwal et al., 2010; Nurmi et al., 2005). These fractures contribute significantly to morbidity and mortality of elderly. As many as 50% of seniors will have permanent functional disabilities after hip fractures, and as many as 20% will die within the first year after the primary event (Bischoff-Ferrari et al., 2008). Supplementation of vitamin D has been shown to reduce the risk of falls (Bischoff-Ferrari et al., 2009a) and hip fractures (Bischoff-Ferrari et al., 2012). One of the first randomized controlled trials investigating the efficacy of vitamin D supplementation to prevent fractures compared the effect of 1200 mg of calcium and 20 μg vitamin D daily versus placebos in 3270 French women averaging 84 years of age. Under supplementation, bone mineral density increased and the risk of hip and nonvertebral fractures was reduced (Chapuy and Meunier, 1996). The Randomized Evaluation of Calcium or Vitamin D (RECORD) study compared the effect of calcium and vitamin D, alone or in combination, and placebos in 5292 community-dwelling older women or men with low-trauma fractures. Over the 62-month follow-up, the authors found no difference in the incidence of hip fractures or other fracture types. A possible explanation for the missing effect of supplementation was found in the extremely poor compliance with supplementation, especially when this included daily calcium (Grant et al., 2005). The women's health initiative study showed an improvement in bone mineral density with the combined supplementation of calcium and vitamin D. Among patients who were compliant with the supplementation scheme there was a significant reduction in the risk of hip fractures (Jackson et al., 2006). A meta-analysis by Bischoff-Ferrari et al. (2009b) suggested that after adjustment of the vitamin D dose the incidence of nonvertebral fractures decreased independently of additional calcium supplementation.

Vertebral fragility fractures are another common type of osteoporosis complication. So far, a distinct correlation between these fractures and vitamin D levels has been described (Cummings et al., 1998; El Maghraoui et al., 2012). Vertebral fractures have direct and indirect effects on quality of life with increased morbidity and mortality (Lyles et al., 1993). Several studies revealed a high rate of hypovitaminosis D in postmenopausal women with osteoporotic vertebral fractures (El Maghraoui et al., 2012; Sakuma et al., 2011). A recent study showed a possible role of vitamin D levels in the occurrence of postkyphoplasty-recurrent vertebral compression fractures in elderly patients undergoing kyphoplasty due to osteoporotic fractures (Zafeiris et al., 2012).

In one of our recent studies, we identified a 89% prevalence of hypovitaminosis D in patients with vertebral fractures. By comparison, a well-matched group of patients with back pain in the absence of fracture who were seen in the same geographical locale (Mainz, Germany, 50 degrees northern latitude) and around the same time of year had a hypovitaminosis D prevalence of 60%. The majority of patients presenting with back pain had low vitamin D levels, regardless of whether or not fractures were present (Maier et al., 2015b). Our results suggest that patients who present with a vertebral fragility fracture are significantly more likely to be vitamin D insufficient or even deficient in comparison to patients without vertebral fractures. These results are in line with the findings of former studies, revealing that higher serum concentrations of vitamin D contribute to healthy bone metabolism and prevent osteoporosis as well as osteoporotic fractures (Bischoff-Ferrari et al., 2006).

Several studies examined the association between fractures in postmenopausal women and low vitamin D levels. Nakamura et al. showed in their 6-year cohort study of 773 community-dwelling elderly Japanese women that patients with sufficient vitamin D concentrations (>71 nmol/L) had a 58% lower risk of developing osteoporotic fractures than those with insufficient serum vitamin D concentrations. They concluded that optimal serum levels of vitamin D could reduce fracture risk (Nakamura et al., 2011). Gerdhem et al. (2005) were able to show that women with serum vitamin D concentrations below 20 ng/mL were twice as likely to sustain osteoporotic fractures compared to women with vitamin D concentrations above this threshold. In 415 elderly Brazilian women assessed with vertebral fragility fracture, vitamin D insufficiency was found to be one of the most important influencing factors (Lopes et al., 2009). El Maghraoui et al. enrolled 178 menopausal Moroccan women in their cohort study to determine serum vitamin D status and assess the association of bone mineral density and vertebral fractures. A widespread rate of vitamin D insufficiency (85% of tested patients) and deficiency (52%) was found. Furthermore, hypovitaminosis D was identified as an independent risk factor for vertebral fractures in postmenopausal women (El Maghraoui et al., 2012).

There is a certain discrepancy in literature regarding the association of gender with vitamin D levels and osteoporosis. Some studies indicate that females have a higher risk to be vitamin D deficient than men (Cooper et al., 1992), but other data identified male sex as a risk factor (Guardia et al., 2008). This conflicting literature indicates that gender may not necessarily be of importance for vitamin D deficiency, which is supported by our data. Both males and females need to be monitored for hypovitaminosis D because both groups are at high risk.

We have shown a mean vitamin D level of 17.1 ng/mL among 1083 patients 70 and older (Maier et al., 2015a). Data on such old geriatric and orthopedic patients is scarce, but they all support a widespread rate of hypovitaminosis D in the elderly (Drinka, 1996). This is an alarming fact, knowing that the official recommendation by the European Society for Clinical and Economic Aspects of Osteoporosis and Osteoarthritis is a minimum serum 25-OH-D level of 30 ng/mL in fragile elderly subjects at an elevated risk of falls and fractures (Rizzoli et al., 2013). Bischoff-Ferrari et al. (2004) showed a 22% reduction in falls of patients taking vitamin D supplements. Gerdhem et al. (2005) evaluated 986 postmenopausal women and showed a twofold increased fracture risk for patients with 25-OH-D levels below 20 ng/mL compared to patients with higher serum vitamin D levels. Moreover, a contributing role of vitamin D deficiency in the occurrence of simultaneous fractures has recently been described in a study of 472 elderly hip fracture patients (Di Monaco et al., 2011).

Nonskeletal Effects of Vitamin D

Besides its regulatory function in bone metabolism, vitamin D has been found by several studies to exert a growing number of nonskeletal effects. In particular, hypovitaminosis D has been linked to a higher risk of cardiovascular diseases, type 2 diabetes, and even mental illness (Giovannucci et al., 2008; Mattila et al., 2007; Menkes et al., 2012). Furthermore, vitamin D also regulates innate and adaptive immune functions by activating macrophages, dendritic cells, and lymphocytes (Hewison, 2010). Hypovitaminosis D has been shown to increase the risk of respiratory tract infection and periprosthetic joint infection, and a recent clinical trial demonstrated that vitamin D supplementation decreases the risk of influenza A infection (Ginde et al., 2009; Maier et al., 2014; Urashima et al., 2010). Dobnig et al. (2008) showed in their prospective cohort study of 3258 patients that patients with deficient vitamin D levels were twice as likely to die over a 7-year follow-up than patients with normal serum 25-OH-D levels. Vitamin D levels below 17.8 ng/mL were shown to increase the risk of death by 26% of all mortalities in the general population. Matthews et al. showed an inverse relation with the length of hospital stay and vitamin D levels in surgical patients admitted to the intensive care unit. With more than 250 patients evaluated, the mean length of stay for patients with severe vitamin D deficiency (<13 ng/mL) was 13.33 days compared to 5.17 days for patients with vitamin D levels above 27 ng/mL (Matthews et al., 2012). The length of stay of 253 patients of a geriatric acute care unit was inversely associated with low vitamin D levels. Helard et al. (2013) reported that patients with vitamin D levels below 50 nmol/L were hospitalized 3 days longer on average than patients with vitamin D levels above 50 nmol/L. Thus, vitamin D not only is important to bone health but also plays an important role in immunomodulation, the regulation of inflammation and cytokines, cell proliferation, cell differentiation, apoptosis, angiogenesis, muscle strength, and muscle contraction.

References

Adams, J.S., Clemens, T.L., Parrish, J.A., Holick, M.F., 1982. Vitamin-D synthesis and metabolism after ultraviolet irradiation of normal and vitamin-D-deficient subjects. N. Engl. J. Med. 306, 722–725.

Annweiler, C., Beauchet, O., 2015. Questioning vitamin D status of elderly fallers and nonfallers: a meta-analysis to address a 'forgotten step'. J. Intern. Med. 277, 16–44.

Annweiler, C., Montero-Odasso, M., Schott, A.M., Berrut, G., Fantino, B., Beauchet, O., 2010. Fall prevention and vitamin D in the elderly: an overview of the key role of the non-bone effects. J. Neuroeng. Rehabil. 7, 50.

Annweiler, C., Pochic, S., Fantino, B., Legrand, E., Bataille, R., Montero-Odasso, M., et al., 2010. Serum vitamin D concentration and short-term mortality among geriatric inpatients in acute care settings. Adv. Ther. 27, 245–249.

Baggerly, C.A., Cuomo, R.E., French, C.B., Garland, C.F., Gorham, E.D., Grant, W.B., et al., 2015. Sunlight and vitamin D: necessary for public health. J. Am. Coll. Nutr. 34, 359–365.

Beauchet, O., Helard, L., Montero-Odasso, M., de Decker, L., Berrut, G., Annweiler, C., 2012. Hypovitaminosis D in geriatric inpatients: a marker of severity of chronic diseases. Aging Clin. Exp. Res. 24, 188–192.

Beauchet, O., Launay, C.P., Maunoury, F., de Decker, L., Fantino, B., Annweiler, C., 2013. Association between vitamin D deficiency and long hospital stay in geriatric acute care unit: results from a pilot cohort study. Aging Clin. Exp. Res. 25, 107–109.

Bischoff-Ferrari, H.A., Dawson-Hughes, B., Willett, W.C., Staehelin, H.B., Bazemore, M.G., Zee, R.Y., et al., 2004. Effect of Vitamin D on falls: a meta-analysis. JAMA 291, 1999–2006.

Bischoff-Ferrari, H.A., Willett, W.C., Wong, J.B., Giovannucci, E., Dietrich, T., Dawson-Hughes, B., 2005. Fracture prevention with vitamin D supplementation: a meta-analysis of randomized controlled trials. JAMA 293, 2257–2264.

Bischoff-Ferrari, H.A., Giovannucci, E., Willett, W.C., Dietrich, T., Dawson-Hughes, B., 2006. Estimation of optimal serum concentrations of 25-hydroxyvitamin D for multiple health outcomes. Am. J. Clin. Nutr. 84, 18–28.

Bischoff-Ferrari, H.A., Can, U., Staehelin, H.B., Platz, A., Henschkowski, J., Michel, B.A., et al., 2008. Severe vitamin D deficiency in Swiss hip fracture patients. Bone 42, 597–602.

Bischoff-Ferrari, H.A., Dawson-Hughes, B., Staehelin, H.B., Orav, J.E., Stuck, A.E., Theiler, R., et al., 2009a. Fall prevention with supplemental and active forms of vitamin D: a meta-analysis of randomised controlled trials. BMJ 339, b3692.

Bischoff-Ferrari, H.A., Willett, W.C., Wong, J.B., Stuck, A.E., Staehelin, H.B., Orav, E.J., et al., 2009b. Prevention of nonvertebral fractures with oral vitamin D and dose dependency: a meta-analysis of randomized controlled trials. Arch. Intern. Med. 169, 551–561.

Bischoff-Ferrari, H.A., Willett, W.C., Orav, E.J., Lips, P., Meunier, P.J., Lyons, R.A., et al., 2012. A pooled analysis of vitamin D dose requirements for fracture prevention. N. Engl. J. Med. 367, 40–49.

Bruyere, O., Malaise, O., Neuprez, A., Collette, J., Reginster, J.Y., 2007. Prevalence of vitamin D inadequacy in European postmenopausal women. Curr. Med. Res. Opin. 23, 1939–1944.

Chapuy, M.C., Meunier, P.J., 1996. Prevention of secondary hyperparathyroidism and hip fracture in elderly women with calcium and vitamin D3 supplements. Osteoporos. Int. 6 (suppl. 3), 60–63.

Clemens, T.L., Adams, J.S., Henderson, S.L., Holick, M.F., 1982. Increased skin pigment reduces the capacity of skin to synthesise vitamin D3. Lancet 1, 74–76.

Cooper, C., Campion, G., Melton 3rd, L.J., 1992. Hip fractures in the elderly: a world-wide projection. Osteoporos. Int. 2, 285–289.

Cummings, S.R., Browner, W.S., Bauer, D., Stone, K., Ensrud, K., Jamal, S., et al., 1998. Endogenous hormones and the risk of hip and vertebral fractures among older women. Study of Osteoporotic Fractures Research Group. N. Engl. J. Med. 339, 733–738.

Dawson-Hughes, B., Heaney, R.P., Holick, M.F., Lips, P., Meunier, P.J., Vieth, R., 2005. Estimates of optimal vitamin D status. Osteoporos. Int. 16, 713–716.

Dhanwal, D.K., Kochupillai, N., Gupta, N., Cooper, C., Dennison, E.M., 2010. Hypovitaminosis D and bone mineral metabolism and bone density in hyperthyroidism. J. Clin. Densitom. 13, 462–466.

Di Monaco, M., Vallero, F., Castiglioni, C., Di Monaco, R., Tappero, R., 2011. Low levels of 25-hydroxyvitamin D are associated with the occurrence of concomitant upper limb fractures in older women who sustain a fall-related fracture of the hip. Maturitas 68, 79–82.

Dobnig, H., Pilz, S., Scharnagl, H., Renner, W., Seelhorst, U., Wellnitz, B., et al., 2008. Independent association of low serum 25-hydroxyvitamin d and 1,25-dihydroxyvitamin d levels with all-cause and cardiovascular mortality. Arch. Intern. Med. 168, 1340–1349.

Dowdy, J.C., Sayre, R.M., Holick, M.F., 2010. Holick's rule and vitamin D from sunlight. J. Steroid. Biochem. Mol. Biol. 121, 328–330.

Drinka, P., 1996. Vitamin D deficiency in older people. J. Am. Geriatr. Soc. 44, 333.

El Maghraoui, A., Ouzzif, Z., Mounach, A., Rezqi, A., Achemlal, L., Bezza, A., et al., 2012. Hypovitaminosis D and prevalent asymptomatic vertebral fractures in Moroccan postmenopausal women. BMC. Womens Health 12, 11.

Gerdhem, P., Ringsberg, K.A., Obrant, K.J., Akesson, K., 2005. Association between 25-hydroxy vitamin D levels, physical activity, muscle strength and fractures in the prospective population-based OPRA Study of Elderly Women. Osteoporos. Int. 16, 1425–1431.

Ginde, A.A., Mansbach, J.M., Camargo Jr., C.A., 2009. Association between serum 25-hydroxyvitamin D level and upper respiratory tract infection in the Third National Health and Nutrition Examination Survey. Arch. Intern. Med. 169, 384–390.

Giovannucci, E., Liu, Y., Hollis, B.W., Rimm, E.B., 2008. 25-hydroxyvitamin D and risk of myocardial infarction in men: a prospective study. Arch. Intern. Med. 168, 1174–1180.

Glowacki, J., Hurwitz, S., Thornhill, T.S., Kelly, M., LeBoff, M.S., 2003. Osteoporosis and vitamin-D deficiency among postmenopausal women with osteoarthritis undergoing total hip arthroplasty. J. Bone Joint Surg. Am. 85-A, 2371–2377.

Godar, D.E., Pope, S.J., Grant, W.B., Holick, M.F., 2011. Solar UV doses of adult Americans and vitamin D(3) production. Dermatoendocrinology 3, 243–250.
Gordon, C.M., DePeter, K.C., Feldman, H.A., Grace, E., Emans, S.J., 2004. Prevalence of vitamin D deficiency among healthy adolescents. Arch. Pediatr. Adolesc. Med. 158, 531–537.
Grant, A.M., Avenell, A., Campbell, M.K., McDonald, A.M., MacLennan, G.S., McPherson, G.C., et al., 2005. Oral vitamin D3 and calcium for secondary prevention of low-trauma fractures in elderly people (Randomised Evaluation of Calcium or vitamin D, RECORD): a randomised placebo-controlled trial. Lancet 365, 1621–1628.
Grant, W.B., Cross, H.S., Garland, C.F., Gorham, E.D., Moan, J., Peterlik, M., et al., 2009. Estimated benefit of increased vitamin D status in reducing the economic burden of disease in western Europe. Prog. Biophys. Mol. Biol. 99, 104–113.
Guardia, G., Parikh, N., Eskridge, T., Phillips, E., Divine, G., Rao, D.S., 2008. Prevalence of vitamin D depletion among subjects seeking advice on osteoporosis: a five-year cross-sectional study with public health implications. Osteoporos. Int. 19, 13–19.
Hamilton, B., 2010. Vitamin D and human skeletal muscle. Scand. J. Med. Sci. Sports 20, 182–190.
Helard, L., Mateus-Hamdan, L., Beauchet, O., Annweiler, C., 2013. Hypovitaminosis D in geriatric acute care unit: a biomarker of longer length of stay. Dis. Markers 35, 525–529.
Hewison, M., 2010. Vitamin D and the immune system: new perspectives on an old theme. Endocrinol. Metab. Clin. North Am. 39, 365–379.
Hill, T.R., Aspray, T.J., Francis, R.M., 2013. Vitamin D and bone health outcomes in older age. Proc. Nutr. Soc. 72, 372–380.
Hintzpeter, B., Mensink, G.B., Thierfelder, W., Muller, M.J., Scheidt-Nave, C., 2008. Vitamin D status and health correlates among German adults. Eur. J. Clin. Nutr. 62, 1079–1089.
Hirani, V., Primatesta, P., 2005. Vitamin D concentrations among people aged 65 years and over living in private households and institutions in England: population survey. Age Ageing 34, 485–491.
Hoffmann, M.R., Senior, P.A., Mager, D.R., 2015. Vitamin D supplementation and health-related quality of life: a systematic review of the literature. J. Acad. Nutr. Diet 115, 406–418.
Holick, M.F., 2007. Vitamin D deficiency. N. Engl. J. Med. 357, 266–281.
Holick, M.F., DeLuca, H.F., 1974. Vitamin D metabolism. Ann. Rev. Med. 25, 349–367.
Jackson, R.D., LaCroix, A.Z., Gass, M., Wallace, R.B., Robbins, J., Lewis, C.E., et al., 2006. Calcium plus vitamin D supplementation and the risk of fractures. N. Engl. J. Med. 354, 669–683.
LeBoff, M.S., Kohlmeier, L., Hurwitz, S., Franklin, J., Wright, J., Glowacki, J., 1999. Occult vitamin D deficiency in postmenopausal US women with acute hip fracture. JAMA 281, 1505–1511.
LeBoff, M.S., Hawkes, W.G., Glowacki, J., Yu-Yahiro, J., Hurwitz, S., Magaziner, J., 2008. Vitamin D-deficiency and post-fracture changes in lower extremity function and falls in women with hip fractures. Osteoporos. Int. 19, 1283–1290.
Lips, P., 2001. Vitamin D deficiency and secondary hyperparathyroidism in the elderly: consequences for bone loss and fractures and therapeutic implications. Endocr. Rev. 22, 477–501.
Lips, P., 2007. Vitamin D status and nutrition in Europe and Asia. J. Steroid. Biochem. Mol. Biol. 103, 620–625.
Lopes, J.B., Danilevicius, C.F., Takayama, L., Caparbo, V.F., Scazufca, M., Bonfa, E., et al., 2009. Vitamin D insufficiency: a risk factor to vertebral fractures in community-dwelling elderly women. Maturitas 64, 218–222.
Lyles, K.W., Gold, D.T., Shipp, K.M., Pieper, C.F., Martinez, S., Mulhausen, P.L., 1993. Association of osteoporotic vertebral compression fractures with impaired functional status. Am. J. Med. 94, 595–601.
Maier, G.S., Jakob, P., Horas, K., Roth, K.E., Kurth, A.A., Maus, U., 2013a. Vitamin D deficiency in orthopaedic patients: a single center analysis. Acta Orthop. Belg. 79, 587–591.
Maier, S., Sidelnikov, E., Dawson-Hughes, B., Egli, A., Theiler, R., Platz, A., et al., 2013b. Before and after hip fracture, vitamin D deficiency may not be treated sufficiently. Osteoporos. Int. 24, 2765–2773.
Maier, G.S., Horas, K., Seeger, J.B., Roth, K.E., Kurth, A.A., Maus, U., 2014. Is there an association between periprosthetic joint infection and low vitamin D levels? Int. Orthop. 38, 1499–1504.
Maier, G.S., Horas, K., Seeger, J.B., Roth, K.E., Kurth, A.A., Maus, U., 2015a. Vitamin D insufficiency in the elderly orthopaedic patient: an epidemic phenomenon. Int. Orthop. 39, 787–792.
Maier, G.S., Seeger, J.B., Horas, K., Roth, K.E., Kurth, A.A., Maus, U., 2015b. The prevalence of vitamin D deficiency in patients with vertebral fragility fractures. Bone Joint J 97-B, 89–93.
Matthews, L.R., Ahmed, Y., Wilson, K.L., Griggs, D.D., Danner, O.K., 2012. Worsening severity of vitamin D deficiency is associated with increased length of stay, surgical intensive care unit cost, and mortality rate in surgical intensive care unit patients. Am. J. Surg. 204, 37–43.
Mattila, C., Knekt, P., Mannisto, S., Rissanen, H., Laaksonen, M.A., Montonen, J., et al., 2007. Serum 25-hydroxyvitamin D concentration and subsequent risk of type 2 diabetes. Diabetes Care 30, 2569–2570.
McCarroll, K.G., Robinson, D.J., Coughlan, A., Healy, M., Kenny, R.A., Cunningham, C., 2012. Vitamin D and orthostatic hypotension. Age Ageing 41, 810–813.
Menkes, D.B., Lancaster, K., Grant, M., Marsh, R.W., Dean, P., du Toit, S.A., 2012. Vitamin D status of psychiatric inpatients in New Zealand's Waikato region. BMC Psychiatry 12, 68.
Mithal, A., Wahl, D.A., Bonjour, J.P., Burckhardt, P., Dawson-Hughes, B., Eisman, J.A., et al., 2009. Global vitamin D status and determinants of hypovitaminosis D. Osteoporos. Int. 20, 1807–1820.
Nakamura, K., Saito, T., Oyama, M., Oshiki, R., Kobayashi, R., Nishiwaki, T., et al., 2011. Vitamin D sufficiency is associated with low incidence of limb and vertebral fractures in community-dwelling elderly Japanese women: the Muramatsu Study. Osteoporos. Int. 22, 97–103.
Nurmi, I., Kaukonen, J.P., Luthje, P., Naboulsi, H., Tanninen, S., Kataja, M., et al., 2005. Half of the patients with an acute hip fracture suffer from hypovitaminosis D: a prospective study in southeastern Finland. Osteoporos. Int. 16, 2018–2024.
Nuti, R., Martini, G., Valenti, R., Gambera, D., Gennari, L., Salvadori, S., et al., 2004. Vitamin D status and bone turnover in women with acute hip fracture. Clin. Orthop. Relat. Res., 208–213.
Perez-Lopez, F.R., Chedraui, P., Fernandez-Alonso, A.M., 2011. Vitamin D and aging: beyond calcium and bone metabolism. Maturitas 69, 27–36.
Pramyothin, P., Holick, M.F., 2012. Vitamin D supplementation: guidelines and evidence for subclinical deficiency. Curr. Opin. Gastroenterol. 28, 139–150.

Priemel, M., von Domarus, C., Klatte, T.O., Kessler, S., Schlie, J., Meier, S., et al., 2010. Bone mineralization defects and vitamin D deficiency: histomorphometric analysis of iliac crest bone biopsies and circulating 25-hydroxyvitamin D in 675 patients. J Bone Miner Res. 25, 305–312.

Rizzoli, R., Boonen, S., Brandi, M.L., Bruyere, O., Cooper, C., Kanis, J.A., et al., 2010. Vitamin D supplementation in elderly or postmenopausal women: a 2013 update of the 2008 recommendations from the European Society for Clinical and Economic Aspects of Osteoporosis and Osteoarthritis (ESCEO). Curr. Med. Res. Opin. 29, 305–313.

Sakuma, M., Endo, N., Hagino, H., Harada, A., Matsui, Y., Nakano, T., et al., 2011. Serum 25-hydroxyvitamin D status in hip and spine-fracture patients in Japan. J. Orthop. Sci. 16, 418–423.

Schilling, S., 2012. Epidemic vitamin D deficiency among patients in an elderly care rehabilitation facility. Dtsch. Arztebl. Int. 109, 33–38.

Soysal, P., Yay, A., Isik, A.T., 2014. Does vitamin D deficiency increase orthostatic hypotension risk in the elderly patients? Arch. Gerontol. Geriatr. 59, 74–77.

Sutra Del Galy, Bertrand, A., Bigot, M., Abraham, F., Thomlinson, P., Paccalin, R., et al., 2009. Vitamin D insufficiency and acute care in geriatric inpatients. J. Am. Geriatr. Soc. 57, 1721–1723.

Urashima, M., Segawa, T., Okazaki, M., Kurihara, M., Wada, Y., Ida, H., 2010. Randomized trial of vitamin D supplementation to prevent seasonal influenza A in schoolchildren. Am. J. Clin. Nutr. 91, 1255–1260.

van Schoor, N.M., Lips, P., 2011. Worldwide vitamin D status. Best Pract. Res. Clin. Endocrinol. Metab. 25, 671–680.

Webb, A.R., Kline, L., Holick, M.F., 1988. Influence of season and latitude on the cutaneous synthesis of vitamin D3: exposure to winter sunlight in Boston and Edmonton will not promote vitamin D3 synthesis in human skin. J. Clin. Endocrinol. Metab. 67, 373–378.

Zafeiris, C.P., Lyritis, G.P., Papaioannou, N.A., Gratsias, P.E., Galanos, A., Chatziioannou, S.N., et al., 2012. Hypovitaminosis D as a risk factor of subsequent vertebral fractures after kyphoplasty. Spine J. 12, 304–312.

CHAPTER

14

Vitamins and Minerals in Older Adults: Causes, Diagnosis, and Treatment of Deficiency

Jennifer Doley

Carondelet St. Mary's Hospital, Tucson, AZ, United States

INTRODUCTION

Micronutrients have been studied for their role in the prevention of many disease states, although evidence for or against routine supplementation is mixed. The US Preventive Services Task Force released a statement specifically on cancer and cardiovascular disease, stating that there is insufficient evidence to assess the harms and benefits of single or multivitamin and mineral supplements, with the exception of vitamin E. The task force concluded that vitamin E has no effect on either disease (Moyer, 2014). This chapter will thus focus on the cause, diagnosis, and treatment of micronutrient deficiencies in older adults rather than on disease prevention.

Vitamins and minerals play an important role in health during aging, and deficiencies can affect both physical and mental functions. Consuming enough micronutrients can be a challenge for some populations, especially the elderly, as a host of physiological and cognitive age-related changes can affect intake, digestion, absorption, and metabolism of these nutrients. Many micronutrient deficiencies can result in impairment of physical and cognitive functions, which can then cause further nutritional decline.

As with any disease or condition, prevention of micronutrient deficiency is ideal; thus, it is important for the clinician to understand micronutrient needs in older adults and to develop the skills necessary to assess dietary intake and identify factors that may impair intake, absorption and utilization of these nutrients. The ability to identify deficiencies and prescribe appropriate food and supplement regimens to treat deficiency is also crucial.

Vitamins

Vitamins are organic compounds required in limited amounts for normal growth and metabolism, and are typically categorized as fat soluble or water soluble. Thirteen compounds are recognized as vitamins; while choline is not technically classified as a vitamin, it is an essential nutrient and will be included in this review (Mahan et al., 2012; Mueller, 2012; NIH, 2016).

Most vitamins are actually groups of structurally related compounds called *vitamers* that have similar activities. For example, vitamin D comprises the vitamers calcitriol, ergocalciferol, and cholecalciferol. Vitamins are necessary for a wide variety of biochemical functions; they function as antioxidants and as cofactors for many enzymatic reactions and serve as regulators of mineral metabolism. See Table 14.1 for a list of common functions of vitamins (Mahan et al., 2012; Mueller, 2012; NIH, 2016).

Nutrition and Functional Foods for Healthy Aging.
DOI: http://dx.doi.org/10.1016/B978-0-12-805376-8.00014-9

TABLE 14.1 Common Functions of Vitamins (Mahan et al., 2012; Mueller, 2012; NIH, 2016)

Vitamin	Common Functions
A	Vision, gene expression, reproduction, immune function
D	Maintenance of serum calcium and phosphorus levels, bone health
E	Antioxidant
K	Synthesis of proteins involved in blood clotting and bone metabolism
B_1 (thiamin)	Carbohydrate and branched-chain amino acid metabolism, nerve function
B_2 (riboflavin)	Carbohydrate, amino acid, and lipid metabolism; conversion of B_6 to its active form
B_3 (niacin)	Carbohydrate, amino acid, and lipid metabolism
B_6 (pyridoxine)	Carbohydrate, amino acid, and lipid metabolism; hemoglobin and neurotransmitter synthesis; immune function
B_{12} (cobalamin)	Nucleic and amino acid metabolism, red blood cell maturation, conversion of folate to active form
C (ascorbic acid)	Collagen, carnitine, and neurotransmitter synthesis; antioxidant and immune functions; absorption of nonheme iron; cholesterol hydroxylation into bile acids
Folic acid	Nucleic and amino acid metabolism, DNA and red blood cell synthesis
Pantothenic acid	Carbohydrate, amino acid, and lipid metabolism; heme and sterol synthesis
Biotin	Carbohydrate, amino acid, and lipid metabolism
Choline	Neurotransmitter and homocysteine synthesis, cell membrane signaling, lipid transport

Minerals

The term *mineral* is a misnomer; dietary minerals are actually chemical elements. The four most common *elements*—hydrogen, carbon, nitrogen, and oxygen—serve organic functions. Other elements known to be necessary for humans include sodium, magnesium, phosphorus, sulfur, chloride, potassium, and calcium. Additional elements considered essential in much smaller amounts are called *trace elements* and include chromium, manganese, iron, cobalt, nickel, copper, zinc, selenium, bromine, molybdenum, and iodine. Some elements are suspected to play a role in human health, although there is insufficient evidence to clearly describe their biochemical functions or needed amounts. These include lithium, boron, fluorine, silicon, vanadium, and arsenic (Mahan et al., 2012; Mueller, 2012; NIH, 2016).

Some elements such as sodium and potassium function primarily as electrolytes; others such as magnesium and calcium serve a structural function in addition to acting as electrolytes. Many minerals are required for the production and function of a wide variety of enzymes necessary for normal metabolic reactions. Other mineral functions include hormone synthesis, antioxidant activity, cell signaling, and energy production. See Table 14.2 for a list of common mineral functions (Mahan et al., 2012; Mueller, 2012; NIH, 2016).

NEEDS

The US Department of Agriculture has established a recommended dietary allowance (RDA) and estimated average requirement (EAR) for most nutrients. The RDA is an estimate of the amount of a nutrient sufficient to meet the needs of 97–98% of a population, while the EAR is the estimated requirement for 50% of a population. There is insufficient evidence to recommend an RDA for some nutrients, thus adequate intakes (AIs) are established, which are quantities believed to be sufficient to meet the needs of most individuals, although inadequate data prevent specificity in determining what percentage of the population would most benefit. RDAs, EARs, and AIs are divided into age and sex categories; see Tables 14.3 and 14.4 for the RDAs and AIs of vitamins and minerals for older adults (USDA, 2016).

Requirements for some micronutrients increase with age, most notably vitamin D and calcium, due in part to the increased incidence and risk for osteopenia and osteoporosis in older adults. Iron requirements decrease for older women because they are no longer of childbearing age. Although the RDAs for other nutrients remain unchanged for older populations, some elders may have needs higher than the RDAs for select micronutrients due to impairments in their absorption or metabolism (USDA, 2016).

TABLE 14.2 Common Functions of Minerals (Mahan et al., 2012; Mueller, 2012; NIH, 2016)

Mineral	Common Functions
Calcium (Ca)	Structural component of bones and teeth, cell membrane integrity, neuromuscular activity, endocrine secretory function, blood coagulation
Chloride (Cl)	Regulation of water distribution, maintenance of acid–base balance, nerve-impulse transmission
Copper (Cu)	Red blood cell formation, iron utilization, energy production, connective tissue synthesis, antioxidation
Iodine (I)	Thyroid hormone synthesis, nerve muscle function, nutrient metabolism
Iron (Fe)	Formation of hemoglobin and myoglobin
Magnesium (Mg)	Structural component of bones; enzyme activation for glucose, DNA, and protein metabolism; fatty acid synthesis; cell membrane potential—muscle and nerve function; cardiovascular excitability
Manganese (Mn)	Constituent of some metalloenzymes; enzyme activation
Molybdenum (Mo)	Enzyme component
Phosphorus (P)	Structural component of bones and cell membranes; pH maintenance; glycolysis; muscle and nerve function
Potassium (K)	Electrolyte, protein, and glycogen synthesis, membrane potential—muscle and nerve function
Selenium (Se)	Cofactor for glutathione and iodine; thyroid function
Sodium (Na)	Regulation of water distribution; membrane potential—muscle and nerve function; active transport of molecules across cell membranes
Zinc (Zn)	Protein synthesis; immunity; growth of genital organs

TABLE 14.3 RDAs or AIs for Vitamins for Older Adults (USDA, 2016)

Fat Soluble	RDA Men	RDA Women
Vitamin A	900 µg	700 µg
Vitamin D	600 IU (50–70 year)	600 IU (50–70 year)
	800 IU (>70 year)	800 IU (>70 year)
Vitamin E	15 mg	15 mg
Vitamin K[a]	120 µg	90 µg
Vitamin B_1	1.2 mg	1.1 mg
Vitamin B_2	1.3 mg	1.1 mg
Vitamin B_3	16 mg	14 mg
Vitamin B_6	1.7 mg	1.5 mg
Vitamin B_{12}	2.4 µg	2.4 µg
Vitamin C	90 mg	75 mg
Folic acid	400 µg	400 µg
Pantothenic acid[a]	5 mg	5 mg
Biotin[a]	30 µg	30 µg
Choline[a]	550 mg	425 mg

[a]*Signifies AI.*

CAUSES OF DEFICIENCY

Micronutrient deficiencies can generally be categorized as primary (caused by inadequate intake) or secondary (caused by a medical condition or medication that interferes with the absorption or metabolism of the vitamin or mineral). However, the origin of deficiency is often multifactorial; a specific disease or host of medical problems can reduce food intake, increase needs, decrease absorption and impair metabolism, all of which can contribute

TABLE 14.4 RDAs or AIs for Minerals for Older Adults (USDA, 2016)

Mineral	RDA Men	RDA Women
Calcium	1000 mg (51–70 year) 1200 mg (>70 year)	1200 mg (≥51 year)
Chloride[a]	2 g	1.8 g
Copper	900 μg	900 μg
Iodine	150 μg	150 μg
Iron	8 mg	8 mg
Magnesium	420 mg	320 mg
Manganese[a]	2.3 mg	1.8 mg
Molybdenum	45 μg	45 μg
Phosphorus	700 mg	700 mg
Potassium[a]	4.7 g	4.7 g
Selenium	55 μg	55 μg
Sodium[a]	1.3 g	1.2 g
Zinc	11 mg	11 mg

[a]*Signifies AI.*

to the development of micronutrient deficiencies. See Tables 14.5 and 14.6 for micronutrient deficiency risk factors (Montgomery et al., 2014).

Insufficient Intake

Micronutrient intake among older adults, as with other populations, can vary significantly. However, in a recent systematic review of 37 studies involving more than 28,000 community-dwelling older adults in 20 Western countries, researchers concluded that a significant percentage of older men and women had inadequate intake of many micronutrients—especially thiamin, riboflavin, vitamin D, calcium, magnesium, and selenium—when compared to the EAR (ter Borg et al., 2015). Nutrient intake assessment methods varied, making study comparisons challenging, but these data are compelling and suggest adequate micronutrient intake is lacking in many older adults.

The most significant factor affecting micronutrient intake, in the United States and worldwide, is socioeconomic status. The elder population suffers more socioeconomic hardships than younger adults (DiMaria-Ghalili, 2014). Both limited income and access to transportation can reduce the ability to purchase and consume a variety of micronutrient-rich foods (Allen et al., 2006).

Older adults face physical barriers to consuming sufficient amounts of micronutrients. Normal or common physiological changes associated with aging often result in reduced intake of nutrient-rich foods, especially fruits, vegetables, and meats. Changes include poor dentition, altered or decreased taste and smell sensations, decreased appetite, and difficulty chewing and swallowing (DiMaria-Ghalili, 2014). Functional limitations leading to decreased ability to obtain and prepare food are also a concern in the aged population. Functional capacity often declines with age, and the cause is usually multifactorial. Medical conditions such as arthritis, pain, neuromuscular dysfunction, and age-related sarcopenia can all contribute to decreased mobility, physical activity, and manual dexterity.

Psychological problems, such as depression and isolation, and cognitive issues such as dementia are more common in elderly populations and contribute to significant reductions in micronutrient consumption. Isolation and depression are associated with reduced appetite, while individuals with dementia often refuse or forget to eat meals (DiFrancesco et al., 2007; DiMaria-Ghalili, 2014).

The incidence of many chronic health conditions such as cancer, diabetes, heart disease, and hypertension increases as people age. Specific medications necessary for the treatment of these conditions, as well as the total volume of medications taken, can contribute to diminished food intake via decreased appetite, early satiety, taste changes, and GI disturbances such as diarrhea, constipation, and nausea. These challenges can result in the reduction of both the quality and total volume of food consumed (DiMaria-Ghalili, 2014). See Table 14.7 for conditions that reduce intake and their potential causes.

TABLE 14.5 Risk Factors for Vitamin Deficiencies (Mueller, 2012; Allen et al., 2006; Mahan et al., 2012; NIH, 2016; Grober and Kisters, 2012)

Vitamin	Deficiency Risk Factors[a]
A	Severe zinc deficiency, chronic alcoholism, severe malnutrition, poor intake of dairy products
D	Limited exposure to sunlight, kidney and liver disease (limits activation of vitamin D), darkly pigmented skin, obesity (vitamin D sequestered in fat cells), medications (antiepileptics, antiretrovirals, glucocorticoids), liver disease, poor intake of dairy products, older age (less ultraviolet exposure, inadequate intake, reduced cutaneous synthesis)
E	Fat malabsorption[a]
K	Fat malabsorption[a]
B_1	Chronic alcoholism, liver disease, AIDS; poor intake of animal and dairy products and legumes; older age (inadequate intake, combination of chronic diseases with concomitant intake of multiple medications, decreased absorption); chronic or high-dose use of diuretic medications
B_2	Chronic alcoholism, liver disease, poor intake of animal and dairy products; usually associated with other B vitamin deficiencies
B_3	Poor intake of animal and dairy products
B_6	Chronic alcoholism, liver disease, poor intake of animal and dairy products, end-stage renal disease or chronic renal insufficiency, autoimmune disorders, long-term use of antiepileptic medications; usually associated with other B vitamin deficiencies
B_{12}	Chronic alcoholism, poor intake of animal and dairy products, decreased or absent gastric acid production (use of proton pump inhibitors, gastrectomy, gastric bypass, *Helicobacter pylori* overgrowth), ileal resection
C	Poor intake of fruits and vegetables rich in vitamin C, smoking (due to increased needs)
Folic acid	Chronic alcoholism, liver disease; poor intake of fruits, vegetables, legumes, and dairy productions; medications (phenytoin, cholestyramine, amphotericin B, metformin)
Pantothenic acid	Severe malnutrition; usually associated with other B vitamin deficiencies
Biotin	Severe malnutrition; usually associated with other B vitamin deficiencies
Choline	Severe malnutrition; usually associated with other B vitamin deficiencies

[a]All micronutrients are affected by gastrointestinal (GI) malabsorptive conditions, including celiac disease, short bowel syndrome, inflammatory bowel disease, pancreatic enzyme insufficiency, and gastric bypass surgery.

TABLE 14.6 Risk Factors for Mineral Deficiencies (Mueller, 2012; Allen et al., 2006; Mahan et al., 2012; NIH, 2016)

Minerals	Deficiency Risk Factors[a]
Calcium	Poor intake of dairy products; older age, especially postmenopausal women; medications (glucocorticoids)
Copper	Increased GI losses (chronic diarrhea), excess iron or zinc supplementation
Iodine	Residence in areas with iodine-poor soil, individuals who do not use iodized salt, long-term administration of iodine-free parenteral nutrition; excess intake of foods high in goitrogens, compounds that inhibit iodine uptake by the thyroid (soy, cassava, and cruciferous vegetables); iron or vitamin A deficiency (also goitrogenic)
Iron	Blood loss, vegetarianism and veganism, decreased or absent gastric acid production, poor vitamin C intake, excess copper or zinc supplementation
Magnesium	Poor intake of magnesium-rich foods, older age, long-term use diuretic medication; acute hypomagnesemia may occur as a result of electrolyte shifts such as those seen in refeeding syndrome
Phosphorus	Poor intake of phosphorus-rich foods, long-term use of phosphorus binders as seen in those with chronic renal disease; acute hypophosphatemia may occur as a result of electrolyte shifts such as those seen in refeeding syndrome
Selenium	HIV disease, residence in areas with selenium-poor soil
Zinc	Trauma, burns, surgery, increased GI losses (chronic diarrhea), chronic alcoholism, poor intake of animal and dairy products, renal disease, excess iron or copper supplementation

[a]All micronutrients are affected by GI malabsorptive conditions, which include celiac disease, short bowel syndrome, inflammatory bowel disease, pancreatic enzyme insufficiency, and gastric bypass.

TABLE 14.7 Common Causes of Decreased Food Intake in Older Adults

Symptom	Potential Causes
Difficulty chewing	Poorly fitting dentures, poor dentition, poor oral hygiene, xerostemia, functional decline
Difficulty swallowing	Weakness, functional decline, dysphagia as a result of neurological dysfunction or injury
Taste and smell changes	Aging, oral infections, poor oral hygiene, zinc deficiency, xerostemia, medications, some chronic diseases, smoking
Poor appetite	Aging, medications, constipation, chronic disease, depression
Self-restriction	Strict adherence to therapeutic diets for disease management; constipation, diarrhea, or other GI symptoms; incontinence

Food Quality

Besides individual conditions that reduce the ability to procure or consume nutrient-rich foods, the other key factor influencing intake is the micronutrient content of the foods consumed. Nutrient content is influenced by food-industry practices, cooking methods, and the environment in which the food is grown.

Food-production practices, including harvesting, transportation, and storage, can subject foods to light and oxygen exposure and time delays between harvest and consumption. Time, light, and oxygen exposure accelerate the ripening process as well as nutrient degradation. Freezing results in minimal micronutrient loss; in addition, produce is typically frozen shortly after harvest, thus maximizing micronutrient content (USDA, 2007). Frozen products may be ideal for some older adults, especially if the frequency with which they can obtain food is limited. Canning may preserve micronutrients if canned shortly after harvest, but minerals can leach from food into surrounding liquid, which is often discarded. Furthermore, adding salt during the canning process may alter the solubility of organometallic compounds, which can affect their bioavailability (Wapnir, 1998).

Other food-industry practices affect micronutrient concentration. Food *enrichment* is the practice of adding micronutrients back to a food product that were lost during processing, while *fortification* adds additional micronutrients not present (or present in small amounts) prior to processing. Food fortification has been practiced in industrialized nations for many years; common fortification practices include B vitamins and folic acid in grains, vitamins A and D in milk, iodine in salt, calcium in orange juice and soy products, and a variety of micronutrients in cereals, bottled water, and other beverages. Although less commonly utilized in developing countries, fortification practices including the use of sugar fortified with vitamin A in Central America and iron-fortified fish and soy sauces in Asia have successfully reduced the prevalence of some micronutrient deficiencies (Allen et al., 2006).

Food-preparation methods that utilize higher temperatures, longer cooking times, and large amounts of water or oil (which is then discarded) will increase the loss of some vitamins and minerals, most notably vitamin C. Other factors affecting nutrient retention include pH and exposure to air and light (Bergstrom, 1994). Because of the short cooking time and limited use of water associated with steaming and microwaving, these methods are recommended to minimize micronutrient losses.

The mineral content of plants depends on the mineral concentration of the soil in which it is grown, thus impacting the micronutrient intake of those who consume the plant. Although data are limited for many minerals, research has shown that soil concentrations of zinc and selenium are low in many areas of the world, including China, Africa, India, and parts of North and South America. Low soil concentrations directly correlate with rates of human zinc and selenium deficiency in developing countries but not in industrialized nations. Scientists believe this is due to the wider dietary variety and use of supplements seen in industrialized countries (Udo de Haes et al., 2012). Thus, individuals in these geographic areas may be more likely to have insufficient intake of these minerals if they do not use supplements and lack variety in their diets.

Impaired Absorption

Absorptive issues render older individuals more vulnerable to micronutrient deficiency, even in those whose intakes are considered sufficient for most adults. Micronutrient absorption is affected by several factors, including age, diseases and conditions that affect the GI tract, medications, and the form and amount of the micronutrient consumed. Most micronutrients are largely absorbed in the duodenum and jejunum, with the exception of vitamin B_{12}, which is absorbed in the ileum; thus conditions affecting the proximal GI tract are more likely to result in micronutrient malabsorption.

Human genetic differences may also result in significant variations in micronutrient absorption, as well as nutrient needs and metabolism. Although growing rapidly, the field of nutrigenetics is still in its infancy and insufficient data preclude any changes to current clinical practice related to micronutrients (Baumler, 2012).

Fat-soluble vitamins are absorbed with dietary fat; malabsorption of these vitamins is rare except in conditions resulting in fat malabsorption. Even in cases of decreased absorption, fat-soluble vitamins, with the exception of vitamin D, are rarely deficient in residents of developed countries because of their long-term storage in fatty tissues (Mahan et al., 2012; Mueller, 2012; NIH, 2016).

Absorption of water-soluble vitamins can be influenced by more factors than that of fat-soluble vitamins, and deficiencies are generally more common as body stores of these vitamins are smaller than that of fat-soluble vitamins. Factors that increase the risk of water-soluble vitamin deficiency include alcohol abuse, malnutrition, poor quality or restrictive diets, and malabsorption (Mahan et al., 2012; Mueller, 2012; NIH, 2016).

Mineral absorption is similarly affected by a number of factors, including concentration, form, and concomitant intake of other specific nutrients and dietary components. Dietary minerals are often found in more than one form, and some forms are more bioavailable than others. For example, iron is more efficiently absorbed in the heme form found in animal-based foods than the nonheme iron found in plant-based foods (Mahan et al., 2012; Mueller, 2012; NIH, 2016).

Absorption can also be affected by the amount of mineral consumed, particularly in supplement form; e.g., the percentage of calcium absorbed decreases in doses of more than 500 mg, so it is recommended that daily supplementation be given in divided doses to maximize absorption (NIH, 2016). Zinc excretion in feces also increases when the amount of zinc absorbed increases, so divided doses of zinc supplements may be beneficial (Hambridge et al., 2010). Iron supplementation has been shown to reduce absorption of nonheme iron consumed in foods but not heme iron. Copper absorption also decreases with an increase in intake (Wapnir, 1998).

Excessive or prolonged supplementation of one mineral may result in deficiency of another due to reduced absorption; in particular, zinc, copper, and iron act competitively in the absorption process. Some dietary elements such as phytic and oxalic acid have been shown to reduce micronutrient absorption, while other dietary components such as vitamin C with iron and vitamin D with calcium actually improve mineral absorption (NIH, 2016).

Common physiological changes in aging can also alter micronutrient absorption. While gastric acid production does not necessarily decrease with normal aging, the negative consequences of chronic gastric conditions will manifest with advancing age. In particular, calcium and B_{12} absorption may be impaired in part due to hypochlorhydria, a common result of atrophic gastritis and the prolonged use of proton pump inhibitors or H_2 antagonists. Gastric acid is needed to cleave vitamin B_{12} from food, and intrinsic factor is needed for B_{12} absorption, both of which are produced by gastric cells. Hypochlorhydria may also reduce folic acid absorption (Holt, 2007; Salles, 2007).

No marked changes have been noted in the structure or function of small intestinal villi and enterocytes in older adults. Likewise, digestive enzyme production generally does not decrease with age—with the exception of lactase. Lactase production is highest in infancy and childhood and decreases steadily in adulthood. Lactose intolerance itself does not inhibit calcium or other micronutrient absorption, but impaired tolerance of lactose may reduce consumption of dairy products, thus limiting the intake of foods rich in Ca, Mg, P, K, and vitamins D and A (Salles, 2007; Corleto et al., 2014).

Diseases or conditions that affect nutrient absorption include short bowel syndrome, which is caused by resection of a significant portion of the small bowel; pancreatic exocrine insufficiency, which is seen in pancreatic resections and cystic fibrosis; total or partial gastrectomy, which is most commonly performed to treat gastric cancer and weight reduction for those who are morbidly obese; untreated celiac disease; an acute phase response typically caused by systemic infections; and genetic disorders resulting in reduced or absent production of specific digestive enzymes. Micronutrient malabsorption is largely influenced by the portion of the GI tract that is dysfunctional or absent. See Tables 14.8 and 14.9 for more details regarding absorption, including physiological and dietary (Mahan et al., 2012; Mueller, 2012; NIH, 2016).

Altered Metabolism

Adequate amounts of micronutrients may be successfully consumed and absorbed, but deficiency can still occur if nutrient utilization is impaired or altered. Some disease states and medications can increase micronutrient losses in the urine or stool, reduce conversion to active forms, and reduce the body's ability to store or transport micronutrients.

Liver disease in particular has a significant effect on micronutrient utilization, as the liver is a primary storage site for some vitamins, produces transport proteins, and serves as a site for such metabolic reactions as hydroxylation or phosphorylation, which are necessary to convert some vitamins to biologically active forms. For example, adequate liver function is necessary for vitamin D to undergo the first of two hydroxylation reactions needed to

TABLE 14.8 Absorption of Vitamins (Mueller, 2012; Allen et al., 2006; Mahan et al., 2012; NIH, 2016)

Vitamin	Approximate % Absorbed	Mechanism	Factors Affecting Absorption
A	90	Proteases hydrolyze proteins needed to release vitamin A; lipases hydrolyze retinyl esters. Fat and bile acids necessary for incorporation into micelles for passive absorption	Decreased absorption with fat malabsorption
D	50	Fat and bile acids necessary for incorporation into micelles for passive absorption	Decreased absorption with fat malabsorption
E	20–50	Fat and bile acids necessary for incorporation into micelles for passive absorption	Absorption decreases as intake increases; at pharmacological doses, absorption can be <10%
K	20–80	Phylloquinones (K_1) absorbed by energy-dependent processes; menaquinones (K_2) and menadione (K_3) absorbed passively	Decreased absorption with fat malabsorption. Vitamin K in free form (from oils or supplements) absorbed at ~80%; much lower absorption from foods
B_1		Phosphatases cleave phosphorylated forms prior to absorption. Energy-dependent active transport mechanism used for absorption with low intake; passive transport used with high intake	Decreased absorption with alcohol consumption (interferes with transport) and folate deficiency (interferes with replication of enterocytes)
B_2	95	HCl and phosphatases cleave B_2 from protein complexes prior to absorption via an energy-dependent carrier-mediated process	Absorption is proportional to intake. Absorption increases in presence of B_2 deficiency. Alcohol consumption and divalent metals (Cu, Zn, Fe, Mn) that form chelates with B_2 may reduce absorption
B_3		Absorption via carrier-mediated facilitated diffusion	Can be synthesized from tryptophan, although process is insufficient to meet needs alone; B_2 and B_6 needed for this process
B_6	75	Phosphatases are needed to cleave phosphorylated forms from protein prior to absorption via passive diffusion	Absorption is pH dependent
B_{12}	50	Pepsin and HCl release B_{12} from food; B_{12} forms a complex in the duodenum with intrinsic factor and is then absorbed via active transport in the ileum. B_{12} is excreted in bile, so it may be reabsorbed via enterohepatic circulation	Absorption is decreased in conditions affecting the function or structure of the stomach or ileum. Absorption decreases for supplemented B_{12} doses above 1–2 μg, as the capacity of intrinsic factor is exceeded
C	80–90	Active transport mechanism	Absorption can decrease to <50% at doses above 1 gm/day
Folic acid	50–100	Zinc-dependent brush border enzymes convert polyglutamate to monoglutamate form before absorption via active transport; passive transport may be used at high doses. Some forms of folate are excreted in bile so they may be reabsorbed via enterohepatic circulation	Absorption of supplemented folate is 80–100%, while approximately 50% of folate naturally occurring in foods is absorbed. Zinc deficiency, alcohol intake, and changes in enteric pH reduce absorption
Pantothenic acid		Dietary CoA form hydrolyzed to pantothenic acid prior to absorption via active and passive transport	Inflammatory bowel disease and alcohol intake may decrease absorption
Biotin		Protease and biotinidase cleave biotin from protein and reduce to free biotin before absorption via carrier-mediated diffusion	Inflammatory bowel disease, achlorhydria, and the biotin-binding protein avidin found in raw egg whites may impair absorption
Choline		Hydrolysis of lecithin by lipases releases choline before carrier-mediated and passive diffusion processes	Endogenous de novo synthesis of choline occurs but alone is insufficient to meet needs

convert it to the active form. Many individuals with advanced liver disease already suffer from malnutrition and insufficient nutrient intake; impairment in storage, metabolism, and transport further compromises micronutrient status (Johnson et al., 2013).

The kidneys are also a site for metabolism of some micronutrients, particularly vitamin D. People with chronic kidney disease are unable to produce sufficient amounts of the biologically active form of vitamin D because the damaged kidney cannot sufficiently perform the second hydroxylation needed for this conversion. Vitamin D deficiency is thus more common in this population (Tsiaras and Weinstock, 2011).

TABLE 14.9 Absorption of Select Minerals (Mueller, 2012; Allen et al., 2006; Mahan et al., 2012; NIH, 2016)

Mineral	Approximate % Absorbed	Mechanism	Factors Affecting Absorption
Calcium	Up to 60 in infants and children ≤15–20 in adults	Active transport used with low luminal Ca concentrations; passive transport with high concentrations	Active transport dependent on vitamin D; vitamin D deficiency decreases absorption. Absorption increases when intake is low or needs are high. Improved absorption at lower pH; achlorhydria reduces absorption. Absorption decreases with age, reduced estrogen production in women, and intake of oxalic and phytic acids
Copper	25–60	HCl and pepsin cleave Cu from food before absorption via active transport when copper intake is low, and passive diffusion is used when intake is high	Absorption decreases as copper intake increases. Absorption decreases with intake of fiber, phytic acid, and other minerals (Zn, Fe, Ca gluconate, Mo)
Iron	Heme 10–30 Nonheme 2–10	HCl cleaves nonheme iron from food and converts it to ferrous form. Heme iron absorbed intact into the enterocyte and converted to its ferrous form intracellularly. Ferrous form requires active transport to leave the enterocyte	Inadequate iron stores or increased needs (growth, pregnancy) increase absorption. Compounds that increase acidity such as vitamin C; lactic, aspartic, and glutamic acids increase absorption. Some dietary components form insoluble complexes with iron and reduce absorption: phytic acid, oxalic acids, Ca, Zn, and Mn
Magnesium	30–40	Active transport used with low luminal Mg concentrations; passive transport with high concentrations	Absorption inversely associated with intake
Manganese	1–5	Absorption process not completely understood but appears to be similar to other minerals	Absorption decreases with increasing intake to prevent toxicity. Nonheme iron intake may reduce absorption due to competition for binding sites
Molybdenum	35–93	Absorbed via active transport when serum molybdenum concentration is low; passive diffusion when concentration is high	
Phosphorus	60–70	Hydrolization with pancreatic or intestinal phosphatases prior to absorption	
Selenium	50–100	Dietary Se in the form of selenoproteins (selomethionine and selenocysteine) is readily absorbed	Absorption increases with Se inadequacy or deficiency
Zinc	20–40	HCl and enteric enzymes hydrolyze Zn from amino acids and nucleic acids before absorption via active transport with low luminal Zn concentrations; passive transport with high concentrations	The protein metallothionein (MT) modulates Zn absorption; inflammation increases MT synthesis, which may reduce Zn absorption. Phytic acid, Ca, and other minerals may also reduce absorption

Individuals who undergo regular renal replacement therapy such as hemodialysis risk water-soluble vitamin and mineral deficiencies due to increased losses during the dialysis process, increased needs, and inadequate intake. It is recommended that those undergoing dialysis receive water-soluble vitamin supplementation in the presence of inadequate intake or deficiency. Water-soluble vitamin supplements have been specifically formulated for this population (K/DOQI, 2000).

The skin is another organ necessary for maintenance of adequate vitamin D stores because skin cells produce the inactive form of vitamin D when exposed to ultraviolet radiation. With sufficient sunlight, those with limited intake or absorption of vitamin D from foods can still produce enough of the vitamin to maintain adequate serum levels. However, because of a greater awareness of cosmetic changes and skin cancer risks associated with ultraviolet radiation, as well as lifestyle changes such as increasing participation in indoor activities, exposure to sunlight has decreased significantly in industrialized nations. Scientists suspect this has contributed to a greater prevalence of vitamin D deficiency. Older populations are particularly at risk because the skin's ability to synthesize vitamin D decreases with age. Furthermore, older individuals, especially those who are residents of long term care facilities, often receive little exposure to sunlight (Tsiaras and Weinstock, 2011).

DIAGNOSIS OF DEFICIENCY

Accurate diagnosis of micronutrient deficiencies can be challenging. Serum levels of many vitamins are typically not reflective of total body stores; in some cases, serum levels remain within normal ranges until the later stages of deficiency. Serum levels of many minerals are also not indicative of deficiency. In particular, phosphorus and calcium homeostasis is maintained via a complex interplay of hormones, which results in mineral release or deposition from the bones to maintain serum levels, regardless of total body stores or intake (Esper, 2015).

Serum levels of other minerals and some vitamins are also greatly affected by disease states. In particular, liver disease and acute illness or injury resulting in inflammation reduces hepatic production of negative acute-phase serum proteins. Many of these proteins serve as micronutrient transporters, thus serum levels tested in the presence of liver disease or inflammation are less likely to be reflective of total body stores (Bresnahan and Tanumihardjo, 2014). Reductions in serum levels of some vitamins such as A, C, and E, as well as such minerals as Se, Cu, Fe, and Zn, are seen in patients with significant trauma or inflammation (Sriram and Lonchyna, 2009).

Experts disagree on the normal or ideal serum level for some micronutrients, which further complicates the issue of deficiency diagnosis. In particular, nutrition experts have not reached a universal consensus regarding recommended serum vitamin D levels, although the vitamin has been widely studied in recent years and is now recognized as commonly deficient worldwide (Brouwer-Brolsma et al., 2013). There is also significant variability in the methods used to perform biochemical tests by various laboratories, thus reference values are not consistent. See Tables 14.10 and 14.11 for commonly utilized reference values for serum vitamin and mineral levels (Mueller, 2012).

B_{12} status can be particularly challenging to assess because serum levels do not clearly reflect body stores. Both B_{12} and folate deficiency can cause megaloblastic anemia, although mean corpuscular volume, which indicates the

TABLE 14.10 Commonly Used Assays for Vitamins (Mueller, 2012)

Vitamin	Assay	Normal Level
A	Serum vitamin A	>30 µg/dL
D	25-hydroxyvitamin D	30–70 ng/mL
E	Alpha-tocopherol	5.5–18 mg/L
K	International normalized ratio	0.8–1.2
	Prothrombin time	10–15 s
B_1	Whole blood thiamin	70–180 nmol/L
	Plasma thiamin	8–30 nmol/L
	Erythrocyte transketolase activity	<1.2 µg/mL/h
B_2	Serum riboflavin	5–50 nmol/L
	Erythrocyte glutathione reductase	<1.2 IU/g
B_3	Serum niacin	0.5–15 ng/mL
	N-methylnicotinamide	>5.8 µmol/day
B_6	Plasma pyridoxal-5 phosphate	20–125 nmol/L
B_{12}	Serum B_{12}	210–911 pg/mL
	Serum methylmalonic acid	0–0.4 µmol/dL
C	Plasma vitamin C	0.2–2 mg/dL
Folic acid	Serum folate	5.4–40 ng/mL
	RBC folate	280–903 ng/mL
Pantothenic acid	Whole blood pantothenic acid	>1 µmol/L
	Urinary excretion	>1 mg/day
Biotin	Serum biotin	100–400 pmol/L
	Urinary excretion	>6 µg/day
Choline	Plasma choline	10 µmol/L

TABLE 14.11 Commonly Used Assays for Select Minerals (Mueller, 2012)

Mineral	Assay	Normal Level
Copper	Serum copper	0.75–1.45 μg/mL
Iodine	Serum iodine	40–92 ng/mL
	Urinary iodine	100–199 μg/L
Iron	Serum iron males	24–336 μg/L
	Serum iron females	11–307 μg/L
	Transferrin	170–340 mg/dL
	Iron-binding capacity	240–450 mg/dL
Manganese	Blood manganese	4.7–18.3 ng/mL
	Serum manganese	0–2 μg/L
Molybdenum	Serum molybdenum	0.58–0.8 μg/L
Selenium	Serum selenium	23–190 μg/L
	Urinary selenium	10–35 μg/day
	Plasma glutathione peroxidase	>10.5 U/mL
Zinc	Plasma zinc	70–120 μg/dL
	RBC zinc	1000–1600 μg/dL

size of the red blood cell, may not necessarily be elevated when B_{12} or folate deficiency is present or if there is a concurrent iron deficiency. Serum methylmalonic acid and homocysteine can be measured; levels of these compounds may be elevated in B_{12} deficiency. It is important to note that treatment of folate deficiency may correct megaloblastic anemia, which will then mask the presence of a B_{12} deficiency; while the anemia is corrected, the neurological effects of B_{12} deficiency may still be present and can become permanent if the deficiency is not treated (Chan and Mike, 2014).

Because of these confounding factors related to diagnosis, the clinician must examine not only biochemical indices but also estimate dietary intake, assess risk factors, and conduct a physical examination to identify possible signs of deficiency. Micronutrient deficiencies are most likely to manifest in body structures that can be easily examined, including the skin, hair, nails, eyes, mouth, and tongue. See Table 14.12 for physical signs of micronutrient deficiency (Esper, 2015; Pogatshnik and Hamilton, 2011).

TREATMENT

Treatment of micronutrient deficiencies should include three key components: (1) identification and treatment of the underlying cause of the deficiency if possible, (2) education and counseling for patients on ways to increase micronutrient consumption and absorption from foods if appropriate, and (3) implementation of an appropriate treatment regimen, including the appropriate chemical form of the supplement, dose, route and timing of administration, and duration of treatment. When determining appropriate treatment regimens, many factors should be considered, including the severity of deficiency, presence of medical conditions that affect nutrient absorption or utilization (especially renal and hepatic function), and reliability and reputation of the supplement manufacturer.

In the presence of untreated fat malabsorption, aqueous forms of fat-soluble vitamins may be used to treat or prevent deficiency. In patients with short bowel syndrome or another malabsorptive condition difficult to treat medically, various forms and doses of water-soluble vitamins are available; increasing the dose, even above the tolerable upper level established by the US Department of Agriculture, may be necessary to effectively treat deficiency. Oral supplementation may be available in tablet, liquid, or chewable forms, especially multivitamin with mineral supplements.

If oral supplementation is ineffective, other forms may be utilized, most notably intravenous solutions, although these are generally used in patients who cannot consume food by mouth and require parenteral nutrition. Vitamin B_{12} is commonly supplemented via a monthly intramuscular injection, especially for those with gastric or ileum resections that prevent B_{12} absorption. B_{12} is also available in the form of nasal sprays or gels.

TABLE 14.12 Physical Signs of Deficiency for Select Micronutrients (Mueller, 2012; Mahan et al., 2012; Pogatshnik and Hamilton, 2011; Esper, 2015)

Micronutrient	Physical Sign or Symptom
Vitamin A	Poor wound healing, abnormally dry skin, follicular hyperkeratosis; pale, mottled, or poor blanching in nails; night blindness, conjunctival xerosis, Bitot's spots, keratomalacia
Vitamin D	Swollen painful joints, rickets, bowleg
Vitamin K	Petechiae, ecchymosis
Vitamin B_1	Stomatitis, pitting edema, motor weakness, peripheral neuropathy
Vitamin B_2	Nasolabial seborrhea, angular palpebritis, stomatitis, cheilosis, angular stomatitis, glossitis, atrophic filiform papillae
Vitamin B_3	Pellagrous dermatitis, nasolabial seborrhea, angular palpebritis, cheilosis, angular stomatitis, glossitis, edematous tongue, dementia
Vitamin B_6	Stomatitis, nasolabial seborrhea, angular palpebritis, cheilosis, angular stomatitis, glossitis, peripheral neuropathy
Vitamin B_{12}	Pale conjunctivae, glossitis, atrophic filiform papillae, peripheral neuropathy, dementia
Vitamin C	Poor wound healing, perifolliculosis, petechiae, ecchymosis; pale, mottled, or poorly blanching nails; splinter hemorrhages on nails, stomatitis, bleeding spongy gums, pitting edema
Folic Acid	Pallor, pale conjunctivae, stomatitis, glossitis, atrophic filiform papillae
Biotin	Pallor, stomatitis, hair loss, dermatitis, glossitis
Copper	Pallor, corkscrew hair, hair loss, depigmentation of hair, peripheral neuropathy
Iodine	Goiter or enlarged thyroid
Iron	General pallor, pale conjunctivae, poor capillary refill, koilonychia, angular stomatitis, atrophic filiform papillae
Zinc	Poor wound healing, generalized dermatitis, impaired night vision, alopecia, dys- and hypogeusia

The chemical form of the nutrient should also be considered when choosing a supplement, especially for minerals. Many forms of Ca and Fe are readily available, and some forms are more easily absorbed than others. It is important to carefully read supplement labels to determine the elemental amount that the product provides, which is the amount expected to be absorbed.

Absorption considerations also need to be addressed when determining a dosing schedule. For some micronutrients, absorption decreases with increasing intake, thus several smaller doses should be taken daily to maximize absorption capacity. Some dietary components can either increase or decrease absorption of specific micronutrients, so prescription instructions should include whether the supplement should be taken with or without food. See Tables 14.8 and 14.9 for more details.

The duration of treatment will depend on the underlying cause of the deficiency; if the primary cause is difficult to treat medically, then long-term supplementation may be necessary. Periodic reassessment of micronutrient status via biochemical assay and physical exam is necessary to determine if signs and symptoms have resolved, and to prevent toxicity. Toxicity is more likely with fat-soluble vitamins because excess amounts of water-soluble vitamins are generally excreted in the urine.

The effect of micronutrient supplementation on the prevention and treatment of numerous disease states has been studied extensively; while an exhaustive review is outside the scope of this chapter, two common conditions seen in older populations bear mention. First, in patients who are critically ill and require nutrition support, it is recommended that antioxidant vitamins be provided—namely, vitamins E and C and some trace minerals such as Se, Zn, and Cu—because evidence indicates that supplementation may reduce overall mortality, although infectious complications and the length of intensive care unit and hospital stays do not appear to be affected (McClave et al., 2016). Iron, however, should not be supplemented in this population as it may contribute to microorganism proliferation (Bresnahan and Tanumihardjo, 2014).

Second, individuals who undergo cancer treatments such as chemotherapy or radiation are advised to avoid supplements that contain antioxidants because some research suggests this antioxidant effect may protect cancer cells, thus reducing the efficacy of cancer therapies. This effect has not been seen with the intake of antioxidant rich foods; individuals should be encouraged to continue consuming nutrient-rich foods (Lawenda et al., 2008). General multivitamin and mineral supplementation may benefit some individuals with cancer, although patients should be advised to consult their oncologist before beginning a micronutrient supplement.

CONCLUSION

The use of multivitamin and mineral supplements in the United States is increasing (Gahche et al., 2011). Despite this, many individuals, especially older adults, are at risk for deficiencies due to poor-quality diets and medical conditions and their treatments that affect the absorption or utilization of micronutrients. Micronutrient deficiencies can result in significant signs and symptoms that further complicate medical conditions and reduce the intake of nutrient-dense foods. It is critical that the health-care practitioner recognize the risk factors for deficiency, screen for deficiencies in high-risk populations, and properly diagnose and treat micronutrient deficiencies.

References

Allen, L., de Benoist, B., Dary, O., Hurrell, R., 2006. Guidelines on food fortification with micronutrients. World Health Organization and Food and Agricultural Organization of the United Nations.

Baumler, M.D., 2012. Nutrigenetics—building a platform for dietitians to offer personalized nutrition. Today's Dietitian 14, 48–50.

Bergstrom, L., 1994. Nutrient Losses and Gains in the Preparation of Foods. National Food Administration, Sweden, Report No. 32/94.

Bresnahan, K.A., Tanumihardjo, S.A., 2014. Undernutrition, the acute phase response to infection and its effects on micronutrient status indicators. Adv. Nutr. 5, 702-211.

Brouwer-Brolsma, E.M., Bishcoff-Ferrari, A., Bouillon, R., Feskens, E.J.M., Gallager, C.J., 2013. Vitamin D: do we get enough? Osteoporos Int. 24, 1567–1577.

Chan, L.-N., Mike, L.A., 2014. The science and practice of micronutrient supplementations in nutritional anemia: an evidence-based review. J. Parenter. Enteral. Nutr. 38, 656–672.

Corleto, V.D., Festa, S., Di Giulio, E., Annibale, B., 2014. Proton pump inhibitor therapy and potential long term harm. Curr. Opin. Endocrinol. Diabetes Obes. 21 (1), 3–8.

DiFrancesco, V., Fantin, F., Omizzolo, F., Residori, L., Bissoli, L., Bosello, O., et al., 2007. Anorexia of aging. Dig. Dis. 25, 129–137.

DiMaria-Ghalili, R.A., 2014. Integrating nutrition in the comprehensive geriatric assessment. Nutr. Clin. Pract. 29, 420–427.

Esper, D.H., 2015. Utilization of nutrition-focused physical assessment in identifying micronutrient deficiencies. Nutr. Clin. Pract. 30, 194–202.

Frank, L.L., 2015. Thiamin in clinical practice. J. Paren. Enteral. Nutr. 39 (5), 503–520.

Gahche, J., Bailey, R., Burt, V., Hughes, J., Yetley, E., Dwyer, J., et al., 2011. Dietary supplement use among U.S. adults has increased since NHANES III (1988–1994). NCHS Data Brief 61, 1–8.

Grober, U., Kisters, K., 2012. Influence of drugs on vitamin D and calcium metabolism. Dermato-Endocrinology 4 (2), 158–266.

Hambridge, K.M., Miller, L.V., Westcott, J.E., Sheng, Z., Krebs, N.F., 2010. Zinc bioavailability and homeostasis. Am. J. Clin. Nutr. 91 (suppl.), 1478S–1483SS.

Holt, P.R., 2007. Intestinal malabsorption in the elderly. Dig. Dis. 25, 144–150.

Johnson, T.M., Overgard, E.B., Cohen, A.E., DiBaise, J.K., 2013. Nutrition assessment and management in advanced liver disease. Nutr. Clin. Pract. 28 (1), 15–29.

K/DOQI National Kidney Foundation Kidney Disease Outcomes Quality Initiative, 2000. Clinical guideline for nutrition in chronic renal failure. Am. J. Kidney Dis. Vol. 35 (No 6), S1–S136. Supplement 2.

Lawenda, B.D., Kelly, K.M., Ladas, E.J., Sagar, S.M., Vickers, A., Blumberg, J., 2008. Should supplemental antioxidant administration be avoided during chemotherapy and radiation therapy? J. Natl. Cancer Inst. 100, 773–783.

Mahan, L.K., Escott-Stump, S., Raymond, J.L. (Eds.), 2012. Krause's Food and the Nutrition Care Process, 13th ed. Saunders, St. Louis, Missouri.

McClave, S.A., Taylor, B.E., Martindale, R.G., Warren, M.M., Johnson, D.R., Braunschweig, C., et al., 2016. Guidelines for the provision and assessment of nutrition support therapy in the adult critically ill patient: Society of Critical Care Medicine and American Society for Parenteral and Enteral Nutrition. J. Pareter. Enteral. Nutr. 40, 159–211.

Montgomery, S.C., Streit, S.M., Beebe, M.L., Maxwell IV, P.J., 2014. Micronutrient needs of the elderly. Nutr. Clin. Pract. 29, 435–444.

Moyer, V.A., 2014. Vitamin mineral and multivitamin supplements for the primary prevention of cardiovascular disease and cancer: U.S. Preventive Services Task Force Recommendation Statement. Ann. Intern. Med. 160, 558–564.

Mueller, C.M. (Ed.), 2012. The ASPEN Adult Nutrition Support Core Curriculum, 2nd edn. Silver Spring, Maryland.

NIH National Institutes of Health Office of Dietary Supplements. https://ods.od.nih.gov/factsheets/list-all/ Accessed February 23, 2016.

Pogatshnik, C., Hamilton, C., 2011. Nutrition-focused physical examination: skin, nails, hair, eyes and oral cavity. Support Line 33 (2), 7–13.

Salles, N., 2007. Basic mechanisms of the aging gastrointestinal tract. Dig. Dis. 25, 112–117.

Sriram, K., Lonchyna, VA., 2009. Micronutrient supplementation in adult nutrition therapy: practical considerations. J Parenter Enteral Nutr 33, 1–15.

ter Borg, S., Verlaan, S., Hemsworth, J., Mijnarends, D.M., Schols, J., Luiking, Y.C., et al., 2015. Micronutrient intakes and potential inadequacies of community-dwelling older adults: a systematic review. Br. J. Nutr. 113, 1195–1206.

Tsiaras, W.G., Weinstock, M.A., 2011. Factors influencing vitamin D status. Acta Derm. Venereol. 91, 115–124.

Udo de Haes, H.A., Voortman, R.L., Bastein, T., Bussink, D.W., Rougoor, C.W., van der Weijden, W.J. 2012. Scarcity of Micronutrients in Soil, Feed, Food and Mineral Reserves—Urgency and Policy Options. Platform for Agriculture, Innovation and Society.

USDA (US Department of Agriculture), 2007. USDA table of nutrient retention factors—release 6.

USDA US Department of Agriculture. Introduction to Dietary Reference Intakes. Accessed January 8, 2016 at http://www.nal.usda.gov/fnic/DRI/DRI_Water/21-36.pdf.

Wapnir, R.A., 1998. Copper absorption and bioavailability. Am J Clin Nutr 67, 1054S–1060SS.

CHAPTER

15

The Role of B Group Vitamins and Choline in Cognition and Brain Aging

Francesco Bonetti, Gloria Brombo and Giovanni Zuliani

University of Ferrara, Ferrara, Italy

INTRODUCTION

Aging is an inescapable process of our body, the cumulative modifications of our organs and systems usually result in a progressive loss of function due to the unbalanced relationship between trophic and homeostatic stimuli and harmful interactions with the environment. Brain aging is no exception. How we age, however, is unique for each individual. Pathological and instrumental exploration of the brain in both demented and nondemented older subjects often shows a mixed pattern of lesions (amyloid plaques, tau protein fibrillary tangles, synucleinopathies, vascular damage, and white matter rarefaction) possibly but not inevitably resulting in cognitive impairment (Fernando and Ince, 2004; Schneider et al., 2007; Kang et al., 2012; Nelson et al., 2012; Seo et al., 2013; Xekardaki et al., 2015; Yu et al., 2015). The finding that cerebral lesions as confirmed by pathology do not always reflect correctly clinical diagnoses and functional status of individuals (Schneider et al., 2007; Jellinger and Attems, 2013; Xekardaki et al., 2015) opens a new window of insight into brain aging, cognitive decline, and dementia. It is imperative to shift from morphological analysis alone to integrated functional evaluations, considering the pathological damage in the context of a system that relies primarily on networks, where on the one hand connections and integrations could somehow survive (even if slightly impaired) in a structurally damaged organ and on the other hand a relatively conserved cellular mass is not surely sufficient to supply loss of interconnections and functional disturbances (Reijmer et al., 2013; Lawrence et al., 2014). Even if individual resilience to pathological brain damage is hardly predictable, possibly due to differences in cognitive reserve (Xekardaki et al., 2015), the global burden of brain lesions correlates with cognitive outcomes for a large number of subjects (Yu et al., 2015; White et al., 2016). Neuroplasticity, in terms of neurogenesis and rearrangement of neural networks, has emerged as one possible target to be enhanced in order to counterbalance the age-related degeneration of the central nervous system (CNS). Sadly, this ability has the tendency to wane even in subjects defined to have "successful aging" (Jellinger and Attems, 2013). Because it is now still impossible to fully revert or compensate neuronal damage when an extensive loss of neurons occurs, to preserve our functional status we need to sustain a tireless and expensive tendency to homeostasis, preventing avoidable brain damage and providing our organism with the essential elements required for normal functioning. One field of growing interest that covers both health promotion and disease prevention with a safe high-impact intervention is nutrition.

Dietary patterns have shown a noteworthy relevance in preventing cognitive decline (Cheung et al., 2014), and it has been known for decades that poor nutritional status, especially in terms of micronutrients deficiency, has a role in the development of neuropsychiatric conditions and neurodegenerative diseases (Bourre, 2006; Del Parigi et al., 2006; Waserman et al., 2015). To better understand the role of micronutrients in neuroprotection and healthy brain aging, it is useful to establish the relationship between a micronutrient intake level and modulation of the physiological events that are regulated, promoted, or contained because of the micronutrient availability. Almost all nutrients have an inverted U-shaped relationship between their concentrations and their physiological functions: the

Nutrition and Functional Foods for Healthy Aging.
DOI: http://dx.doi.org/10.1016/B978-0-12-805376-8.00015-0

optimal effect occurs over a variable range of intake levels, while both deficiency and excess of the substance could result in detrimental and even life-threatening effects (Morris, 2011; Morris, 2015). Moreover, the dietary requirements and the maximum tolerable intake levels can vary among individuals on the basis of constitutional, clinical, and physiological characteristics. These basic rules are determinant in understanding why there is no "standardized approach" that perfectly fits the requirements of an entire population. However, an estimation of the population needs based on epidemiological data united with a documented knowledge of the risk-benefit ratio could allow planning for a fairly safe and potentially beneficial intervention at the population level. Clear examples are dietary recommendations implemented for health-promotion and food-fortification programs. To accurately analyze the amount of substances needed to maintain a normal metabolic function, it is necessary to introduce the concepts of estimated average requirement (EAR), or intake with 50% risk of inadequacy; recommended dietary allowance (RDA), or intake with about 3% risk of inadequacy; and tolerable upper intake level (UL), or intake with a clinically relevant risk of toxicity. The adequate intake (AI) represents the span of intake of a nutrient that almost certainly satisfies the physiological requirements of an individual with a low risk of developing toxic effects; theoretically, the AI is higher than RDA (almost certainly sufficient) and lower than UL (possibly toxic). AI is the reference value if sufficient scientific evidence is not available to establish an EAR on which to base an RDA.

Many micronutrients have a role in modulating brain activity or in neurodegeneration, so we will focus here on B group vitamins (BGVs), a group that is essential for normal cognitive development and is supposed to be helpful in preventing cognitive decline, as well as on choline, a precursor of membrane lipids that share BGV metabolic pathways.

ROLE OF B GROUP VITAMINS AND CHOLINE IN NORMAL BRAIN FUNCTIONING AND NEUROPROTECTION

BGVs are a heterogeneous group of hydrosoluble vitamins whose chemical and functional diversity is associated with an equally varied pool of food sources. Almost all deficiency syndromes related to the compounds that belong to BGVs have neurological manifestations, either as direct effects of deficiency or as consequences of the accumulation of neurotoxic metabolites (Lanska, 2010; Abdou and Hazell, 2015; Nardone et al., 2013; Bowman et al., 2012; Powers, 2003; Ghavanini and Kimpinski, 2014; Gerlach et al., 2011; Said, 2012). Before detailing the possible mechanisms underlying BGV-related neuronal damage and subsequent protective activities, we remind readers of the physiological role of each vitamin for a better understanding of their contribution in complex metabolic processes (often the same detrimental condition involves more than one micronutrient metabolism, which makes interactions between micronutrients essential for broadly seeing the phenomenon). Piridoxyne (vB6), folate (vB9), cobalamin (vB12), and choline will be discussed together because they share biochemical pathways that are highly relevant to normal brain functioning and common neurodegenerative processes. Dietary recommendations for each micronutrient are summarized in Table 15.1.

Thiamin

Thiamin (vB1), the first BGV identified, is an essential nutrient involved in carbohydrate and amino acid metabolism and in energy production (El-Sohemy et al., 2013). The vB1 active form, thiamine diphosphate, acts as a cofactor of three step-limiting enzymes of carbohydrate metabolism (transketolase in the pentose phosphate pathway and pyruvate dehydrogenase and α-ketoglutarate dehydrogenase in the Krebs cycle) (Zhao et al., 2009). The RDA for vB1 is set at 1.2 mg/day for adult men and 1.1 mg/day for adult women. These values do not vary for people aged 50 and older but can be affected by energy-demanding situations such as physical activity or diseases with increased energy metabolism (e.g., hyperthyroidism) (Institute of Medicine, 1998; El-Sohemy et al., 2013). It is absorbed in the jejunum through active carriers at low doses (with about 90% of absorption at administration up to 5 mg) (El-Sohemy et al., 2013) and via passive diffusion with lower rates of absorption at higher doses (Institute of Medicine, 1998). Since the intake of several hundred mg of vB1 gave no measurable adverse effects, no UL for this nutrient has been established (Institute of Medicine, 1998; El-Sohemy et al., 2013). The European Food Safety Authority (EFSA) states that even if vB1 is an essential contributor to normal cognitive functioning, a balanced diet should easily meet the daily requirements of the nutrient (in the absence of pathological conditions) (EFSA, 2010a). Historically, a vB1 deficiency was identified with beriberi, a disease known for centuries: deficiency-related symptoms are anorexia, weight loss, apathy, short-term memory loss, confusion, irritability, muscle weakness (El-Sohemy et al., 2013), and cardiovascular effects such as an enlarged heart and heart failure (Azizi-Namini et al., 2012). Today vB1 deficiency

TABLE 15.1 Summary of Multiple-Source Dietary Recommendations for BGVs and Choline

Micronutrient	Nonfortified Food Source[a]	RDA: M/F (Elderly[d])	AI: M/F	UL	UL/RDA[b]: M/F (Elderly[d])
Vitamin B_1	Lean pork, legumes, and cereal grains (germ fraction)	1.2/1.1 mg/day IOM[f]	—	NA	NA; presumably very high
Vitamin B_2	Especially yeast and liver but also milk, egg white, fish roe, kidney, and leafy vegetables	1.3/1.1 mg/day IOM[f]	—	NA	NA; presumably very high
Vitamin B_3	Meat, fish, or poultry, roasted coffee	16/14 mg/day IOM[f]	—	35 mg/day IOM[f]	2.2/2.5
Vitamin B_5	Chicken, beef, potatoes, oat cereals, tomato products, liver, kidney, yeast, egg yolk, broccoli, and whole grains	NA	5 mg/day,[e] IOM[f]	NA	NA; presumably very high
Vitamin B_6	Fish and meat, seeds, noncitrus fruits (bananas, watermelons)	1.3/1.4 mg/day IOM[f] (1.5/1.7) IOM[f]	—	25 mg/day EFSA[g]	19.2/17.8 (16.6/14.7)
Vitamin B_7	Liver, kidney, egg yolk, soybeans, nuts, spinach, mushrooms, lentils	NA	30 µg/day,[e] IOM[f]	NA	NA; presumably very high
Vitamin B_9	Fruits and green leafy vegetables, yeast, liver	400 µg/day,[e] IOM[f]	—	1 mg/day IOM[f]	2.2[e]
Vitamin B_{12}	Meat, fish, liver, dairy products	2.4 µg/day,[e] IOM[f]	4 µg/day,[e] EFSA[g]	NA	NA; presumably extremely high
Choline	Milk, liver, eggs, peanuts	NA	550/425 mg/day IOM[f]	3500 g/day IOM[f]	6.4/8.2[c]

This table is derived from data obtained by NDA panels (EFSA, 2006) and Institute of Medicine (1998) statements on dietary references and tolerable upper limits of the listed micronutrients. If the two considered statements presented different recommendations, we chose on the basis of our clinical and scientific knowledge on the possible clinical efficacy of neuroprotection and benefit–risk considerations.RDA, recommended daily allowance; AI, adequate intake; UL, tolerable upper intake level; NA, not available; M, male; F, female.

[a]*These lists of food sources are not complete but represent examples of foods with relatively high contents of each micronutrient.*

[b]*When possible, we indicated the ratio between UL and RDA (or AI if RDA was not available) to quantify the safety span of a possible integration into the diet.*

[c]*AI was used instead of RDA (lack of sufficient quality evidences).*

[d]*Reference values for elderly individuals when available.*

[e]*No gender differences.*

[f]*IOM derived value (Institute of Medicine, 1998).*

[g]*EFSA value derived by European NDA panel statement (EFSA, 2006).*

is mainly associated with alcoholism and malnutrition (such as in obese patients, both during weight loss in preparation for bariatric surgery and after surgery if not adequately treated, and in elderly people in different countries) (Kerns et al., 2015; de Carvalho et al., 1996; Yang et al., 2005). Wernike encephalopathy (vision and muscle coordination impairment) and Korsakoff syndrome (memory loss, confabulation, hallucination) are vB1-related neurological manifestations that occur more frequently in alcoholic patients (Morris et al., 2006). The neuropsychological symptoms of Wernike–Korsakoff syndrome (confusion, episodic memory deficit with relatively spared working memory, confabulation, impairment in verbal fluency and flexibility, perseverative responding with strong frontal signs) seem caused by a severe impairment in the cholinergic networks, primarily due to neuronal cell loss (Nardone et al., 2013). These neurological manifestations are supported by the fact that vB1 deficiency has been proposed to lead to mitochondrial dysfunction, impaired cellular metabolism, glutamate excitotoxicity, and oxidative stress (OS) in deep brain structures (thalamus, mammillary bodies, and other diencephalic sites) (Nardone et al., 2013). Concern is rising over the possibility that vB1 could contribute to other chronic diseases even in general population subjects. In particular, some authors suggest that vB1 deficiency could impair neuroplasticity via inhibition of hippocampal neurogenesis (Zhao et al., 2009); this finding places vB1 deficiency in the pool of harmful conditions that theoretically could hasten or worsen Alzheimer's disease (AD) symptoms in predisposed individuals. The report of reduced thiamin plasma levels in AD patients supports the latter theory (Gold et al., 1995, 1998). Moreover, abnormal vB1-related enzyme activity has been observed in both brain and peripheral tissues in AD patients (Gibson et al., 1988; Butterworth and Besnard, 1990; Héroux et al., 1996), and vB1 deficiency in preclinical models seems to be able to promote β-amyloid (Aβ) deposition and tau protein hyperphosphorylation in the brain (Zhao et al., 2011), possibly via increased β-secretase activity (Zhang et al., 2011) and OS promotion (Karuppagounder et al., 2009).

Riboflavin

Riboflavin (vB2) is a yellow fluorescent compound whose biological role is as an integral component of two coenzymes—flavin mononucleotide (FMN) and flavin-adenine dinucleotide (FAD)—that are involved in several redox reactions including important steps in energy production. In addition, these flavocoenzymes regulate crucial intersections between other vitamins pathways, the most relevant being their impact on neuronal damage through the FMN-mediated generation of pyridoxal 5′-phosphate (a vitamin B_6–derived coenzyme) and the FAD-dependent reduction of 5,10-methylene-tetrahydrofolate to 5′-methyl-tetrahydrofolate, which reacts with vB12 in homocysteine (Hcy) remethylation to metionine (Met) (Institute of Medicine, 1998). RDA for men and women between ages 30 and 70 is set at 1.3 and 1.1 mg/day, respectively; on the basis of few studies, the same amount seems to be reasonably sufficient even for individuals older than 70 (Institute of Medicine, 1998). No UL has been set for vB2. The majority of vB2 of food origin is from flavocoenzymes complexed with proteins that require a normal gastric acid environment to be separated; riboflavin is then released from coenzymes via nonspecific enzymatic activity in the upper gut (Institute of Medicine, 1998). vB2 is absorbed primarily in the proximal small intestine via a saturable transport system while a small amount is subject to enterohepatic circulation or is absorbed in the large intestine (Institute of Medicine, 1998). The absorption is proportional to intake and is facilitated by concomitant ingestion of other food (Institute of Medicine, 1998). The main signs of vB2 deficiency are dermatological alterations, edema, and mucosal alterations of the larynx and oral cavity and possible interference with iron handling and hemopoiesis. However, as previously stated, vB2 deficiency may exert some of its effects by reducing the metabolism of other BGVs (folate and vB6), raising concerns about possible Hcy metabolism perturbation (Powers, 2003) (see the later section "The Homocysteine Cycle: Biochemistry and Clinical Implications"). Moreover, laboratory data from animal experiments suggest a possible neurological involvement in severe deficiencies, but little evidence is available for humans (Powers, 2003). On these bases, EFSA declared vB2 as essential for maintenance of normal nervous system function (EFSA, 2010b).

Niacin

Niacin (vB3) is defined as a group of compounds with biological activities similar to nicotinamide (nicotinic acid amide itself, nicotinic acid, and other molecules with similar structures and functions) (Institute of Medicine, 1998). Nicotinamide adenine dinucleotide (NAD) and nicotinamide adenine dinucleotide phosphate (NADP) are niacin-derived coenzymes fundamental for a wide range of redox reactions. NAD is also involved in reactions crucial to DNA repair and calcium signaling (Institute of Medicine, 1998). RDA for vB3 is set at 16 mg/day for men and 14 mg/day for women; these values are the same for both adult and elderly individuals. Tryptophan can be transformed into niacin, so its intake could reduce the requirements of vB3, but because vB2, vB6, and iron are needed in the tryptophan to niacin conversion pathway, a multiple deficiency of these nutrients could impair this alternative endogenous supply route (Institute of Medicine, 1998). The UL for adult individuals is set at 35 mg/day of niacin on the basis of the onset of flushing (vasodilation of face and extremities that produces red skin changes along with tingling, burning, or itching), which is the first adverse effect presented at low doses (recently other authors suggested a safer threshold at 10 mg/day) (Scientific Committee on Food, 2002). Higher doses could induce ocular and gastrointestinal disturbances and, at dosages of 3 g/day of nicotinamide (1.5 g/day of nicotinic acid), severe and possibly life-threatening hepatotoxicity (Institute of Medicine, 1998). In addition, individual susceptibility to niacin and the assumed form of the vitamin could greatly influence the genesis of adverse effects; in fact, severe forms of hepatitis have been observed for dosages as low as 500 mg/day (Eeuwijk et al., 2012).

Vitamin B_3 is absorbed readily by the stomach and small intestine, with an active transport prevalent at low doses overruled by passive diffusion at higher doses (Institute of Medicine, 1998). The main manifestation of deficiency is pellagra, which consists of skin pigmentation, gastrointestinal symptoms, and neurasthenia followed by psychosis, disorientation, memory loss, and confusion. Nowadays pellagra has almost disappeared in industrialized countries, but niacin deficiency is still a possible problem in long-term alcoholism or malabsorption conditions and severe malnutrition (Hegyi et al., 2004), which is more likely to occur in older patients. Niacin acts as a lipid-lowering drug and is able to reduce cardiovascular risk in hypercholesterolemic patients (Lavigne and Karas, 2013), but it is less effective than statins and not the therapy of choice for dyslipidemia, being relegated as an option for patients with multiple drug intolerances (Sando and Knight, 2015). That said, on the basis of preclinical data, some authors have suggested that vB3 activity in preventing the progression of atherosclerosis does not rely only on reduction of cholesterol (Lavigne and Karas, 2013). An antiinflammatory activity observed on vasal walls cells (Su et al., 2015), adipocytes (Digby et al., 2010), and macrophages (Digby, 2012) could be partially responsible for vB3 effects, opening a frame of possible multilevel interactions between vB3 and CNS damage, not only contributing to cerebrovascular prevention (known also to affect AD progression) (Saito and Ihara, 2016) but also reducing the systemic inflammatory burden, which is known to be related to cognitive decline and dementia (Zuliani et al., 2007; Marsland et al., 2015).

The antiinflammatory effects of niacin are probably mediated by the GPR109a nicotinic acid receptor; its activation in macrophages results in reduced production of interleukin-6 (IL-6), tumor necrosis factor-α (TNF-α), and monocyte chemoattractant protein-1 along with inhibition of chemotaxis and adhesion in experimental conditions (Digby, 2012). Recent findings suggest a role for niacin and the nicotinic acid GPR109a receptor in Parkinson's disease (PD): vB3 levels were lower in PD patients compared to age-matched controls, and they correlated with a rise in inflammation markers and clinical reports of higher body pain and more pronounced sleep disturbances (Wakade et al., 2014).

Other authors have explored the possible impact of 1-g extended-release niacin on cholesterol metabolism in the CNS of AD patients (Vega et al., 2003). This suggests that an investigation might be worth conducting into the possible mechanisms underlying the debated reduced incidence of AD in previously healthy subjects treated with lipid-lowering drugs (reported in an observational study but at the moment not confirmed by good quality evidences) (McGuinness et al., 2016). Anyway, Vega and colleagues demonstrated a reduction in plasma 24S-hydroxycholesterol concentrations in niacin-treated AD patients (Vega et al., 2003). As a marker of neurodegeneration with hypothesized neurotoxic properties, 24S-hydroxycholesterol (Bogdanovic et al., 2001; Lütjohann et al., 2002) has been found to be higher in the plasma and cerebrospinal fluid of AD patients compared to the general population (Zuliani et al., 2011; Lütjohann and von Bergmann, 2003) and is possibly implicated in Aβ pathology (Lütjohann and von Bergmann, 2003). Even if there are rational bases to hypothesize a possible role for vB3 in modulating neuronal damage, the literature data are scant and come from studies with low qualities of evidence. Lower niacin plasma levels have been observed in demented patients in respect to controls (along with multiple deficiencies of other nutrients in a small sample) (Thomas et al., 1986), and a possible role for niacin dietary intake levels in AD prevention has been postulated on the basis of observational data (findings with a high risk of bias due to the many possible confounders) (Morris et al., 2004). In our opinion, better-designed studies are needed to clarify this subject. Alas, a main bias of nutritional investigations in demented patients is that dementia is often a cause of malnutrition itself, so even longitudinal data should be critically considered.

Pantothenic Acid

Pantothenic acid (vB5) is involved in the synthesis of coenzyme A (CoA) and acyl carrier proteins. CoA in its different forms is an essential cofactor in a wide range of biological reactions, including the regulation of lipid metabolism, the production of molecules fundamental for the structure of the body machinery (such as amino acids, cholesterol, and membrane phospholipids), and the synthesis of substances with high-impact functional roles such as steroid hormones, vitamin D, and neurotransmitters (El-Sohemy et al., 2013). Acetyl-CoA and succinyl-CoA have a key role in the tricarboxylic acid cycle. Pantothenate kinase is the enzyme that transforms pantothenate in CoA, and it is regulated by its end product (CoA), so CoA concentrations do not exactly reflect the pantothenate availability for the body (Institute of Medicine, 1998).

The RDA for vB5 has not been established due to the lack of scientific data to support it, but an AI of 5 mg/day for both adult and elderly men and women has been considered sufficient on the basis of the balance between intake and excretion (Institute of Medicine, 1998; El-Sohemy et al., 2013). No adverse effects have been associated with high intakes of pantothenic acid, so no UL has been set (Institute of Medicine, 1998). Even if vB5 is not synthesized in humans, deficiency is unlikely to occur because vB5 itself and its derivatives are widely available in food; moreover, it is probable that resident microbiota of the intestine contribute to the pantothenic acid supply (an active synthesis has been observed in mice, but it is not clear whether the phenomenon is relevant to humans) (Institute of Medicine, 1998). Pantothenic acid absorption is mediated by a saturable active transport system at low concentrations and with greater contribution of passive diffusion at higher levels of intake (Institute of Medicine, 1998).

Data on deficiency-related clinical manifestations are deduced by historical reports of plausible peripheral neuropathy ("burning feet") reversible with vB5 administration in war prisoners in Asia during World War II (Glusman, 1947). Moreover, it has been observed that patients fed a diet poor in vB5 or treated with a pantothenate antagonist (Hodges et al., 1958, 1959; Fry et al., 1976) exhibited irritability, restlessness, fatigue, apathy, sleep disturbances, gastrointestinal manifestations (nausea, vomiting, abdominal pain), and neurological symptoms involving the peripheral nervous system (numbness, paresthesias, muscle cramps, and gait disturbances). Preclinical data suggest that pantothenate could have a role in cellular protection from apoptosis at a subsequent OS exposure (Wojtczak and Slyshenkov, 2003), plausibly via mitochondrial activity optimization and increased glutathione synthesis (Slyshenkov et al., 2004). A striking example of a possible neurological repercussion with severe impairment in pantothenic acid metabolism on CNS is pantothenate kinase–associated neurodegeneration (PKAN), the most frequent of a group of neurodegenerative disorders characterized by high iron accumulation in the brain, which has as major clinical expression in extrapyramidal symptoms and cognitive impairment. PKAN is secondary to rare autosomal recessive mutations (about 1:500 carriers in the general population) of the gene pantothenate kinase type 2, which is a mitochondrial protein necessary to CoA biosynthesis (Brunetti et al., 2012). The depletion in CoA availability due to impaired vB5 metabolism (and subsequent disturbances in mitochondrial bioenergetics and cellular metabolic reactions) has been proposed as a possible explanation of this disease (Shumar et al., 2015).

PKAN has a marginal role in adult onset neurodegenerative diseases, considering that it is a rare syndrome with usual onset during childhood and rapid progression, but adult variants with slower progression have been documented (Doi et al., 2010). Pantethine, a vB5-related molecule composed of two molecules of pantothenic acid linked by cysteamine bridging groups, seems able to bypass pantothenate kinase impairment in animal models of PKAN (Rana et al., 2010; Brunetti et al., 2014). These considerations open a possible future perspective in investigating the eventual role of dietary pantothenic acid or vB5 derivative supplements in brain containment of OS and optimization of energy metabolism, two key points in normal brain function maintenance often suggested to be contributors in age-related neurodegenerative diseases.

Biotin

Biotin (vB7) is a structural part of enzymes involved in bicarbonate-dependent carboxylation reactions, some of which are of exclusive mitochondrial pertinence (namely, pyruvate carboxylase, methylcrotonyl-CoA carboxylase, and propionyl-CoA carboxylase), while others are found also in the cytosol (acetyl-CoA carboxylase 1 and 2) (Institute of Medicine, 1998; Zempleni et al., 2012). Holocarboxylase synthetase (HLCS), a chromatin protein, catalyzes the covalent binding of biotin to carboxylases, while biotinidase releases biotin, which disrupts the covalent bond in enzymes to render it available for recycling (Zempleni et al., 2012). These enzymatic reactions are linked to tricarboxylic acid cycle, gluconeogenesis, fatty acid elongation, and branch-chained amino-acids (leucine) degradation (Institute of Medicine, 1998). Moreover, biotin seems to have a role in DNA stability maintenance and gene expression (Zempleni et al., 2011, 2012; Liu and Zempleni, 2014). HLCS is able to covalently bind biotin to histones; biotinylated histones play a role in transcriptional repression of genes and are particularly represented in long terminal repeats, although in humans <0.001% of histones are biotinylated (Li et al., 2013). Derepression of long terminal repeats in biotin-depleted cell cultures is associated with genome instability (Zempleni et al., 2011). Some authors suggest that an epigenomic synergy between biotinylation and methylation reactions on histones could significantly amplify the relative selectivity of histone biotinylation and render this phenomenon more relevant in gene expression (Li et al., 2013). Furthermore, it seems that biotin and folate can act in concert to promote the suppression of long terminal repeats via interactions between HLCS and other chromatin proteins (Xue and Zempleni, 2013).

Due to the lack of data on biotin requirements, a RDA cannot be deduced, although an AI has been set at 30 μg/day for both men and women of all ages as a weight-adjusted estimation based on inferred infant requirements: biotin intake from exclusive human milk feeding. For similar reasons (scant data on possible toxic effects), it is not possible to establish a UL (Institute of Medicine, 1998). Hemodialysis, inborn errors of enzymes involved in vB7 absorption or metabolism, dietary habits (heavy raw egg white consumption), and lactation could represent conditions with higher requirements for biotin (Institute of Medicine, 1998). Doses up to 200 mg orally and 20 mg intravenously were administered to treat human patients with biotin-responsive inborn errors of metabolism or acquired biotin deficiency without reports of toxicity (Mock, 1996). Preclinical data on pregnant rats reported a possible risk of implant prevention or miscarriage at very high doses of vB7 (about 100 mg/kg). The data could be severely biased because this dose is more than 108 times the estimated AI and vB7 was coadministered along with toxic substances via an unusual route (subcutaneous); a 10-mg daily administration in a woman at the ninth month of pregnancy did not measurably affect either mother or infant (Institute of Medicine, 1998).

Vitamin B_7 is absorbed in its free form in the small intestine and possibly in the proximal colon with both active and passive mechanisms (Institute of Medicine, 1998). Vitamin B7 is partially produced by colonic microflora, but its real role in supplying vitamins in humans is not clear. In food, vB7 is found as both free biotin and protein bound; biotinidase is essential to release biotin from proteins to get it ready to absorption (and to recycle endogenous biotin bound to proteins). Patients deficient in this enzyme usually require a vB7 supplement in its unbound form to meet daily requirements. Other conditions observed to be at risk of deficiency are short gut syndrome, inadequate total parenteral nutrition, and diets characterized by high prolonged consumption of raw egg white (Baugh et al., 1968), which contains avidin, a protein able to sequester biotin in the small intestine and prevent its absorption (Institute of Medicine, 1998). Low biotin plasma levels have also been reported in patients with glucose metabolism dysfunctions such as type 2 diabetes, and an inverse correlation between biotin and fasting plasma glucose has been observed (Kennedy, 2016). The clinical findings of biotin deficiency include dermatitis (periorificial red scaly skin rash), conjunctivitis, alopecia, and neurological abnormalities (depression, lethargy, hallucinations, and paresthesia of the extremities) (Institute of Medicine, 1998).

In an animal model of biotinidase deficiency, the neurological symptoms were associated with demyelination and axonal degeneration in the CNS. Confirmation that these pathological manifestations are subsequent to biotin deficiency itself and not to the accumulation of biotinylated products was supported by rapid regression of both neurological symptoms and pathology after free biotin supplementation (Pindolia et al., 2012). It is not completely understood if the neurological manifestations of vB7 deficiency are consequent to epigenetic modifications or impaired glucose metabolism and energy production or to other unknown causes; neither is it clear if a marginal deficiency of this vitamin could have a clinically relevant impact on aging adults nor if exceeding the normal daily requirements with supplements could ameliorate energy metabolism in healthy individuals. Considering that vB7 seems safe even when administered at high dosages and that prolonged deficiency of this vitamin has sure neurological consequences, it would be recommended to treat promptly in case of suspected deficiency.

Pyridoxine (and Related Compounds), Folate, Cobalamin, and Choline

The link between BGVs and choline is the Met metabolism and Hcy cycle. Specifically, pyridoxine, folate, and cobalamin (with an indirect contribution of riboflavin) are the BGV that intersect one of the numerous metabolic pathways of choline metabolism. After a brief summary for each micronutrient and its function, we will discuss such interactions (see "The Homocysteine Cycle: Biochemistry and Clinical Implications" later in this chapter).

Pyridoxine and Related Compounds

Pyridoxine, pyridoxal, pyridoxamine, and their 5′-phosphate forms are all grouped under the definition of vitamin B6 (vB6) because interconversion between forms is possible (Bender, 1989), and they can be transformed to pyridoxal-phosphate, the main active form of vB6 in the human body (Institute of Medicine, 1998). Vitamin B_6 is a coenzyme in reactions involved in the metabolism of amino acids, glycogen, and sphingoid bases. Relevant biochemical reactions in which vB6 plays a fundamental role are heme biosynthesis and transsulfuration reactions that transform Hcy to cysteine (Cys) via cystathionine β-synthase and cystathionine γ-lyase activity (Institute of Medicine, 1998). Moreover, pyridoxine is an essential cofactor in monoamine synthesis, mediating a step in the conversion of tryptophan and tyrosine in serotonin and dopamine, respectively (Rotstein and Kang, 2009). The RDA for vB6 is set at 1.3 and 1.4 mg/day for adult men and women, rising to 1.5 and 1.7 mg/day in elderly men and women (Institute of Medicine, 1998). The EFSA reported a possible adjustment for daily protein intake because it has been observed that vB6 plasma values tend to decrease more rapidly in individuals with higher protein intake. The suggested RDA in relation to dietary protein load would be 15 μ g of vB6 per gram of protein, reaching an average RDA in adults of 2–3 g/day (EFSA, 2006). Absorption in the gut is mediated by a not saturable passive diffusion system for nonphosphorylated forms of vB6 (a phosphatase hydrolyze 5 ′ -phosphate forms of vB6, no saturation effect has been seen even for extremely high doses) (Institute of Medicine, 1998). Bioavailability varies among different vitamers of vB6 group; in a mixed diet, the mean absorption of the vitamers has been estimated to reach values of 75% of the ingested dose. The absorbed part of dietary source is phosphorylated in the liver and stored bound to proteins (Institute of Medicine, 1998). Vitamin B_6 is the BGV with the most established and relevant adverse effect; the UL has been set at 100 mg/day due to onset of neurotoxicity, consisting mainly in a symptomatic peripheral neuropathy (Institute of Medicine, 1998). Concerns of possible neurotoxicity associated to prolonged intake of lower daily doses impose a critical approach to supplementation, and some authors suggest caution in choosing dosages (Ghavanini and Kimpinski, 2014). Because this side effect is dependent on individual susceptibility, dose, and time of exposure, the EFSA suggested a safer UL: 25 mg/day (EFSA, 2006). Clinical signs of deficiency are retarded growth, acrodynia, hair loss and thinning, bone abnormalities, and microcytic anemia (Institute of Medicine, 1998; EFSA, 2006). On the neurological side, the perturbation of neurotransmission (depletion of dopamine, serotonin, norepinephrine, tryptamine, tyramine, histamine, gamma-aminobutyric acid, and taurine) probably contributes to psychological and cognitive alterations and seizures (EFSA, 2006). The link between vB6 deficiency and high Hcy plasma levels will be discussed separately in the section "The Homocysteine Cycle: Biochemistry and Clinical Implications").

Folate

Folate (vB9) is a generic name for a group of vitamers (compounds with similar vitamin biological activities). Naturally occurring folates have a chain of molecules of glutamate joined to a γ-carboxyl site in peptide linkage; variable in their numbers of molecules, these vitamers are defined pteroylpolyglutamates (Institute of Medicine, 1998). Not all the vitamers have the same bioavailability, but all can be converted to tetrahydrofolate (the main biologically active form). Folic acid (pteroylmonoglutamic acid) is the vitamer most used in supplements and fortified foods due to its stability, but it is scarcely represented in foods of natural origin; it has nearly 1.7 times the availability of natural occurring folates (Gregory, 2012). Folate participates in DNA synthesis and one-carbon metabolisms (methylation reactions); folate-dependent enzymatic steps are also described in amino acid interconversion reactions (histidine to glutamic acid, serine to glycine, and Met to Hcy) (Institute of Medicine, 1998).

The RDA for folates has been set at 400 μg/day for both adult men and women; it has been decided to maintain this threshold even for elderly individuals (Institute of Medicine, 1998). More recently, a lower RDA has been proposed by the EFSA (250 μg/day) (EFSA, 2014), but in our opinion, thinking at the good therapeutic index of folates, probably 400 μg/day is a more suitable RDA. Absorption in the small intestines is favored by a proximal active saturable transport system that is overcome by distal passive diffusion at higher dosages (EFSA, 2014). To be internalized by the gut mucosa, polyglutamic forms must be hydrolyzed to monoglutamates by γ-glutamyl carboxypeptidase (an enzyme of the intestinal brush border membrane), then it is mainly transported in this form bound to plasma proteins and finally retransformed in a functional form in target organs (EFSA, 2014). Several situations could increase the requirements of folates. Probably one of the most clinically relevant is a mutation of the methylenetetrahydrofolate reductase (MTHFR) gene. MTHFR mutation reduces the enzyme activity inhibiting the normal folate metabolism (with consequent raise Hcy concentration and reduction of methyl donors). The most common variant reduces enzymatic activity up to 45% of the wild type (Leclerc et al., 2000). It consists of an amino acid substitution of an alanine with a valine (a cytosine in position 677 into thymine—MTHFR C677T). The frequency of the mutated gene varies greatly geographically: about 30% in Europe and Japan and only about 11% in African Americans (Clarke and Armitage, 2000). In the homozygote condition, it is associated with a mild to moderate rise in Hcy plasma levels (Carmel et al., 2003) and low red blood cell folates (Molloy et al., 1997). In Asian populations, MTHFR C677T polymorphism has been linked by epidemiological data to vascular dementia (Liu et al., 2010), AD (Hua et al., 2011), and depression (Jiang et al., 2015). In individuals carriers of MTHFR C677T homozygous mutation, a higher daily dose of folic acid supplement may be useful to force the enzymatic pathway and reduce the detrimental effects of this condition (Jacques et al., 1999; Ashfield-Watt et al., 2002; de Bree et al., 2003). A second polymorphism of MTHFR at base pair (bp) 1298, resulting in a substitution of a glutamate with an alanine (MTHFR A1298C), has lower clinical significance. The enzyme mutated at bp 1298 shows a minor reduction in its activity (68% of wild type vs, 45% of the one mutated in bp 677), and homozygous individuals (about 8% in European populations) are reported to have near normal Hcy levels. Individuals who are compound heterozygotes for the MTHFR

A1298C and MTHFR C677T alleles tend to have a biochemical profile closer to that seen among MTHFR C677T homozygotes (Leclerc et al., 2000). Moreover, some authors suggest that the *cis configuration of mutation A1298C and C677T is rarely observed; even in this case, it seems that the colocalization of both alleles on the same chromosome would not significantly affect enzyme activity compared to MTHFR C677T alone* (Leclerc et al., 2000).

High intake of folates of food origin do not seem to cause severe adverse effects, while folic acid supplements gave rise to concerns about possible masking of vB12 deficiency and induction of neurotoxicity and carcinogenesis. The so-called folate trap is a major concern, especially in nations in which isolated folate fortification of foods has been implemented. It consists of masking the hematological consequences of cobalamin deficiency (macrocytic anemia) without reversing the neurological damage (or enhancing it) (EFSA, 2014). The subsequent delay in diagnosis due to the initially paucisymptomatic onset of cognitive, psychological, and sensory impairment (subacute combined degeneration) secondary to cobalamin deficiency can impede a full recovery (Martin, 1992; Abyad, 2002). Some authors also reported concerns of possible direct neurotoxic effect of high dosage supplements with folic acid (>400 μ g/day) (Morris et al., 2005). These concerns are apparently open to discussion since the same authors later identified the signs of vB12 deficiency as the strongest risk factors for cognitive decline in a subgroup of the same population (exposed to folic acid fortification and consequently to a high risk of undetected progression of vB12 deficiency-related neurological complications) (Tangney et al., 2009). Other authors have found similar results in a different cohort of individuals subjected to folate fortification, in which low vB12 in presence of normal folate was associated to cognitive decline, while high folic acid intake in individuals with normal vB12 status emerged as a protective factor (Morris et al., 2007). Adequate folate intake is reported to reduce the risk of colon and breast cancer (EFSA, 2014), but some contrasting evidences seem to correlate folate intake and cancer development or recurrence (Cole et al., 2007; Figueiredo et al., 2009). This has been sustained by the hypothesis that folate can be protective for normal tissue but has, on the other hand, the ability to fuel ongoing neoplastic foci (EFSA, 2014; Ulrich, 2006). A recent meta-analysis confuted the hypothesized relationship between folate intake and cancer development (Mackerras et al., 2014), but the topic is still widely debated and caution in general is suggested (Choi et al., 2014).

In conclusion, there is no sufficient strength of evidence to express a solid statement on this matter (EFSA, 2014). The UL has been set at 1 mg/day from fortified foods and supplements because of the described concerns about possible carcinogenic properties and most of all disease masking and neurotoxic effects in the case of vB12 deficiency (Institute of Medicine, 1998; EFSA, 2014). It should be a fairly safe dosage even in the latter case (EFSA, 2014). Folate deficiency syndrome shares multiple features with cobalamin deficiency: macrocytic anemia and neuronal symptoms (psychiatric and cognitive disorders and less commonly peripheral neuropathy) are the main manifestations (Young and Ghadirian, 1989; Reynolds, 2014). The observation of higher prevalence of folate deficiency in psychiatric patients and the (partial) reversibility of psychiatric symptoms in deficient patients confirms that folate deficiency alone could induce neurological symptoms (Young and Ghadirian, 1989) without the contribution of a concomitant vB12 deficiency (in this case, a folate supplement would have had no effect or could even have a detrimental contribution). A partial explanation of the neurological impact of folate deficiency probably resides in an elevation of Hcy plasma levels (see "The Homocysteine Cycle: Biochemistry and Clinical Implications" later in this chapter).

Cobalamin

Cobalamin (vB12) is a generic description of compounds characterized by a corrinic ring structure (a cobalt atom bound to six ligands) with similar biological activity. The upper (or β-axial) ligand varies and defines the vitamer of vB12 (cyano, hydroxo, aquo, methyl, sulfito, nitrite, glutathionyl, or adenosyl group). The bioactive forms of the vitamin are methylcobalamin and 5′-deoxyadenosylcobalamin. Cyanocobalamin is a stable synthetic compound usually found in supplements and drugs. Cobalamin is known to participate as a coenzyme in two biochemical reactions in humans: (1) remethylation of Hcy to Met via methionine synthase in the cytosol and (2) rearrangement of methylmalonyl-CoA to succinyl-CoA in mitochondria via methylmalonyl-CoA mutase (EFSA, 2015). Globally, vB12 contributes to DNA regulation via epigenetic modifications and to amino acids and fatty acid metabolism. Succinyl-CoA is directly involved in the tricarboxylic acid cycle, while remethylation of Hcy is fundamental for recycling this neurotoxic sulfur-containing nonessential amino acid (see "The Homocysteine Cycle: Biochemistry and Clinical Implications" later in the chapter) and for Met pool maintenance and subsequent *S*-adenosyl-methionine (SAM) synthesis. As better described later, SAM is a methyl donor involved in genetic regulation (see the later section "Epigenetic Theory of BGV Deficiency-Related Neurodegeneration") and neurotransmitter synthesis (see "Impact of BGV and Choline on Neurotransmission") along with many other methylation reactions (EFSA, 2015). In 1998, the US Institute of Medicine set the RDA for vB12 at 2.4 μg/day for both men and women older than 19 (Institute of Medicine, 1998). Recently, the EFSA, given a reported lack of information necessary to calculate the average requirement for vB12, only set an AI at 4 μg/day for both adults and the elderly without gender differences (EFSA, 2015).

The absorption process of vB12 is quite different from other BGVs; indeed, being a complex molecule, its transport into the blood stream from the intestinal lumen necessitates an active system at normal dietary intake levels. Effective passive diffusion occurs only with very high dosages of the micronutrient, up to 1–2g, but can be a viable alternative to parenteral administration for supplements in patients with vB12 malabsorption due to inactivity of the normal facilitated transport (Vidal-Alaball et al., 2005; Stabler, 2013). The absorption process initiates in the proximal digestive tract with haptocorrin (or transcobalamin 1) production. Haptocorrin is a glycoprotein secreted by the salivary glands that binds vB12 in the stomach after it has been released from food proteins by acid and enzymatic processes. The vB12–haptocorrin complex is able to resist the gastric acid environment and then in the duodenum, haptocorrin is digested by pancreatic enzymes and substituted by intrinsic factor (a transport glycoprotein produced by gastric parietal cells) to form the complex that is able to be absorbed in the ileum by a specific transport system. This complex system is particularly prone to inefficiency due to its multiple step-limiting passages. Different conditions (especially prevalent in elderly individuals) can lead to gastric pH modifications and lower intrinsic factor production that affects vB12 availability (antacid medications for increments in pH, autoimmune processes such as pernicious anemia for intrinsic factor-limited production, and chronic gastritis for both mechanisms) (Andrès et al., 2008). Moreover, integrity of the distal ileum is essential to reach a good absorption rate at intake levels normally reached with food (Institute of Medicine, 1998). Only about 1.2% of vB12 is absorbed via passive diffusion (Vidal-Alaball et al., 2005). No adverse effects have ever been related to cobalamin administration, even at high dosages, so it is impossible at the moment to establish an UL.

A vB12 deficiency develops after a prolonged inadequate cobalamin intake, since usually the biological stores of the vitamin in a healthy subject without prior deficient intake are sufficient for several months (Loew et al., 1999). The main clinical manifestations of deficiency are a macrocytic anemia that is very similar to the one observable in folate deficiency and which evolves to pancytopenia at later stages (leukopenia associated with typical hypersegmented neutrophils and thrombocytopenia; elevated lactic dehydrogenase may be found due to ineffective erythropoiesis), neurological abnormalities (spinal cord degeneration, depression, and cognitive impairment), and gastrointestinal symptoms (even if the latter are debated because the cause of vB12 deficiency itself often can be responsible for the symptoms) (Institute of Medicine, 1998).

The neurological consequences of vB12 deficiency can be the only clinical manifestations of the disease (Stabler, 2013). In some cohorts of patients with neuropsychiatric disorders secondary to vB12 deficiency, macrocytosis, and anemia were absent in about one-third of subjects (Lindenbaum et al., 1988). At early stages, neurological symptoms can be subtle and difficult to diagnose because of the possible polymorphic presentation symptoms ranging from sensory alterations (paresthesias, dysesthesias, hypoesthesias, hypopallesthesia, and altered proprioception) to mild cognitive impairment and mood changes. In advanced stages, patients could present ataxia, double incontinence, impotence, optic-nerve atrophy, severe cognitive impairment or frank dementia, and various psychiatric disorders (depression, psychosis, and abnormal behavior) (Stabler et al., 1990). The *spongy degeneration* (swelling of myelin sheets that subsequently evolves to full demyelination) historically observed in the dorsolateral columns of the spinal cord is now known to occur systemically (subacute combined degeneration). Magnetic resonance imaging (MRI) scans can observe signs of spinal cord degeneration early in the disease (Senol et al., 2008), but leukoencephalopathy and peripheral nerves demyelination has also been described (Pacheco et al., 2015). A possible sequential involvement due to regional differences in myelin composition and resilience to vB12 deficiency in central and peripheral nervous system has been postulated (Minn et al., 2012). Part of the neurotoxic effect of vB12 deficiency is probably due to a rise in plasma Hcy with subsequent associated damage (see the later section "The Homocysteine Cycle: Biochemistry and Clinical Implications"). It has been observed that symptoms related to cobalamin deficiency can be found also in individuals with near-normal vB12 plasmatic levels; this could be a sign of scarce utilization of the micronutrient. Surrogate markers have been proposed for confirmation of suspected deficiency even in the presence of normal vitamin levels; one of these is Hcy, even if it has low specificity due to its multifactorial biochemistry (vB9 and vB6 deficits, glomerular filtration-rate reduction, many drugs and illnesses can cause a rise in Hcy plasma levels). Methylmalonic acid instead seems to be more reliable: some authors suggest that subjects with normal vB12 and raised levels of Hcy and methylmalonic acid should be considered functionally deficient and that surrogate markers of deficiency have a higher sensibility and specificity than vB12 plasma levels themselves (Carmel, 2000; Carmel et al., 2003; Ulrich et al., 2015).

Choline

Choline pool is balanced by both endogenous synthesis and exogenous supply. Usually the normal choline biosynthesis is not sufficient to support the numerous physiological functions for which it is required (Institute of Medicine, 1998), so generally dietary intake assumes a notable importance even if the micronutrient is not formally considered a vitamin. Phosphatidylcholine (PC) accounts for about 95% of the body storage of choline in mammalians; the remaining pool is divided by free choline, phosphocholine, glycerophosphocholine, cytidine 5-diphosphocholine, and acetylcholine (Ach) (Ueland, 2011). Choline is present in food as free choline and in its esterified forms—mainly as lecithin, Ach, and citicoline (El-Sohemy et al., 2013). Lecithin, in which PC is usually the most represented phospholipid, is a common supplement also used for its amphipathic properties as an emulsifier in foods (Institute of Medicine, 1998).

To understand the wide metabolic implications of choline, it is to consider that it is involved in membrane structure maintenance, lipid metabolism, neurotransmission, methylation reactions, and Hcy balance (Institute of Medicine, 1998; Ueland, 2011). Choline intake accelerates the synthesis and release of Ach, thus affecting global brain functions (with special reference to memory storage and recall), autonomic nervous system regulation, and muscle activity (Institute of Medicine, 1998). Betaine (Bet), a choline metabolite, is an important methyl donor involved in the Hcy cycle (the remethylation of Hcy to Met via betaine-homocysteine *S*-methyltransferase, a non-BGV–dependent shunt for BGV-dependent reactions in the Hcy cycle) with osmotic properties essential for normal renal physiology (Institute of Medicine, 1998). De novo biosynthesis of PC (the most used form of choline in the body and obtained by the methylation of phosphoethanolamide) is strictly bound to SAM availability, so indirectly Met, vB9, and vB12 intake and metabolism regulate the requirements of exogenous choline provision (Institute of Medicine, 1998). PC synthesis is probably the most demanding SAM-dependent methylation reaction in human body, so this reaction is a candidate to be the principal source of Hcy in human metabolism once deprived of the methyl group SAM, which becomes *S*-adenosyl-homocysteine (SAH) and then Hcy (Stead et al., 2006).

The AI for choline has been set at 550 mg/day for men and 425 mg/day for women of all ages (19 and older) (Institute of Medicine, 1998). Folate restriction or MTHFR polymorphisms with reduced enzymatic activity along with intense physical activity can increase the daily choline requirements (Institute of Medicine, 1998; El-Sohemy et al., 2013). The UL has been set at 3.5 g/day for choline. The main manifestation of excessive intake are hypotension at high dosages (observed for 7.5 g/day supplements in AD patients), gastrointestinal symptoms, and sweating with a fishy odor (probably due to increased vagal tone and trimethylamine production) (Institute of Medicine, 1998). Choline deficiency, although rare in subjects with a varied diet, has been associated with liver damage, including elevated alanine aminotransferase and the development of fatty liver. Moreover, insufficient choline intake can result in increased Hcy plasma levels, especially in folate poor diets (Ueland, 2011) (see "The Homocysteine Cycle: Biochemistry and Clinical Implications" section). This may be attributable to Bet promoting remethylation of homocysteine to methionine in the liver (El-Sohemy et al., 2013).

THE HOMOCYSTEINE CYCLE: BIOCHEMISTRY AND CLINICAL IMPLICATIONS

In the last few decades, clinical research in the fields of brain aging and dementia treatment and prevention has focused mostly on two BGVs—namely, vB9 and vB12 (Morris, 2006)—mainly because epidemiological data reported a possible association with cognition and dementia development (Hinterberger and Fischer, 2013; O'Leary et al., 2012). These results are still controversial, and some interventional clinical trials did not show any benefit from vB9 or vB12 supplementation in terms of cognition (Malouf and Areosa Sastre, 2003; Malouf and Grimley Evans, 2008; Ford and Almeida, 2012; Clarke et al., 2014). A hypothesized path of neuronal damage involved in BGV-related defects in cognition is related to an intermediate product of Met metabolism: Hcy. Hcy is a sulfur amino acid with several interactions with the vascular and neuronal systems (Selhub et al., 1996; Kalmijn et al., 1999; Seshadri et al., 2002; Hassan et al., 2004; Martí-Carvajal et al., 2009; Ford and Flicker, 2012) that accumulates in conditions of vB9 and vB12 deficiency. Another key micronutrient in Hcy metabolism is vB6, and for this reason it has been proposed as having a possible role in determining Hcy-related neuronal damage. As for the other two just cited BGVs, studies about vB6 supplementation still have not shown any benefit in terms of cognition (Malouf and Grimley Evans, 2003). As a precursor of Bet, choline seems to be useful in partially compensating for the Hcy rise (Ueland, 2011). To better understand the possible role of vB6, vB9, vB12, and choline in Hcy-mediated neuronal damage, we will discuss the metabolic interconnections among these molecules and the supposed mechanisms that underlie their detrimental effects on the CNS. Met metabolism has a crucial role in methylation processes, via *S*-adenosyl-methionine synthase it generates SAM, one of the main methyl donors in the human body. Methylation processes regulate DNA synthesis and are essential in a large number of enzymatic reactions. Losing a methyl group, SAM becomes SAH, which is then hydrolyzed in Hcy. Hcy represents a juncture between remethylation reactions that restore the Met pool and transsulfuration reactions that transform Hcy in Cys. The remethylation pathway requires vB9 and vB12 (Carmel et al., 2003). In conditions where one of the aforementioned vitamins is deficient, it can only be partially shunted via betaine–homocysteine–methyltransferase, which requires Bet as a cofactor (Ueland, 2011). The transsulfuration enzymatic pathway, on the other hand, requires vB6 as a cofactor. Moreover, as previously described (see the riboflavin in the section titled "Riboflavin"), vB2 is necessary for both vB9 and vB6 metabolism.

It is simple to deduce that a deficit of vB6, vB9, vB12 (and vB2 indirectly), or choline results in hyperhomocysteinemia (HHcy), which is defined as a plasma concentration higher than 15 μmol/L. In animal models, HHcy is clearly related to a rapid and massive development of cognitive impairment and pathological findings of microvascular damage and tissue phlogosis in the brain (Sudduth et al., 2013). Even if the HHcy-induced damage seems to be incontrovertible in preclinical models (Sudduth et al., 2013), the experimental conditions used to simulate a HHcy exposure are far from the prevalent forms of human clinical expression of HHcy, which is usually a mild or moderate increase of the metabolite. Currò and colleagues demonstrated that also prolonged exposure to mildly elevated Hcy levels can be toxic in neuronal cell cultures promoting genotoxicity and OS (Currò et al., 2014). HHcy can reach a severe degree (values of 100 μmol/L or more) in rare cases of genetic defects (homocystinuria), long standing multiple BGV deficiency and/or severe renal disease (Carmel et al., 2003). In humans it is reported a higher rate of microvascular brain damage, on CT and MRI scans, in hyperhomocysteinemic patients (Vermeer et al., 2002; Tangney et al., 2011), the instrumental findings of leukoaraiosis and small white matter infarcts, though, did not seem to fully explain the decline in cognitive performance observed in HHcy (Nilsson et al., 2012; Dufouil et al., 2003). Numerous epidemiological studies also associate HHcy with neurodegenerative diseases and neuropsychiatric manifestations in elderly patients (Lehmann et al., 1999; Seshadri et al., 2002; Quadri et al., 2004). The possible relation between HHcy and AD (the neurodegenerative dementia with the highest prevalence in elderly people) or other types of dementia is supported by epidemiological correlation (Seshadri et al., 2002; Ford and Flicker, 2012). Even if AD symptoms could be anticipated and worsened by brain vascular damage (Snowden et al., 1997), recent evidence has shown that HHcy also contributes to AD development with other mechanisms (Fuso et al., 2012). Since HHcy is a consequence of low BGV intake or activity, it is difficult to separate the neurological effects of raised Hcy plasma levels and BGV deficiencies, but it has been reported that HHcy is correlated to cognitive decline and dementia independently of BGV status (Bonetti et al., 2015). Preclinical studies linked HHcy to many detrimental effects with possible neurological repercussions that deserve a detailed description.

Excitotoxicity, Endoplasmatic Reticulum Stress, and Reactive Oxygen Species Production

In both acute ischemic brain damage and chronic neurodegenerative disorders (including AD and PD), a common activation of glutamatergic receptors induces or worsens cellular dysfunction, which leads ultimately to cell death (Prentice et al., 2015). Hcy is a potent agonist of *N*-methyl-D-aspartate (NMDA) glutamatergic receptors (McCully, 2009). Activation of NMDA receptors results in intracellular calcium overload and mitochondrial dysfunction (Prentice et al., 2015). A heavy activation of NMDA receptors brings intracellular calcium concentrations at levels scarcely compatible with cell survival (oxidative phosphorylation inhibition, phosphate depletion, and even deposition of insoluble salts of calcium and phosphate). The degree and the time of exposure to this dysfunctional process influence the type of damage: tissutal necrosis when it is intense and acute or programmed cellular death if it does not completely overcome the essential cellular reactions (McCully, 2009; Prentice et al., 2015). Impaired mitochondrial activity determines a reduction in energy production with subsequent dysfunction of cellular machinery due to depletion of adenosine triphosphate and augmented production of reactive oxygen species. Furthermore, NMDA activation induces neuronal nitric oxide synthase, which accelerates nitric oxide production, and OS is increased by interaction of nitric oxide with superoxide with the generation of reactive nitrogen species (Prentice et al., 2015). Moreover, the altered cytosolic ambient and the strong OS insult result in protein misfolding and activation of endoplasmatic reticulum stress reactions defined as an unfolded protein response (UPR) (Doyle et al., 2011; Prentice et al., 2015). If prolonged over time, UPR contributes to the induction of apoptotic pathways and has been postulated as an etiological contributor to neurodegenerative diseases (Zhang et al., 2001; Doyle et al., 2011; Penke et al., 2016). HHcy has been linked to apoptosis and prolonged UPR activation, which seems to be one of the mechanisms that underlie this correlation (Zhang et al., 2001; Perla-Kajan et al., 2007).

Protein Homocysteinylation

Circulating Hcy is mainly found bound to proteins. One particularly relevant form of covalent modification of circulating proteins occurs as a consequence of the high reactivity of a Hcy derivative: homocysteine thiolactone (Htl) (Sharma et al., 2015). Htl is a cyclic thioester that results from an error-editing reaction by methionyl–tRNA synthetase (Jakubowski and Goldman, 1993; Jakubowski et al., 2000). One possible mechanism of Htl toxicity is the nonenzymatic formation of amide bonds with ε-amino groups of protein lysine residues; this reaction is a defined protein *N*-homocysteinylation (Sharma et al., 2014). Htl production and the subsequent protein homocysteinylation rate depend on Hcy concentration and result in enzyme inactivation, protein denaturation, aggregation, and precipitation (Sharma et al., 2015). On the basis of these observations, it has been postulated a role of Htl-mediated homocysteinylation in AD progression via promotion of amyloid deposition in the brain and tau protein aggregation (Sharma et al., 2015) and enhancement of Aβ peptide neurotoxicity via stabilization of its oligomeric form (the most reactive and dangerous) (Khodadadi et al., 2012). Moreover, homocysteinylation produces new epitopes on proteins usually recognized as self (Undas et al., 2004), and it has been postulated that autoantibodies versus homocysteinylated proteins could contribute to immunomediated damage to vessels walls and the promotion of atherosclerosis (Sharma et al., 2015). Furthermore, homocysteinylation of low-density lipoproteins (LDLs) renders them more prone to oxidation (augmented also due to Hcy-induced OS) and to uptake by macrophages to form foam cells and promote atherosclerotic plaque progression (Bełtowski, 2005; McCully, 2009).

Endothelial Damage and Atherothrombosis

Early atherosclerosis and thrombotic events are the hallmarks of vascular damage in homocystinuria, an inherited disorder in Met metabolism due to a cystathionine beta synthase deficiency that results in markedly high Hcy. Endothelial dysfunction is initially represented by impaired vasodilation capability, probably due to reduction in nitric oxide availability (McCully, 2009). Later stages exhibit various pathological manifestations such as vacuolization, cytoplasmic swelling, and hyperplasia of endothelial cells (McCully, 2009), vascular smooth cells growth, and enhanced collagen deposition in arterial intima and media (Tsai et al., 1994; Majors et al., 1997). So atherogenesis is promoted and sustained by endothelial dysfunction, OS and protein homocysteinylation consequences (especially oxidized homocysteinylated LDLs), and phlogistic or immunologic processes (activation of macrophages and production of IL-1, IL-6, and TNF-α) (McCully, 2009). A pronounced intimal damage in the absence of significant lipid deposition in vessel walls of young homocystinuric patients suggests that inflammatory modifications are the primary movers of Hcy-induced arterial alterations (McCully, 1969). Another Hcy effect able to further mine the stability of these severely phlogistic plaques is the promotion of platelet aggregation (McCully, 1969; Harker et al., 1974) and thrombosis (Genoud, 2014). Thus, vascular brain damage subsequent to prolonged exposure to HHcy can lead to stroke and vascular cognitive impairment or favor the progression of other neurodegenerative diseases (e.g., AD and PD).

The Epigenetic Theory of BGV Deficiency-Related Neurodegeneration

In the last decades, epigenetics gained noteworthy attention in the field of brain health maintenance and neurodegeneration (Fuso, 2013). DNA methylation is essential to the regulation of gene expression and genome stability, and recently growing evidence seems to suggest a relationship with neurodegenerative diseases such as AD and PD (Kwok, 2010). Methylated sequences are silenced, but the silencing could interfere with both inhibitory and promoting genes, resulting in a complex and varied, although specific, modified DNA expression. Numerous environmental factors could affect DNA expression; nutritional factors in particular have a potentially critical role (Fuso, 2013). SAM is the main substrate of DNA-methyl-transferases (DNMT), a class of enzymes responsible for the transposition of methyl groups from SAM to DNA cytosine, leaving SAH as a by-product of the reaction, which is then transformed to Hcy (Fuso et al., 2011). DNA-demethylase (DDM) conversely demethylates DNA, delineating a finely regulated equilibrium that depends on DNMTs and DDM activity and the availability of their substrates (Fuso et al., 2011). The SAM-to-SAH ratio defines the methylation potential (MP) of the body. Reduced SAM synthesis (due to Met or BGV deficiency) or SAH clearance (e.g., the inhibited transformation of SAH in Hcy even simply due to excess product) determines a reduction of the MP, resulting in DNA hypomethylation and aberrant gene expression (Fuso et al., 2011). SAM synthesis requires Met, and Hcy remethylation promotes an increment in MP in two ways: (1) by increasing Met availability (and as a consequence SAM availability) and (2) by scavenging Hcy (that, as already said, favors SAH degradation). Hcy remethylation is a key point in methyl donors synthesis, so it is clear that both the enzymatic pathways mediated by betaine–homocysteine–methyltransferase (which requires Bet, a metabolite of choline) and methionine synthase (which uses 5′-methylene-tetrahydrofolate as a substrate and cobalamin as cofactor) have repercussions for DNA methylation processes. Moreover, as previously described, vB2 could also be considered to have an impact in SAM synthesis by being a cofactor for MTHFR in the transformation of 5,10-methylene-tetrahydrofolate to 5′-methyl-tetrahydrofolate. Finally, though via mechanisms not completely understood, vB7-mediated histone biotinylation could also interfere with DNA methylation and further modify DNA expression.

Fuso and colleagues demonstrated with preclinical models of HHcy, obtained with BGV deficiency, that SAM depletion and SAH accumulation inhibit DNMTs and promote DDM activity. That results in DNA hypomethylation of the presenilin 1 gene promoter and increased γ-secretase synthesis (Fuso et al., 2011). Increased amyloidogenesis via γ-secretase cleavage of amyloid precursor protein into Aβ delineates the final steps of the complex relationship between BGV deficiency epigenetic consequences and AD development. Even if not studied in relation to BGV deficiency specific hypomethylation pattern, some authors have hypothesized that similar epigenetic mechanisms (in particular, DNA methylation pattern modifications) could be the expression of both "normal" age-related brain changes and neurodegeneration with variations in the entity and topography of DNA alterations (Keleshian et al., 2013). Other authors report that similar hypomethylation patterns have been observed in AD and AD-like syndromes such as in PD and Lewy body dementia (Sanchez-Mut et al., 2016). In conclusion, BGV deficiency seems to have epigenetic repercussions that could interfere with normal brain aging by promoting AD-like pathology and possibly other neurodegenerative pathways. More research is needed to confirm and eventually clarify these relationships.

An observation that could have an enormous impact on BGV fortification policies is that recent evidence from animal models supports the transmission of a hypomethylation pattern induced by BGV deficiency in pregnant rats to the brain cells of their offspring with permanent consequences until adult age (Sable, 2015). If such findings are observed and confirmed in humans, then new perspectives will open in the field of nutritional programs for disease prevention and health promotion on a generational level. An adequate fortification of foods with all of the BGV involved in one-carbon metabolism would reduce drastically the consequences of the detrimental genetic processes just described, possibly modifying the clinical landscape of neurodegenerative diseases as we know it.

Impact of B Group Vitamins and Choline on Neurotransmission

A balanced activity of neural networks sustained by different neurotransmitters is essential for normal brain functioning. Disturbances in the availability of neurotransmitters have been recognized as etiological in many neuropsychiatric and neurological disorders. Nowadays, therapies that directly or indirectly substitute or enhance the activity of neurotransmitters remain cornerstones for the treatment of depression, PD, AD, and other neurological conditions. The synthesis of monoamines (dopamine, serotonin, noradrenaline) depends on vB6 availability, and SAM is a cofactor in their metabolism (Bottiglieri, 1996; Rotstein and Kang, 2009). SAM administration or promotion of its synthesis via BGV has been reported as effective in increasing CNS monoaminergic systems and in treating depressive disorders (Bottiglieri, 1996, 1997). Moreover, the observation that SAM administration also enhances cholinergic neurotransmission (increased brain concentrations of acetylcholine and the expression of muscarinic receptors) led to the finding that it could be beneficial in treating the cognitive symptoms of major depression (Levkovitz et al., 2012) and to the hypothesis that it, along with the BGV implicated in its maintenance levels, could also have a role in treating demented patients (Bottiglieri, 2013). Being the cholinergic system strongly related to attention, learning, memory, and motivation (Luchicchi et al., 2014), it has been selected as main target for nootropic drugs, and its augmentation remains the main therapeutic strategy in AD patients (Allgaier and Allgaier, 2014). Both dietary choline (Hollenbeck, 2012) and its pharmacological derivatives (Gareri et al., 2015) promote acetylcholine synthesis. Moreover, in combination with other micronutrients (uridine monophosphate and omega-3 fatty acids), it has been proposed to modulate synaptic plasticity and consequently neurotransmission efficacy (Engelborghs et al., 2014; Wurtman, 2014).

CONCLUSIONS

BGV and choline are certainly essential nutrients for adequate brain development, function, and protection. A balanced diet rich in fruits and vegetables and minimal intake of foods of animal origin, in the absence of malabsorption and severe comorbidities, should ensure a sufficient provision of the necessary micronutrients for the maintenance of normal neurological functions. Elderly individuals often require a higher intake of BGVs, probably because of an expected reduced absorption capability and the onset of concomitant age-related conditions (e.g., increased OS, burden of acquired organ damage, and impaired buffer mechanisms due to abnormal metabolic activity). Most BGVs (with vB3, vB6, and perhaps vB9 as exceptions) are almost surely safe even at intake levels reached with food fortification or supplements. In the latter case, considering the complex interaction between all BGVs and choline, a complete supplementation of all of these micronutrients is safer and surely more effective than the administration of a single vitamin. In the presence of initial cognitive decline or, even worse, frank dementia, supplementation is probably useful but with limited rate of efficacy in the absence of a severe deficiency of the micronutrients supplemented. A neuroprotective dietary pattern should be adopted as soon as possible (even in early adulthood) to obtain the maximum result when all of the systems are still functional. Moreover, given the repercussion of systemic state on brain aging, a global approach that also contemplates regular physical activity and the adoption of a stimulating and challenging but healthy lifestyle is recommended.

References

Abdou, E., Hazell, A.S., 2015. Thiamine deficiency: an update of pathophysiologic mechanisms and future therapeutic considerations. Neurochem. Res. 40 (2), 353–361.

Abyad, A., 2002. Prevalence of vitamin B_{12} deficiency among demented patients and cognitive recovery with cobalamin replacement. J. Nutr. Health Aging 6 (4), 254–260.

Allgaier, M., Allgaier, C., 2014. An update on drug treatment options of Alzheimer's disease. Front. Biosci. (Landmark Ed) 19, 1345–1354.

Andrès, E., Vogel, T., Federici, L., Zimmer, J., Ciobanu, E., Kaltenbach, G., 2008. Cobalamin deficiency in elderly patients: a personal view. Curr. Gerontol. Geriatr. Res., 848267. http://dx.doi.org/10.1155/2008/848267.

Ashfield-Watt, P.A., Pullin, C.H., Whiting, J.M., Clark, Z.E., Moat, S.J., Newcombe, R.G., et al., 2002. Methylenetetrahydrofolate reductase 677C- > T genotype modulates homocysteine responses to a folate-rich diet or a low-dose folic acid supplement: a randomized controlled trial. Am. J. Clin. Nutr. 76 (1), 180–186.

Azizi-Namini, P., Ahmed, M., Yan, A.T., Keith, M., 2012. The role of B vitamins in the management of heart failure. Nutr. Clin. Pract. 27 (3), 363–374.

Baugh, C.M., Malone, J.H., Butterworth Jr, C.E., 1968. Human biotin deficiency. A case history of biotin deficiency induced by raw egg consumption in a cirrhotic patient. Am. J. Clin. Nutr. 21, 173–182.

Bełtowski, J., 2005. Protein homocysteinylation: a new mechanism of atherogenesis? Postepy. Hig. Med. Dosw. (Online) 59, 392–404.

Bender, D.A., 1989. Vitamin B6 requirements and recommendations. Eur. J. Clin. Nutr. 43, 289–309.

Bonetti, F., Brombo, G., Magon, S., Zuliani, G., 2015. Cognitive status according to homocysteine and B-group vitamins in elderly adults. J. Am. Geriatr. Soc. 63 (6), 1158–1163.

Bogdanovic, N., Bretillon, L., Lund, E.G., Diczfalusy, U., Lannfelt, L., Winblad, B., et al., 2001. On the turnover of brain cholesterol in patients with Alzheimer's disease: abnormal induction of the cholesterol-catabolic enzyme CYP46 in glial cells. Neurosci. Lett. 314 (1–2), 45–48.

Bottiglieri, T., 1996. Folate, vitamin B12, and neuropsychiatric disorders. Nutr. Rev. 54 (12), 382–390.

Bottiglieri, T., 1997. Ademetionine (S-adenosylmethionine) neuropharmacology: implications for drug therapies in psychiatric and neurological disorders. Exp. Opin. Investig. Drugs 6 (4), 417–426.

Bottiglieri, T., 2013. Folate, vitamin B_{12}, and S-adenosylmethionine. Psychiatr. Clin. North Am. 36 (1), 1–13.

Bourre, J.M., 2006. Effects of nutrients (in food) on the structure and function of the nervous system: update on dietary requirements for brain. Part 1: micronutrients. J. Nutr. Health Aging 10 (5), 377–385.

Bowman, G.L., Silbert, L.C., Howieson, D., Dodge, H.H., Traber, M.G., Frei, B., et al., 2012. Nutrient biomarker patterns, cognitive function, and MRI measures of brain aging. Neurology 78 (4), 241–249.

Brunetti, D., Dusi, S., Morbin, M., Uggetti, A., Moda, F., D'Amato, I., et al., 2012. Pantothenate kinase-associated neurodegeneration: altered mitochondria membrane potential and defective respiration in Pank2 knock-out mouse model. Hum. Mol. Genet. 21 (24), 5294–5305.

Brunetti, D., Dusi, S., Giordano, C., Lamperti, C., Morbin, M., Fugnanesi, V., et al., 2014. Pantethine treatment is effective in recovering the disease phenotype induced by ketogenic diet in a pantothenate kinase-associated neurodegeneration mouse model. Brain 137 (Pt 1), 57–68.

Butterworth, R.F., Besnard, A.M., 1990. Thiamine-dependent enzyme changes in temporal cortex of patients with Alzheimer's disease. Metab. Brain Dis. 5 (4), 179–184.

Carmel, R., 2000. Current concepts in cobalamin deficiency. Ann. Rev. Med. 51, 357–375.

Carmel, R., Green, R., Rosenblatt, D.S., Watkins, D., 2003. Update on cobalamin, folate, and homocysteine. Hematol. Am. Soc. Hematol. Educ. Program 2003, 62–81.

Cheung, B.H., Ho, I.C., Chan, R.S., Sea, M.M., Woo, J., 2014. Current evidence on dietary pattern and cognitive function. Adv. Food Nutr. Res. 71, 137–163.

Choi, J.H., Yates, Z., Veysey, M., Heo, Y.R., Lucock, M., 2014. Contemporary issues surrounding folic Acid fortification initiatives. Prev. Nutr. Food Sci. 19 (4), 247–260.

Clarke, R., Armitage, J., 2000. Vitamin supplements and cardiovascular risk: review of the randomized trials of homocysteine-lowering vitamin supplements. Semin. Thromb. Hemost. 26, 341–348.

Clarke, R., Bennett, D., Parish, S., Lewington, S., Skeaff, M., Eussen, S.J., et al., 2014. B-Vitamin Treatment Trialists' Collaboration. Effects of homocysteine lowering with B vitamins on cognitive aging: meta-analysis of 11 trials with cognitive data on 22,000 individuals. Am. J. Clin. Nutr. 100 (2), 657–666.

Cole, B.F., Baron, J.A., Sandler, R.S., Haile, R.W., Ahnen, D.J., Bresalier, R.S., et al., 2007. Folic acid for the prevention of colorectal adenomas—a randomized clinical trial. JAMA 297, 2351–2359.

Currò, M., Gugliandolo, A., Gangemi, C., Risitano, R., Ientile, R., Caccamo, D., 2014. Toxic effects of mildly elevated homocysteine concentrations in neuronal-like cells. Neurochem. Res. 39 (8), 1485–1495.

de Bree, A., Verschuren, W.M.M., Bjorke-Monsen, A., van der Put, N.M., Heil, S.G., Trijbels, F.J., et al., 2003. Effect of the methylenetetrahydrofolate reductase 677C→T mutation on the relation among folate intake and plasma folate and homocysteine concentrations in a general population sample. Am. J. Clin. Nutr. 77, 687–693.

de Carvalho, M.J., Guilland, J.C., Moreau, D., Boggio, V., Fuchs, F., 1996. Vitamin status of healthy subjects in Burgundy (France). Ann. Nutr. Metab. 40 (1), 24–51.

Del Parigi, A., Panza, F., Capurso, C., Solfrizzi, V., 2006. Nutritional factors, cognitive decline, and dementia. Brain Res. Bull. 69 (1), 1–19.

Digby, J.E., McNeill, E., Dyar, O.J., Lam, V., Greaves, D.R., Choudhury, R.P., 2010. Anti-inflammatory effects of nicotinic acid in adipocytes demonstrated by suppression of fractalkine, RANTES, and MCP-1 and upregulation of adiponectin. Atherosclerosis 209 (1), 89–95.

Digby, J.E., Martinez, F., Jefferson, A., Ruparelia, N., Chai, J., Wamil, M., et al., 2012. Anti-inflammatory effects of nicotinic acid in human monocytes are mediated by GPR09A dependent mechanisms. Arterioscler. Thromb. Vasc. Biol. 32 (3), 669–676.

Doi, H., Koyano, S., Miyatake, S., Matsumoto, N., Kameda, T., Tomita, A., et al., 2010. Siblings with the adult-onset slowly progressive type of pantothenate kinase-associated neurodegeneration and a novel mutation, Ile346Ser, in PANK2: clinical features and (99m)Tc-ECD brain perfusion SPECT findings. J. Neurol. Sci. 290 (1–2), 172–176.

Doyle, K.M., Kennedy, D., Gorman, A.M., Gupta, S., Healy, S.J., Samali, A., 2011. Unfolded proteins and endoplasmic reticulum stress in neurodegenerative disorders. J. Cell Mol. Med. 15 (10), 2025–2039.

Dufouil, C., Alpe´rovitch, A., Ducros, V., Tzourio, C., 2003. Homocysteine, White Matter Hyperintensities, and Cognition in Healthy Elderly People. Ann. Neurol. 53, 214–221.

Eeuwijk, J., Oordt, A., Terzikhan, N., Noordegraaf-Schouten, M.V., 2012. Pallas health research and consultancy; Literature search and review related to specific preparatory work in the establishment of Dietary Reference Values for Niacin, Biotin and Vitamin B_6. Supporting Publications EN-365. [474 pp.]. Available online: www.efsa.europa.eu/publications.

EFSA Panel on Dietetic Products, Nutrition and Allergies (NDA), 2006 Scientific Commitee on Food. Tolerable Upper Intake Levels for Vitamins and Minerals. Available online: www.efsa.europa.eu/sites/default/files/assets/ndatolerableuil.pdf.

EFSA Panel on Dietetic Products, Nutrition and Allergies (NDA), 2010a. Scientific Opinion on the substantiation of health claims related to thiamin and reduction of tiredness and fatigue (ID 23) and contribution to normal psychological functions (ID 205) pursuant to Article 13(1) of Regulation (EC) No 1924/2006. EFSA Journal 8(10), 1755 [13 pp.]. Available online: www.efsa.europa.eu/efsajournal.htm.

EFSA Panel on Dietetic Products, Nutrition and Allergies (NDA), 2010b. Scientific Opinion on the substantiation of health claims related to riboflavin (vitamin B_2) and contribution to normal energy-yielding metabolism (ID 29, 35, 36, 42), contribution to normal metabolism of iron (ID 30, 37), maintenance of normal skin and mucous membranes (ID 31,33), contribution to normal psychological functions (ID 32), maintenance of normal bone (ID 33), maintenance of normal teeth (ID 33), maintenance of normal hair (ID 33), maintenance of normal nails (ID 33), maintenance of normal vision (ID 39), maintenance of normal red blood cells (ID 40), reduction of tiredness and fatigue (ID 41), protection of DNA, proteins and lipids from oxidative damage (ID 207), and maintenance of the normal function of the nervous system (ID 213) pursuant to Article 13(1) of Regulation (EC) No 1924/2006. EFSA Journal 8(10), 1814. [28 pp.]. Available online: www.efsa.europa.eu/efsajournal.htm.

EFSA Panel on Dietetic Products, Nutrition and Allergies (NDA), 2014. Scientific Opinion on Dietary Reference Values for folate. EFSA Journal 12(11), 3893. [59 pp]. Available online: www.efsa.europa.eu/efsajournal.

EFSA Panel on Dietetic Products, Nutrition and Allergies (NDA), 2015. Scientific Opinion on Dietary Reference Values for cobalamin (vitamin B_{12}). EFSA Journal 13(7), 4150. [64 pp]. Available online: www.efsa.europa.eu/efsajournal.

El-Sohemy, A., Xanthakos, H., Beaulieu, F., Allaire, L., Fournier, V., 2013. Fondation INITIA. Literature search and review related to specific preparatory work in the establishment of Dietary Reference Values for thiamin, pantothenic acid and choline. Supporting Publications EN-443. [229 pp.]. CFT/EFSA/NUTRI/2011/01, LOT 1. Available online: www.efsa.europa.eu/en/publications.htm.

Engelborghs, S., Gilles, C., Ivanoiu, A., Vandewoude, M., 2014. Rationale and clinical data supporting nutritional intervention in Alzheimer's disease. Acta Clin. Belg. 69 (1), 17–24.

Fernando, M.S., Ince, P.G., 2004. MRC Cognitive Function and Ageing Neuropathology Study Group. Vascular pathologies and cognition in a population-based cohort of elderly people. J. Neurol. Sci. 226 (1-2), 13–17.

Figueiredo, J.C., Grau, M.V., Haile, R.W., Sandler, R.S., Summers, R.W., Bresalier, R.S., et al., 2009. Folic acid and risk of prostate cancer: results from a randomized clinical trial. J. Natl. Cancer Inst. 101, 432–435.

Ford, A.H., Almeida, O.P., 2012. Effect of homocysteine lowering treatment on cognitive function: a systematic review and meta-analysis of randomized controlled trials. J. Alzheimers Dis. 29 (1), 133–149.

Ford, A.H., Flicker, L., Alfonso, H., Hankey, G.J., Norman, P.E., van Bockxmeer, F.M., et al., 2012. Plasma homocysteine and MTHFRC677T polymorphism as risk factors for incident dementia. J. Neurol. Neurosurg. Psychiatry 83 (1), 70–75.

Fry, P.C., Fox, H.M., Tao, H.G., 1976. Metabolic response to a pantothenic acid deficient diet in humans. J. Nutr. Sci. Vitaminol. (Tokyo) 22, 339–346.

Fuso, A., 2013. The 'golden age' of DNA methylation in neurodegenerative diseases. Clin. Chem. Lab. Med. 51 (3), 523–534.

Fuso, A., Nicolia, V., Cavallaro, R.A., Scarpa, S., 2011. DNA methylase and demethylase activities are modulated by one-carbon metabolism in Alzheimer's disease models. J. Nutr. Biochem. 22, 242–251.

Fuso, A., Cavallaro, R.A., Nicolia, V., Scarpa, S., 2012. PSEN1 promoter demethylation in hyperhomocysteinemic TgCRND8 mice is the culprit, not the consequence. Curr. Alzheimer. Res. 9 (5), 527–535.

Gareri, P., Castagna, A., Cotroneo, A.M., Putignano, S., De Sarro, G., Bruni, A.C., 2015. The role of citicoline in cognitive impairment: pharmacological characteristics, possible advantages, and doubts for an old drug with new perspectives. Clin. Interv. Aging 10, 1421–1429.

Gerlach, A.T., Thomas, S., Stawicki, S.P., Whitmill, M.L., Steinberg, S.M., Cook, C.H., 2011. Vitamin B6 deficiency: a potential cause of refractory seizures in adults. JPEN J. Parenter. Enteral. Nutr. 35 (2), 272–275.

Genoud, V., Lauricella, A.M., Kordich, L.C., Quintana, I., 2014. Impact of homocysteine-thiolactone on plasma fibrin networks. J. Thromb. Thrombolysis 38 (4), 540–545.

Ghavanini, A.A., Kimpinski, K., 2014. Revisiting the evidence for neuropathy caused by pyridoxine deficiency and excess. J. Clin. Neuromuscul. Dis. 16 (1), 25–31.

Gibson, G.E., Sheu, K.F., Blass, J.P., Baker, A., Carlson, K.C., Harding, B., et al., 1988. Reduced activities of thiamine-dependent enzymes in the brains and peripheral tissues of patients with Alzheimer's disease. Arch. Neurol. 45 (8), 836–840.

Gold, M., Chen, M.F., Johnson, K., 1995. Plasma and red blood cell thiamine deficiency in patients with dementia of the Alzheimer's type. Arch. Neurol. 52 (11), 1081–1086.

Gold, M., Hauser, R.A., Chen, M.F., 1998. Plasma thiamine deficiency associated with Alzheimer's disease but not Parkinson's disease. Metab. Brain Dis. 13 (1), 43–53.

Glusman, M., 1947. The syndrome of "burning feet" (nutritional melagia) as a manifestation of nutritional deficiency. Am. J. Med. 3, 211–223.

Gregory 3rd, J.F., 2012. Accounting for differences in the bioactivity and bioavailability of vitamers. Food Nutr. Res., 56. http://dx.doi.org/10.3402/fnr.v56i0.5809.

Harker, L.,A., Slichter, S.J., Scott, C.R., Ross, R., 1974. Homocystinemia. Vascular injury and arterial thrombosis. N. Engl. J. Med. 291 (11), 537–543.

Hassan, A., Hunt, B.J., O'Sullivan, M., Bell, R., D'Souza, R., Jeffery, S., et al., 2004. Homocysteine is a risk factor for cerebral small vessel disease, acting via endothelial dysfunction. Brain 127 (Pt1), 212–219.

Hegyi, J., Schwartz, R.A., Hegyi, V., 2004. Pellagra: Dermatitis, dementia, and diarrhea. Inter. J. Dermatol. 43, 1–5.

Héroux, M., Raghavendra Rao, V.L., Lavoie, J., Richardson, J.S., Butterworth, R.F., 1996. Alterations of thiamine phosphorylation and of thiamine-dependent enzymes in Alzheimer's disease. Metab. Brain Dis. 11 (1), 81–88.

Hinterberger, M., Fischer, P., 2013. Folate and Alzheimer: when time matters. J. Neural. Transm. 120 (1), 211–224.

Hodges, R.E., Ohlson, M.A., Bean, W.B., 1958. Pantothenic acid deficiency in man. J. Clin. Invest. 37, 1642–1657.

Hodges, R.E., Bean, W.B., Ohlson, M.A., Bleiler, R., 1959. Human pantothenic acid deficiency produced by omega-methyl pantothenic acid. J. Clin. Invest. 38, 1421–1425.

Hollenbeck, C.B., 2012. An introduction to the nutrition and metabolism of choline. Cent. Nerv. Syst. Agents Med. Chem. 12 (2), 100–113.

Hua, Y., Zhao, H., Kong, Y., Ye, M., 2011. Association between the MTHFR gene and Alzheimer's disease: a meta-analysis. Int. J. Neurosci. 121 (8), 462–471.

Institute of Medicine (US): Standing Committee on the Scientific Evaluation of Dietary Reference Intakes and its Panel on Folate, Other B Vitamins, and Choline, 1998. Dietary Reference Intakes for Thiamin, Riboflavin, Niacin, Vitamin B6, Folate, Vitamin B12, Pantothenic Acid, Biotin, and Choline. National Academies Press (US), Washington (DC).

Jacques, P.F., Selhub, J., Bostom, A.G., Wilson, P.W.F., Rosenberg, I.H., 1999. The effect of folic acid fortification on plasma folate and total homocysteine concentrations. N. Engl. J. Med. 340, 1449–1454.

Jakubowski, H., Goldman, E., 1993. Synthesis of homocysteine thiolactone by methionyl-tRNA synthetase in cultured mammalian cells. FEBS Lett. 317, 237–240.

Jakubowski, H., Zhang, L., Bardeguez, A., Aviv, A., 2000. Homocysteine thiolactone and protein homocysteinylation in human endothelial cells: implications for atherosclerosis. Circ. Res. 87, 45–51.

Jellinger, K.A., Attems, J., 2013. Neuropathological approaches to cerebral aging and neuroplasticity. Dialogues Clin. Neurosci. 15 (1), 29–43.

Jiang, W., Xu, J., Lu, X.J., Sun, Y., 2015. Association between MTHFR C677T polymorphism and depression: a meta-analysis in the Chinese population. Psychol. Health Med. 17, 1–11.

Kalmijn, S., Launer, L.J., Lindemans, J., Bots, M.L., Hofman, A., Breteler, M.M., 1999. Total homocysteine and cognitive decline in a community-based sample of elderly subjects: the Rotterdam Study. Am. J. Epidemiol. 150 (3), 283–289.

Kang, S.J., Park, B.J., Shim, J.Y., Lee, H.R., Hong, J.M., Lee, Y.J., 2012. Mean platelet volume (MPV) is associated with leukoaraiosis in the apparently healthy elderly. Arch. Gerontol. Geriatr. 54 (2), e118–e121.

Karuppagounder, S.S., Xu, H., Shi, Q., Chen, L.H., Pedrini, S., Pechman, D., et al., 2009. Thiamine deficiency induces oxidative stress and exacerbates the plaque pathology in Alzheimer's mouse model. Neurobiol. Aging 30 (10), 1587–1600.

Keleshian, V.L., Modi, H.R., Rapoport, S.I., Rao, J.S., 2013. Aging is associated with altered inflammatory, arachidonic acid cascade, and synaptic markers, influenced by epigenetic modifications, in the human frontal cortex. J. Neurochem. 125 (1), 63–73.

Kennedy, D.O., 2016. B vitamins and the brain: mechanisms, dose and efficacy-a review. Nutrients 8 (2) pii: E68.

Kerns, J.C., Arundel, C., Chawla, L.S., 2015. Thiamin deficiency in people with obesity. Adv. Nutr. 6 (2), 147–153.

Khodadadi, S., Riazi, G.H., Ahmadian, S., Hoveizi, E., Karima, O., Aryapour, H., 2012. Effect of N-homocysteinylation on physicochemical and cytotoxic properties of amyloid β-peptide. FEBS Lett. 586 (2), 127–131.

Kwok, J.B., 2010. Role of epigenetics in Alzheimer's and Parkinson's disease. Epigenomics 2 (5), 671–682.

Lanska, D.J., 2010. Chapter 30: historical aspects of the major neurological vitamin deficiency disorders: the water-soluble B vitamins In: Aminoff, M.J. Bolier, F. Swaab, D.F. (Eds.), Handb Clin Neurol—History of Neurology, vol. 95. Elsevier B. V, pp. 445–476.

Lavigne, P.M., Karas, R.H., 2013. The current state of niacin in cardiovascular disease prevention: a systematic review and meta-regression. J. Am. Coll. Cardiol. 61 (4), 440–446.

Lawrence, A.J., Chung, A.W., Morris, R.G., Markus, H.S., Barrick, T.R., 2014. Structural network efficiency is associated with cognitive impairment in small-vessel disease. Neurology 83 (4), 304–311.

Leclerc, D., Sibani, S., Rozen, R., 2000. Molecular Biology of Methylenetetrahydrofolate Reductase (MTHFR) and Overview of Mutations/Polymorphisms. In: Madame Curie Bioscience Database [Internet]. Austin (TX): Landes Bioscience. Available online: http://www.ncbi.nlm.nih.gov/books/NBK6561/.

Lehmann, M., Gottfries, C.G., Regland, B., 1999. Identification of cognitive impairment in the elderly: homocysteine is an early marker. Dem. Geriatr. Cogn. Disord. 10, 12–20.

Levkovitz, Y., Alpert, J.E., Brintz, C.E., Mischoulon, D., Papakostas, G.I., 2012. Effects of S-adenosylmethionine augmentation of serotonin-reuptake inhibitor antidepressants on cognitive symptoms of major depressive disorder. J. Affect Disord. 136 (3), 1174–1178.

Li, Y., Hassan, Y., Moriyama, H., Zempleni, J., 2013. Holocarboxylasesynthetase interacts physically with euchromatic histone-lysine N-methyltransferase, linking histone biotinylation with methylation events. J. Nutr. Biochem. 24 (8), 1446–1452.

Liu, H., Yang, M., Li, G.M., Qiu, Y., Zheng, J., Du, X., et al., 2010. The MTHFR C677T polymorphism contributes to an increased risk for vascular dementia: a meta-analysis. J. Neurol. Sci. 294 (1-2), 74–80.

Liu, D., Zempleni, J., 2014. Holocarboxylase synthetase interacts physically with nuclear receptor co-repressor, histone deacetylase 1 and a novel splicing variant of histone deacetylase 1 to repress repeats. Biochem. J. 461 (3), 477–486.

Lindenbaum, J., Healton, E.B., Savage, D.G., Brust, J.C., Garrett, T.J., Podell, E.R., et al., 1988. Neuropsychiatric disorders caused by cobalamin deficiency in the absence of anemia or macrocytosis. N. Engl. J. Med. 318 (26), 1720–1728.

Loew, D., Wanitschke, R., Schroedter, A., 1999. Studies on vitamin B12 status in the elderly—prophylactic and therapeutic consequences. Int. J. Vitam. Nutr. Res. 69 (3), 228–233.

Luchicchi, A., Bloem, B., Viaña, J.N., Mansvelder, H.D., Role, L.W., 2014. Illuminating the role of cholinergic signaling in circuits of attention and emotionally salient behaviors. Front. Synap. Neurosci. 24, 1–10.

Lütjohann, D., Brzezinka, A., Barth, E., Abramowski, D., Staufenbiel, M., von Bergmann, K., et al., 2002. Profile of cholesterol-related sterols in aged amyloid precursor protein transgenic mouse brain. J. Lipid. Res. 43, 1078–1085.
Lütjohann, D., von Bergmann, K., 2003. 24S-hydroxycholesterol: a marker of brain cholesterol metabolism. Pharmacopsychiatry 36 (suppl. 2), S102–S106.
Mackerras, D., Tan, J., Larter, C., 2014. Folic acid, selected cancers and all-cause mortality: a meta-analysis. Inter. Food Risk Analys. J. 4, 1–27.
Majors, A., Ehrhart, L.A., Pezacka, E.H., 1997. Homocysteine as a risk factor for vascular disease. Enhanced collagen production and accumulation by smooth muscle cells. Arterios. Thromb. Vasc. Biol. 17 (10), 2074–2081.
Malouf, R., Areosa Sastre, A., 2003. Vitamin B12 for cognition. Cochrane Database Syst. Rev. (3), CD004326.
Malouf, R., Grimley Evans, J., 2003. The effect of vitamin B6 on cognition. Cochrane Database Syst. Rev. (4), CD004393.
Malouf, R., Grimley Evans, J., 2008. Folic acid with or without vitamin B12 for the prevention and treatment of healthy elderly and demented people. Cochrane Database Syst. Rev. (4), CD004514.
Marsland, A.L., Gianaros, P.J., Kuan, D.C., Sheu, L.K., Krajina, K., Manuck, S.B., 2015. Brain morphology links systemic inflammation to cognitive function in midlife adults. Brain Behav. Immun. 48, 195–204.
Martí-Carvajal, A.J., Solà, I., Lathyris, D., Salanti, G., 2009. Homocysteine lowering interventions for preventing cardiovascular events. Cochrane Database Syst. Rev. (4), CD006612.
Martin, D.C., 1992. Time dependency of cognitive recovery with cobalamin replacement: report of a pilot study. J. Am. Geriatr. Soc. 40 (2), 168–172.
McGuinness, B., Craig, D., Bullock, R., Passmore, P., 2016. Statins for the prevention of dementia. Cochrane Database Syst. Rev. (1), CD003160.
McCully, K.S., 1969. Vascular pathology of homocysteinemia: implications for the pathogenesis of arteriosclerosis. Am. J. Pathol. 56, 111–128.
McCully, K.S., 2009. Chemical pathology of homocysteine. IV. Excitotoxicity, oxidative stress, endothelial dysfunction, and inflammation. Ann. Clin. Lab. Sci. 39 (3), 219–232.
Minn, Y.K., Kim, S.M., Kim, S.H., Kwon, K.H., Sunwoo, I.N., 2012. Sequential involvement of the nervous system in subacute combined degeneration. Yonsei Med. J. 53 (2), 276–278.
Mock, D.M., 1996. Biotin. In: Ziegler, E.E., Filer Jr, L.J. (Eds.), Present Knowledge in Nutrition, 7th ed. ILSI Nutrition Foundation, Washington, DC, pp. 220–235.
Molloy, A.M., Daly, S., Mills, J.L., Kirke, P.N., Whitehead, A.S., Ramsbottom, D., et al., 1997. Thermolabile variant of 5,10-methylenetetrahydrofolate reductase associated with low red-cell folates: implications for folate intake recommendations. Lancet 349, 1591–1593.
Morris, M.C., Tagney, C.C., 2011. A potential design flaw of randomized trials of vitamin supplements. JAMA 305 (13), 1348–1349.
Morris, M.C., 2012. Nutritional determinants of cognitive aging and dementia. Proc. Nutr. Soc. 71 (1), 1–13.
Morris, M.C., Evans, D.A., Bienias, J.L., Scherr, P.A., Tangney, C.C., Hebert, L.E., et al., 2004. Dietary niacin and the risk of incident Alzheimer's disease and of cognitive decline. J. Neurol. Neurosurg. Psychiatry 75 (8), 1093–1099.
Morris, M.C., Evans, D.A., Bienias, J.L., Tangney, C.C., Hebert, L.E., Scherr, P.A., et al., 2005. Dietary folate and vitamin B12 Intake and cognitive decline among community-dwelling older persons. Arch. Neurol. 62 (4), 641–645.
Morris, M.C., Schneiderd, J.A., Tangney, C.C., 2006. Thoughts on B-vitamins and dementia. J. Alzheimers Dis. 9 (4), 429–433.
Morris, M.S., Jacques, P.F., Rosenberg, I.H., Selhub, J., 2007. Folate and vitamin B-12 status in relation to anemia, macrocytosis, and cognitive impairment in older Americans in the age of folic acid fortification. Am. J. Clin. Nutr. 85 (1), 193–200.
Morris, H.A., 2015. Vitamin D: can you have too much of a good thing in chronic kidney disease? Kidney Int 88 (5), 936–938.
Nardone, R., Höller, Y., Storti, M., Christova, M., Tezzon, F., Golaszewski, S., et al., 2013. Thiamine deficiency induced neurochemical, neuroanatomical, and neuropsychological alterations: a reappraisal. Sci. World J. 2013, 309143.
Nelson, P.T., Alafuzoff, I., Bigio, E.H., Bouras, C., Braak, H., Cairns, N.J., et al., 2012. Correlation of Alzheimer disease neuropathologic changes with cognitive status: a review of the literature. J. Neuropathol. Exp. Neurol. 71 (5), 362–381.
Nilsson, K., Gustafson, L., Hultberg, B., 2012. Plasma homocysteine, brain imaging and cognition in older patients with mental illness. Int. J. Geriatr. Psychiatry 27 (4), 409–414.
O'Leary, F., Allman-Farinelli, M., Samman, S., 2012. Vitamin B12 status, cognitive decline and dementia: a systematic review of prospective cohort studies. Br. J. Nutr. 108 (11), 1948–1961.
Pacheco, F.T., Scoppetta, T.L., Sznirer, M., Paes, R.A., Rocha, A.J., 2015. Acute demyelination with leukoencephalopathy and cerebellar involvement in vitamin B12 deficiency. Arq. Neuropsiquiatr. 73 (3), 257.
Penke, B., Bogár, F., Fülöp, L., 2016. Protein folding and misfolding, endoplasmic reticulum stress in neurodegenerative diseases: in trace of novel drug targets. Curr. Protein Pept. Sci. 17 (2), 169–182.
Perla-Kajan, J., Twardowski, T., Jakubowski, H., 2007. Mechanisms of homocysteine toxicity in humans. Amino Acids 32, 561–572.
Pindolia, K., Chen, J., Cardwell, C., Cui, X., Chopp, M., Wolf, B., 2012. Neurological deficits in mice with profound biotinidase deficiency are associated with demylination and axonal degeneration. Neurobiol. Dis. 47 (3), 428–435.
Powers, H.J., 2003. Riboflavin (vitamin B-2) and health. Am. J. Clin. Nutr. 77 (6), 1352–1360.
Prentice, H., Modi, J.P., Wu, J.Y., 2015. Mechanisms of neuronal protection against excitotoxicity, endoplasmic reticulum stress, and mitochondrial dysfunction in stroke and neurodegenerative diseases. Oxid Med. Cell Longev. 2015, 964518.
Quadri, P., Fragiacomo, C., Pezzati, R., Zanda, E., Forloni, G., Tettamanti, M., et al., 2004. Homocysteine, folate and vitamin B-12 in mild cognitive impairment, Alzheimer's disease and vascular dementia. Am. J. Clin. Nutr. 80, 114–122.
Rana, A., Seinen, E., Siudeja, K., Muntendam, R., Srinivasan, B., van der Want, J.J., et al., 2010. Pantethine rescues a Drosophila model for pantothenate kinase-associated neurodegeneration. Proc. Natl. Acad. Sci. U S A 107 (15), 6988–6993.
Reijmer, Y.D., Leemans, A., Caeyenberghs, K., Heringa, S.M., Koek, H.L., Biessels, G.J., 2013. Utrecht Vascular Cognitive Impairment Study Group. Disruption of cerebral networks and cognitive impairment in Alzheimer disease. Neurology 80 (15), 1370–1377.
Reynolds, E.H., 2014. The neurology of folic acid deficiency. Handb. Clin. Neurol. 120, 927–943.
Rotstein, M., Kang, U.J., 2009. Consideration of gene therapy for paediatric neurotransmitter diseases. J. Inherit Metab. Dis. 32 (3), 387–394.
Said, H.M., 2012. Biotin: biochemical, physiological and clinical aspects. Subcell Biochem. 56, 1–19.
Sable, P., Randhir, K., Kale, A., Chavan-Gautam, P., Joshi, S., 2015. Maternal micronutrients and brain global methylation patterns in the offspring. Nutr. Neurosci. 18 (1), 30–36.
Saito, S., Ihara, M., 2016. Interaction between cerebrovascular disease and Alzheimer pathology. Curr. Opin. Psychiatry 29 (2), 168–173.

Sanchez-Mut, J.V., Heyn, H., Vidal, E., Moran, S., Sayols, S., Delgado-Morales, R., et al., 2016. Human DNA methylomes of neurodegenerative diseases show common epigenomic patterns. Transl. Psychiatry 6, e718.

Sando, K.R., Knight, M., 2015. Nonstatin therapies for management of dyslipidemia: a review. Clin. Ther. 37 (10), 2153–2179.

Seo, S.K., Jung, I., Lee, S.M., Cho, S., Choi, Y.S., Chung, T.S., et al., 2013. Relationship between leukoaraiosis and menopause in healthy middle-aged women. Fertil Steril 100 (2), 500–504.

Schneider, J.A., Arvanitakis, Z., Bang, W., Bennett, D.A., 2007. Mixed brain pathologies account for most dementia cases in community-dwelling older persons. Neurology 69 (24), 2197–2204.

Scientific Committee on Food, 2002. Opinion of the Scientific Committee on Food on the Tolerable Upper Intake Levels of Nicotinic Acid and Nicotinamide (Niacin). Brussels: EUROPEAN COMMISSION. Available online: http://ec.europa.eu/food/fs/sc/scf/out80j_en.pdf.

Selhub, J., Jacques, P.F., Bostom, A.G., D'Agostino, R.B., Wilson, P.W., Belanger, A.J., et al., 1996. Relationship between plasma homocysteine, vitamin status and extracranial carotid-artery stenosis in the Framingham Study population. Nutrition 126 (suppl. 4), 1258S.

Senol, M.G., Sonmez, G., Ozdag, F., Saracoglu, M., 2008. Reversible myelopathy with vitamin B12 deficiency. Singapore Med. J. 49 (11), e330–e332.

Seshadri, S., Beiser, A., Selhub, J., Jacques, P.F., Rosenberg, I.H., D'Agostino, R.B., et al., 2002. Plasma homocysteine as a risk factor for dementia and Alzheimer's disease. N. Engl. J. Med. 346 (7), 476–483.

Sharma, G.S., Kumar, T., Singh, L.R., 2014. N-Homocysteinylation Induces Different Structural and Functional Consequences on Acidic and Basic Proteins. PLoS One 9 (12), e116386.

Sharma, G.S., Kumar, T., Dar, T.A., Singh, L.R., 2015. Protein N-homocysteinylation: From cellular toxicity to neurodegeneration. Biochim. Biophys. Acta 1850 (11), 2239–2245.

Shumar, S.A., Fagone, P., Alfonso-Pecchio, A., Gray, J.T., Rehg, J.E., Jackowski, S., et al., 2015. Induction of Neuron-Specific Degradation of Coenzyme A Models Pantothenate Kinase-Associated Neurodegeneration by Reducing Motor Coordination in Mice. PLoS One 10 (6), e0130013.

Slyshenkov, V.S., Dymkowska, D., Wojtczak, L., 2004. Pantothenic acid and pantothenol increase biosynthesis of glutathione by boosting cell energetics. FEBS Lett. 569 (1-3), 169–172.

Snowden, D.A., Greiner, L.H., Mortimer, J.A., Riley, K.P., Greiner, P.A., Markesbery, W.R., 1997. Brain infarction and the clinical expression of Alzheimer disease: the Nun Study. JAMA 277, 813–817.

Stabler, S.P., 2013. Clinical practice. Vitamin B12 deficiency. N. Engl. J. Med. 368 (2), 149–160.

Stabler, S.P., Allen, R.H., Savage, D.G., Lindembaum, J., 1990. Clinical spectrum and diagnosis of cobalamin deficiency. Blood 76 (5), 871–881.

Stead, L.M., Brosnan, J.T., Brosnan, M.E., Vance, D.E., Jacobs, R.L., 2006. Is it time to reevaluate methyl balance in humans? Am. J. Clin. Nutr. 83, 5–10.

Su, G., Sun, G., Liu, H., Shu, L., Zhang, J., Guo, L., et al., 2015. Niacin suppresses progression of atherosclerosis by inhibiting vascular inflammation and apoptosis of vascular smooth muscle cells. Med. Sci. Monit. 21, 4081–4089.

Sudduth, T.L., Powell, D.K., Smith, C.D., Greenstein, A., Wilcock, D.M., 2013. Induction of hyperhomocysteinemia models vascular dementia by induction of cerebral microhemorrhages and neuroinflammation. J. Cereb. Blood Flow Metab. 33 (5), 708–715.

Tangney, C.C., Tang, Y., Evans, D.A., Morris, M.C., 2009. Biochemical indicators of vitamin B12 and folate insufficiency and cognitive decline. Neurology 72 (4), 361–367.

Tangney, C.C., Aggarwal, N.T., Li, H., Wilson, R.S., Decarli, C., Evans, D.A., et al., 2011. Vitamin B_{12}, cognition, and brain MRI measures: a cross-sectional examination. Neurology 77 (13), 1276–1282.

Thomas, D.E., Chung-A-O, K.O., Dickerson, J.W., Tidmarsh, S.F., Shaw, D.M., 1986. Tryptophan and nutritional status of patients with senile dementia. Psychol. Med. 16, 297–305.

Tsai, J.C., Perrella, M.A., Yoshizumi, M., Hsieh, C.M., Haber, E., Schlegel, R., et al., 1994. Promotion of vascular smooth muscle cell growth by homocysteine: a link to atherosclerosis. Proc. Natl. Acad. Sci. U S A 91 (14), 6369–6373.

Ueland, P.M., 2011. Choline and betaine in health and disease. J. Inherit. Metab. Dis. 34 (1), 3–15.

Ulrich, C.M., Potter, J.D., 2006. Folate supplementation: too much of a good thing? Cancer Epidemiol. Biomarkers Prev. 15 (2), 189–193.

Ulrich, A., Müller, D., Linnebank, M., Tarnutzer, A.A., 2015. Pitfalls in the diagnostic evaluation of subacute combined degeneration. BMJ Case Rep. 2015 May 14.

Undas, A., Perła, J., Lacinski, M., Trzeciak, W., Kaźmierski, R., Jakubowski, H., 2004. Autoantibodies against N-homocysteinylated proteins in humans: implications for atherosclerosis. Stroke 35 (6), 1299–1304.

Vega, G.L., Weiner, M.F., Lipton, A.M., Von Bergmann, K., Lutjohann, D., Moore, C., et al., 2003. Reduction in levels of 24S-hydroxycholesterol by statin treatment in patients with Alzheimer disease. Arch. Neurol. 60 (4), 510–515.

Vermeer, S.E., Van Dijk, E.J., Koudstaal, P.J., Oudkerk, M., Hofman, A., Clarke, R., et al., 2002. Homocysteine, silent brain infarcts, and white matter lesions: the Rotterdam scan study. Ann. Neurol. 51, 285–289.

Vidal-Alaball, J., Butler, C.C., Cannings-John, R., Goringe, A., Hood, K., McCaddon, A., et al., 2005. Oral vitamin B12 versus intramuscular vitamin B12 for vitamin B12 deficiency. Cochrane Database Syst. Rev. (3), CD004655.

Wakade, C., Chong, R., Bradley, E., Thomas, B., Morgan, J., 2014. Upregulation of GPR109A in Parkinson's disease. PLoS One 9 (10), e109818.

Waserman, J.E., Hategan, A., Bourgeois, J.A., 2015. Neuropsychiatric features associated with nutritional and metabolic status in a gastric bypass patient. Gen. Hosp. Psychiatry 37 (1) 98. e1–3.

White, L.R., Edland, S.D., Hemmy, L.S., Montine, K.S., Zarow, C., Sonnen, J.A., et al., 2016. Neuropathologic comorbidity and cognitive impairment in the Nun and Honolulu-Asia Aging Studies. Neurology. [Epub ahead of print: 2016 Feb 17].

Wojtczak, L., Slyshenkov, V.S., 2003. Protection by pantothenic acid against apoptosis and cell damage by oxygen free radicals--the role of glutathione. Biofactors 17 (1-4), 61–73.

Wurtman, R.J., 2014. A nutrient combination that can affect synapse formation. Nutrients 6 (4), 1701–1710.

Xekardaki, A., Kövari, E., Gold, G., Papadimitropoulou, A., Giacobini, E., Herrmann, F., et al., 2015. Neuropathological changes in aging brain. Adv. Exp. Med. Biol. 821, 11–17.

Xue, J., Zempleni, J., 2013. Epigenetic synergies between biotin and folate in the regulation of pro-inflammatory cytokines and repeats. Scand. J. Immunol. 78 (5), 419–425.

Yang, F.L., Liao, P.C., Chen, Y.Y., Wang, J.L., Shaw, N.S., 2005. Prevalence of thiamin and riboflavin deficiency among the elderly in Taiwan. Asia Pac. J. Clin. Nutr. 14 (3), 238–243.

Young, S.N., Ghadirian, A.M., 1989. Folic acid and psychopathology. Prog. Neuropsychopharmacol. Biol. Psychiatry 13 (6), 841–863.

Yu, L., Boyle, P.A., Leurgans, S., Schneider, J.A., Kryscio, R.J., Wilson, R.S., et al., 2015. Effect of common neuropathologies on progression of late life cognitive impairment. Neurobiol. Aging 36 (7), 2225–2231.

Zempleni, J., Li, Y., Xue, J., Cordonier, E.L., 2011. The role of holocarboxylase synthetase in genome stability is mediated partly by epigenomic synergies between methylation and biotinylation events. Epigenetics 6 (7), 892–894.

Zempleni, J., Camara Teixeira, D., Kuroishi, T., Cordonier, E.L., Baier, S., 2012. Biotin requirements for DNA damage prevention. Mutat. Res. 733 (1-2), 58–60.

Zhang, C., Cai, Y., Adachi, M.T., Oshiro, S., Aso, T., Kaufman, R.J., et al., 2001. Homocysteine induces programmed cell death in human vascular endothelial cells through activation of the unfolded protein response. J. Biol. Chem. 276, 35867–35874.

Zhang, Q., Yang, G., Li, W., Fan, Z., Sun, A., Luo, J., et al., 2011. Thiamine deficiency increases β-secretase activity and accumulation of β-amyloid peptides. Neurobiol. Aging 32 (1), 42–53.

Zhao, Y., Pan, X., Zhao, J., Wang, Y., Peng, Y., Zhong, C., 2009. Decreased transketolase activity contributes to impaired hippocampal neurogenesis induced by thiamine deficiency. J. Neurochem. 111 (2), 537–546.

Zhao, J., Sun, X., Yu, Z., Pan, X., Gu, F., Chen, J., et al., 2011. Exposure to pyrithiamine increases β-amyloid accumulation, tau hyperphosphorylation, and glycogen synthase kinase-3 activity in the brain. Neurotox. Res. 19 (4), 575–583.

Zuliani, G., Guerra, G., Ranzini, M., Rossi, L., Munari, M.R., Zurlo, A., et al., 2007. High interleukin-6 plasma levels are associated with functional impairment in older patients with vascular dementia. Int. J. Geriatr. Psychiatry 22 (4), 305–311.

Zuliani, G., Donnorso, M.P., Bosi, C., Passaro, A., Dalla Nora, E., Zurlo, A., et al., 2011. Plasma 24S-hydroxycholesterol levels in elderly subjects with late onset alzheimer's disease or vascular dementia: a case-control study. BMC Neurol. 11, 121.

C H A P T E R

16

Vitamin B_{12} Deficiency in the Elderly

Chit Wai Wong

Caritas Medical Centre, Kowloon, Hong Kong

INTRODUCTION

Vitamin B_{12} and cobalamin are generally used interchangeable. Acquiring vitamin B_{12} for human body's cell metabolism involves dietary intake of vitamin B_{12}-enriched foods and the absorption of vitamin B_{12} into our body. The main dietary sources of vitamin B_{12} are animal products because animals obtain vitamin B_{12} through microbial symbiosis. Our dietary requirement of vitamin B_{12} is 2–3 μg, and around 3–30 μg daily can be obtained from our normal diet. There is 2–3 mg of vitamin B_{12} reserve in our bodies, mainly stored in the liver. Thus, even if vitamin B_{12} were to be completely depleted in the diet, it might not result in low serum vitamin B_{12} levels in a healthy adult for several years.

The prevalence of vitamin B_{12} deficiency appears to increase with age, which varies between 5% and 40% in the elderly, depending on the definition of vitamin B_{12} deficiency used and the population groups studied (Lindenbaum et al., 1994; Baik and Rusell, 1999; Carmel, 2000; Chui et al., 2001; Clarke et al., 2003, 2004; Loikas et al., 2007). Elderly people are particularly at risk of vitamin B_{12} deficiency because of the increased prevalence of pernicious anemia (PA) and the high prevalence of gastric atrophy that impairs the release of vitamin B_{12} from food protein for absorption (Baik and Rusell, 1999; Carmel, 1995). Besides, multiple comorbidities with multiple drugs intake and increasing dependency associated with aging can lead to inadequate intake and malabsorption of vitamin B_{12}, thus leaving a vitamin B_{12} deficiency.

Vitamin B_{12} is essential for cell metabolism and function, so a deficiency has significant effects on the body, especially organ systems with high cell turnover and metabolism such as bone marrow, the gastrointestinal tract, the brain, and the nervous system. Clinical features of vitamin B_{12} deficiency can be subtle and nonspecific, which creates a challenge in diagnosis. Although vitamin B_{12} deficiency can be readily treated by vitamin B_{12} replacement, damage to the organ system can be extensive and irreversible if diagnosis and treatment are delayed.

VITAMIN B_{12} ABSORPTION

Absorption of vitamin B_{12} into the body is complex. Vitamin B_{12} in animal food is bound to protein. After ingestion, it is broken down by pepsin and hydrochloric acid in the stomach to release free vitamin B_{12}, which is then bound to R protein (also known as *haptocorrin* or *transcobalamin I*) secreted from the salivary gland and stomach to protect vitamin B_{12} from degradation in the stomach's acidic environment. On traveling to the duodenum, the vitamin B_{12}–R protein complex is degraded by pancreatic enzyme to release free vitamin B_{12}. The free vitamin B_{12} is then bound to an intrinsic factor secreted from the parietal cells of the stomach to protect vitamin B_{12} from catabolism by intestinal bacteria and to facilitate absorption of vitamin B_{12} in the terminal ileum. These vitamin B_{12}–intrinsic factor complexes travel undisturbed until distal 80 cm of the ileum, where they bind to the receptors on enterocytes. Subsequently, vitamin B_{12} is carried by a transport protein, transcobalamin II, via the portal system to all cells in the body for use. About 60% of vitamin B_{12} in food is absorbed through this pathway. There is enterohepatic circulation

Nutrition and Functional Foods for Healthy Aging.
DOI: http://dx.doi.org/10.1016/B978-0-12-805376-8.00016-2

of vitamin B_{12} in which most of the vitamin B_{12} (in the form of a vitamin B_{12}–R protein complex) excreted from the liver via the bile to the duodenum is carried by the intrinsic factor to be reabsorbed at the terminal ileum. Because of this efficient enterohepatic circulation, it takes several years for vitamin B_{12} deficiency to develop even if there is a complete depletion of vitamin B_{12} in diet, provided that the above absorption mechanism is intact.

In addition to the classic route which involves intrinsic factor produced by the stomach and transport system in the terminal ileum, around 1% of free vitamin B_{12} can be absorbed along the entire intestine by passive diffusion (Berlin et al., 1968).

VITAMIN B_{12} METABOLISM AND FUNCTION

Vitamin B_{12} plays a significant role in the metabolism of all cells in the body, including energy production, myelin synthesis, and DNA synthesis. In humans, two enzymatic reactions depend on vitamin B_{12}: 5-methyltetrahydrofolate-homocysteine methyltransferase (MTR) (also known as *methionine synthase*) reaction and methylmalonyl coenzyme A mutase (MUT) reaction.

5-Methyltetrahydrofolate-Homocysteine Methyltransferase (MTR) or Methionine Synthase Reaction

Methylcobalamin, a cofactor form of vitamin B_{12}, together with folate is required for the conversion of homocysteine to methionine by MTR (Fig. 16.1). Methionine is needed to make S-adenosylmethionine (SAM), which is necessary for the methylation of numerous biochemical reactions, including myelin sheath production and the synthesis of

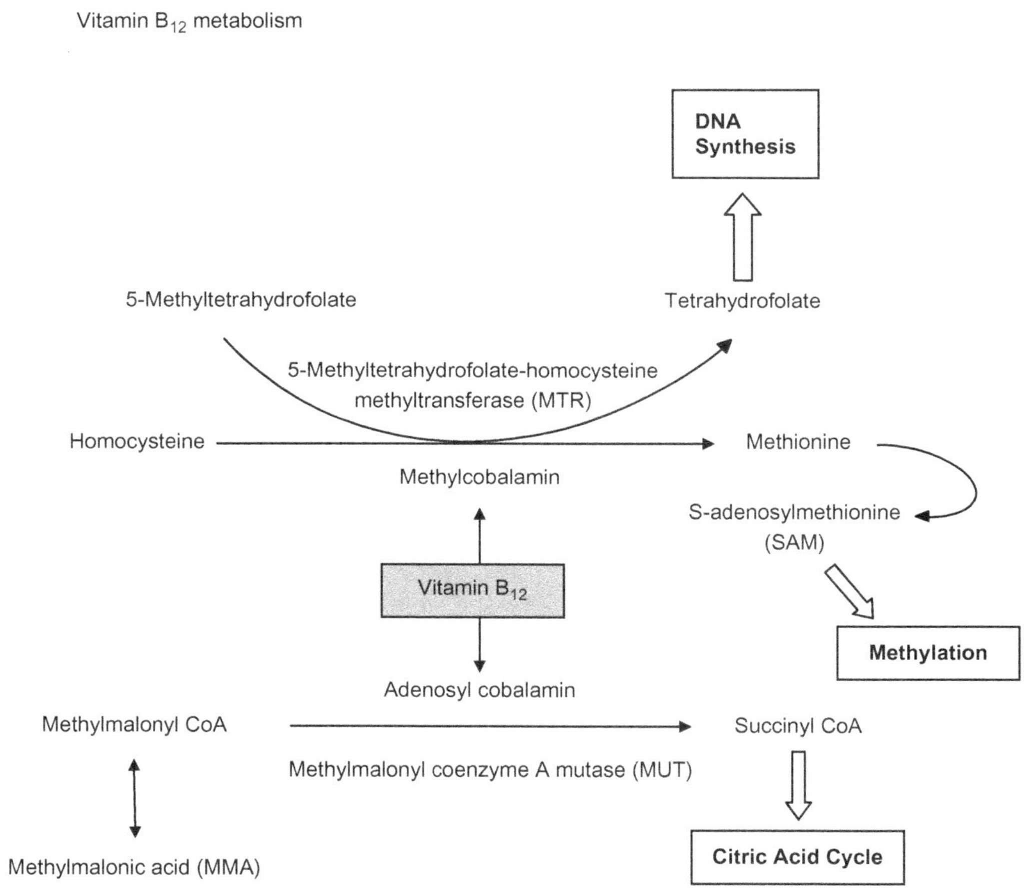

FIGURE 16.1 Metabolism of vitamin B_{12} *(Wong, 2015, with permission from Hong Kong Med. J).*

certain neurotransmitters, for maintaining brain and nervous system function. Besides, in the MTR reaction, vitamin B_{12} also helps to regenerate tetrahydrofolate (THF), an active form of folate involved in DNA synthesis. In vitamin B_{12} deficiency, the conversion of homocysteine to methionine and 5-methyltetrahydrofolate to tetrahydrofolate are affected, which in turn lead to the buildup of homocysteine and 5-methytetrahydrofolate in the body. Fortunately, both methionine and THF can be obtained from the diet or from dietary supplements. Therefore, even with a vitamin B_{12} deficiency that causes an MTR reaction dysfunction, both the SAM production and DNA synthesis can be maintained if there is enough methionine and folate from an external source. However, they cannot correct the underlying vitamin B_{12} deficiency and the accumulation of homocysteine with hyperhomocysteinemia will continue.

Methylmalonyl Coenzyme A Mutase (MUT) Reaction

Adenosylcobalamin, another cofactor form of vitamin B_{12}, is essential for the conversion of methylmalonyl coenzyme A (a coenzyme A–linked form of methylmalonic acid (MMA)) to succinyl coenzyme A by MUT. This is an important step in the extraction of energy from protein and fat in the mitochondrial citric acid cycle. This function is lost in vitamin B_{12} deficiency and results in the elevation of MMA level. MMA may prevent normal fatty acid synthesis, which may interfere with the formation of myelin sheaths and thus results in neurological damage. Unlike the MTR, the MUT reaction totally depends on vitamin B_{12} and cannot be corrected by external supplements other than vitamin B_{12}.

CAUSES OF VITAMIN B_{12} DEFICIENCY IN THE ELDERLY

A vitamin B_{12} deficiency can have a variety of causes, but impaired absorption of vitamin B_{12} and inadequate dietary intake are more common in the elderly (Table 16.1).

Food-Cobalamin Malabsorption

Vitamin B_{12} deficiency can be seen even among elderly people who consume animal protein. Food-cobalamin (vitamin B_{12}) malabsorption, which was first described by Carmel (1995), is the most common cause of vitamin B_{12} deficiency in the elderly and accounts for 40–70% of all cases (Carmel, 1997; Andrès et al., 2004, 2005). It is characterized by the body's inability to extract vitamin B_{12} from food or its binding protein, and this prevents vitamin B_{12}

TABLE 16.1 Causes of Vitamin B_{12} Deficiency

Cause	Particulars
Inadequate intake	Alcohol consumption
	Vegetarian diet
Malabsorption	Food vitamin B_{12} malabsorption
	Pernicious anemia
	Atrophic gastritis
	Postgastrectomy
	Ileal malabsorption • Ileal resection • Crohn's disease
	Pancreatic insufficiency • Chronic alcohol consumption • Cystic fibrosis
Drugs	Proton pump inhibitor, histamine H_2 blocker, metformin, cholestyramine
Others	*Helicobacter pylori* infection, intestinal bacterial overgrowth, transcobalamin II deficiency (genetic)

from being taken up by intrinsic factor for absorption. Elderly people are particular vulnerable because increasing age often brings atrophic gastritis, which affects from 20% to 50% of the elderly (Kransinski et al., 1986; Selhub et al., 2000; Andrès et al., 2005). Atrophic gastritis with a reduction in gastric acid and pepsin secretion prevents vitamin B_{12} from being released from food for absorption, and it also promotes intestinal bacterial overgrowth that competes for vitamin B_{12} uptake; both factors lead to a decline in vitamin B_{12} level in the body. Chronic *Helicobacter pylori* infection, which is strongly associated with atrophic gastritis (Blaser and Parsonnet, 1994), seems to be prevalent in patients with vitamin B_{12} deficiency and was found in 56% of people with vitamin B_{12} deficiency in one study (Kaptan et al., 2000). Other factors that decrease the gastric acid or pancreatic enzyme production can cause food-cobalamin malabsorption, including long-term consumption of proton pump inhibitors or histamine H_2 blockers (Valuck and Ruscin, 2004), gastrectomy, gastric bypass surgery, and pancreatic insufficiency in patients with chronic alcoholic consumption or cystic fibrosis. Food-cobalamin malabsorption often produces a slow, progressive depletion of vitamin B_{12} compared with the more complete malabsorption caused by PA. The clinical manifestation tends to be subtle and mild, although progression to the severe form can still occur in the minority. It can be corrected simply with an oral vitamin B_{12} supplement since free vitamin B_{12} absorption is not affected.

Pernicious Anemia

PA was considered a classical cause of vitamin B_{12} deficiency in the elderly before the discovery of food-cobalamin malabsorption. It accounts for 15–25% of deficiency in the elderly (Dali-Youcef and Andrè, 2009) and involves the autoimmune destruction of gastric mucosa and autoantibodies blockage of the vitamin B_{12} binding site of the intrinsic factor. The two antibodies found in PA are anti-parietal cell antibody, which is more sensitive (>90%) but less specific (50%) for PA, and an anti-intrinsic factor antibody that is less sensitive (50%) but more specific (98%) for diagnosis of PA (Toh et al., 1997; Andrè et al., 2004). The resultant gastric atrophy and depletion of intrinsic factors lead to poor absorption of food-bound, free, and biliary vitamin B_{12} and thus a more complete and severe vitamin B_{12} malabsorption and deficiency. Although PA is associated with an excess risk of gastric carcinoma and gastric carcinoid tumor (Hsing et al., 1993), the benefit of endoscopic surveillance has still not been established. There is a recommendation that a single endoscopy should be considered to identify gastric cancer or carcinoid tumor once the patient is diagnosed with pernicious anemia (Hirota et al., 2006). However, there is insufficient data to support the subsequent routine endoscopic surveillance.

Other Causes

Contrary to common belief that the most common cause of vitamin B_{12} deficiency in the elderly of developed countries is inadequate dietary intake, studies have shown that this is not the truth. A French study showed that among 172 elderly patients with vitamin B_{12} deficiencies, only 2% were affected by inadequate intake (Andrès et al., 2005), while in a hospital-based Chinese study on 52 patients, only 3.8% of patients with megaloblastic anemia (98% had vitamin B_{12} deficiency) had inadequate dietary intake (Chan et al., 1998). However, this can be a problem for strict vegans because animal products are the only dietary source of vitamin B_{12}. According to a local study on 119 older Chinese vegetarian women, the prevalence of deficiency was 42% (Kowk et al., 2002). Besides, factors such as poor health conditions with poor nutrition and vitamin B_{12} intake can contribute to vitamin B_{12} deficiency.

Long-term use of medications for comorbidities can interfere or reduce vitamin B_{12} absorption in the elderly. These include proton pump inhibitors and histamine H_2 blockers, which suppress gastric acid secretion and prevent the release of vitamin B_{12} from food (Schumann, 1999); metformin, which reduces the intestinal availability of free calcium ions for the uptake of the vitamin B_{12}–intrinsic factor complex by ileal cell membrane receptors (Bausman et al., 2000); and cholestyramine, which interferes with vitamin B_{12} absorption from the intestine (Desouza et al., 2002).

CLINICAL MANIFESTATIONS OF VITAMIN B_{12} DEFICIENCY

Since vitamin B_{12} is essential for metabolism (through MTR and MUT reactions) of all cells in the body, multiple organ systems can be affected by a vitamin B_{12} deficiency and exhibit a wide spectrum of clinical manifestations. Those manifestations of vitamin B_{12} deficiency are usually nonspecific and highly varied in severity or in the organ system involved (Dali-Youcef and Andrè, 2009). No one clinical feature is unique to all patients with vitamin B_{12} deficiency. Nonspecific symptoms and signs include loss of appetite, diarrhea, fatigue and weakness, shortness of breath, low blood pressure, confusion, and changes in mental state. Classic manifestations include Hunter's glossitis, megaloblastic anemia, and subacute combined degeneration of the spinal cord. Some have postulated that the expression of clinical manifestations in an individual is governed by genetic factors (Herbet, 1994; Carmel, 2000). Since the food-cobalamin malabsorption as a cause of vitamin B_{12} deficiency is common in the elderly, frequently the elderly have mild, subclinical deficiency that is usually asymptomatic; on the other hand, clinically overt deficiency with classical features of macrocytic anemia and neuropathy is infrequently seen (Carmel, 2000; Wong et al., 2015).

Macrocytic Anemia

A classical finding of macrocytic anemia may not be present with a vitamin B_{12} deficiency. There are observations that macrocytosis cannot predict the presence of a vitamin B_{12} deficiency (Oosterhuis et al., 2000; Chui et al., 2001; Kowk et al., 2002). The macrocytosis has been shown to have low sensitivity of 17–30% for the detection of vitamin B_{12} deficiency and up to 84% of deficiency would be undetected if macrocytosis is used to screen for deficiency (Oosterhuis et al., 2000). Although macrocytosis cannot be an indicator of vitamin B_{12} deficiency, it seems that severe vitamin B_{12} deficiency is associated with more macrocytosis (Wong et al., 2015). Herbet (1994) described four stages of vitamin B_{12} deficiency: (1) serum depletion with low holotranscobalamin level, (2) cell store depletion with low holohaptocorrin and red cell vitamin B_{12} levels, (3) biochemical deficiency with elevated serum homocysteine and MMA levels, and (4) clinical deficiency with anemia and macrocytosis. Thus, macrocytosis and anemia occur late despite biochemical tests showing a deficiency, especially if there is an external supply of folate. Besides, the influence of genetic factors on the functionality in different cell lines could play a role in the clinical expression of a vitamin B_{12} deficiency (Herbet, 1994; Carmel, 2000).

Neuropsychiatric Illness

Neuropsychiatric manifestations without hematological abnormality are common among the elderly (Lindenbaum et al., 1988; Hin et al., 2006) and include paresthesia, weakness, gait abnormalities, cognitive or behavioral changes, psychosis, and depression. Both vitamin B_{12}–dependent reactions—MTR and MUT—may play a role in the pathogenesis of neuropsychiatric disorders, but the exact mechanism is unclear. Vitamin B_{12} deficiency may have an association with Alzheimer's disease because a high prevalence of low serum vitamin B_{12} levels and other indicators of vitamin B_{12} deficiency have been reported among people with Alzheimer's disease (Malouf and Areosa Sastre, 2003). Although vitamin B_{12} replacement helps to reverse the hematological abnormalities and psychiatric disorder, the ability to reverse the cognitive impairment or neurological disorder is not promising (Lindenbaum et al., 1988; Malouf and Areosa Sastre, 2003; Sabeen and Holroyd, 2009; Vogel et al., 2009). The longer the time the cognitive impairment or neurological disorder presents before treatment, the less likely it can be reversed. It is suggested that prompt correction of deficiency should be done within 6–12 months of the disorder in order to obtain a maximum response (Martin et al., 1992).

DIAGNOSIS OF VITAMIN B_{12} DEFICIENCY

There is no gold standard test to diagnose vitamin B_{12} deficiency. The diagnosis is usually based on identifying a low serum level of vitamin B_{12} with clinical evidence of a deficiency that would respond to a vitamin B_{12} replacement. The most frequently reported serum vitamin B_{12} threshold level is 150 pmol/L (200 pg/mL). It is based on the level below which the metabolites (serum homocysteine, and serum and urine MMA) become elevated; it is endorsed by the World Health Organization (De Benoist, 2008; Selhub et al., 2008). However, serum vitamin B_{12} level is known to lack both sensitivity and specificity in diagnosing vitamin B_{12} deficiency. For example, neurological symptoms can occur even if a serum vitamin B_{12} level is above 150 pmol/L. Note that not all the vitamin B_{12} circulating in the serum is in metabolically active form. Furthermore, different quantities of vitamin B_{12} are stored in different organs, so not all organ systems are at the same stage of deficiency simultaneously (e.g., vitamin B_{12} stored in the nervous system is depleted earlier than that stored in bone marrow) (Herbet, 1994). Thus, a simple cutoff point is not practical to identify genuine or tissue vitamin B_{12} deficiency in the body.

Elevated serum homocysteine and MMA levels are more sensitive markers for vitamin B_{12} deficiency and have sensitivities of 95.9% and 98.4%, respectively (Salvage et al., 1994; Snow, 1999; Klee, 2000). Serum homocysteine level rises before the increase in MMA, so an increased homocysteine level is an earlier indicator of vitamin B_{12} deficiency. However, it is less specific than an elevated MMA level because elevated homocysteine can occur also in vitamin B_6 and folate deficiencies. Both serum homocysteine and MMA levels can also be elevated by renal insufficiency, hypovolemia, and inherited metabolic defects (Snow, 1999). Elevated serum MMA and homocysteine levels seem to increase with age, and the prevalence of elevated MMA and homocysteine levels is higher than the prevalence of low vitamin B_{12} or clinically evident vitamin B_{12} deficiency in the elderly (Pennypacker et al., 1992; Joosten et al., 1993, 1996; Chanarin and Metz, 1997). This leads to the concern about overdiagnosis and overtreatment if assays for these metabolites are used alone. Thus, using estimations of these metabolites is not recommended as an initial test to diagnose a vitamin B_{12} deficiency. They are suggested only when serum vitamin B_{12} results are normal but clinical suspicion remains.

Holotranscobalamin is composed of vitamin B_{12} attached to a transport protein (transcobalamin II); it is a biologically active fraction of vitamin B_{12} and represents 6–20% of total serum vitamin B_{12} (Hermann et al., 2003). A reduced serum holotranscobalamin level is considered the most sensitive and an early marker for vitamin B_{12} deficiency as the serum level of holotranscobalamin decreases even before the elevation of homocysteine and MMA (Herbet, 1994; Hermann et al., 2003; Nexo and Holffmann-Lückeu, 2011). Holotranscobalamin levels also cannot be tested in renal patients because its level increases in renal impairment (Hermann et al., 2003). Like homocysteine and MMA, holotranscobalamin testing is more expensive and less readily available than tests for total serum vitamin B_{12}, which limits their use in clinical practice.

VITAMIN B_{12} DEFICIENCIES IN THE INSTITUTIONALIZED ELDERLY

Institutionalized elderly people with multiple comorbidities and increasing dependency seem to be particular at risk of vitamin B_{12} deficiency, and the prevalence has been estimated at 30–40% (Matthews, 1995; Dali-Youcef and Andrè, 2009). In our study on around 2000 institutionalized Chinese residents 65 years and older, the prevalence of vitamin B_{12} deficiency, defined as a serum vitamin B_{12} level $<150\,pmol/L$, was 34.9% (Wong et al., 2015). The prevalence was higher than the studies performed with free-living elderly using similar definitions for vitamin B_{12} deficiency in which the prevalence was between 5.3% and 20% (Lindenbaum et al., 1994; Clarke et al., 2003, 2004; Loikas et al., 2007). Furthermore, in another local study conducted on free-living Chinese elderly people older than 70, the prevalence of vitamin $B_{12}<140\,pmol/L$ was only 6.6% (Chui et al., 2001).

Institutionalized elderly people tend to have poor health status and are more frail and dependent on others for their daily living activities. They are frequently encouraged to drink milk or nutritional supplements that are supposedly associated with a lower prevalence of vitamin B_{12} deficiency. However, multiple comorbidities and chronic disease state are detrimental to the body's nutritional status and may increase the body's vitamin requirements (Rajan et al., 2002; Obeid et al., 2004). Anorexia and dysphagia with poor dietary intake can further compromise the vitamin status. Long-term usage of medications may also impair appetite and some used to treat comorbidities such as proton pump inhibitors, histamine H_2 blockers, and metformin can interfere with or reduce vitamin B_{12} absorption. Moreover, the level of skilled nursing care provided and the amount of care residents receive can also affect their vitamin B_{12} status (Baik and Rusell, 1999). As a result, the institutionalized elderly are more prone to vitamin B_{12} deficiencies with the exception of those given tube feeding. Tube feeding residents rarely have vitamin B_{12} deficiencies but have rather high serum vitamin B_{12} levels (Wong et al., 2015) because the feeding formula contains recommended daily requirements of vitamin B_{12} or even higher levels in the form of cyanocobalamin (crystalline vitamin B_{12}), which can be readily absorbed into the body.

THERAPEUTIC MANAGEMENT

The classical treatment for vitamin B_{12} deficiency is parenteral administration, usually intramuscular injection, to correct the deficiency and build up the body's stores. The regimen for vitamin B_{12} replacement varies across countries and between individual practices. Generally, the schedule for vitamin B_{12} replacement is 1 mg daily for a week or 1 mg 3 times a week for 2 weeks followed by 1 mg per week for 1 month and then 1 mg per month as a maintenance dose.

Around 1% of free vitamin B_{12} can be absorbed along the entire intestine by passive diffusion (Berlin et al., 1968). Oral vitamin B_{12} replacement is theoretically as effective as parenteral administration even in patients with PA or ileal disease provided the dosage is high (Vidal-Alaball et al., 2005). However, the unpredictable absorption by passive diffusion makes the recommendation of a standard dose difficult. The recommendation for oral replacement is 1 mg daily for a month and then 125–250 μ g as maintenance dose for patients with dietary insufficiency and food-cobalamin malabsorption while for PA the maintenance dose is 1 mg daily (Andrè et al., 2004).

Vitamin B_{12} replacement does not have side effects even when prescribed in large doses (Food and Nutrition Board, 1998). However, hypokalemia, as a complication of vitamin B_{12} replacement that results from the uptake of circulating potassium by newly growing and dividing hematopoietic cells, can be severe and even life-threatening. Transient potassium supplement in the initial stage of vitamin B_{12} replacement, especially in patients with low-normal serum potassium, can prevent subsequent hypokalemia.

In addition to vitamin B_{12} replacement, the correction of risk factors associated with vitamin B_{12} deficiency—e.g., antibiotics to treat *H. pylori* infections and intestinal bacterial overgrowth, and stopping or replacing the offending medications—may also be useful in managing or preventing the development of vitamin B_{12} deficiency.

SCREENING FOR VITAMIN B_{12} DEFICIENCY IN THE ELDERLY

Currently, there is no formal screening recommendation for vitamin B_{12} deficiency in the asymptomatic elderly. However, vitamin B_{12} deficiency is common in the elderly because of the increasing prevalence of age-related atrophic gastritis associated food-cobalamin malabsorption, pernicious anemia, and drugs taken to treat comorbidities. Symptoms and signs of vitamin B_{12} deficiency are usually vague and unrecognized, and there is no useful clinical indicator for the deficiency. Furthermore, early detection with prompt treatment is needed before the damage becomes extensive and irreversible. Both oral and parenteral administration of vitamin B_{12} are effective and without untoward side effects. All of these support screening for vitamin B_{12} deficiency in the elderly (Wong, 2015), although the diagnosis is not straightforward because laboratory tests have their limitations and there is no consensus for diagnosis. Nonetheless, more liberal testing for vitamin B_{12} status or universal vitamin supplementation to the elderly may be warranted, but the cost-effectiveness of detecting and treating the deficiency, especially for those with subclinical or asymptomatic vitamin B_{12} deficiency, remains to be determined.

References

Andrès, E., Loukili, N.H., Noel, E., Kaltonbach, G., Abdelgheni, M.B., Perrin, A.E., et al., 2004. Vitamin B_{12} (cobalamin) deficiency in elderly patients. CMAJ 171, 251–259.

Andrès, E., Affenberger, S., Vinzio, S., Kurtz, J.E., Noel, E., Kaltenbach, G., et al., 2005. Food-cobalamin malabsorption in elderly patients: clinical manifestations and treatment. Am. J. Med. 118, 1154–1159.

Baik, H.W., Rusell, R.M., 1999. Vitamin B_{12} deficiency in the elderly. Annu. Rev. Nutr. 19, 357–377.

Bausman, W.A., Shaw, S., Jayatilleke, E., Spungen, A.M., Herbert, V., 2000. Increased intake of calcium reverse vitamin B_{12} malabsorption induced by metfaormin. Diabetes Care 23, 1227–1231.

Berlin, H., Berlin, R., Brante, G., 1968. Oral treatment of pernicious anaemia with high doses of vitamin B_{12} without intrinsic factor. Acta Med. Scand. 184, 247–258.

Blaser, M.J., Parsonnet, J., 1994. Parasitism by the "slow" bacterium *Helicobacter pylori* leads to altered gastric homeostasis and neoplasia. J. Clin. Invest. 94, 4–8.

Carmel, R., 1995. Malabsorption of food cobalmin. Baillieres Clin. Haematol. 8, 639–655.

Carmel, R., 1997. Cobalamin, the stomach, and aging. Am. J. Clin. Nutr. 66, 750–759.

Carmel, R., 2000. Current concept in cobalamin deficiency. Annu. Rev. Med. 51, 357–375.

Chan, J.C.W., Liu, H.S.Y., Kho, B.C.S., Chu, R.W., Ma, E.S.K., Ma, K.M., et al., 1998. Megaloblastic anaemia in Chinese patients: a review of 52 cases. Hong Kong Med. J. 4, 269–274.

Chanarin, I., Metz, J., 1997. Diagnosis of cobalamin deficiency: the old and the new. Br. J. Haematol. 97, 695–700.

Chui, C.H., Lau, F.Y., Wong, R., Soo, O.Y., Lam, C.K., Lee, P.W., et al., 2001. Vitamin B_{12} deficiency—need for a new guideline. Nutrition 17, 917–920.

Clarke, R., Refsum, H., Birks, J., Evans, J.G., Jognson, C., Sheriker, P., et al., 2003. Screening for vitamin B_{12} and folate deficiency in older persons. Am. J. Clin. Nutr. 77, 1241–1247.

Clarke, R., Eveans, J.G., Schneede, J., Nexo, E., Bates, C., Fletcher, A., et al., 2004. Vitamin B_{12} and folate deficiency in later life. Age Ageing 33, 34–41.

Dali-Youcef, N., Andrès, E., 2009. An update on cobalamin deficiency in adults. QMJ 102, 17–28.

De Benoist, B., 2008. Conclusion of a WHO technical consultation on folate and vitamin B_{12} deficiencies. Food Nutr. Bull. 29, S238–S244.

Desouza, C., Keebler, M., McNamara, D B., Fonseca, V., 2002. Drugs affecting homocysteine metabolism: impact on cardiovascular risk. Drugs 62, 605–616.

Food and Nutrition Board, Institute of Medicine, 1998. Dietary References Intakes for Thiamine, Riboflavin, Niacin, Vitamin B_6, Folate, Vitamin B_{12}, Pantothenic Acid, Biotin, and Choline. National Academy Press, Washington, DC.

Herbet, V., 1994. Staging vitamin B_{12} (cobalamin) status in vegetarians. Am. J. Clin. Nutr. 59, 1213S–1222S.

Hermann, W., Obeid, R., Schorr, H., Geisel, J., 2003. Functional vitamin B_{12} deficiency and determination of holotranscobalamin in populations at risk. Clin. Chem. 46, 1277–1283.

Hin, H., Clarke, R , Sherliker, P., Atoyerbi, W., Emmens, K., Birks, J., et al., 2006. Clinical relevance of low serum vitamin B_{12} concentrations in older people: the Banbury B_{12} study. Age Ageing 35, 416–422.

Hirota, W.K., Zuckerman, M.J., Adler, D.G., Davila, R.E., Egan, J., Leighton, J.A., Standards of Practice Committee. American Society for Gastrointestinal Endoscopy, 2006. ASGE guideline: the role of endoscopy in the surveillance of premalignant conditions of upper GI tract. Gastrointest. Endosc. 63, 570–580.

Hsing, A.W., Hansson, L.E., McLaughlin, J.K., Nyren, O., Blot, W.J., Ekbom, A., et al., 1993. Pernicious anaemia and subsequent cancer. A population-based cohort study. Cancer 71, 745–750.

Joosten, E., Van den Berg, A., Riezier, R., Naurath, H.J., Lindenbaum, J., Stabler, S.P., et al., 1993. Metabolic evidecne that difference of vitamin B-12 (cobalamin), folate, and vitamin-6 occur commonly in elderly people. Am. J. Clin. Nutr. 58, 468–476.

Joosten, E., Lesaffre, E., Riezier, R., 1996. Are different reference intervals for methylmalonic acid and total homocysteine necessary in elderly people? Eur. J. Haematol. 57, 222–226.

Kaptan, K., Beyan, C., Ural, A.U., Cetin, T., Avcu, F., Gulsen, M., et al., 2000. *Helicobacter pylori*—is it a novel causative agent in Vitamin B_{12} deficiency? Arch. Intern. Med. 160, 1349–1353.

Klee, G.C., 2000. Cobalamin and folate evaluation: measurement of methylmalonic acid and homocysteine vs vitamin B_{12} and folate. Clin. Chem. 46, 1277–1283.

Kowk, T., Cheng, G., Woo, J., Lai, W.K., Pang, C.P., 2002. Independent effect of vitamin B_{12} deficiency on haematological status in older Chinese vegetarian women. Am. J. Hematol. 70, 186–190.

Kransinski, S.D., Russell, R.M., Samloff, I.M., Jacob, R.A., Dallal, G.E., McGandy, R.B., et al., 1986. Fundi atrophic gastritis in an elderly population. Effect on hemoglobin and several serum nutritional indicators. J. Am. Geriatr. Soc. 34, 800–806.

Lindenbaum, J., Rosenberg, L.H., Wilson, P.W., Stabler, S.P., Allen, R.H., 1994. Prevalence of cobalamin deficiency in the Framingham elderly population. Am. J. Clin. Nutr. 60, 2–11.

Lindenbaum, J., Healton, E.B., Savage, D.G., Brust, J.C., Garrett, T.J., Podell, E.R., et al., 1988. Neuropsychiatric disorders caused by cobalamin deficiency in the absence of anaemia or macrocytosis. N. Engl. Med 318, 1720–1728.

Loikas, S., Koskinen, P., Pirjala, K., Löppönen, M., Isoaho, R., Kivelä, S.L., et al., 2007. Vitamin B_{12} deficiency in the aged: a population-based study. Age Ageing 36, 177–183.

Malouf, R., Areosa Sastre, A., 2003. Vitamin B_{12} for cognition. Cochrane Database Syst. Rev. 3, CD004326.

Martin, D.C., France, J., Protech, J., Huff, F.J., 1992. Time dependency of cognitive recovery with cobalamin replacement: report of a pilot study. J. Am. Geriatr. Soc. 40, 168–172.

Matthews, J.H., 1995. Cobalamin and folate deficiency in the elderly. Bailleres Clin. Haematol. 8, 679–697.

Nexo, E., Holffmann-Lückeu, E., 2011. Holotrancobalamin, a marker of vitamin B_{12} status: analytical aspects and clinical utility. Am. J. Clin. Nutr. 94, 359S–365S.

Obeid, R., Schorr, H., Eckert, R., Hermann, W., 2004. Vitamin B_{12} status in the elderly as judged by available biochemical markers. Clin. Chem. 7, 467–472.

Oosterhuis, W.P., Niessen, R.W., Rossuyt, P.M., Sanders, G.T., Sturk, A., 2000. Diagnostic values of the main corpuscular volume in the detection of vitamin B_{12} deficiency. Scand. J. Clin. Lab. Invest 60, 9–18.

Pennypacker, L.C., Allen, R.H., Kelly, J.P., Matthews, L.M., Grigsby, J., Kaye, K., et al., 1992. High prevalence of cobalamin deficiency in elderly outpatients. J. Am. Geriatr. Soc. 40, 1197–1204.

Rajan, S., Wallace, J.I., Brodkin, K.I., Beresford, S.A., Allen, R.H., Stabler, S.P., 2002. Response of elevated methylmalonic acid to three dose levels of oral cobalamin in older adults. J. Am. Geriatr. Soc 50, 1789–1795.

Sabeen, S., Holroyd, S., 2009. Vitamin B12 and psychiatric illness. Ann. Longterm Care 17, 32–36.

Salvage, D.G., Lindenbaum, J., Stabler, S.P., Allen, R.H., 1994. Sensitivity of serum methylmalonic acid and total homocysteine determinations for diagnosing cobalamin and folate deficiencies. Am. J. Med. 96, 239–246.

Schumann, K., 1999. Interactions between drugs and vitamins at advanced age. Int. J. Vitam. Nutr. Res. 69, 173–178.

Selhub, J., Bagley, L.C., Miller, J., Rosenberg, I.H., 2000. B vitamins, homocysteine, and neurocognitive function in the elderly. Am. J. Clin. Nutr. 71, 614S–620S.

Selhub, J., Jacus, P.F., Dallal, G., Choumenkovitch, S., Rogers, G., 2008. The use of a combination of blood concentrations of vitamins and their respective functional indicators to define folate and vitamin B_{12} status. Food Nutr. Bull. 29, S67–S73.

Snow, C.F., 1999. Laboratory diagnosis of vitamin B_{12} and folate deficiency: a guide for the primary care physician. Arch. Intern. Med. 159, 1289–1298.

Toh, B.H., Van Driel, I.R., Gleeson, P.A., 1997. Pernicious anaemia. N. Engl. J. Med. 337, 1441–1448.

Valuck, R.J., Ruscin, J.M., 2004. A case-control study on adverse effects: H2 blocker or proton pump inhibitor use and risk of vitamin B_{12} deficiency in older adults. J. Clin. Epidermiol. 57, 422–428.

Vidal-Alaball, J., Butler, C.C., Cannings-John, R., goringe, A., Hood, K., McCaddon, A., et al., 2005. Oral vitamin B_{12} verses intramuscular vitamin B_{12} for vitamin B_{12} deficiency. Cochrane Database Syst. Rev. 3, CD004655.

Vogel, T., Dali-Youcef, N., Kaltenbach, G., Andrè, E., 2009. Homocysteine, vitamin B_{12}, folate and cognitive functions: a systematic and critical review of the literature. Int. J. Clin. Pract. 63, 1061–1067.

Wong, C.W., 2015. Vitamin B_{12} deficiency in the elderly: is it worth screening? Hong Kong Med. J. 21, 155–164.

Wong, C.W., Ip, C.Y., Leung, C.P., Leung, C.S., Cheng, J.N., Siu, C.Y., 2015. Vitamin B_{12} deficiency in the institutionalized elderly: a regional study. Exp. Gerontol. 69, 221–225.

CHAPTER

17

Vitamin E Isoform-Specific Functions in Allergic Inflammation and Asthma

Joan M. Cook-Mills

Northwestern University, Chicago, IL, United States

INTRODUCTION

Asthma manifests as a heterogeneous disease that results from complex interactions of environmental and genetic factors (Martinez, 2007). The World Health Organization reported that the prevalence of asthma from 1950 to the present has increased in many countries, including those with high, intermediate, and low rates of asthma (Friebele, 1996; Vollmer et al., 1998; Bousquet et al., 2005). The marked rise in rates of asthma over a few decades and the differences in rates among countries and in migrating populations suggest an important role of the local environment, such as diet, in the development of asthma. One environmental change over the past 40 years has been an increase in the γ-tocopherol isoform of vitamin E in the diet and in infant formulas that contain soybean oil, a rich source of γ-tocopherol (Cook-Mills and McCary, 2010; Uauy et al., 1994). In a model of allergic asthma in adult mice, α-tocopherol decreases and γ-tocopherol increases allergic lung inflammation in mice. Moreover, maternal supplementation of α-tocopherol decreases and maternal supplementation of γ-tocopherol increases offspring development of allergic lung inflammation (Abdala-Valencia et al., 2014, 2016). In humans, increasing α-tocopherol levels are associated with better lung function and high plasma γ-tocopherol levels are associated with lower lung function (Berdnikovs et al., 2009; Cook-Mills and McCary, 2010; Marchese et al., 2014; McCary et al., 2011). In this chapter, we discuss the complex and opposing functions of α-tocopherol and γ-tocopherol on asthma in humans and in animal models of lung inflammation. We will discuss how the variation in global prevalence of asthma may be influenced, at least in part, by country-specific plasma γ-tocopherol concentrations.

VITAMIN E ISOFORMS, SOURCES, AND FUNCTIONS

Vitamin E consists of natural isoforms and synthetic racemic isoforms. The eight natural isomers are D-α-, D-β-, D-γ-, and D-δ-tocopherol and D-α-, D-β-, D-γ-, and D-δ-tocotrienol (Fig. 17.1). Plants synthesize the natural isoforms from tyrosine and chlorophyll (Hunter and Cahoon, 2007). These isoforms are consumed in the diet primarily from plant lipids in food and cooking oils and in vitamin supplements. After consumption of the tocopherols, they are taken up from the intestine, transported via the lymph to the blood, and then enter the liver. Mammals do not synthesize or interconvert the tocopherol isoforms. The most abundant isoforms of vitamin E are α-tocopherol and γ-tocopherol, which differ by one methyl group on the chromanol ring (Fig. 17.1). There are 10-fold higher tissue concentrations of α-tocopherol than γ-tocopherol (Wolf, 2006) because there is preferential loading of α-tocopherol on high-density lipoprotein (HDL) and low-density lipoprotein (LDL) particles in the liver by α-tocopherol transfer protein (αTTP) and because there is a higher rate of degradation of γ-tocopherol into its metabolites for excretion (Bella et al., 2006; Leonard et al., 2005). Human genetic variants of liver α-TTP affect α-tocopherol concentrations, resulting in α-tocopherol deficiency (Cavalier et al., 1998). Moreover, αTTP is also expressed by trophoblasts, fetal

Nutrition and Functional Foods for Healthy Aging.
DOI: http://dx.doi.org/10.1016/B978-0-12-805376-8.00017-4

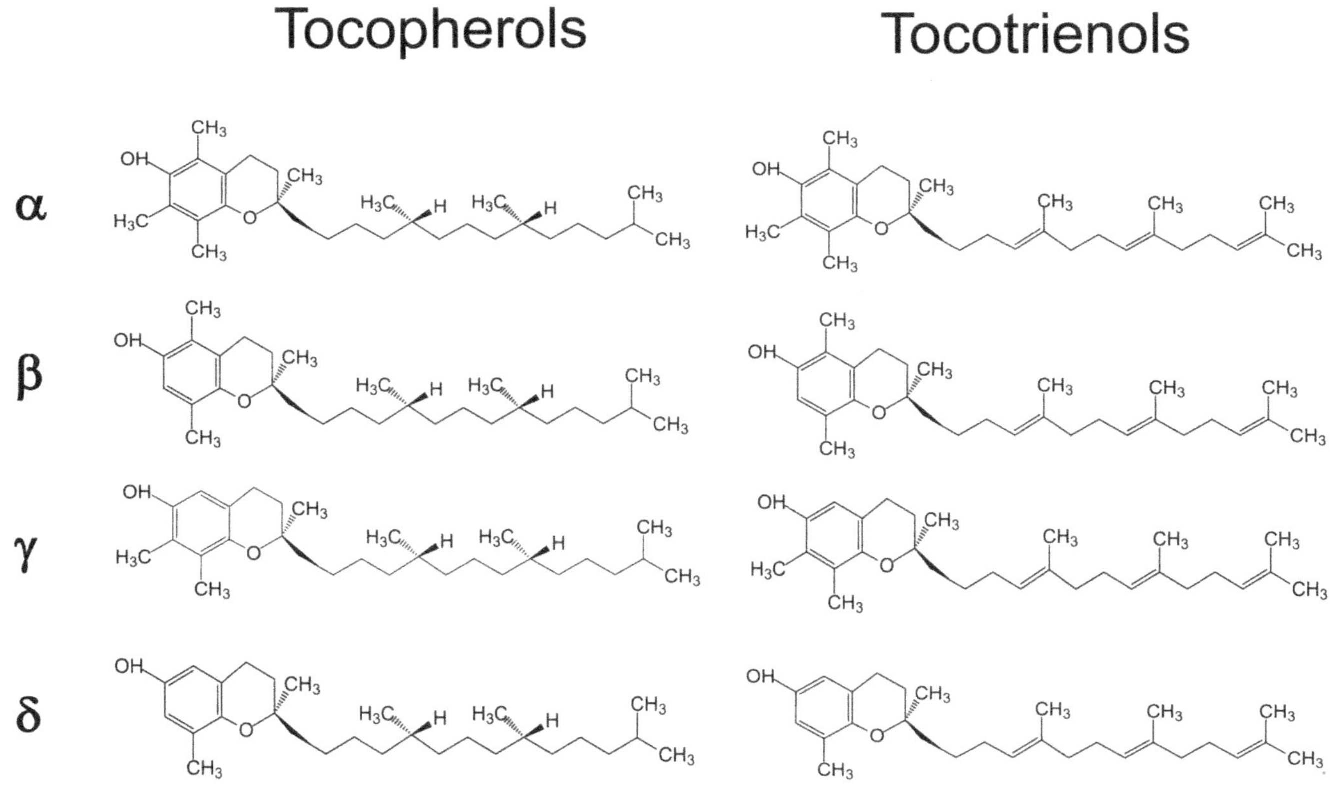

FIGURE 17.1 Vitamin E isoforms.

endothelium, and amnion epithelium of the placenta (Muller-Schmehl et al., 2004). This localization of α-TTP is important because basal levels of α-tocopherol are required for placental development (Jishage et al., 2005; Muller-Schmehl et al., 2004). In addition, other diet components may influence tocopherol absorption, including dietary L-carnitine, which enhances absorption of α-tocopherol in rats (Zou et al., 2005). It is also reported that human plasma levels of α-tocopherol but not γ-tocopherol are increased in male adults and children by the apolipoprotein A5 1131 T > C gene polymorphism (Guardiola et al., 2010; Sundl et al., 2007). In mice, apoE4 mice have lower plasma α-tocopherol levels than do apoE3 mice (Huebbe et al., 2009). Tocopherols in plasma lipid particles are transferred to cells by plasma phospholipid transfer protein, scavenger receptors, or the lipoprotein lipase pathway. After uptake, the tocopherols are found in cell membranes because they are lipid vitamins.

Within tissues, tocopherol isoforms have antioxidant and nonantioxidant functions. Tocopherols are antioxidants. Both α-tocopherol and γ-tocopherol at equal molar concentrations have a relatively similar capacity to scavenge reactive oxygen species (ROS) during lipid peroxidation in vitro and in cells (Nishio et al., 2013; Yoshida et al., 2007). Thus, because α-tocopherol is at a 10-fold higher concentration in tissues than γ-tocopherol, there is 10-fold more scavenging of ROS by α-tocopherol than by γ-tocopherol in vivo. Besides scavenging ROS, γ-tocopherol, in contrast to α-tocopherol, also reacts with reactive nitrogen species (RNS) such as peroxynitrite forming 5-nitro-γ-tocopherol (Patel et al., 2007). The γ-tocopherol scavenging of RNS may be beneficial for inflammation with increases in RNS such as neutrophilic inflammation induced by ozone or by endotoxins in mice (Fakhrzadeh et al., 2004). In the endotoxin-induced lung-inflammation model, administration of aerosol α-tocopherol (30 μg/rat) immediately before inhalation of a lipopolysaccharide (LPS) reduces lung neutrophilia, TNF-α, and cytokine-induced neutrophil chemoattractant-1 (Hybertson et al., 1995). However, in these studies, the source and purity of the α-tocopherol, as well as the lung tissue levels of tocopherols, were not determined. Lung neutrophilia is also reduced in an LPS inflammation model when liposomes containing α-tocopherol (50 mg α-tocopherol/kg mouse) were administered; however, there was no effect on blood neutrophil numbers, TNF-α, IL-1β, or MIP-1α (Rocksen et al., 2003). In asthmatic children exposed to ozone, vitamin E and C supplementation reduces IL-6 in nasal lavages, although the isoform of vitamin E was not indicated (Barthel et al., 2008). Nebulized γ-tocopherol reduces neutrophilia, IL-8, and IL-6 in burn and smoke inhalation injury models in sheep (Wardlaw, 2004). Consistent with this, supplementation with a mixture of tocopherols enriched for γ-tocopherol blocks acute endotoxin-stimulated or ozone-stimulated neutrophil inflammation in the rat and human lung (Hernandez et al., 2013; Wagner et al., 2009; Wiser et al., 2008). In another study, γ-tocopherol supplementation reduced antigen induction of rat lung inflammation in which there was several fold more neutrophils than eosinophils (Wagner et al., 2008). Therefore, γ-tocopherol may be of benefit for acute neutrophilic inflammation. In a study with ex vivo treatment of human macrophages, 300 μM γ-tocopherol decreased macrophage phagocytosis via modulation of surface receptor activity (Wardlaw, 2004). However, such highly elevated γ-tocopherol levels are not achievable in vivo. An important point to note is that although high levels of tocopherols have been used clinically, they can have adverse effects on the brain in animals and humans (Wardlaw, 2004). In contrast to reports of γ-tocopherol benefits in neutrophilic inflammation, it is reported that plasma γ-tocopherol associates with lower lung function in humans (Marchese et al., 2014) and with increased lung eosinophilia and airway hyper-responsiveness in mouse models of allergic asthma (Marchese et al., 2014). Therefore, chronic consumption of γ-tocopherol may be detrimental during lung development or chronic inflammatory diseases such as allergies and asthma. Further mechanistic clinical studies of tocopherol regulation of allergic lung inflammation are needed.

Tocopherol isoforms also have nonantioxidant functions that regulate cell signaling. Tocopherols have a relatively similar capacity to inhibit activation of protein kinase B (Akt) in cancer cells in vitro (Huang et al., 2013), and α-tocopherol inhibits activation of protein kinase Cα (PKCα) in cell systems or cell extracts (Mahoney and Azzi, 1988). Moreover, it is demonstrated that α-tocopherol and γ-tocopherol can directly regulate enzyme activity (McCary et al., 2012). For example, α-tocopherol and γ-tocopherol bind to PKCα at the C1a regulatory domain of PKCα (McCary et al., 2012). On binding, γ-tocopherol increases recombinant PKCα activity whereas α-tocopherol decreases recombinant PKCα activity (McCary et al., 2012), thereby demonstrating opposing regulatory functions for these tocopherol isoforms during cell signaling. Thus, α-tocopherol functions as an antagonist of PKCα activity and γ-tocopherol functions as an agonist of PKCα activity (McCary et al., 2012).

ASTHMA AND ALLERGIC LUNG INFLAMMATION

The World Health Organization has reported a worldwide increase in asthma and allergies ever since 1950 (Friebele, 1996; Vollmer et al., 1998). In 2012–13, the US Centers for Disease Control and Prevention reported asthma and allergy prevalence as 10–20% and affecting about 26 million people and costing $56 million/year and averaging nine deaths per day (CDC, 2012; Akinbami et al., 2012). Current therapies, including corticosteroids, have serious side effects, so it is critical to determine mechanisms for regulating inflammation in allergies and asthma in order to identify novel approaches for interventions. In humans, measurements of lung function include forced expiratory volume (FEV) in 1 s (FEV1: forced volume blown out in 1 s) and forced vital capacity (FVC), which is forced volume when all air is blown out. Asthma is characterized by inflammatory processes with T-helper (Th) cell responses of the Th2 phenotype being considered crucial for the initiation and perpetuation of the inflammatory responses (Palli et al., 2003). Important mediators of asthma and allergic inflammation are cytokines such as the interleukins IL-4, IL-5, and IL-13. Asthmatic and allergic inflammation is characterized by elevated immunoglobulin E, mast cell degranulation, and eosinophilic inflammation (Fiscus et al., 2001). Recruitment of eosinophils is a consistent feature of allergic inflammation and allergic asthma (Chin et al., 1997; Hakugawa et al., 1997; Sagara et al., 1997). A crucial component of recruitment of eosinophils during inflammation is leukocyte migration from the blood and across the endothelium and into the tissue (transendothelial migration) (Cook-Mills and Deem, 2005; Muller, 2011; Vestweber, 2012). Mechanisms for this eosinophil recruitment involve the coordinated actions of adhesion molecules, chemokines, and cytokines (Mould et al., 2000; Yang et al., 1998). Tocopherol isoform regulation of allergic inflammation has been studied in humans, animal models, and cell systems.

The increase in allergic inflammation and asthma may in part be influenced by the increase in γ-tocopherol consumption. In the past 50 years, there has been an increase in the γ-tocopherol isoform in the diet, in infant formulas containing soybean oil that is rich in γ-tocopherol, and in vitamin supplements (Cook-Mills and McCary, 2010; Uauy et al., 1994). Moreover, it has been suggested that early exposures to environmental factors increase the risk of allergic disease (Bousquet et al., 2011). Maternal exposure to environmental factors, including high fat diets, can alter neonatal hematopoietic or metabolic functions (Burke et al., 2009; Fedulov et al., 2008; Izzotti et al., 2003; Lim et al., 2010; Odaka et al., 2010; Rebholz et al., 2011; Vanhees et al., 2011; Woollett, 2005). In reports examining human maternal and paternal asthma associations with development of allergies in offspring, most associations are with maternal asthma (Lim and Kobzik, 2009a). In animal studies, the offspring of allergic mothers have increased responses to suboptimal doses of allergens (Lim and Kobzik, 2009a), and tocopherol isoforms regulate development of offspring responses (Abdala-Valencia et al., 2014, 2016). Therefore, studies of the regulation of adult allergies and asthma as well as the development of allergic disease and asthma early in life are critical to generating approaches to limit these diseases.

CLINICAL STUDIES OF ASTHMA AND TOCOPHEROL ISOFORMS

Most clinical studies on vitamin E include mixed forms of natural and synthetic tocopherols from supplementation or diet. Some studies have reported what seem to be conflicting outcomes for vitamin E on allergies and other inflammatory diseases, but these differences are consistent with the differences in levels of tocopherol isoforms present in the study supplements, vehicles, and diets in the studies (Cook-Mills, 2012; Cook-Mills et al., 2011b; Cook-Mills and McCary, 2010) and consistent with mechanistic studies demonstrating that γ-tocopherol elevates allergic inflammation and that α-tocopherol reduces allergic inflammation (Abdala-Valencia et al., 2012a; Berdnikovs et al., 2009; Cook-Mills et al., 2011b; Marchese et al., 2014; McCary et al., 2011, 2012). In humans and mice, the tocopherol concentrations in plasma correlate with those in the lung tissue (Berdnikovs et al., 2009; McCary et al., 2011; Redlich et al., 1996). An interesting note is that countries with the highest prevalence rate of asthma tend to have higher plasma levels of γ-tocopherol (Cook-Mills et al., 2013; Cook-Mills and Avila, 2014). In the Unites States, the average human plasma γ-tocopherol levels are two to five times higher than those of many European and Asian countries, whereas the average levels of human plasma α-tocopherol is similar among all countries (Cook-Mills et al., 2013; Cook-Mills and Avila, 2014). The high human plasma γ-tocopherol levels in the United States are consistent with soybean oil consumption, which is high in γ-tocopherol (Abdala-Valencia et al., 2013; Cook-Mills et al., 2013; Cook-Mills and Avila, 2014; Jiang et al., 2001; Talegawkar et al., 2007). Most of the vitamin E consumed in the diet in the United States is γ-tocopherol in vegetable oils such as soybean oil, corn oil, and canola oil (Bieri and Evarts, 1973, 1975). Therefore, the high human plasma γ-tocopherol levels in the US population are consistent with high levels of γ-tocopherol in these oils (Table 17.1) (Choo et al., 2003; Davenpeck et al., 2000; Jiang et al., 2001; Miller et al., 2001). It has been demonstrated that soybean oil administration to humans and hamsters increases the plasma γ-tocopherol levels two- to fivefold (Meydani et al., 1987; Myou et al., 2002). In murine models of asthma with a two- to fivefold increase in plasma γ-tocopherol levels, there is an exacerbation of lung inflammation and suppression of the anti-inflammatory functions of α-tocopherol (Berdnikovs et al., 2009).

In contrast to its high levels in soybean oil, γ-tocopherol is low in other oils such as sunflower, safflower, and olive oil (Table 17.1), which are commonly used across Europe (Abdala-Valencia et al., 2013; Berdnikovs et al., 2009; Cook-Mills et al., 2013; Cook-Mills and Avila, 2014). These oils contain predominantly the α-tocopherol isoform (Abdala-Valencia et al., 2013; Cook-Mills et al., 2013; Cook-Mills and Avila, 2014). Also, in a study in which olive oil or soybean oil was administered to preterm human infants starting 24h after birth, there was a significant 1.5-fold increase in plasma α-tocopherol after feeding with olive oil as compared to feeding with soybean oil, but unfortunately γ-tocopherol was not reported (Gobel et al., 2003). In countries with preferential consumption of safflower oil or olive oil, α-tocopherol supplementation of asthmatic patients in Italy and Finland was beneficial for outcomes of physician-diagnosed asthma and lung function as measured by FEV1 or wheeze (Dow et al., 1996; Smit et al., 1999; Tabak et al., 1999; Troisi et al., 1995; Weiss, 1997). Disappointingly, α-tocopherol was not beneficial

TABLE 17.1 Tocopherol Isoforms in Dietary Oils

	Tocopherol (mg/100g of oil)		
Oils	**α-T**	**γ-T**	**δ-T**
Sunflower	56.27 ± 2.95[a]	1.22 ± 0.10	0.22 ± 0.02
Safflower	49.33 ± 6.88	3.85 ± 0.45	ND
Olive	6.13 ± 0.61	0.08 ± 0.004	ND
Grapeseed	7.58 ± 0.54	2.07 ± 0.12	0.11 ± 0.01
Soybean	7.82 ± 0.20	53.87 ± 0.09	15.99 ± 0.25
Corn	29.01 ± 3.21	46.69 ± 0.07	5.07 ± 1.38
Canola	16.45 ± 0.19	21.92 ± 0.05	0.13 ± 0.01
Peanut	14.41 ± 0.19	9.66 ± 0.27	0.80 ± 0.23
Sesame	77.68 ± 6.07	75.41 ± 4.82	56.27 ± 0.45

Source: Adapted from Cook-Mills, J.M., Abdala-Valencia, H., Hartert, T., 2013. Two faces of vitamin E in the lung. Am. J. Respir. Crit. Care Med. 188, 279–284.
ND, not detected.
[a]*Mean ± standard deviation.*

for asthmatic patients in the United States or the Netherlands (Dow et al., 1996; Smit et al., 1999; Tabak et al., 1999; Troisi et al., 1995; Weiss, 1997), which have high plasma levels of γ-tocopherol and high intake of soybean oil. In contrast, administration of acetate-conjugated α-tocopherol oral supplementation at a very high dose (1500 IU, which is 1006 mg) to mild atopic asthmatics in the United States for 16 weeks resulted in increased plasma α-tocopherol, decreased plasma γ-tocopherol, and improved airway responsiveness to methacholine challenge (Hoskins et al., 2012). A meta-analysis study indicated that vitamin E has no association with asthma outcome measures of lung function and wheeze (Devaraj et al., 2007), but this did not take into account the opposing functions of α-tocopherol and γ-tocopherol. We interpret the results of this meta-analysis (Allen et al., 2009) as a combination of data across studies that included marked variation of vitamin E isoforms that have opposing functions and that were present in the diets, supplements, and supplement vehicles.

As countries assume Western lifestyles, diets may change and this would include an increased consumption of soybean oil (Devereux and Seaton, 2005). In two Scottish cohorts, it was reported that reduced maternal intake of vitamin E (likely referring to α-tocopherol) was associated with increased asthma and wheezing in children up to 5 years old (Devereux, 2007; Martindale et al., 2005). In Devereaux's review of these data and changes in the environment in Scotland (Devereux, 2007) from 1967 to 2004, there was a significant increase in vegetable oil intake by Scottish residents, and we suggest that this would at least result in an increase in γ-tocopherol since vegetable oil (soybean oil) is rich in γ-tocopherol. In a study in England, dietary supplementation with α-tocopherol in soy oil to asthmatics had no impact on FEV1, asthma symptom scores, or bronchodilator use, but the γ-tocopherol in the soy oil may have opposed the benefit of the α-tocopherol (Pearson et al., 2004). Also, in a study in the United Kingdom, α-tocopherol administration in soybean oil to asthmatics did not have benefits (Hernandez et al., 2009) consistent with opposing functions of α-tocopherol and γ-tocopherol. There are also differences in asthma prevalence among racial and ethnic groups (Zahran and Bailey, 2013). However, studies examining tocopherol association with clinical outcomes generally adjust for several known confounding factors such as gender, age, body mass index, race, and smoking. Although there may be other differences regarding the environment and genetics of people in different countries, the outcomes for tocopherol isoforms and asthma in clinical studies are consistent with the studies demonstrating inhibitory functions of α-tocopherol and agonist functions of γ-tocopherol. Thus, the differences in outcomes of clinical reports mirror the opposing regulatory functions of α- and γ-tocopherol forms of vitamin E consumed in diets, supplements, and supplement vehicles (Berdnikovs et al., 2009). Our interpretation, supported by animal studies, is that the γ-tocopherol in soybean oil or other vehicles ablates the benefit of α-tocopherol supplementation in asthma. Therefore, differences in outcomes from clinical reports on the associations of vitamin E and asthma may, in part, reflect the opposing regulatory effects of α-tocopherol and γ-tocopherol in the supplements, the vehicles for the supplements, and diets in the individuals.

We reported that the findings of opposing regulatory functions of tocopherol isoforms in animal models can be translated to human lung function. In a prospective clinical study, 4526 adults were included in the United States in the Coronary Artery Risk Development in Young Adults (CARDIA) multicenter cohort with data for spirometry and serum tocopherol isoforms. In this cohort, there were equal numbers of blacks and whites and equal numbers of females and males by study design. Interestingly, increasing serum concentrations of γ-tocopherol were associated with lower FEV1 or FVC, whereas increasing serum concentrations of α-tocopherol were associated with higher FEV1 or FVC (Marchese et al., 2014). Since these two tocopherols have opposing functions, the analysis of opposing functions of tocopherol isoforms in clinical studies should include quartiles of plasma tocopherols with a determination of whether there is an association of a tocopherol isoform with the clinical outcome when the concentration of the opposing tocopherol is low and presenting the least competing opposing effects. Using this approach, in the analysis of the CARDIA cohort, plasma γ-tocopherol associates with lower lung function (FEV1) and plasma α-tocopherol associates with better lung function (FEV1) in nonasthmatics and asthmatics (Marchese et al., 2014) with adjustments for several known confounding factors such as gender, age, body mass index, race, and smoking. In the CARDIA cohort, a fivefold higher human plasma γ-tocopherol (>10 μM γ-tocopherol) was associated with reduced FEV1 and FVC in all participants (asthmatics and nonasthmatics) by ages 21–27. The γ-tocopherol-associated decreases in FEV1 and FVC before age 21 may occur during development and lung responses to environmental pollutants, allergens, or infections because tocopherols can directly regulate PKCα (Berdnikovs et al., 2009; Cook-Mills et al., 2011b; Cook-Mills and McCary, 2010; McCary et al., 2011). For the asthmatic group with plasma γ-tocopherol >10 μM, the participants had 350–570 mL lower FEV1 or FVC as compared to the low to moderate γ-tocopherol concentrations (<10 μM γ-tocopherol) at ages 21–27 (Marchese et al., 2014). This 10–17% decrease in FEV1 with >10 μM plasma γ-tocopherol in asthmatics is similar to the 5–10% reduction in FEV1 reported for other environmental factors. For example, individuals with occupational allergen exposure have a 5–8% decrease in FEV1 compared to nonasthmatics, and this decrease is associated with dyspnea, chest tightness, chronic bronchitis, and chronic cough

(Jacobs et al., 1993). Responders to particulate matter have a 2–6% decrease in FEV1 (Delfino et al., 2004), responders to cold or exercise have a 5–11% decrease in FEV1 (Koskela et al., 1994), and responders to house dust mite or dog or cat dander have a 2–8% decrease in FEV1 (Blanc et al., 2005). Moreover, based on the 2% prevalence of serum γ-tocopherol >10 μM in adults in CARDIA and the adult US population in the 2010 Census, we expect that the lower FEV1 and FVC at >10 μM serum γ-tocopherol occur in up to 4.5 million adults in the US population. Thus, there are opposing outcomes for associating plasma α-tocopherol and γ-tocopherol with lung function in humans. This is consistent with mechanistic preclinical studies demonstrating opposing functions for α-tocopherol and γ-tocopherol (Abdala-Valencia et al., 2012a, 2014, 2016; Berdnikovs et al., 2009; Hess et al., 1997; McCary et al., 2011, 2012).

Adults and children with asthma have low plasma α-tocopherol levels (Al-Abdulla et al., 2010; Kalayci et al., 2000; Kelly et al., 1999; Schunemann et al., 2001). Plasma and tissue tocopherols correlate (Berdnikovs et al., 2009; McCary et al., 2011; Redlich et al., 1996). It is reported that patients with asthma have reduced α-tocopherol and ascorbic acid in airway fluid, but the average plasma concentration of α-tocopherol and ascorbic acid in these patients is normal (Kalayci et al., 2000; Kelly et al., 1999). Similarly, α-tocopherol and ascorbic acid levels are decreased in bronchoalveolar lavage of guinea pigs sensitized with ovalbumin (OVA) (Ratnasinghe et al., 2000). Tocopherol isoforms are also reduced in mice with allergic inflammation (Abdala-Valencia et al., 2014, 2016). Therefore, since α-tocopherol levels are low in asthmatics and α-tocopherol can reduce allergic inflammation, supplementation with physiological levels of natural α-tocopherol and maintenance of low dietary levels of γ-tocopherol in combination with other regimens may be an attractive strategy to either prevent or improve control of allergic disease or asthma. Based on average human plasma tocopherol isoforms in studied countries (Cook-Mills et al., 2013), prevalence of asthma in studied countries (Cook-Mills et al., 2013), and low α-tocopherol in asthma (Al-Abdulla et al., 2010; Kalayci et al., 2000; Kelly et al., 1999; Schunemann et al., 2001), a potential target for balancing tocopherol isoforms during allergic disease and asthma may be about 1–1.4 μM plasma γ-tocopherol and 22–30 μM plasma α-tocopherol (Fig. 17.2). Further intervention studies with analysis of the tocopherol isoforms in plasma are necessary to examine tocopherol isoform regulation of allergic lung inflammation and asthma in humans.

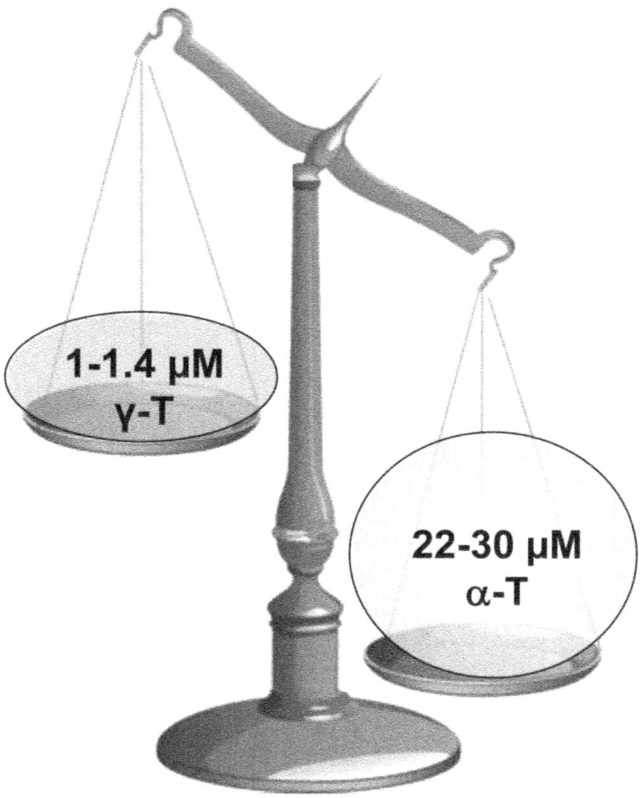

FIGURE 17.2 Potential target for balance of human plasma α-tocopherol (α-T) and γ-tocopherol (γ-T) during allergic inflammation. Further studies are needed.

COMPARING TOCOPHEROL DOSES IN HUMANS AND PRECLINICAL MOUSE STUDIES

For mouse models of disease, it is important to consider tocopherol doses for mice that might be relevant for humans. Ultimately, comparing doses for mice and humans is difficult because of differences in rates of metabolism. Relevant doses of tocopherol isoforms for studies in mice is a physiologic, nontoxic dose that achieves fold changes in mouse tissues similar to fold changes in human tissues. Basal α-T is necessary for mouse and human placental development (Jishage et al., 2005; Muller-Schmehl et al., 2004). For healthy adult humans, the recommended daily allowance of α-tocopherol is 15 mg/day. Doses of γ-tocopherol have not been addressed. Furthermore, whether doses higher than 15 mg α-tocopherol/day are necessary during disease has not been established. For mice, the standard basal mouse chow diet contains about 45 mg α-tocopherol/kg of diet and 45 mg γ-tocopherol/kg of diet (Abdala-Valencia et al., 2014, 2016). This results in about a 10-fold higher tissue α-tocopherol concentration than γ-tocopherol concentration (Abdala-Valencia et al., 2014, 2016) because of the preferential transfer of α-tocopherol by α-TTP in the liver.

Converting mouse doses to human doses is complex, so we briefly discuss translations of mouse α-tocopherol doses to human tocopherol doses. The basal mouse diet of 45 mg α-tocopherol/kg of diet is translated as follows:

[(45 mg α-tocopherol/kg of diet) × (1 kg/1000 g) × (6 g diet eaten/mouse/day)]/(28 g body weight for an adult mouse) × 65,000 g human adult) = 627 mg α-tocopherol/day for human adult

However, mouse metabolism is about eightfold less efficient, and mice have a higher metabolic turnover rate per unit of body weight than humans (Kleiber, 1975; Terpstra, 2001). Thus, mice require about eightfold higher intake per gram of body weight. Furthermore, mice eat one-sixth their body weight in food/day (Bachmanov et al., 2002), which is considerably higher than the average amount of food/day for adult humans. Thus, to adjust for metabolic rate:

(627 mg/day for adult human)/(8 for metabolic rate difference) = 78 mg α-tocopherol/day for human adults

For supplementation levels, a three- to fivefold increase in α-tocopherol for supplementation of mice during studies of inflammation (150 or 250 mg α-T/kg of diet for mice) is then 235–392 mg α-tocopherol/day for human adults (calculation: 78 mg/day × (3 or 5)). These supplemental doses are well below upper safety limits of 1,000 mg α-tocopherol/day in human pregnancy and near clinical levels in preeclampsia pregnancy trials of 268 mg (400 IU) α-tocopherol (Greenough et al., 2010; Gungorduk et al., 2014; Hauth et al., 2010; Kalpdev et al., 2011; McCance et al., 2010; Villar et al., 2009). Also, a supplemented mouse diet with 150 or 250 mg α-tocopherol/kg of diet is 30–60 times lower than the rodent maternal α-tocopherol diet dose that reduces rodent hippocampus function (Betti et al., 2011). The doses of 150 or 250 mg α-tocopherol/kg of diet for mice achieves a two- to threefold increase in tissue concentrations of α-tocopherol, which is similar to the fold tissue changes achievable in humans (Abdala-Valencia et al., 2012a; Berdnikovs et al., 2009; Cook-Mills et al., 2011a; Cook-Mills and McCary, 2010; McCary et al., 2011, 2012).

ALPHA-TOCOPHEROL AND GAMMA-TOCOPHEROL REGULATE ALLERGIC INFLAMMATION AND AIRWAY HYPER-RESPONSIVENESS IN PRECLINICAL ADULT ANIMAL STUDIES

Differences among reports for tocopherol regulation of eosinophilic lung inflammation may reflect differences in the intake of tocopherol isoforms and doses of tocopherols. Also, discrepancies among reports for tocopherol regulation of lung inflammation may be explained by an important parameter such as tocopherol isoforms used in the oil vehicle during supplementation. The levels of α-tocopherol and γ-tocopherol are different among dietary oils (Table 17.1) (Berdnikovs et al., 2009; Jiang et al., 2001; Wagner et al., 2004). High levels of γ-tocopherol are found in soybean, corn, canola, and sesame oils, so the administration of supplemental tocopherols in any of these vehicles would lead to misinterpretations. For example, Suchankova et al. (2006) reported that the administration of purified α-tocopherol in soy oil by gavage had no major effect on immune parameters or lung airway responsiveness in mice challenged with OVA. An interpretation is that high γ-tocopherol in the soy oil vehicle opposed the effect of the α-tocopherol, although tissue and plasma tocopherol levels were not reported for these studies. Okamoto et al. (2006) found that feeding mice α-tocopherol starting 2 weeks before antigen sensitization did not affect immunoglobulin E (IgE) levels but did reduce the number of eosinophils in the bronchoalveolar lavage, although the form and purity of α-tocopherol were not indicated. Mabalirajan et al. (2009) reported that oral administration of α-tocopherol in ethanol after antigen sensitization blocked OVA-induced lung inflammation and airway hyper-responsiveness. In this report, α-tocopherol treatment reduced airway hyper-responsiveness and mediators of inflammation, including

IL-4, IL-5, IL-13, OVA-specific IgE, eotaxin, transforming growth factor beta (TGF-β), 12/15-LOX, lipid peroxidation, and lung nitric oxide metabolites (Mamdouh et al., 2009). Thus, supplementation with α-tocopherol alleviated allergic inflammation. For interpretation of studies with tocopherol isoforms, the vehicle, diet, and tissue concentrations of tocopherol isoforms need to be measured.

In mouse models of allergic lung responses to house dust mites, a mouse diet supplemented with 250mg of α-tocopherol/kg during house dust mite challenges reduces eosinophilia in the lung (Cook-Mills et al., 2016). In contrast, a mouse diet supplemented with 250mg γ-tocopherol/kg of diet elevated house dust mite–induced eosinophilia in the lung (Cook-Mills et al, 2016). Another mouse model of allergic lung inflammation is induced by sensitization with chicken egg OVA in adjuvant and followed by challenging the lung with inhaled OVA. In a study with the OVA model, the focus was on supplementation with tocopherols after OVA sensitization to determine whether tocopherol isoforms modulate the OVA antigen-challenge phase (Berdnikovs et al., 2009); this is relevant because patients are already sensitized. In this study, tocopherols were administered by daily injections after sensitization but before the allergen challenge (Berdnikovs et al., 2009). Subcutaneous administration of tocopherols achieves a plateau in levels of tissue tocopherols in a few days whereas dietary supplementation of tocopherols takes a couple of weeks to achieve a plateau in tissue tocopherol levels (Meydani et al., 1987; Mustacich et al., 2006). Administration of α-tocopherol or γ-tocopherol subcutaneously to allergic adult mice during challenge with OVA raises lung and plasma concentrations of the tocopherol isoform four- to fivefold without affecting body or lung weight (Berdnikovs et al., 2009). This fold change is achievable in humans. When tocopherols are administered subcutaneously or in the diet, the tocopherols enter the lymph and then the thoracic duct and the liver where the tocopherols are loaded on lipoproteins that enter circulation. Subcutaneous administration of γ-tocopherol elevates lung eosinophil recruitment by 175%, and α-tocopherol reduces lung eosinophil recruitment by 65% after challenge with OVA. Furthermore, in these mice, α-tocopherol blocks and γ-tocopherol increases airway hyper-responsiveness (Berdnikovs et al., 2009). The levels of tocopherols in these studies did not alter numbers of blood eosinophils, indicating that a sufficient number of eosinophils was available for recruitment (Berdnikovs et al., 2009). Also, the expression of adhesion molecules, cytokines, and chemokines required for the leukocyte recruitment was not compromised by tocopherol supplementation (Berdnikovs et al., 2009). This modulation of leukocyte infiltration in allergic inflammation without alteration of adhesion molecules, cytokines, or chemokines is similar to several other reports of in vivo inhibition of lung inflammation by inhibition of intracellular signals in endothelial cells (Abdala-Valencia et al., 2007, 2012b; Keshavan et al., 2005). The competing functions of tocopherol isoforms have important implications for the interpretation of clinical and animal studies of vitamin E regulation of inflammation.

Interestingly, γ-tocopherol negates the antiinflammatory benefit of α-tocopherol (Berdnikovs et al., 2009; McCary et al., 2011). Administration of both α-tocopherol and γ-tocopherol during challenge with OVA results in numbers of lung eosinophils and airway responses similar to those of the vehicle control treated allergic mice, suggesting that these two tocopherols have competing opposing functions. This strong opposing function of γ-tocopherol occurs even though γ-tocopherol is about 5–10 times lower in concentration in vivo than α-tocopherol. The proinflammatory allergic effects of γ-tocopherol in mice are partially reversed by switching supplements from γ-tocopherol to α-tocopherol for 4 weeks (McCary et al., 2011). It was also demonstrated that γ-tocopherol elevation of inflammation is fully reversible by highly elevated levels (10 times supplemental levels) of α-tocopherol (McCary et al., 2011). However, carefully considered should be the implications and adverse effects of high doses of tocopherols that may significantly increase the incidence of hemorrhagic stroke, elevated blood pressure, and increased all-cause mortality (Barthel et al., 2008; Wagner et al., 2004, 2008). Consequently, administration of very-high-dose α-tocopherol may be a potentially risky approach for reversing the proinflammatory effects of supplemental levels of γ-tocopherol. An alternative may be longer supplementation with modest levels of α-tocopherol.

In summary, the isoform α-tocopherol is antiinflammatory and blocks airway hyper-reactivity, and a fivefold increase in the isoform γ-tocopherol is proinflammatory and increases airway hyper-reactivity during eosinophilic allergic lung inflammation in adult mice (Abdala-Valencia et al., 2012a; Berdnikovs et al., 2009; Cook-Mills and McCary, 2010; McCary et al., 2011, 2012). These studies are consistent with the human studies, demonstrating that a fivefold increase in human plasma γ-tocopherol associated with a reduction in lung function in humans (Marchese et al., 2014). Furthermore, a fivefold difference in γ-tocopherol concentrations is consistent with fivefold higher γ-tocopherol in Americans versus Western Europeans and Asians and higher prevalence of asthma in Americans (Cook-Mills et al., 2013; Cook-Mills and Avila, 2014).

In allergic inflammation in the lung, eosinophil migration is dependent on the vascular cell adhesion molecule-1 (VCAM-1) whereas the other leukocytes can migrate on the intercellular adhesion molecule 1 (ICAM-1) (Chin et al., 1997; Sagara et al., 1997). These adhesion molecules signal through PKCα that can be directly regulated by tocopherol isoforms (McCary et al., 2012) as discussed previously. Thus, a mechanism for the opposing regulatory functions for α-tocopherol and γ-tocopherol on allergic inflammation in the mouse lung is, in part, a result of tocopherol regulation of signals for leukocyte transendothelial migration from the blood into the lung.

TOCOPHEROL REGULATION OF LEUKOCYTE RECRUITMENT

During allergic inflammation, leukocytes are recruited from the blood into the tissues by migrating across the vascular endothelial cells. The migration of leukocytes across endothelial cells is inhibited by pretreatment of the endothelial cells with α-tocopherol and elevated by pretreatment of the endothelial cells with γ-tocopherol (Berdnikovs et al., 2009). Endothelial cells pretreated with α-tocopherol plus γ-tocopherol result in an intermediate phenotype that is not different from the vehicle-treated control endothelial cells, indicating that α-tocopherol and γ-tocopherol have opposing regulatory functions during leukocyte recruitment (Berdnikovs et al., 2009). The opposing functions of α-tocopherol and γ-tocopherol on endothelial cells during leukocyte transendothelial migration can occur through direct regulation of mediators of signal transduction. Briefly, the recruitment of eosinophils to sites of allergic inflammation requires eosinophil binding to adhesion molecules on endothelial cells such as VCAM-1 and ICAM-1 (Chin et al., 1997). These adhesion molecules signal through protein kinase Cα (PKCα) for the recruitment of leukocytes (Abdala-Valencia et al., 2012a; Berdnikovs et al., 2009; Jourd'heuil et al., 1997).

On loading the endothelial cells with physiological tocopherol concentrations that are at the same concentrations of tocopherols in lung tissues in mice, it was demonstrated that α-tocopherol inhibits VCAM-1 and ICAM-1 activation of PKCα in endothelial cells, and this inhibition is opposed by pretreatment of endothelial cells with γ-tocopherol (Abdala-Valencia et al., 2012a; Berdnikovs et al., 2009; Jourd'heuil et al., 1997). Alpha-tocopherol is an antagonist of PKCα and γ-tocopherol is an agonist of PKCα on binding to the C1A regulatory domain of PKCα (McCary et al., 2012). Alpha-tocopherol has been also reported to inhibit PKCα activation in other cell systems or cell extracts, but the mechanisms for inhibition in these systems were not demonstrated (de Luis et al., 2005). In summary, PKCα is differentially regulated by tocopherol isoforms in endothelial cells, which is critical for leukocyte recruitment in allergic lung inflammation and airway hyper-responsiveness.

MATERNAL TOCOPHEROLS AND OFFSPRING DEVELOPMENT OF ALLERGY

Clinical Studies of Maternal Tocopherols and Allergies and Asthma

The prevalence of allergies has increased in just a few decades, suggesting that environmental factors likely impact allergies and asthma because this is too short a time span for genetic alterations in whole populations. Environmental factors that regulate allergy and asthma in the mother could then affect the risk of development of allergy and asthma in offspring. Exposure to environmental factors such as chemical irritants or nutrients during pregnancy has been associated with allergic disease in offspring. An environmental change over the past 40 years that may contribute to elevating allergic responses has been an increase in the D-γ-tocopherol isoform of vitamin E in the diet and in infant formulas that contain soybean oil (Berdnikovs et al., 2009; Boyle et al., 1996; Cook-Mills and McCary, 2010; Nelson et al., 1996; Uauy et al., 1994).

Some studies suggest that development of allergen responsiveness may occur prenatally (Blumer et al., 2005; Devereux et al., 2002; Uthoff et al., 2003). In reports examining human maternal and paternal asthma associations with development of allergies in offspring, most associations are with maternal allergies or asthma (Celedon et al., 2002; Folsgaard et al., 2012; Kurukulaaratchy et al., 2003, 2005; Latzin et al., 2007; Lim et al., 2010; Litonjua et al., 1998; Martinez et al., 1995), suggesting that sensitization can occur prenatally or early postnatally. It is suggested that in utero and early exposures to environmental factors are critical for increased risk of allergic disease (Bousquet et al., 2011). There is an association of higher risk of eczema, wheezing, and lower respiratory tract infections in early life with increases in human maternal and cord blood C-reactive protein, which is an acute phase protein produced during inflammation (Sonnenschein-van der Voort et al., 2013).

Tocopherol isoforms may influence development of allergies early in life. It was demonstrated in a 20-year prospective study in the United States that by age 21 human plasma α-tocopherol associates with better lung spirometry and human plasma γ-tocopherol associates with worse lung spirometry (Marchese et al., 2014). This suggests that during human development prior to age 21, tocopherols may have regulatory functions on responsiveness to allergen. Thus, the balance of α-tocopherol and γ-tocopherol in women may regulate adult allergic responses (Marchese et al., 2014), and the balance of tocopherol isoforms in pregnant females may influence the development of risk of allergies in her children. It was demonstrated that maternal α-tocopherol dietary intake was inversely associated with cord blood mononuclear cells proliferative responses to allergen challenges (Devereux et al., 2002; Wassall et al., 2013). Also, maternal α-tocopherol supplementation of rats during pregnancy results in larger lungs with normal structure in offspring (Islam et al., 1999). Also, from ultrasound studies of the fetus, maternal α-tocopherol levels are reported to associate with fetal growth (Turner et al., 2010). In other clinical studies, α-tocopherol did not associate with asthma (Erkkola et al., 2001; Maslova et al., 2014; West et al., 2012), but these studies did not measure tocopherol isoforms or include analysis of potential opposing functions of γ-tocopherol.

Preclinical Studies of Maternal Contribution to Development of Offspring Allergy and Asthma

A mouse model for maternal transfer of risk of allergy to offspring reflects many of the parameters of development of allergic disease in humans, including increased risk for development of allergies in offspring of allergic mothers (Celedon et al., 2002; Fedulov and Kobzik, 2011; Fedulov et al., 2007; Folsgaard et al., 2012; Hamada et al., 2003; Kurukulaaratchy et al., 2003, 2005; Latzin et al., 2007; Leme et al., 2006; Lim and Kobzik, 2009a; Lim et al., 2010; Litonjua et al., 1998; Martinez et al., 1995). Moreover, as in humans, in this mouse model the allergic responses of the offspring are not specific to the allergen of the mother (Hamada et al., 2003). In the mouse model of maternal transfer of risk of allergy to offspring, allergy is induced in female mice by sensitizing with OVA in the adjuvant alum in the first 2 weeks and then challenging with OVA three times on weeks 4, 8, and 12 (Fedulov and Kobzik, 2011; Fedulov et al., 2007; Hamada et al., 2003). After the last OVA challenge in week 12, these female mice are mated. Therefore, the female mice have allergic lung inflammation during the first half of the pregnancy because it takes about 2 weeks for a resolution of allergic lung inflammation, which is the majority of the 3 weeks of mouse gestation. This is consistent with humans who have allergen-challenged pregnancies. Additional challenge of mice with OVA during pregnancy is not necessary for induction of risk of allergy in the offspring (Hamada et al., 2003). To determine allergen responsiveness in the offspring, all of the offspring from allergic mothers and nonallergic mothers are treated with a suboptimal OVA protocol. The suboptimal protocol includes neonates receiving only one instead of two OVA–alum treatments at postnatal days 3–5; then starting 7 days later, the neonates are challenged with aerosolized OVA for three consecutive days. The offspring of these allergic mothers develop allergic lung inflammation and airway responsiveness, whereas pups from nonallergic mothers do not develop inflammation in response to the allergen challenge. Moreover, this ability of the offspring of allergic mothers to respond to allergen is sustained for up to 8 weeks of age in the mouse (Fedulov et al., 2007). The magnitude of the offspring response to an initial allergen challenge declines in the offspring after 8 weeks (Fedulov et al., 2007). Allergic responses are inhibited in the mother by anti–IL-4 antibody administration to the mothers at preconception, and this maternal anti–IL-4 treatment blocks development of responsiveness of offspring to suboptimal allergen (Hamada et al., 2003). These data suggest that an IL-4–dependent allergic response in the mother is involved in the transmission of risk to the offspring. However, IL-4 and IgE do not pass to the fetus from the mother (Leme et al., 2006; Lim and Kobzik, 2009b; Uthoff et al., 2003). Th2 cytokines (IL-4, IL-5, and IL-13) are elevated in the placenta, but transplacental crossing of these cytokines has not been demonstrated (Bowen et al., 2002; Ostojic et al., 2003; Zourbas et al., 2001). It is reported that only 2% of maternal granulocyte macrophage–colony stimulating factor (GM-CSF) crosses the human placenta in ex vivo perfusate studies (Gregor et al., 1999). Whether maternal GM-CSF increases risk of offspring for allergic responses is not known. It was reported that antibody depletion of T cells in allergic mothers modulates the development of responsiveness of offspring to allergen (Hubeau et al., 2007). In other studies, adoptive transfer of allergen-specific T cells from OVA TCR transgenic mice DO11.10 mice to females prior to mating results in offspring with responsiveness to suboptimal challenge of antigen (Hubeau et al., 2006). These data suggest that maternal Th2 responses induce maternal signals that induce development of allergen responsiveness in offspring. Thus, female mice that are allergic before conception and develop a Th2 response during pregnancy produce offspring that have augmented responsiveness to suboptimal allergen challenge. Understanding mechanisms of maternal transfer of risk for allergy to offspring and mechanisms for regulation of this risk will have impact on limiting the development of allergic disease early in life.

The responses of the offspring from allergic mothers are not specific to the allergen to which the mother responds. Uthoff et al. (2003) reported that allergens can cross the placenta but that offspring are responsive to β-lactoglobulin whereas mothers were stimulated with OVA, suggesting that the process is antigen-independent. The antigen-independent maternal transfer of risk of allergy to offspring was also demonstrated (Hamada et al., 2003). In their report, offspring are responsive to casein, whereas the mothers were sensitized and challenged at preconception with OVA (Hamada et al., 2003). An antigen-independent effect of maternal allergy on allergen responsiveness in pups has also been demonstrated in canines (Barrett et al., 2003). Similarly, in humans, children respond to different allergens than the allergic mother. Thus, the offspring responses are not specific to the allergen that the mother responds to; instead, the offspring have an increased responsiveness to sensitization to allergens.

The sensitization to allergens and allergic responses are dependent on dendritic cells (DCs) which produce regulatory cytokines (van Rijt and Lambrecht, 2005; Williams et al., 2013). Interestingly, there are functional changes in the DCs from offspring of allergic mothers (Fedulov and Kobzik, 2011). Offspring from allergic mothers have increased allergic responsiveness to suboptimal allergen challenge (Abdala-Valencia et al., 2014; Fedulov and Kobzik, 2011; Hamada et al., 2003; Lim et al., 2007; Lim and Kobzik, 2009a), and this increased responsiveness of the offspring occurs through changes in pup DCs but not in pup macrophages (Fedulov and Kobzik, 2011). In these studies, the transfer of splenic DCs from nonchallenged neonates of allergic mothers into neonates from nonallergic mothers confers increased allergic susceptibility in recipient neonates (Fedulov and Kobzik, 2011). In contrast, the transfer of macrophages from nonchallenged neonates of allergic mothers into neonates from nonallergic mothers does not confer increased allergic susceptibility in recipient neonates (Fedulov and Kobzik, 2011). This is suggestive of a functional change in neonatal DCs in offspring from allergic mothers. Changes in DCs are consistent with the antigen-independent transfer of risk from allergic mothers to offspring in humans and in animal models.

Offspring of allergic mothers have an increase in a distinct subset of DCs. The fetal livers from allergic mothers and the OVA-challenged pup lungs from the offspring of allergic mothers have increased numbers of CD11b + subsets of CD11c + DCs (Abdala-Valencia et al., 2014), a DCs subset that is critical for generating allergic responses (Williams et al., 2013). In contrast, in these tissues, there are no changes in CD11b–regulatory DC subsets, including plasmacytoid DCs and CD103 + DCs (Abdala-Valencia et al., 2014). Furthermore, before antigen challenge of the pups, the DCs of pups from allergic mothers had little transcriptional changes but extensive DNA methylation changes (Mikhaylova et al., 2013). Then, after allergen challenge, there were many transcriptional changes in the DCs (Mikhaylova et al., 2013). These studies suggest that mediators, that do not confer allergen specificity, may be transferred from the mother to the offspring and these mediators regulate offspring DCs and heighten the responsiveness of offspring to challenge with suboptimal doses of allergens. This is consistent with the clinical reports demonstrating that the risk for allergy in children has been associated with mothers with existing allergic disease before conception (Celedon et al., 2002; Folsgaard et al., 2012; Kurukulaaratchy et al., 2003, 2005; Latzin et al., 2007; Lim et al., 2010; Litonjua et al., 1998; Martinez et al., 1995).

It has been reported that there is a role of breast milk of allergic mother mice on development of offspring allergic responses. However, the milk of allergic mothers is not necessary for the offspring allergic responses because the in utero maternal effects are sufficient for allergic responses by the offspring of allergic mothers. This was demonstrated by cross-fostering the offspring. Briefly, pups from allergic mothers that are nursed by nonallergic mothers still have an allergic response to suboptimal challenge with OVA (Leme et al., 2006). Therefore, maternal effects in utero mediate development of allergen responsiveness in the offspring of allergic mothers (Leme et al., 2006). Breast milk is sufficient, but not necessary, for maternal transmission of asthma risk in the offspring because when pups from nonallergic mothers are nursed by allergic mothers, the pups exhibit a response to suboptimal allergen challenge (Leme et al., 2006). In this study, the breast milk from allergic and nonallergic mothers contained no detectable interferon-γ (IFN-γ), IL-2, IL-4, IL-5, IL-13, or TNF-α, suggesting that other mediators increase the risk of offspring allergy through breast milk (Leme et al., 2006). In clinical studies, it is reported that the mediators, omega-3 and omega-6 polyunsaturated fatty acids, in human milk associate with asthma and atopy, but the mechanism is not known (Reichardt et al., 2004; Stoney et al., 2004). It is also reported that omega-3 fatty acids during pregnancy associates with lower infantile wheeze (Miyake et al., 2011).

In contrast to studies in which the mother mice were allergic before conception, the function of breast milk has been studied in female mothers that were not allergic at preconception. In these models, the nonallergic mother mice were exposed during pregnancy or lactation to an allergen or an antigen tolerance protocol. In mouse models in which the mother was not allergic at preconception but then exposed during pregnancy or lactation to an allergen or an antigen tolerance protocol, there was protection of offspring responses to allergen sensitization and challenge. Briefly, it is reported that the exposure of normal female mice during lactation to OVA results in the transfer of antigen and TGF-β in milk, and this inhibited allergic inflammation in offspring treated later as adults (6–8 weeks old) with two sensitizations with OVA–alum and five OVA challenges (Verhasselt et al., 2008). These adult offspring also had elevated regulatory CD4 + T cells, and the increase in T regulatory cells was dependent on milk TGF-β but not milk immunoglobulins (Verhasselt et al., 2008). In another approach, it was demonstrated that sensitization of females before mating and then extensive antigen challenges (10 OVA challenges) during lactation resulted in the transfer of IgG immune complexes in the milk and the induction of regulatory T cells and tolerance in the offspring when offspring were challenged with OVA at 6–8 weeks old; in this model, immune complexes but not TGF-β in the milk was required for tolerance (Mosconi et al., 2010). In summary, depending on timing, doses, and the number of antigen challenges, factors in breast milk can contribute mediators that either increase or decrease offspring responses to allergen.

One endogenous transplacental maternal mediator in mice may contribute to the increased responsiveness in the offspring to a suboptimal OVA challenge (Lim et al., 2014). This mediator is increased but is still low-level maternal corticosterone (Lim et al., 2014). In adult mice and rats, OVA sensitization and challenge increases stress (Costa-Pinto et al., 2005, 2006; Portela Cde et al., 2001, 2002, 2007; Tonelli et al., 2009) and increases endogenous serum corticosterone (Chida et al., 2007; Lu et al., 2010). Moreover, it is reported that symptoms of stress or anxiety are commonly associated with allergy or asthma in adult mice and in humans (Cheung et al., 2009; Cordina et al., 2009; Di Marco et al., 2010; Sansone and Sansone, 2008; Strine et al., 2008). When maternal corticosterone is elevated during pregnancy, the maternal cortisol can cross the placenta and affect fetal cortisol levels (Huang et al., 2012; von Hertzen, 2002). Other researchers have reported that maternal corticosterone crosses the placenta to the fetus and is a strong inducer of Th2 responses (Norbiato et al., 1997; Ramirez et al., 1996). Cortisol is also present in human breast milk (Groer et al., 1994) and has the potential to affect allergic responses in neonates. Consistent with the mechanistic studies in mouse models, in pregnant asthmatic women without treatment for asthma, a deficiency in the placenta of a cortisol-metabolizing enzyme 11-beta-hydroxysteroid dehydrogenase 2 leads to increased fetal cortisol and low birth weight, which is predictive of lower lung function later in life (Murphy et al., 2002, 2003).

It has been reported that stress in adult 4-week-old mice exacerbates OVA-induced allergic responses and that this stress-induced effect is blocked by pretreatment with a glucocorticoid receptor antagonist (Chida et al., 2007). It has also been demonstrated that subjecting pregnant female mice to stress increases endogenous corticosterone, offspring allergic responses to suboptimal allergen, and offspring airway responsiveness after suboptimal allergen challenge (Lim et al., 2014; von Hertzen, 2002). Furthermore, glucocorticoid during pregnancy is sufficient for allergic responses in offspring because administration of a low dose of glucocorticoid to nonallergic mothers on day 15 of gestation increases offspring allergic responsiveness to suboptimal allergen challenges (Lim et al., 2014). In addition, when these mothers are subjected to stress and treated during pregnancy with an inhibitor of endogenous corticosterone synthesis, there is a reduction in the allergic response by the offspring (Lim et al., 2014). Therefore, elevated corticosterone in allergic pregnant mice might be a mediator that is transferred from the mother to the fetus or in the breast milk to the neonate, resulting in enhanced responses of offspring to suboptimal allergen challenge. This mechanism is consistent with the antigen-independent transfer of risk from mother to offspring for allergic responsiveness (Barrett et al., 2003; Hamada et al., 2003).

A maternal effect on offspring allergic responses has also been demonstrated for maternal exposure to environmental irritants. Maternal inhalation of titanium oxide or diesel exhaust particles during pregnancy increased responses of offspring to allergen challenges (Fedulov et al., 2008). Also, skin sensitization to toluene diisocyanate (TDI) induces a Th2 response in the mother; when the mother was mated after a second dose of TDI, the offspring had increased allergic responses to suboptimal OVA (Lim et al., 2007). In contrast, a Th1 response in the mother may protect the offspring from developing allergic responses. When females are sensitized to dinitrochlorobenzene which induces a Th1 response, and then mated, the offspring do not develop an allergic response to suboptimal OVA (Lim et al., 2007). Also, offspring are protected from development of asthma by prenatal challenge of the mother with LPS, which induces a Th1 inflammation, an increase in IFN-γ, and a decrease in IL-5 and IL-13 (Gerhold et al., 2002, 2003, 2006; Tulic et al., 2001). Injection of nonallergic mothers with IFN-γ on gestational day 6.5 protects against the development of allergic responses in offspring (Lima et al., 2005). Fedolov et al. (2005) demonstrated that treatment of the offspring from allergic mothers on postnatal day 4 with cytosine guanine oligonucleotides, a toll-like receptor-9 agonist and Th1-type stimulant, (de Brito et al., 2010) protected the offspring from development of allergic responses to suboptimal OVA challenges. Therefore, exposure of mothers, allergic mothers, or offspring from allergic mothers to a Th1 stimuli inhibited offspring responses to allergen challenge.

Maternal α-Tocopherol Supplementation Reduces Allergic Responses in Offspring in Preclinical Models

In mice, α-tocopherol supplementation of allergic female mice during pregnancy or lactation decreases neonate development of allergic lung inflammation in response to suboptimal allergen challenges (Abdala-Valencia et al., 2014). In these studies, allergic responses to OVA were induced in adult female mice, who were then mated while receiving α-tocopherol–supplemented diets (250 mg α-tocopherol/kg diet) or a basal α-tocopherol diet (45 mg α-tocopherol/kg diet) (Abdala-Valencia et al., 2014). A basal α-tocopherol diet is used as the control because adequate α-tocopherol levels are required for placental development (Jishage et al., 2005; Muller-Schmehl et al., 2004).

Then, the 3-day-old neonates received a suboptimal allergen sensitization with OVA–alum and OVA-challenge on days 10–12 (Abdala-Valencia et al., 2014). The α-tocopherol–supplemented diet significantly increases liver α-tocopherol in the saline-treated mothers threefold compared to basal diet controls. The OVA-induced allergic response reduces the α-tocopherol tissue concentrations in the α-tocopherol–supplemented mothers, which is consistent with reduced α-tocopherol levels in asthmatics (Kalayci et al., 2000; Kelly et al., 1999; Schunemann et al., 2001; Shvedova et al., 1995), suggesting that α-tocopherol supplementation may be especially necessary for asthmatic mothers. Maternal α-tocopherol supplementation increases pup liver α-tocopherol 2.5-fold (Abdala-Valencia et al., 2014). The α-tocopherol supplementation of allergic mothers during pregnancy and lactation results in a dose-dependent inhibition of lung eosinophils (Abdala-Valencia et al., 2014) in the OVA-stimulated pups from allergic mothers as compared to OVA-challenged pups from nonallergic mothers (Abdala-Valencia et al., 2014). There is no effect of tocopherol or OVA treatments on pup weight, pup numbers, or pup gender distribution (Abdala-Valencia et al., 2014). OVA-treated pups from allergic mothers increase serum IgE, but α-tocopherol supplementation does not alter the IgE (Abdala-Valencia et al., 2014). Maternal α-tocopherol supplementation of allergic female mothers inhibits OVA-induced pup lung mRNA expression of cytokines that regulate allergic inflammation (IL-33 and IL-4) and chemokines for eosinophil recruitment (CCL11 and CCL24) (Abdala-Valencia et al., 2014). Therefore, α-tocopherol supplementation of allergic mothers inhibits allergic inflammation and cytokine or chemokine mediators of allergic inflammation in OVA-challenged pups from these allergic mothers.

In studies to determine the regulatory effect of α-tocopherol in utero and in the milk, pups were cross-fostered at birth. Cross-fostering pups from allergic mothers with 250 mg α-tocopherol/kg diet to allergic mothers with a basal diet (45 mg α-tocopherol/kg diet) indicated that α-tocopherol supplementation of the allergic mother during pregnancy was sufficient to inhibit the OVA-induced increase in neonate lung eosinophils (Abdala-Valencia et al., 2014). In addition, α-tocopherol supplementation during lactation reduces the allergic responses in the neonates (Abdala-Valencia et al., 2014), suggesting a contribution of α-tocopherol after birth (Abdala-Valencia et al., 2014). In summary, α-tocopherol supplementation of allergic mothers during pregnancy is sufficient to reduce development of allergic responses in the offspring.

Supplementation with α-tocopherol starting at conception of a second pregnancy of allergic female mice also inhibits development of allergic lung inflammation in their offspring. The offspring from allergic mothers that were supplemented with α-tocopherol at the time of the second mating had >90% inhibition of lung lavage eosinophils in the OVA-challenged pups (Abdala-Valencia et al., 2014). Moreover, in OVA-challenged pups from allergic mothers, α-tocopherol reduces pup lung mRNA expression of several mediators of allergic inflammation: the cytokines IL-4, IL-33, and thymic stromal lymphopoietin and the chemokines CCL11 and CCL24 (Abdala-Valencia et al., 2014). This is consistent with α-tocopherol regulation of the development of allergic inflammation. There are no effects of maternal α-tocopherol supplementation on pup low levels of the Th1 cytokine IFN-γ or the regulatory cytokine IL-10 (Abdala-Valencia et al., 2014), which indicates that α-tocopherol does not switch the response to OVA to a Th1 response.

Maternal Gamma-Tocopherol Supplementation Elevates Allergic Responses in Offspring in Preclinical Models

In studies with maternal diets supplemented with a 250-mg γ-tocopherol/kg diet, maternal γ-tocopherol raises the maternal liver γ-tocopherol level twofold and the pup liver γ-tocopherol fivefold, which is consistent with the fold tocopherol changes in human and mouse tissues after supplementation (Abdala-Valencia et al., 2012a; Berdnikovs et al., 2009; Cook-Mills et al., 2011a; Cook-Mills and McCary, 2010; McCary et al., 2011, 2012). Supplementation of allergic female mice with γ-tocopherol elevates neonatal development of lung eosinophils in offspring challenged with suboptimal doses of allergen (Abdala-Valencia et al., 2016). The γ-tocopherol does not induce allergic inflammation because it does not increase allergic inflammation in the pups from nonallergic mothers. In pups from allergic mothers, maternal d-γ-tocopherol supplementation increases inflammatory mediators, including the Th2 mediator amphiregulin, IL-5, CCL11, CCL24, activin A, and GM-CSF. Of potential relevance and concern, maternal γ-tocopherol supplementation also decreases the numbers of mated females that had pups, but it did not affect the numbers of pups per litter or pup body weight. Basal levels of α-tocopherol are required for placentation (Jishage et al., 2005; Muller-Schmehl et al., 2004), but it is not known whether γ-tocopherol influences placentation. Whether γ-tocopherol regulates placenta development or other functions during development is not known. Nevertheless, the reduced numbers of mothers with pups and increased pup allergic responses with γ-tocopherol supplementation has potential important implications for allergic mothers consuming γ-tocopherol in their diet or prenatal vitamins and for infants consuming infant formulas supplemented with γ-tocopherol.

Maternal Gamma-Tocopherol Supplementation Elevates and Maternal α-Tocopherol Supplementation Reduces Dendritic Cell Development

It has been reported that the transfer of DCs but not macrophages from pups born to allergic mothers to the pups of nonallergic mothers are sufficient for the development of the allergic responses in recipient pups in response to suboptimal OVA challenge (Fedulov and Kobzik, 2011). Furthermore, lungs of allergen-challenged offspring from allergic mothers have elevated numbers of a distinct subsets of lung DCs (CD11b+ CD11c + resident and alveolar DCs) but there are no changes in numbers of CD11b–CD11c + DCs (plasmacytoid DCs and CD103 + DCs) (Abdala-Valencia et al., 2014). During fetal development, hematopoiesis occurs in the fetal liver. In gestational day 18 fetal livers of allergic mothers, there is an increase in DCs of the phenotype of CD11b+ CD11c + resident DCs (Abdala-Valencia et al., 2014). Therefore, there is an effect of maternal allergy on the development of distinct subsets of DCs in the fetus.

The increase in the numbers of DC subsets in offspring of allergic mothers is regulated by α-tocopherol. Maternal supplementation with α-tocopherol significantly reduces the OVA-stimulated pup lung numbers of CD11b + subsets of CD11c + DCs, including resident DCs, myeloid DCs, and CD11b + alveolar DCs, without altering CD11b– subsets of CD11c + DCs, including plasmacytoid DCs, CD103 + DCs, CD11b– alveolar DCs, and alveolar macrophages (Abdala-Valencia et al., 2014). It is interesting that α-tocopherol supplementation does not completely deplete CD11b + DCs; instead, α-tocopherol supplementation of allergic mothers reduces the numbers of pup CD11b + DCs to the numbers of these DCs in pups from nonallergic mothers (Abdala-Valencia et al., 2014). For all DCs subsets, the cell surface mediators MHCII, CD80, and CD86 are not different among the groups in the pup lungs (Abdala-Valencia et al., 2014). Furthermore, in the fetus on gestational day 18, α-tocopherol supplementation of allergic mothers reduces the number of fetal liver CD11b + subsets of CD11c + DCs, including those of the phenotype of myeloid DCs and phenotype of resident DCs without altering expression of MHCII, CD80 or CD86 (Abdala-Valencia et al., 2014). The fetal liver CD11b- subsets of CD11c + DCs are not altered by maternal supplementation of α-tocopherol (Abdala-Valencia et al., 2014). Thus, the specificity of tocopherol regulation of the CD11b+ DC subsets in the fetus suggests that tocopherols may regulate signals for DC differentiation of these DC subsets or regulate signals for expression of CD11b.

In contrast to maternal α-tocopherol supplementation, maternal supplementation with γ-tocopherol increases development of CD11c+ CD11b+ DCs but not the numbers of pup lung CD11b–DC subsets in allergen-challenged lungs of neonates (Abdala-Valencia et al., 2016). In addition, there is an increase in neonatal cytokines, chemokines, and lung CD11b+ IRF4+ DC subsets that are critical to development of allergic responses. The γ-tocopherol supplementation of allergic mothers also increases the generation of IRF4+ CD11c+ CD11b+ DCs in the fetal liver on GD18 (Abdala-Valencia et al., 2016). In the gestational day 18 fetal livers of γ-tocopherol–supplemented mothers, there are fewer regulatory CD11b–CD11c+ pDCs (Abdala-Valencia et al., 2016), suggesting that γ-tocopherol supplementation may see a reduced control of magnitude of responses to allergen challenge early in life. However, in the postnatal day 13 OVA-challenged pup lung, the number of pDCs was not altered with γ-tocopherol supplementation (Abdala-Valencia et al., 2016).

Maternal supplementation of allergic mothers with γ-tocopherol also partially increases mediators of allergic inflammation and DC subsets in the offspring of nonallergic mothers. Maternal D-γ-tocopherol supplementation partially increases the numbers of resident DCs in the fetus and OVA-challenged pup lung from nonallergic mothers but not to the extent as in the OVA-challenged pups from D-γ-tocopherol–supplemented allergic mothers (Abdala-Valencia et al., 2016). This is consistent with the increased GM-CSF with γ-tocopherol supplementation in pup lungs from allergic mothers (Abdala-Valencia et al., 2016). γ-tocopherol also increased activin A in pups from nonallergic and allergic mothers (Abdala-Valencia et al., 2016). Activin A is a member of the TGF-β superfamily of cytokines and regulates allergic inflammation (Hardy et al., 2015). Activin A is produced by several cell types including epithelium, endothelium, mast cells, fibroblasts and DCs and it can induce differentiation of monocytes to mDCs and recruitment of DCs (Hedger et al., 2011). Therefore, with maternal γ-tocopherol activin A may function in concert with other mediators to increase the numbers of DCs and allergic inflammation. In fact, γ-tocopherol increases CCL11 in pups from allergic and nonallergic mothers, and it increases CCL24 and IL-5 in the pups from nonallergic mothers (Abdala-Valencia et al., 2016). An OVA challenge in pups from allergic mothers with D-γ-tocopherol does not result in further increases in CCL24 or IL-5 (Abdala-Valencia et al., 2016), which may indicate that a maximum response was achieved with an OVA challenge. Nevertheless, the pups from the allergic mothers with D-γ-tocopherol have elevated CCL11 and amphiregulin, which suggests that, in combination, these signals as well as the presence of GM-CSF, CCL24, IL-5, and activin A may function to amplify recruitment of eosinophils in pups from allergic mothers with D-γ-tocopherol–supplemented diets.

There may be at least a direct effect of tocopherols on bone marrow DC differentiation. When bone marrow from 10-day-old mouse neonates from nonallergic mothers with basal diets are incubated with GM-CSF for 8 days in vitro in the presence of α-tocopherol, α-tocopherol supplementation of the culture reduces the number of CD45+ CD11b+ CD11c+ DCs and the number of cells with resident DC phenotype (CD45+ CD11b+ CD11c+ Ly6c-MHCII DCs) without affecting the percent of viable cells in the culture (Abdala-Valencia et al., 2014). Gamma-tocopherol has at least a direct effect on hematopoietic development of DCs because D-γ-tocopherol increases the generation of IRF4+ CD11c+ CD11b+ bone marrow–derived DCs in vitro (Abdala-Valencia et al., 2016). In addition, D-γ-tocopherol decreased the numbers of inhibitory PDCA+ plasmacytoid CD11c+ CD11b–DCs in the fetal liver (Abdala-Valencia et al., 2016). There was no effect of D-γ-tocopherol on the level of expression of MHCII, CD80, or IRF4 by the fetal liver and pup lung DCs (Abdala-Valencia et al., 2016).

Thus, γ-tocopherol and α-tocopherol regulate generation of DCs and signals for allergic inflammation during development. Maternal supplementation with γ-tocopherol in mouse models increases allergic responses in offspring from allergic mothers and increases development of CD11c+ CD11b+ DC types in utero, in antigen-challenged neonate lungs, and in bone marrow cultures. Moreover, there is specificity of regulation of DCs by γ-tocopherol because γ-tocopherol supplementation increases the number of CD11c+ CD11b+ but not CD11c+ CD11b– DC types in pup lungs. There is also specificity of regulation of DCs in utero because maternal γ-tocopherol increases fetal liver CD11c+ CD11b+ DCs and decreases the numbers of plasmacytoid regulatory DCs in the fetal liver. Supplementation with γ-tocopherol elevated several mediators of inflammation without altering OVA-specific IgE. Studies of γ-tocopherol regulation of inflammation provide a basis for designing drugs, supplements, and diets that more effectively modulate these pathways in allergic disease. Further studies are needed for the design of future clinical studies with vitamin E isoforms and on our understanding of vitamin E isoform regulation of DC function during allergic inflammation. The function of tocopherol isoforms on allergic inflammation and asthma may have implications for dietary impact on the risk of allergic disease in future generations. More studies are needed in humans to examine short-term versus long-term outcomes of a range of plasma concentrations of tocopherol isoforms.

ALPHA-TOCOPHEROL AND GAMMA-TOCOPHEROL: OPPOSING FUNCTIONS IN OTHER CHRONIC INFLAMMATORY DISEASES

In addition to opposing functions of tocopherol isoforms in allergic disease, α-tocopherol and γ-tocopherol may have opposing outcomes for other diseases, including arthritis and cardiovascular. However, as with asthma, there are conflicting outcomes for vitamin E in these diseases. Briefly, human plasma γ-tocopherol positively associates with osteoarthritis, whereas plasma α-tocopherol negatively associates with osteoarthritis (Jordan et al., 2004). In coronary heart disease and stroke, studies of tocopherols and heart disease are complex because different dietary oils contain different lipids that affect heart disease. Nevertheless, for plasma γ-tocopherol, it is either not associated with heart disease or is associated with an increase in risk for myocardial infarction (Dietrich et al., 2006). In contrast, for α-tocopherol, it is either not associated with heart disease or is associated with reduced death from heart disease (Dutta and Dutta, 2003; Meydani, 2004; Munteanu and Zingg, 2007; Siekmeier et al., 2007). Therefore, for those reports with effects on heart disease, γ-tocopherol associates with an increase and α-tocopherol associates with a decrease in heart disease.

CONCLUSIONS

Epidemiological studies and randomized prevention trials have demonstrated the potential of a number of protective dietary factors for asthma, including α-tocopherol. However, these reports have seemingly varied outcomes regarding the benefits of supplementation with the α-tocopherol and γ-tocopherol isoforms of vitamin E. These discrepancies in clinical results are consistent with mechanistic studies of differential regulatory functions of these tocopherol isoforms in animal asthma models and in cell cultures with physiological doses of the tocopherol isoforms. Tocopherols also function beyond their antioxidant capacity and regulate signaling pathways essential in the inflammatory process. Specifically, supplementation with physiological levels of purified α-tocopherol and γ-tocopherol has opposing regulatory functions during inflammation such that α-tocopherol is antiinflammatory and γ-tocopherol is proinflammatory. Understanding the differential regulations of inflammation by isoforms of vitamin E provides a basis for designing drugs and diets that more effectively modulate inflammatory pathways and improve lung function in disease.

The marked differences in rates of asthma across the world, changes in disease prevalence over short periods, and changes with migrating populations means that environment influences the development and responses to triggers that worsen asthma and allergic inflammation. This means that changes in diet or lifestyle or both could modify disease. Going forward, studies in preclinical models and clinical studies need to be designed to include measurements of the tocopherol isoforms in the supplements, vehicles for the supplements, and the plasma or tissues. Moreover, in preclinical animal and clinical studies, tocopherol isoforms need to be measured prior to intervention and after interventions with tocopherol isoform-specific supplementation. These tocopherol measurements are necessary to clearly interpret study outcomes. Understanding the epidemiology, biology, and regulation of asthma inception by environmental factors will lead to approaches that could reduce the development of allergy and asthma. Further studies are necessary to define and provide a basis for recommendations for doses for tocopherol isoforms in normal and, more important, inflammatory disease states in adult human females and males as well as ethnic groups that differ in the prevalence of asthma (Kim et al., 2016; Sheikh et al., 2016). The therapeutic potential of dietary manipulation and supplementation in allergic pregnant mothers and children with asthma requires further work. The investigation of early life diet in relation to childhood asthma raises the possibility of early life dietary interventions.

Sources of Support: This study was supported by National Institutes of Health Grants R01 AT004837 and R01 HLB111624, and the Ernest S. Bazley Grant.

References

Abdala-Valencia, H., Earwood, J., Bansal, S., Jansen, M., Babcock, G., Garvy, B., et al., 2007. Nonhematopoietic NADPH oxidase regulation of lung eosinophilia and airway hyperresponsiveness in experimentally induced asthma. Am. J. Physiol. Lung Cell Mol. Physiol. 292, L1111–L1125.

Abdala-Valencia, H., Berdnikovs, S., Cook-Mills, J.M., 2012a. Vitamin E isoforms differentially regulate intercellular adhesion molecule-1 activation of PKCalpha in human microvascular endothelial cells. PLoS One 7, e41054.

Abdala-Valencia, H., Berdnikovs, S., McCary, C.A., Urick, D., Mahadevia, R., Marchese, M.E., et al., 2012b. Inhibition of Allergic Inflammation by Supplementation with 5-hydroxytryptophan. Am. J. Physiol. Lung Cell Mol. Physiol. 303, L642–L660.

Abdala-Valencia, H., Berdnikovs, S., Cook-Mills, J.M., 2013. Vitamin E isoforms as modulators of lung inflammation. Nutrients 5, 4347–4363.

Abdala-Valencia, H., Berdnikovs, S., Soveg, F., Cook-Mills, J.M., 2014. Alpha-tocopherol supplementation of allergic female mice inhibits development of CD11c+ CD11b+ dendritic cells in utero and allergic inflammation in neonates. Am. J. Physiol. Lung Cell Mol. Physiol. 307, L482–L496.

Abdala-Valencia, H., Soveg, F., Cook-Mills, J.M., 2016. γ-Tocopherol Supplementation of Allergic Female Mice Augments Development of CD11c+ CD11b+ Dendritic Cells in Utero and Allergic Inflammation in Neonates. Am. J. Physiol. Lung Cell Mol. Physiol. 310, L759–L771.

Akinbami, L.J., Moorman, J.E., Bailey, C., Zahran, H.S., King, M., Johnson, C.A., et al., 2012. Trends in asthma prevalence, health care use, and mortality in the United States, 2001-2010. NCHS Data Brief 94, 1–8.

Al-Abdulla, N.O., Al Naama, L.M., Hassan, M.K., 2010. Antioxidant status in acute asthmatic attack in children. J. Pak. Med. Assoc. 60, 1023–1027.

Allen, S., Britton, J.R., Leonardi-Bee, J.A., 2009. Association between antioxidant vitamins and asthma outcome measures: systematic review and meta-analysis. Thorax 64, 610–619.

Bachmanov, A.A., Reed, D.R., Beauchamp, G.K., Tordoff, M.G., 2002. Food intake, water intake, and drinking spout side preference of 28 mouse strains. Behav. Genet. 32, 435–443.

Barrett, E.G., Rudolph, K., Bowen, L.E., Bice, D.E., 2003. Parental allergic status influences the risk of developing allergic sensitization and an asthmatic-like phenotype in canine offspring. Immunology 110, 493–500.

Barthel, S.R., Johansson, M.W., McNamee, D.M., Mosher, D.F., 2008. Roles of integrin activation in eosinophil function and the eosinophilic inflammation of asthma. J. Leukoc. Biol. 83, 1–12.

Bella, D.L., Schock, B.C., Lim, Y., Leonard, S.W., Berry, C., Cross, C.E., et al., 2006. Regulation of the alpha-tocopherol transfer protein in mice: lack of response to dietary vitamin E or oxidative stress. Lipids 41, 105–112.

Berdnikovs, S., Abdala-Valencia, H., McCary, C., Somand, M., Cole, R., Garcia, A., et al., 2009. Isoforms of vitamin E have opposing immunoregulatory functions during inflammation by regulating leukocyte recruitment. J. Immunol. 182, 4395–4405.

Betti, M., Ambrogini, P., Minelli, A., Floridi, A., Lattanzi, D., Ciuffoli, S., et al., 2011. Maternal dietary loads of alpha-tocopherol depress protein kinase C signaling and synaptic plasticity in rat postnatal developing hippocampus and promote permanent deficits in adult offspring. J. Nutr. Biochem. 22, 60–70.

Bieri, J.G., Evarts, R.P., 1973. Tocopherols and fatty acids in American diets. The recommended allowance for vitamin E. J. Am. Diet. Assoc. 62, 147–151.

Bieri, J.G., Evarts, R.P., 1975. Vitamin E adequacy of vegetable oils. J. Am. Diet. Assoc. 66, 134–139.

Blanc, P.D., Eisner, M.D., Katz, P.P., Yen, I.H., Archea, C., Earnest, G., et al., 2005. Impact of the home indoor environment on adult asthma and rhinitis. J. Occup. Environ. Med. 47, 362–372.

Blumer, N., Herz, U., Wegmann, M., Renz, H., 2005. Prenatal lipopolysaccharide-exposure prevents allergic sensitization and airway inflammation, but not airway responsiveness in a murine model of experimental asthma. Clin. Exp. Allergy 35, 397–402.

Bousquet, J., Bousquet, P.J., Godard, P., Daures, J.P., 2005. The public health implications of asthma. Bull. World Health Organ. 83, 548–554.

Bousquet, J., Anto, J., Auffray, C., Akdis, M., Cambon-Thomsen, A., Keil, T., et al., 2011. MeDALL (Mechanisms of the Development of ALLergy): an integrated approach from phenotypes to systems medicine. Allergy 66, 596–604.

Bowen, J.M., Chamley, L., Mitchell, M.D., Keelan, J.A., 2002. Cytokines of the placenta and extra-placental membranes: biosynthesis, secretion and roles in establishment of pregnancy in women. Placenta 23, 239–256.

Boyle, F.G., Yuhas, R.J., Lien, E.L., 1996. Red blood cell and tissue phospholipid fatty acid profiles of weanling rats fed infant formula fat blends containing soy and/or corn oil. Ann. Nutr. Metab. 40, 234–242.

Burke, K.T., Colvin, P.L., Myatt, L., Graf, G.A., Schroeder, F., Woollett, L.A., 2009. Transport of maternal cholesterol to the fetus is affected by maternal plasma cholesterol concentrations in the golden Syrian hamster. J. Lipid. Res. 50, 1146–1155.

Cavalier, L., Ouahchi, K., Kayden, H.J., Di Donato, S., Reutenauer, L., Mandel, J.L., et al., 1998. Ataxia with isolated vitamin E deficiency: heterogeneity of mutations and phenotypic variability in a large number of families. Am. J. Hum. Genet. 62, 301–310.

Celedon, J.C., Litonjua, A.A., Ryan, L., Platts-Mills, T., Weiss, S.T., Gold, D.R., 2002. Exposure to cat allergen, maternal history of asthma, and wheezing in first 5 years of life. Lancet 360, 781–782.

CDC National Asthma Control Program. 2012. http://www.cdc.gov/asthma/impacts_nation/asthmafactsheet.pdf.

Cheung, T.K., Lam, B., Lam, K.F., Ip, M., Ng, C., Kung, R., et al., 2009. Gastroesophageal reflux disease is associated with poor asthma control, quality of life, and psychological status in Chinese asthma patients. Chest 135, 1181–1185.

Chida, Y., Sudo, N., Sonoda, J., Hiramoto, T., Kubo, C., 2007. Early-life psychological stress exacerbates adult mouse asthma via the hypothalamus-pituitary-adrenal axis. Am. J. Respir. Crit. Care Med. 175, 316–322.

Chin, J.E., Hatfield, C.A., Winterrowd, G.E., Brashler, J.R., Vonderfecht, S.L., Fidler, S.F., et al., 1997. Airway recruitment of leukocytes in mice is dependent on alpha4-integrins and vascular cell adhesion molecule-1. Am. J. Physiol. 272, L219–L229.

Choo, J.H., Nagata, M., Sutani, A., Kikuchi, I., Sakamoto, Y., 2003. Theophylline attenuates the adhesion of eosinophils to endothelial cells. Int. Arch. Allergy Immunol. 131 (suppl. 1), 40–45.

Cook-Mills, J.M., 2012. Eosinophil-endothelial cell interactions. Eosinophils in health and disease. In: Lee, J.J., Rosenberg, H.F. (Eds.), Eosinophils in Health and Disease. Elsevier, Amsterdam, pp. 139–153.

Cook-Mills, J.M., Avila, P.C., 2014. Vitamin E and D regulation of allergic asthma immunopathogenesis. Int. Immunopharmacol. 29, 007.

Cook-Mills, J.M., Deem, T.L., 2005. Active participation of endothelial cells in inflammation. J. Leukoc. Biol. 77, 487–495.

Cook-Mills, J.M., McCary, C.A., 2010. Isoforms of Vitamin E Differentially Regulate Inflammation. Endocr. Metab. Immune Disord. Drug Targets 10, 348–366.

Cook-Mills, J.M., Marchese, M., Abdala-Valencia, H., 2011a. Vascular Cell adhesion molecule-1 expression and signaling during disease: regulation by reactive oxygen species and antioxidants. Antioxid Redox Signal 15, 1607–1638.

Cook-Mills, J.M., Marchese, M.E., Abdala-Valencia, H., 2011b. Vascular cell adhesion molecule-1 expression and signaling during disease: regulation by reactive oxygen species and antioxidants. Antioxid Redox Signal 15, 1607–1638.

Cook-Mills, J.M., Abdala-Valencia, H., Hartert, T., 2013. Two faces of vitamin e in the lung. Am. J. Respir. Crit. Care Med. 188, 279–284.

Cook-Mills, J., Gebretsadik, T., Abdala-Valencia, H., Green, J., Larkin, E.K., Dupont, W.D., et al., 2016. Brief research report: interaction of vitamin E isoforms on asthma and allergic airway disease. Thorax 71, 954–956.

Cordina, M., Fenech, A.G., Vassallo, J., Cacciottolo, J.M., 2009. Anxiety and the management of asthma in an adult outpatient population. Ther. Adv. Respir. Dis. 3, 227–233.

Costa-Pinto, F.A., Basso, A.S., Britto, L.R., Malucelli, B.E., Russo, M., 2005. Avoidance behavior and neural correlates of allergen exposure in a murine model of asthma. Brain Behav. Immun. 19, 52–60.

Costa-Pinto, F.A., Basso, A.S., De Sa-Rocha, L.C., Britto, L.R., Russo, M., Palermo-Neto, J., 2006. Neural correlates of IgE-mediated allergy. Ann. N Y Acad. Sci. 1088, 116–131.

Davenpeck, K.L., Berens, K.L., Dixon, R.A., Dupre, B., Bochner, B.S., 2000. Inhibition of adhesion of human neutrophils and eosinophils to P-selectin by the sialyl Lewis antagonist TBC1269: preferential activity against neutrophil adhesion in vitro. J. Allergy Clin. Immunol. 105, 769–775.

de Brito, C.A., Fusaro, A.E., Victor, J.R., Rigato, P.O., Goldoni, A.L., Muniz, B.P., et al., 2010. CpG-induced Th1-type response in the downmodulation of early development of allergy and inhibition of B7 expression on T cells of newborn mice. J. Clin. Immunol. 30, 280–291.

Delfino, R.J., Quintana, P.J., Floro, J., Gastanaga, V.M., Samimi, B.S., Kleinman, M.T., et al., 2004. Association of FEV1 in asthmatic children with personal and microenvironmental exposure to airborne particulate matter. Environ. Health Perspect. 112, 932–941.

de Luis, D.A., Armentia, A., Aller, R., Asensio, A., Sedano, E., Izaola, O., et al., 2005. Dietary intake in patients with asthma: a case control study. Nutrition 21, 320–324.

Devaraj, S., Tang, R., Adams-Huet, B., Harris, A., Seenivasan, T., de Lemos, J.A., et al., 2007. Effect of high-dose alpha-tocopherol supplementation on biomarkers of oxidative stress and inflammation and carotid atherosclerosis in patients with coronary artery disease. Am. J. Clin. Nutr. 86, 1392–1398.

Devereux, G., 2007. Early life events in asthma—diet. Pediatr. Pulmonol. 42, 663–673.

Devereux, G., Seaton, A., 2005. Diet as a risk factor for atopy and asthma. J. Allergy Clin. Immunol. 115, 1109–1117.

Devereux, G., Barker, R.N., Seaton, A., 2002. Antenatal determinants of neonatal immune responses to allergens. Clin. Exp. Allergy 32, 43–50.

Dietrich, M., Traber, M.G., Jacques, P.F., Cross, C.E., Hu, Y., Block, G., 2006. Does gamma-tocopherol play a role in the primary prevention of heart disease and cancer? A review. J. Am. Coll. Nutr. 25, 292–299.

Di Marco, F., Verga, M., Santus, P., Giovannelli, F., Busatto, P., Neri, M., et al., 2010. Close correlation between anxiety, depression, and asthma control. Respir. Med. 104, 22–28.

Dow, L., Tracey, M., Villar, A., Coggon, D., Margetts, B.M., Campbell, M.J., et al., 1996. Does dietary intake of vitamins C and E influence lung function in older people? Am. J. Respir. Crit. Care Med. 154, 1401–1404.

Dutta, A., Dutta, S.K., 2003. Vitamin E and its role in the prevention of atherosclerosis and carcinogenesis: a review. J. Am. Coll. Nutr. 22, 258–268.

Erkkola, M., Karppinen, M., Javanainen, J., Rasanen, L., Knip, M., Virtanen, S.M., 2001. Validity and reproducibility of a food frequency questionnaire for pregnant Finnish women. Am. J. Epidemiol. 154, 466–476.

Fakhrzadeh, L., Laskin, J.D., Laskin, D.L., 2004. Ozone-induced production of nitric oxide and TNF-alpha and tissue injury are dependent on NF-kappaB p50. Am. J. Physiol. Lung Cell Mol. Physiol. 287, L279–L285.

Fedulov, A.V., Kobzik, L., 2011. Allergy risk is mediated by dendritic cells with congenital epigenetic changes. Am. J. Respir. Cell Mol. Biol. 44, 285–292.

Fedulov, A., Silverman, E., Xiang, Y., Leme, A., Kobzik, L., 2005. Immunostimulatory CpG oligonucleotides abrogate allergic susceptibility in a murine model of maternal asthma transmission. J. Immunol. 175, 4292–4300.

Fedulov, A.V., Leme, A.S., Kobzik, L., 2007. Duration of allergic susceptibility in maternal transmission of asthma risk. Am. J. Reprod. Immunol. 58, 120–128.

Fedulov, A.V., Leme, A., Yang, Z., Dahl, M., Lim, R., Mariani, T.J., et al., 2008. Pulmonary exposure to particles during pregnancy causes increased neonatal asthma susceptibility. Am. J. Respir. Cell Mol. Biol. 38, 57–67.

Fiscus, L.C., Van Herpen, J., Steeber, D.A., Tedder, T.F., Tang, M.L., 2001. L-Selectin is required for the development of airway hyperresponsiveness but not airway inflammation in a murine model of asthma. J. Allergy Clin. Immunol. 107, 1019–1024.

Folsgaard, N.V., Chawes, B.L., Rasmussen, M.A., Bischoff, A.L., Carson, C.G., Stokholm, J., et al., 2012. Neonatal cytokine profile in the airway mucosal lining fluid is skewed by maternal atopy. Am. J. Respir. Crit. Care Med. 185, 275–280.

Friebele, E., 1996. The attack of asthma. Environ. Health Perspect. 104, 22–25.

Gerhold, K., Blumchen, K., Bock, A., Seib, C., Stock, P., Kallinich, T., et al., 2002. Endotoxins prevent murine IgE production, T(H)2 immune responses, and development of airway eosinophilia but not airway hyperreactivity. J. Allergy Clin. Immunol. 110, 110–116.

Gerhold, K., Bluemchen, K., Franke, A., Stock, P., Hamelmann, E., 2003. Exposure to endotoxin and allergen in early life and its effect on allergen sensitization in mice. J. Allergy Clin. Immunol. 112, 389–396.

Gerhold, K., Avagyan, A., Seib, C., Frei, R., Steinle, J., Ahrens, B., et al., 2006. Prenatal initiation of endotoxin airway exposure prevents subsequent allergen-induced sensitization and airway inflammation in mice. J. Allergy Clin. Immunol. 118, 666–673.

Gobel, Y., Koletzko, B., Bohles, H.J., Engelsberger, I., Forget, D., Le Brun, A., et al., 2003. Parenteral fat emulsions based on olive and soybean oils: a randomized clinical trial in preterm infants. J. Pediatr. Gastroenterol. Nutr. 37, 161–167.

Greenough, A., Shaheen, S.O., Shennan, A., Seed, P.T., Poston, L., 2010. Respiratory outcomes in early childhood following antenatal vitamin C and E supplementation. Thorax 65, 998–1003.

Gregor, H., Egarter, C., Levin, D., Sternberger, B., Heinze, G., Leitich, H., et al., 1999. The passage of granulocyte-macrophage colony-stimulating factor across the human placenta perfused in vitro. J. Soc. Gynecol. Investig. 6, 307–310.

Groer, M.W., Humenick, S., Hill, P.D., 1994. Characterizations and psychoneuroimmunologic implications of secretory immunoglobulin A and cortisol in preterm and term breast milk. J. Perinat Neonatal. Nurs. 7, 42–51.

Guardiola, M., Ribalta, J., Gomez-Coronado, D., Lasuncion, M.A., de Oya, M., Garces, C., 2010. The apolipoprotein A5 (APOA5) gene predisposes Caucasian children to elevated triglycerides and vitamin E (Four Provinces Study). Atherosclerosis 212, 543–547.

Gungorduk, K., Asicioglu, O., Gungorduk, O.C., Yildirim, G., Besimoglu, B., Ark, C., 2014. Does vitamin C and vitamin E supplementation prolong the latency period before delivery following the preterm premature rupture of membranes? A randomized controlled study. Am. J. Perinatol. 31, 195–202.

Hakugawa, J., Bae, S.J., Tanaka, Y., Katayama, I., 1997. The inhibitory effect of anti-adhesion molecule antibodies on eosinophil infiltration in cutaneous late phase response in Balb/c mice sensitized with ovalbumin (OVA). J. Dermatol. 24, 73–79.

Hamada, K., Suzaki, Y., Goldman, A., Ning, Y.Y., Goldsmith, C., Palecanda, A., et al., 2003. Allergen-independent maternal transmission of asthma susceptibility. J. Immunol. 170, 1683–1689.

Hardy, C.L., Rolland, J.M., O'Hehir, R.E., 2015. The immunoregulatory and fibrotic roles of activin A in allergic asthma. Clin. Exp. Allergy 45, 1510–1522.

Hauth, J.C., Clifton, R.G., Roberts, J.M., Spong, C.Y., Myatt, L., Leveno, K.J., et al., 2010. Vitamin C and E supplementation to prevent spontaneous preterm birth: a randomized controlled trial. Obstet. Gynecol. 116, 653–658.

Hedger, M.P., Winnall, W.R., Phillips, D.J., de Kretser, D.M., 2011. The regulation and functions of activin and follistatin in inflammation and immunity. Vitam. Horm. 85, 255–297.

Hernandez, M., Zhou, H., Zhou, B., Robinette, C., Crissman, K., Hatch, G., et al., 2009. Combination treatment with high-dose vitamin C and alpha-tocopherol does not enhance respiratory-tract lining fluid vitamin C levels in asthmatics. Inhal. Toxicol. 21, 173–181.

Hernandez, M.L., Wagner, J.G., Aline Kala, R., Mills, K., Wells, H.B., Alexis, N.E., et al., 2013. Vitamin E gamma-tocopherol reduces airway neutrophil recruitment after inhaled endotoxin challenge in rats and in healthy volunteers. Free Radic. Biol. Med. 8 00054-00053.

Hess, K.L., Babcock, G.F., Askew, D.S., Cook-Mills, J.M., 1997. A Novel Flow Cytometric Method for Quantifying Phagocytosis of Apoptotic Cells. Cytometry 27, 145–152.

Hoskins, A., Roberts 2nd, J.L., Milne, G., Choi, L., Dworski, R., 2012. Natural-source d-alpha-tocopheryl acetate inhibits oxidant stress and modulates atopic asthma in humans in vivo. Allergy 67, 676–682.

Huang, C.C., Shih, M.C., Hsu, N.C., Chien, Y., Chung, B.C., 2012. Fetal glucocorticoid synthesis is required for development of fetal adrenal medulla and hypothalamus feedback suppression. Endocrinology 153, 4749–4756.

Huang, P.H., Chuang, H.C., Chou, C.C., Wang, H., Lee, S.L., Yang, H.C., et al., 2013. Vitamin E Facilitates the Inactivation of the Kinase Akt by the Phosphatase PHLPP1. Sci. Signal 6, ra19.

Hubeau, C., Apostolou, I., Kobzik, L., 2006. Adoptively transferred allergen-specific T cells cause maternal transmission of asthma risk. Am. J. Pathol. 168, 1931–1939.

Hubeau, C., Apostolou, I., Kobzik, L., 2007. Targeting of CD25 and glucocorticoid-induced TNF receptor family-related gene-expressing T cells differentially modulates asthma risk in offspring of asthmatic and normal mother mice. J. Immunol. 178, 1477–1487.

Huebbe, P., Jofre-Monseny, L., Rimbach, G., 2009. Alpha-tocopherol transport in the lung is affected by the apoE genotype—studies in transgenic apoE3 and apoE4 mice. IUBMB Life 61, 453–456.

Hunter, S.C., Cahoon, E.B., 2007. Enhancing vitamin E in oilseeds: unraveling tocopherol and tocotrienol biosynthesis. Lipids 42, 97–108.

Hybertson, B.M., Leff, J.A., Beehler, C.J., Barry, P.C., Repine, J.E., 1995. Effect of vitamin E deficiency and supercritical fluid aerosolized vitamin E supplementation on interleukin-1-induced oxidative lung injury in rats. Free Radical Biol. Med. 18, 537–542.

Islam, S., Narra, V., Cote, G.M., Manganaro, T.F., Donahoe, P.K., Schnitzer, J.J., 1999. Prenatal vitamin E treatment improves lung growth in fetal rats with congenital diaphragmatic hernia. J. Pediatr. Surg. 34, 172–176.

Izzotti, A., Balansky, R.M., Cartiglia, C., Camoirano, A., Longobardi, M., De Flora, S., 2003. Genomic and transcriptional alterations in mouse fetus liver after transplacental exposure to cigarette smoke. FASEB J. 17, 1127–1129.

Jacobs, R.R., Boehlecke, B., van Hage-Hamsten, M., Rylander, R., 1993. Bronchial reactivity, atopy, and airway response to cotton dust. Am. Rev. Respir. Dis. 148, 19–24.

Jiang, Q., Christen, S., Shigenaga, M.K., Ames, B.N., 2001. gamma-tocopherol, the major form of vitamin E in the US diet, deserves more attention. Am. J. Clin. Nutr. 74, 714–722.

Jishage, K., Tachibe, T., Ito, T., Shibata, N., Suzuki, S., Mori, T., et al., 2005. Vitamin E is essential for mouse placentation but not for embryonic development itself. Biol. Reprod. 73, 983–987.

Jordan, J.M., De Roos, A.J., Renner, J.B., Luta, G., Cohen, A., Craft, N., et al., 2004. A case-control study of serum tocopherol levels and the alpha- to gamma-tocopherol ratio in radiographic knee osteoarthritis: the Johnston County Osteoarthritis Project. Am. J. Epidemiol. 159, 968–977.

Jourd'heuil, D., Morise, Z., Conner, E.M., Kurose, I., Grisham, M.B., 1997. Oxidant-regulation of gene expression in the chronically inflamed intestine. Keio J. Med. 46, 10–15.

Kalayci, O., Besler, T., Kilinc, K., Sekerel, B.E., Saraclar, Y., 2000. Serum levels of antioxidant vitamins (alpha tocopherol, beta carotene, and ascorbic acid) in children with bronchial asthma. Turkish J. Pediatr. 42, 17–21.

Kalpdev, A., Saha, S.C., Dhawan, V., 2011. Vitamin C and E supplementation does not reduce the risk of superimposed PE in pregnancy. Hypert. Preg. 30, 447–456.

Kelly, F.J., Mudway, I., Blomberg, A., Frew, A., Sandstrom, T., 1999. Altered lung antioxidant status in patients with mild asthma. Lancet 354, 482–483.

Keshavan, P., Deem, T.L., Schwemberger, S.J., Babcock, G.F., Cook-Mills, J.M., Zucker, S.D., 2005. Unconjugated bilirubin inhibits VCAM-1-mediated transendothelial leukocyte migration. J. Immunol. 174, 3709–3718.

Kim, H.B., Zhou, H., Kim, J.H., Habre, R., Bastain, T.M., Gilliland, F.D., 2016. Lifetime prevalence of childhood eczema and the effect of indoor environmental factors: analysis in Hispanic and non-Hispanic white children. Allergy Asthma Proc. 37, 64–71.

Kleiber, M., 1975. Metabolic turnover rate: a physiological meaning of the metabolic rate per unit body weight. J. Theor. Biol. 53, 199–204.

Koskela, H., Tukiainen, H., Kononoff, A., Pekkarinen, H., 1994. Effect of whole-body exposure to cold and wind on lung function in asthmatic patients. Chest 105, 1728–1731.

Kurukulaaratchy, R.J., Matthews, S., Waterhouse, L., Arshad, S.H., 2003. Factors influencing symptom expression in children with bronchial hyperresponsiveness at 10 years of age. J. Allergy Clin. Immunol. 112, 311–316.

Kurukulaaratchy, R.J., Waterhouse, L., Matthews, S.M., Arshad, S.H., 2005. Are influences during pregnancy associated with wheezing phenotypes during the first decade of life? Acta Paediatr. 94, 553–558.

Latzin, P., Frey, U., Roiha, H.L., Baldwin, D.N., Regamey, N., Strippoli, M.P., et al., 2007. Prospectively assessed incidence, severity, and determinants of respiratory symptoms in the first year of life. Pediatr. Pulmonol. 42, 41–50.

Leme, A.S., Hubeau, C., Xiang, Y., Goldman, A., Hamada, K., Suzaki, Y., et al., 2006. Role of breast milk in a mouse model of maternal transmission of asthma susceptibility. J. Immunol. 176, 762–769.

Leonard, S.W., Paterson, E., Atkinson, J.K., Ramakrishnan, R., Cross, C.E., Traber, M.G., 2005. Studies in humans using deuterium-labeled alpha- and gamma-tocopherols demonstrate faster plasma gamma-tocopherol disappearance and greater gamma-metabolite production. Free Radic. Biol. Med. 38, 857–866.

Lim, R.H., Kobzik, L., 2009a. Maternal transmission of asthma risk. Am. J. Reprod. Immunol. 61, 1–10.

Lim, R.H., Kobzik, L., 2009b. Transplacental passage of interleukins 4 and 13? PLoS One 4, e4660.

Lim, R.H., Arredouani, M.S., Fedulov, A., Kobzik, L., Hubeau, C., 2007. Maternal allergic contact dermatitis causes increased asthma risk in offspring. Respir. Res. 8, 56.

Lim, R.H., Kobzik, L., Dahl, M., 2010. Risk for asthma in offspring of asthmatic mothers versus fathers: a meta-analysis. PLoS One 5, e10134.

Lim, R., Fedulov, A.V., Kobzik, L., 2014. Maternal stress during pregnancy increases neonatal allergy susceptibility: role of glucocorticoids. Am. J. Physiol. Lung Cell Mol. Physiol. 307, L141–L148.

Lima, C., Souza, V.M., Faquim-Mauro, E.L., Hoshida, M.S., Bevilacqua, E., Macedo, M.S., et al., 2005. Modulation of the induction of lung and airway allergy in the offspring of IFN-gamma-treated mother mice. J. Immunol. 175, 3554–3559.

Litonjua, A.A., Carey, V.J., Burge, H.A., Weiss, S.T., Gold, D.R., 1998. Parental history and the risk for childhood asthma. Does mother confer more risk than father? Am. J. Respir. Crit. Care Med. 158, 176–181.

Lu, Y., Liu, M., Shi, S., Jiang, H., Yang, L., Liu, X., et al., 2010. Effects of stress in early life on immune functions in rats with asthma and the effects of music therapy: early-life psychological stress exacerbates adult mouse asthma via the hypothalamus-pituitary-adrenal axis. J. Asthma 47, 526–531.

Mabalirajan, U., Aich, J., Leishangthem, G.D., Sharma, S.K., Dinda, A.K., Ghosh, B., 2009. Effects of vitamin E on mitochondrial dysfunction and asthma features in an experimental allergic murine model. J. Appl. Physiol. 107, 1285–1292.

Mahoney, C.W., Azzi, A., 1988. Vitamin E inhibits protein kinase C activity. Biochem. Biophys. Res. Commun. 154, 694–697.

Mamdouh, Z., Mikhailov, A., Muller, W.A., 2009. Transcellular migration of leukocytes is mediated by the endothelial lateral border recycling compartment. J. Exp. Med. 206, 2795–2808.

Marchese, M.E., Kumar, R., Colangelo, L.A., Avila, P.C., Jacobs Jr, D.R., Gross, M., et al., 2014. The vitamin E isoforms alpha-tocopherol and gamma-tocopherol have opposite associations with spirometric parameters: the CARDIA study. Respir. Res. 15, 31.

Martindale, S., McNeill, G., Devereux, G., Campbell, D., Russell, G., Seaton, A., 2005. Antioxidant intake in pregnancy in relation to wheeze and eczema in the first two years of life. Am. J. Respir. Crit. Care Med. 171, 121–128.

Martinez, F.D., 2007. Genes, environments, development and asthma: a reappraisal. Eur. Respir. J. 29, 179–184.

Martinez, F.D., Wright, A.L., Taussig, L.M., Holberg, C.J., Halonen, M., Morgan, W.J., 1995. Asthma and wheezing in the first six years of life. The Group Health Medical Associates. N. Engl. J. Med. 332, 133–138.

Maslova, E., Hansen, S., Strom, M., Halldorsson, T.I., Olsen, S.F., 2014. Maternal intake of vitamins A, E and K in pregnancy and child allergic disease: a longitudinal study from the Danish National Birth Cohort. Br. J. Nutr. 111, 1096–1108.

McCance, D.R., Holmes, V.A., Maresh, M.J., Patterson, C.C., Walker, J.D., Pearson, D.W., et al., 2010. Vitamins C and E for prevention of pre-eclampsia in women with type 1 diabetes (DAPIT): a randomised placebo-controlled trial. Lancet 376, 259–266.

McCary, C.A., Abdala-Valencia, H., Berdnikovs, S., Cook-Mills, J.M., 2011. Supplemental and highly elevated tocopherol doses differentially regulate allergic inflammation: reversibility of alpha-tocopherol and gamma-tocopherol's effects. J. Immunol. 186, 3674–3685.

McCary, C.A., Yoon, Y., Panagabko, C., Cho, W., Atkinson, J., Cook-Mills, J.M., 2012. Vitamin E isoforms directly bind PKCalpha and differentially regulate activation of PKCalpha. Biochem. J. 441, 189–198.

Meydani, M., 2004. Vitamin E modulation of cardiovascular disease. Ann. N Y Acad. Sci. 1031, 271–279.

Meydani, S.N., Shapiro, A.C., Meydani, M., Macauley, J.B., Blumberg, J.B., 1987. Effect of age and dietary fat (fish, corn and coconut oils) on tocopherol status of C57BL/6Nia mice. Lipids 22, 345–350.

Mikhaylova, L., Zhang, Y., Kobzik, L., Fedulov, A.V., 2013. Link between epigenomic alterations and genome-wide aberrant transcriptional response to allergen in dendritic cells conveying maternal asthma risk. PLoS One 8, e70387.

Miller, M., Sung, K.L., Muller, W.A., Cho, J.Y., Roman, M., Castaneda, D., et al., 2001. Eosinophil tissue recruitment to sites of allergic inflammation in the lung is platelet endothelial cell adhesion molecule independent. J. Immunol. 167, 2292–2297.

Miyake, Y., Okubo, H., Sasaki, S., Tanaka, K., Hirota, Y., 2011. Maternal dietary patterns during pregnancy and risk of wheeze and eczema in Japanese infants aged 16-24 months: the Osaka Maternal and Child Health Study. Pediatr. Allergy Immunol. 22, 734–741.

Mosconi, E., Rekima, A., Seitz-Polski, B., Kanda, A., Fleury, S., Tissandie, E., et al., 2010. Breast milk immune complexes are potent inducers of oral tolerance in neonates and prevent asthma development. Mucosal. Immunol. 3, 461–474.

Mould, A.W., Ramsay, A.J., Matthaei, K.I., Young, I.G., Rothenberg, M.E., Foster, P.S., 2000. The effect of IL-5 and eotaxin expression in the lung on eosinophil trafficking and degranulation and the induction of bronchial hyperreactivity. J. Immunol. 164, 2142–2150.

Muller, W.A., 2011. Mechanisms of leukocyte transendothelial migration. Ann. Rev. Pathol. 6, 323–344.

Muller-Schmehl, K., Beninde, J., Finckh, B., Florian, S., Dudenhausen, J.W., Brigelius-Flohe, R., et al., 2004. Localization of alpha-tocopherol transfer protein in trophoblast, fetal capillaries' endothelium and amnion epithelium of human term placenta. Free Radic. Res. 38, 413–420.

Munteanu, A., Zingg, J.M., 2007. Cellular, molecular and clinical aspects of vitamin E on atherosclerosis prevention. Mol. Aspects Med. 28, 538–590.

Murphy, V.E., Zakar, T., Smith, R., Giles, W.B., Gibson, P.G., Clifton, V.L., 2002. Reduced 11beta-hydroxysteroid dehydrogenase type 2 activity is associated with decreased birth weight centile in pregnancies complicated by asthma. J. Clin. Endocrinol. Metab. 87, 1660–1668.

Murphy, V.E., Gibson, P.G., Giles, W.B., Zakar, T., Smith, R., Bisits, A.M., et al., 2003. Maternal asthma is associated with reduced female fetal growth. Am. J. Respir. Crit. Care Med. 168, 1317–1323.

Mustacich, D.J., Leonard, S.W., Devereaux, M.W., Sokol, R.J., Traber, M.G., 2006. Alpha-tocopherol regulation of hepatic cytochrome P450s and ABC transporters in rats. Free Radic. Biol. Med. 41, 1069–1078.

Myou, S., Zhu, X., Boetticher, E., Myo, S., Meliton, A., Lambertino, A., et al., 2002. Blockade of focal clustering and active conformation in beta 2-integrin-mediated adhesion of eosinophils to intercellular adhesion molecule-1 caused by transduction of HIV TAT-dominant negative Ras. J. Immunol. 169, 2670–2676.

Nelson, S.E., Rogers, R.R., Frantz, J.A., Ziegler, E.E., 1996. Palm olein in infant formula: absorption of fat and minerals by normal infants. Am. J. Clin. Nutr. 64, 291–296.

Nishio, K., Horie, M., Akazawa, Y., Shichiri, M., Iwahashi, H., Hagihara, Y., et al., 2013. Attenuation of lipopolysaccharide (LPS)-induced cytotoxicity by tocopherols and tocotrienols. Redox Biol. 1, 97–103.

Norbiato, G., Bevilacqua, M., Vago, T., Clerici, M., 1997. Glucocorticoids and Th-1, Th-2 type cytokines in rheumatoid arthritis, osteoarthritis, asthma, atopic dermatitis and AIDS. Clin. Exp. Rheumatol. 15, 315–323.

Odaka, Y., Nakano, M., Tanaka, T., Kaburagi, T., Yoshino, H., Sato-Mito, N., et al., 2010. The influence of a high-fat dietary environment in the fetal period on postnatal metabolic and immune function. Obesity 18, 1688–1694.

Okamoto, N., Murata, T., Tamai, H., Tanaka, H., Nagai, H., 2006. Effects of alpha tocopherol and probucol supplements on allergen-induced airway inflammation and hyperresponsiveness in a mouse model of allergic asthma. Int. Arch. Allergy Immunol. 141, 172–180.

Ostojic, S., Dubanchet, S., Chaouat, G., Abdelkarim, M., Truyens, C., Capron, F., 2003. Demonstration of the presence of IL-16, IL-17 and IL-18 at the murine fetomaternal interface during murine pregnancy. Am. J. Reprod. Immunol. 49, 101–112.

Palli, D., Masala, G., Vineis, P., Garte, S., Saieva, C., Krogh, V., et al., 2003. Biomarkers of dietary intake of micronutrients modulate DNA adduct levels in healthy adults. Carcinogenesis 24, 739–746.

Patel, A., Liebner, F., Netscher, T., Mereiter, K., Rosenau, T., 2007. Vitamin E chemistry. Nitration of non-alpha-tocopherols: products and mechanistic considerations. J. Org. Chem. 72, 6504–6512.

Pearson, P.J., Lewis, S.A., Britton, J., Fogarty, A., 2004. Vitamin E supplements in asthma: a parallel group randomised placebo controlled trial. Thorax 59, 652–656.

Portela Cde, P., Massoco Cde, O., de Lima, W.T., Palermo-Neto, J., 2001. Stress-induced increment on total bronchoalveolar cell count in OVA-sensitized rats. Physiol. Behav. 72, 415–420.

Portela Cde, P., Tiberio Ide, F., Leick-Maldonado, E.A., Martins, M.A., Palermo-Neto, J., 2002. Effects of diazepam and stress on lung inflammatory response in OVA-sensitized rats. Am. J. Physiol. Lung Cell Mol. Physiol. 282, L1289–L1295.

Portela, C.P., Leick-Maldonado, E.A., Kasahara, D.I., Prado, C.M., Calvo-Tiberio, I.F., Martins, M.A., et al., 2007. Effects of stress and neuropeptides on airway responses in ovalbumin-sensitized rats. Neuroimmunomodulation 14, 105–111.

Ramirez, F., Fowell, D.J., Puklavec, M., Simmonds, S., Mason, D., 1996. Glucocorticoids promote a TH2 cytokine response by CD4+ T cells in vitro. J. Immunol. 156, 2406–2412.

Ratnasinghe, D., Tangrea, J.A., Forman, M.R., Hartman, T., Gunter, E.W., Qiao, Y.L., et al., 2000. Serum tocopherols, selenium and lung cancer risk among tin miners in China. Cancer Causes Control 11, 129–135.

Rebholz, S.L., Burke, K.T., Yang, Q., Tso, P., Woollett, L.A., 2011. Dietary fat impacts fetal growth and metabolism: uptake of chylomicron remnant core lipids by the placenta. Am. J. Physiol. Endocrinol. Metab. 301, E416–E425.

Redlich, C.A., Grauer, J.N., Van Bennekum, A.M., Clever, S.L., Ponn, R.B., Blaner, W.S., 1996. Characterization of carotenoid, vitamin A, and alpha-tocopheral levels in human lung tissue and pulmonary macrophages. Am. J. Respir. Crit. Care Med. 154, 1436–1443.

Reichardt, P., Muller, D., Posselt, U., Vorberg, B., Diez, U., Schlink, U., et al., 2004. Fatty acids in colostrum from mothers of children at high risk of atopy in relation to clinical and laboratory signs of allergy in the first year of life. Allergy 59, 394–400.

Rocksen, D., Ekstrand-Hammarstrom, B., Johansson, L., Bucht, A., 2003. Vitamin E reduces transendothelial migration of neutrophils and prevents lung injury in endotoxin-induced airway inflammation. Am. J. Respir. Cell Mol. Biol. 28, 199–207.

Sagara, H., Matsuda, H., Wada, N., Yagita, H., Fukuda, T., Okumura, K., et al., 1997. A monoclonal antibody against very late activation antigen-4 inhibits eosinophil accumulation and late asthmatic response in a guinea pig model of asthma. Intl. Arch. Allergy Immunol. 112, 287–294.
Sansone, R.A., Sansone, L.A., 2008. Asthma: wheezing, woes, and worries. Psychiatry 5, 48–52.
Schunemann, H.J., Grant, B.J., Freudenheim, J.L., Muti, P., Browne, R.W., Drake, J.A., et al., 2001. The relation of serum levels of antioxidant vitamins C and E, retinol and carotenoids with pulmonary function in the general population. Am. J. Respir. Crit. Care Med. 163, 1246–1255.
Sheikh, A., Steiner, M.F., Cezard, G., Bansal, N., Fischbacher, C., Simpson, C.R., et al., 2016. Ethnic variations in asthma hospital admission, readmission and death: a retrospective, national cohort study of 4.62 million people in Scotland. BMC Med. 14, 3.
Shvedova, A.A., Kisin, E.R., Kagan, V.E., Karol, M.H., 1995. Increased lipid peroxidation and decreased antioxidants in lungs of guinea pigs following an allergic pulmonary response. Toxicol. Appl. Pharmacol. 132, 72–81.
Siekmeier, R., Steffen, C., Marz, W., 2007. Role of oxidants and antioxidants in atherosclerosis: results of in vitro and in vivo investigations. J. Cardiovasc. Pharmacol. Ther. 12, 265–282.
Smit, H.A., Grievink, L., Tabak, C., 1999. Dietary influences on chronic obstructive lung disease and asthma: a review of the epidemiological evidence. Proc. Nutr. Soc. 58, 309–319.
Sonnenschein-van der Voort, A.M., Jaddoe, V.W., Moll, H.A., Hofman, A., van der Valk, R.J., de Jongste, J.C., et al., 2013. Influence of maternal and cord blood C-reactive protein on childhood respiratory symptoms and eczema. Pediatr. Allergy Immunol. 24, 469–475.
Stoney, R.M., Woods, R.K., Hosking, C.S., Hill, D.J., Abramson, M.J., Thien, F.C., 2004. Maternal breast milk long-chain n-3 fatty acids are associated with increased risk of atopy in breastfed infants. Clin. Exp. Allergy 34, 194–200.
Strine, T.W., Mokdad, A.H., Balluz, L.S., Gonzalez, O., Crider, R., Berry, J.T., et al., 2008. Depression and anxiety in the United States: findings from the 2006 Behavioral Risk Factor Surveillance System. Psychiatr. Serv. 59, 1383–1390.
Suchankova, J., Voprsalova, M., Kottova, M., Semecky, V., Visnovsky, P., 2006. Effects of oral alpha-tocopherol on lung response in rat model of allergic asthma. Respirology 11, 414–421.
Sundl, I., Guardiola, M., Khoschsorur, G., Sola, R., Vallve, J.C., Godas, G., et al., 2007. Increased concentrations of circulating vitamin E in carriers of the apolipoprotein A5 gene—1131T> C variant and associations with plasma lipids and lipid peroxidation. J. Lipid Res. 48, 2506–2513.
Tabak, C., Smit, H.A., Rasanen, L., Fidanza, F., Menotti, A., Nissinen, A., et al., 1999. Dietary factors and pulmonary function: a cross sectional study in middle aged men from three European countries. Thorax 54, 1021–1026.
Talegawkar, S.A., Johnson, E.J., Carithers, T., Taylor Jr, H.A., Bogle, M.L., Tucker, K.L., 2007. Total alpha-tocopherol intakes are associated with serum alpha-tocopherol concentrations in African American adults. J. Nutr. 137, 2297–2303.
Terpstra, A.H., 2001. Differences between humans and mice in efficacy of the body fat lowering effect of conjugated linoleic acid: role of metabolic rate. J. Nutr. 131, 2067–2068.
Tonelli, L.H., Katz, M., Kovacsics, C.E., Gould, T.D., Joppy, B., Hoshino, A., et al., 2009. Allergic rhinitis induces anxiety-like behavior and altered social interaction in rodents. Brain Behav. Immun. 23, 784–793.
Troisi, R.J., Willett, W.C., Weiss, S.T., Trichopoulos, D., Rosner, B., Speizer, F.E., 1995. A prospective study of diet and adult-onset asthma. Am. J. Respir. Crit. Care Med. 151, 1401–1408.
Tulic, M.K., Knight, D.A., Holt, P.G., Sly, P.D., 2001. Lipopolysaccharide inhibits the late-phase response to allergen by altering nitric oxide synthase activity and interleukin-10. Am. J. Respir. Cell Mol. Biol. 24, 640–646.
Turner, S.W., Campbell, D., Smith, N., Craig, L.C., McNeill, G., Forbes, S.H., et al., 2010. Associations between fetal size, maternal α-tocopherol and childhood asthma. Thorax 65, 391–397.
Uauy, R., Hoffman, D.R., Birch, E.E., Birch, D.G., Jameson, D.M., Tyson, J., 1994. Safety and efficacy of omega-3 fatty acids in the nutrition of very low birth weight infants: soy oil and marine oil supplementation of formula. J. Pediatr. 124, 612–620.
Uthoff, H., Spenner, A., Reckelkamm, W., Ahrens, B., Wolk, G., Hackler, R., et al., 2003. Critical role of preconceptional immunization for protective and nonpathological specific immunity in murine neonates. J. Immunol. 171, 3485–3492.
Vanhees, K., Coort, S., Ruijters, E.J., Godschalk, R.W., van Schooten, F.J., Barjesteh van Waalwijk van Doorn-Khosrovani, S., 2011. Epigenetics: prenatal exposure to genistein leaves a permanent signature on the hematopoietic lineage. FASEB J. 25, 797–807.
van Rijt, L.S., Lambrecht, B.N., 2005. Dendritic cells in asthma: a function beyond sensitization. Clin. Exp. Allergy 35, 1125–1134.
Verhasselt, V., Milcent, V., Cazareth, J., Kanda, A., Fleury, S., Dombrowicz, D., et al., 2008. Breast milk-mediated transfer of an antigen induces tolerance and protection from allergic asthma. Nat. Med. 14, 170–175.
Vestweber, D., 2012. Novel insights into leukocyte extravasation. Curr. Opin. Hematol. 19, 212–217.
Villar, J., Purwar, M., Merialdi, M., Zavaleta, N., Thi Nhu Ngoc, N., Anthony, J., et al., 2009. World Health Organisation multicentre randomised trial of supplementation with vitamins C and E among pregnant women at high risk for pre-eclampsia in populations of low nutritional status from developing countries. BJOG 116, 780–788.
Vollmer, W.M., Osborne, M.L., Buist, A.S., 1998. 20-year trends in the prevalence of asthma and chronic airflow obstruction in an HMO. Am. J. Respir. Crit. Care Med. 157, 1079–1084.
von Hertzen, L.C., 2002. Maternal stress and T-cell differentiation of the developing immune system: possible implications for the development of asthma and atopy. J. Allergy Clin. Immunol. 109, 923–928.
Wagner, J.G., Jiang, Q., Harkema, J.R., Ames, B.N., Illek, B., Roubey, R.A., et al., 2008. Gamma-tocopherol prevents airway eosinophilia and mucous cell hyperplasia in experimentally induced allergic rhinitis and asthma. Clin. Exp. Allergy 38, 501–511.
Wagner, J.G., Harkema, J.R., Jiang, Q., Illek, B., Ames, B.N., Peden, D.B., 2009. Gamma-tocopherol attenuates ozone-induced exacerbation of allergic rhinosinusitis in rats. Toxicol. Pathol. 37, 481–491.
Wagner, K.H., Kamal-Eldin, A., Elmadfa, I., 2004. Gamma-tocopherol—an underestimated vitamin? Ann. Nutr. Metab. 48, 169–188.
Wardlaw, A., 2004. Eosinophil trafficking: new answers to old questions. Clin. Exp. Allergy 34, 676–679.
Wassall, H.J., Devereux, G., Seaton, A., Barker, R.N., 2013. Complex effects of vitamin E and vitamin C supplementation on in vitro neonatal mononuclear cell responses to allergens. Nutrients 5, 3337–3351.
Weiss, S.T., 1997. Diet as a risk factor for asthma. Ciba Found. Symp. 206, 244–257.
West, C.E., Dunstan, J., McCarthy, S., Metcalfe, J., D'Vaz, N., Meldrum, S., et al., 2012. Associations between maternal antioxidant intakes in pregnancy and infant allergic outcomes. Nutrients 4, 1747–1758.

Williams, J.W., Tjota, M.Y., Clay, B.S., Van der Lugt, B., Bandukwala, H.S., Hrusch, C.L., et al., 2013. Transcription factor IRF4 drives dendritic cells to promote Th2 differentiation. Nat. Commun. 4, 2990.

Wiser, J., Alexis, N.E., Jiang, Q., Wu, W., Robinette, C., Roubey, R., et al., 2008. In vivo gamma-tocopherol supplementation decreases systemic oxidative stress and cytokine responses of human monocytes in normal and asthmatic subjects. Free Radic. Biol. Med. 45, 40–49.

Wolf, G., 2006. How an increased intake of alpha-tocopherol can suppress the bioavailability of gamma-tocopherol. Nutr. Rev. 64, 295–299.

Woollett, L.A., 2005. Maternal cholesterol in fetal development: transport of cholesterol from the maternal to the fetal circulation. Am. J. Clin. Nutr. 82, 1155–1161.

Yang, L., Cohn, L., Zhang, D.H., Homer, R., Ray, A., Ray, P., 1998. Essential role of nuclear factor kappaB in the induction of eosinophilia in allergic airway inflammation. J. Exp. Med. 188, 1739–1750.

Yoshida, Y., Saito, Y., Jones, L.S., Shigeri, Y., 2007. Chemical reactivities and physical effects in comparison between tocopherols and tocotrienols: physiological significance and prospects as antioxidants. J. Biosci. Bioeng. 104, 439–445.

Zahran, H.S., Bailey, C., 2013. Factors associated with asthma prevalence among racial and ethnic groups-United States, 2009-2010 Behavioral Risk Factor Surveillance System. J. Asthma 11, 11.

Zou, W., Noh, S.K., Owen, K.Q., Koo, S.I., 2005. Dietary L-carnitine enhances the lymphatic absorption of fat and alpha-tocopherol in ovariectomized rats. J. Nutr. 135, 753–756.

Zourbas, S., Dubanchet, S., Martal, J., Chaouat, G., 2001. Localization of pro-inflammatory (IL-12, IL-15) and anti-inflammatory (IL-11, IL-13) cytokines at the foetomaternal interface during murine pregnancy. Clin. Exp. Immunol. 126, 519–528.

PART III

DIETARY SUPPLEMENTS AND HERBS, FUNCTIONAL FOODS, IN HEALTH IN AGING ADULTS

CHAPTER

18

Polyphenols and Intestinal Health

Kristina B. Martinez[1], *Jessica D. Mackert*[2] and *Michael K. McIntosh*[2]

[1]University of Chicago, Chicago, IL, United States [2]UNC-Greensboro, Greensboro, NC, United States

INTRODUCTION

Recent studies indicate that intestinal dysbiosis contributes to a multitude of intestinal (e.g., ulcers and inflammatory bowel) and systemic diseases (e.g., obesity, hepatic steatosis, and diabetes) that are associated with aging. Modulating specific populations of gut microbes by prebiotic (e.g., indigestible carbohydrates), probiotic (e.g., *Bifidobacteria* and *Lactobacilli*), or antibiotic treatments protects against or resolves the development of several of these disorders. However, less is known about the ability of dietary polyphenols to alter populations of commensal and pathogenic bacteria and their metabolic products that influence intestinal health. Therefore, this chapter examines the influence of dietary polyphenols and their metabolites on intestinal health, focusing on their antioxidant and antiinflammatory properties.

ROLE OF GUT MICROBIOTA IN INTESTINAL AND SYSTEMIC HEALTH

The Gut Microbiota

The gut microbial ecosystem is increasingly appreciated for its role in influencing intestinal and systemic diseases. The collection of microorganisms in the gastrointestinal (GI) tract is known as the *gut microbiota*. The collection of microbial genes is referred to as the *gut microbiome*. The gut microbiota consists largely of bacteria including two major phylotypes—Bacteroidetes and Firmicutes—and others such as Proteobacteria, Verrucomicrobia, and Actinobacteria (Eckburg et al., 2005). Colonization of these bacteria occurs immediately after birth and further develops within the first few years of life, contributing to the development of the host immune system. Intestinal and autoimmune diseases such as inflammatory bowel disease (IBD) and type 1 diabetes mellitus as well as other metabolic disorders are often associated with gut microbial dysbiosis. A dysbiotic microbiota is characterized by a (1) loss in microbial diversity; (2) change in composition, including blooms of pathogenic bacteria and decreases in commensal or potentially beneficial bacteria; or (3) change in metabolic function that ultimately leads to adverse consequences for the host (Schaubeck and Haller, 2015). Advances in sequencing technology have enabled researchers to interrogate the structure or relative abundance of the gut microbiota through 16s rRNA sequencing as well as their functional characteristics through metagenomic and metatranscriptomic analyses. Thus, the wealth of information regarding host–microbe interactions is rapidly increasing (Lagier et al., 2012). The human gut microbiota maintain resilience and stability over time but also shifts in response to acute changes in the environment, disease state, or diet (Berry et al., 2015). For instance, David et al. (2014) demonstrated that a diet consisting of animal products such as meat and cheese can rapidly alter microbial structure compared to a plant-based diet. However, resilience in microbial communities has also been demonstrated in studies following long-term dietary patterns

Nutrition and Functional Foods for Healthy Aging.
DOI: http://dx.doi.org/10.1016/B978-0-12-805376-8.00018-6

(Wu et al., 2011). Due to the relationships established between gut microbes and disease, it is of particular interest to understand how modulating gut microbial communities through diet or dietary supplements such as probiotics, prebiotics, or other functional food components like dietary polyphenols reassemble the gut microbiota structure and functional characteristics to promote better health.

Gut Microbes and Intestinal Health

The GI tract is a major site of host–microbe interactions. The human gut is populated by 10^{1-7} bacteria in the small intestine and 10^{10-13} in the colon, constituting a larger amount than in any other part of the body (Hartstra et al., 2015). Thus, it is not surprising that communication between microbes inhabiting the gut and the host significantly contributes to the development and progression of IBD, including Crohn's disease and ulcerative colitis. Crohn's disease is characterized by transmural intestinal inflammation that can occur throughout the length of the GI tract, whereas colitis is characterized by more superficial inflammation specific to the colon. Typically, inflammatory states are associated with a decrease in microbial diversity or richness, meaning a decrease in the total number of bacterial species present. In IBD, these changes correspond to increases in the relative abundance of Proteobacteria and reductions in Bacteroidetes and Firmicutes, specifically Clostridium cluster XIVa and IV, including *Faecalibacterium prausnitzii* and other butyrate-producing bacteria (Schaubeck and Haller, 2015). The direct interaction between microbes and IBD is strongly exemplified by the finding that genetically susceptible interleukin (IL)-$10^{-/-}$ mice are resistant to colitis when raised germ free. Exposure of IL$10^{-/-}$ mice to specific pathogens such as *Helicobacter hepaticus*, *Helicobacter rodentium*, and *Helicobacter typhlonius* or other pathobionts may lead to 100% penetrance of colitis (Kaur et al., 2011). Genetically susceptible hosts have aberrant immune responses to microbial dysbiosis or even commensal bacteria that lead to chronic inflammation (Sartor, 2016). However, it is still unclear whether the inflammatory state of the host precedes microbial dysbiosis or whether the dysbiotic communities initiate inflammation in the host.

Gut Microbes and Systemic Health

Microbes residing in the gut influence host metabolism and have been linked to obesity, nonalcoholic fatty liver disease, diabetes, and metabolic syndrome. Obesity afflicts more than one-third of the adult population (Flegal et al., 2010) and is often thought to result from sedentary lifestyles and consumption of Western diets, which are high in saturated fats and simple sugars. However, advancing research on the gut microbiota has convincingly established host–microbe interactions in the development of obesity and associated disorders (Ojeda et al., 2016). Obese humans and mice exhibit altered community structure such as decreased abundance of Bacteroidetes and increased abundance of Firmicutes compared to lean subjects (Ley et al., 2005, 2006). Transfer of obese microbiota to germ-free (GF) mice leads to increased adiposity, suggesting that microbiota alone can induce transferability of an obeselike phenotype (Turnbaugh et al., 2008). The inverse scenario has also been demonstrated because fecal transplantations of lean donor stool have shown improved insulin sensitivity in patients with metabolic syndrome (Vrieze et al., 2012). Furthermore, Roux-en-Y gastric bypass surgery, which dramatically improves glucose homeostasis and results in the rapid loss of 65–75% of body weight and fat mass, distinctly alters the community structure of intestinal microbiota in humans and rodents, namely by increasing the abundance of Gammaproteobacteria and Verrucomicrobia. In addition, fecal transplants from Roux-en-Y-treated mice cause decreased weight and fat mass in GF recipient mice (Liou et al., 2013). Taken together, gut microbes may directly improve the state of obesity and associated comorbidities. It is expected that therapeutic approaches such as the use of prebiotics, probiotics, and fecal microbiota transplantation (FMT) can be employed to promote restructuring of microbial communities leading to improved intestinal and systemic health for those suffering from IBD or systemic metabolic disease.

Therapies Targeting Gut Microbiota in Intestinal and Metabolic Disease

Current therapies targeting the gut microbiota to combat IBD and metabolic disease include antibiotics, probiotics, prebiotics, and FMT. These therapies directly target the GI microorganisms, the host, or both. These therapies are discussed in the following sections.

Antibiotics

Classic therapies for IBD include those targeting gut bacteria such as antibiotics and the host immune system such as immunomodulators (e.g., glucocorticoids) and biologics (e.g., antitumor necrosis factor (TNF) therapy;

Martinez et al., 2015). However, the use of antibiotics presents with inconsistent effectiveness in patients with Crohn's disease and ulcerative colitis and have limitations such as the length of treatment, bacterial resistance, and systemic responses (Sartor, 2016). However, antibiotics in combination with probiotics have been shown as effective in *Clostridium difficile* infection and pouchitis (Sartor, 2016). Thus, there is a need for unique individual or additive therapies targeting the gut microbiota that might improve health outcome in IBD patients and avoid the adverse consequence of antibiotic therapy.

Prebiotics

Prebiotics are foods that promote the growth of beneficial bacteria and include indigestible carbohydrates such as inulin and oligofructose. Prebiotics are classified based on resistance to gastric acidity, passage through the small intestine without digestion, fermentation by bacteria, and promotion of healthy gut microbial communities (Viladomiu et al., 2013). Recently, polyphenols from blueberries, cranberries, and grapes have been attributed with prebiotic characteristics given their poor bioavailability to the host, bacterial fermentation in the distal intestine, and growth promotion of commensal microbes (Anhe et al., 2015). Mechanisms explaining the beneficial action of prebiotics for IBD and metabolic disease include (1) increased expression of antimicrobial peptides against deleterious bacteria; (2) short-chain fatty acid (SCFA) production and SCFA-mediated stimulation of intestinal gluconeogenesis and increased epithelial integrity; (3) increased satiety and insulin sensitivity via release of gut peptide hormones, including polypeptide YY (PYY) and glucagon-like peptide (GLP)-1, respectively; and (4) restructured microbial communities, including the decreased relative abundance of pathogenic bacteria and the increased abundance of commensal bacteria (reviewed in Shen et al., 2014; Ojeda et al., 2016).

Probiotics

Probiotics have been given less favorable attention by the scientific community due to the lack of colonization or ineffectiveness, especially when provided as only one bacterial species (Ettinger et al., 2014). Thus, more recent recommendations have been provided for the classification of probiotics, including (1) isolated from a human subject, (2) generally recognized as safe with no harmful effects after prolonged use, (3) preparations yielding viable and active bacteria, (4) resistance to low gastric pH, (5) adherence to intestinal lining, (6) production of antimicrobial compounds against pathogens, (7) safe consumption when given as a food component, and (8) safety and efficacy supported by randomized controlled clinical trials (Martinez et al., 2015). Other important considerations for consumers include the type, duration, and amount of probiotic to consume and, most important, the intended purpose of the probiotic. For IBD, probiotics are often used in combination with other therapeutics. For instance, the commercially available probiotic formula VSL3, which contains *Bifidobacterium breve*, *Bifidobacterium longum*, *Bifidobacterium infantis*, *Lactobacillus acidophilus*, *Lactobacillus plantarum*, *Lactobacillus paracasei*, and *Lactobacillus bulgaricus* was given in combination with corticosteroid treatment in ulcerative colitis patients and was effective in reducing proinflammatory cytokines and increasing dendritic cell function (Ng et al., 2010). Less evidence supports a role for therapeutic effects of probiotics in Crohn's disease (Ghouri et al., 2014). Regarding systemic metabolic diseases, VSL3 has also been shown to decrease the severity of nonalcoholic fatty liver disease in obese children (Alisi et al., 2014) as well as reduce the risk of hepatic encephalitis in patients with cirrhosis (Dhiman et al., 2014). Overall, more research is warranted to identify dietary energy sources, bioactive food components, and probiotic species that benefit patients with IBD.

Fecal Microbiota Transplantation

Fecal microbiota transplantation (FMT) is the therapeutic transplantation of fecal contents from a healthy donor to a recipient via enema, nasogastric, nasoenteric, or endoscopic routes. The use of FMT dates back to 4th-century China, but only recently has it become a popular treatment in modern medicine. Fecal enema was used in 1958 and 1983 to treat pseudomembranous colitis and *C. difficile* infections, respectively (Brandt and Aroniadis, 2013). More than 400 cases of FMT were documented worldwide in 2011, a trend that is not surprising given the evidence that FMT is protective against *C. difficile* infection in approximately 90% of cases (Bakken, 2009). However, FMT is less commonly used or studied in the treatment of IBD and metabolic disease. The first case report of FMT for ulcerative colitis was published in 1989 by Drs. Justin D. Bennet and Brinkman after Bennet treated himself for severe ulcerative colitis. Three months following treatment, no active inflammation was evident and Bennet remained in remission (Borody and Khoruts, 2012). More recently, FMT from anonymous donors was shown to be effective in 24% of ulcerative colitis patients (9 out of 38) versus only 5% (2 out of 39) who received placebo enemas. While there were significantly more patients who achieved remission from FMT versus placebo control, the remaining 29 patients in the FMT group did not (Moayyedi et al., 2015). Thus, human trials have shown that some but not all patients achieve remission following FMT for IBD.

Human studies demonstrating the effectiveness of FMT for metabolic disease in particular are lacking. However, the reported use of FMT in the study by Vrieze et al. (2012) shows promise for improving insulin sensitivity in patients with metabolic syndrome. Not surprisingly, FMT must be closely monitored, and appropriate screening tools for donors and recipients are necessary. Donors are screened for an array of diseases, including HIV, hepatitis, inflammatory bowel disorders, and others (Brandt and Aroniadis, 2013; exclusion criteria reviewed in Bakken et al., 2011). Nutritional implications of FMT also deserve attention as the metabolic characteristics of the donor are transmissible. Nevertheless, in IBD, FMT is an attractive option for patients who are not responsive to classical treatment regimens. Overall, the newly gained knowledge in this field is expected to result in therapeutic strategies that target the gut microbiota for improved intestinal and systemic health.

In summary, intestinal microbes distinctly impact intestinal and systemic health. Ingested foods and beverages markedly alter gut microbes, with some causing dysbiosis and others enhancing the growth of healthy types of microbes. A number of plant-derived prebiotics have been identified. However, because less is known about the beneficial effects of plant polyphenols, they are examined in the following sections.

CLASSES, SUBCLASSES, EXAMPLES, AND SOURCES OF DIETARY POLYPHENOLS

Phytochemicals

Phytochemicals or chemicals in plants play important roles in their growth and development. They protect plants from harmful agents such as insects and microbes as well as stressful events such as ultraviolet (UV) irradiation and extreme temperatures. They also attract beneficial birds and insects that promote pollination, germination, and seed dispersal. Phytochemicals provide colors to plants and an array of flavors both pleasant and unpleasant when consumed. They are unique to specific plants and parts of plants, and they usually increase in abundance during stressful events. Phytochemicals also provide health benefits when consumed. They consist of nutrients essential for optimal health (e.g., proteins, carbohydrates, vitamins, and minerals) and other chemicals (e.g., phenolic acids, flavonoids, and other phenolics) (Fig. 18.1) (Bohn, 2014) with lesser known roles in health promotion or disease prevention. A number of these phytochemicals are recognized as bioactive components in traditional herbal medicines (e.g., salicylates (aspirin) found in willow bark used to reduce inflammation, quinine in cinchona bark used to treat malaria, and proanthocyanidins in cranberries used to treat urinary tract infections). Polyphenols represent the largest category of phytochemicals and serve as powerful antioxidants due to their multiple hydroxyl groups (Pietta, 2000), so they will be the focus of this chapter.

Phenolic Phytochemicals

Polyphenols or compounds containing multiple phenol ring structures represent at least 4000 known plant chemicals that are particularly abundant in fruits, vegetables, and beverages made from fruits (Cao et al., 1997). They are defined based on the nature of their carbon skeletons, patterns of hydroxylations, existence of stereoisomers, and states of oxidation, glycosylation (of flavonoids), and acylation (of phenolic acids) of heterocyclic rings. The polyphenol content in plants varies between 1 and 3 mg/kg and is influenced by cultivar, maturity, part of the plant, growing conditions, processing, and storage. There are three main classes of polyphenols: (1) phenolic acids (i.e., hydroxybenzoic and hydoxycinnamic acids), (2) flavonoids (e.g., flavones, flavonols, flavan-3-ols, isoflavones, flavanones, and anthocyanidins or anthocyanins), and (3) other phenolics (e.g., stibenes, lignans, tannins, xanthones, lignins, chromones, and anthraquinones) (Fig. 18.1).

Phenolic Acids

These aromatic acids represent approximately 30% of all dietary polyphenols, depending on the geographical location, food-harvesting techniques, processing practices, and cultural considerations inherent to the region of origin. The two major subclasses of phenolic acids are listed in the following sections, and their structures are shown in Fig. 18.2.

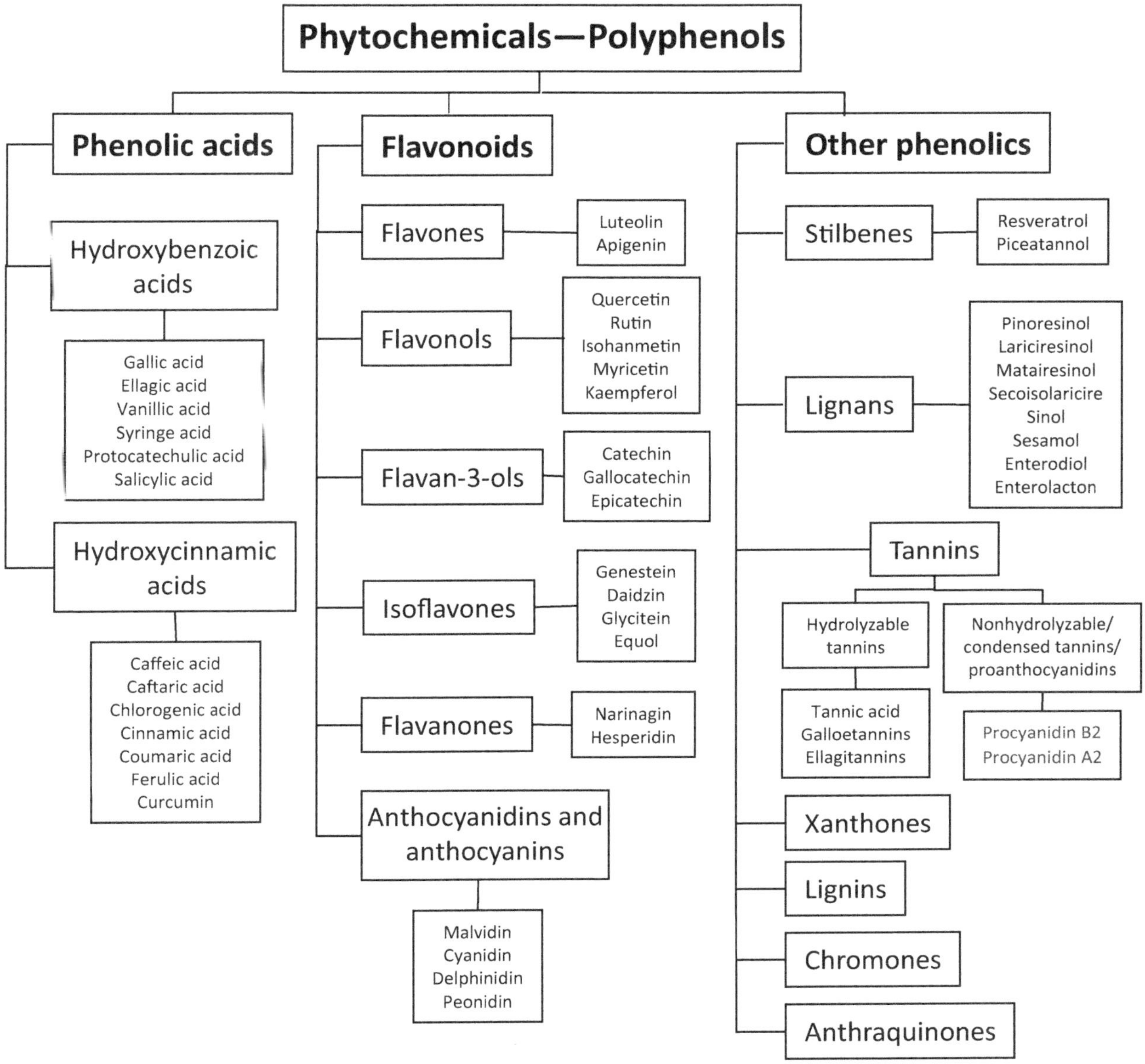

FIGURE 18.1 Types of polyphenols.

Hydroxybenzoic Acids

Structurally, hydroxybenzoic acids are common metabolites of flavonoids and several hydroxycinnamic acids (e.g., chlorogenic acid) and contain as many as four hydroxyl groups surrounding a single benzene ring (C6). Most fruits, especially berries, contain hydroxybenzoic acid. Gallic, ellagic (esterified to glucose in hydrolyzable tannins), protocatechuic, salicylic, syringic, and vanillic acids are plentiful in blackberries, cranberries, grapefruit, grapes, mangos, pomegranate, raspberries, rhubarb, strawberries, juices made from these fruits, tea, and red and white wines (Costain, 2001; Selma et al., 2009). Hydroxybenzoic acids are also found in chestnuts, peanuts, pecans, walnuts, and wheat, and in select herbs and spices.

Hydroxycinnamic Acids

Structurally, hydroxycinnamic acids are hydroxy metabolites of cinnamic acid with a C6–C3 backbone. Subclasses of these acids include caffeic, caftaric, (neo)chlorogenic, cinnamic, coumaric, and ferulic acids (often linked with dietary fibers that form esters with hemicellulose), and curcumin. Dietary sources include apples

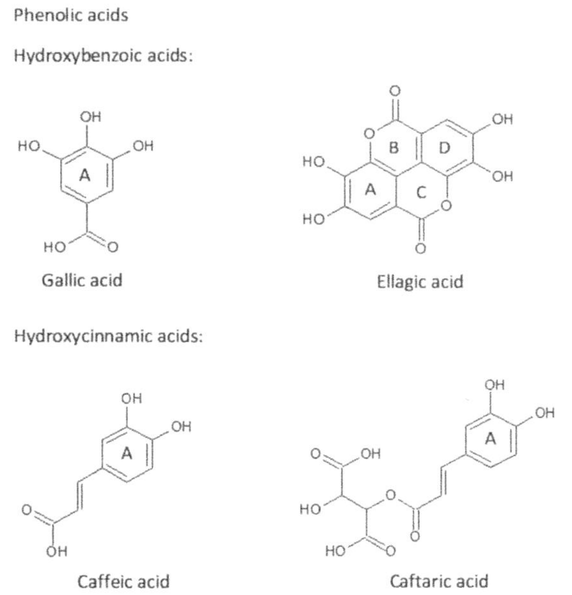

FIGURE 18.2 Structures of phenolic acids.

(and juice), blueberries, cereal grains and bran, cherries, cinnamon (cinnamic acid), coffee, ginger, grapes (and juice), lettuce, olives, oranges, pears, pineapples, plums, potatoes, prunes, spinach, strawberries, sunflower seeds, and turmeric, as well as select herbs (e.g., basal, marjoram, oregano, rosemary, sage, and thyme) (Costain, 2001; Selma et al., 2009).

Flavonoids

Flavonoids represent approximately 60% of all dietary polyphenols. They share a common chemical structure (e.g., C6–C3–C6) having at least 15 carbons with two benzene rings (A and B) and a heterocylic ring (C). Classifications are based on variations in the heterocyclic (C) ring. Major subclasses and structures of flavonoids are described in the following sections and shown in Fig. 18.3.

Flavones

Examples of flavones (2-phenylchromen-4-one structure) include luteolin in artichokes, beets, carrots, and red and chili peppers; and apigenin in celery, chamomile, olives, parsley, and thyme (Costain, 2001; Selma et al., 2009).

Flavonols

Examples of flavonols (3-hydroxy-2-phenylchromen-4-one structure) include isorhamnetin, kaempferol, myricetin, quercetin, and rutin. They are commonly found in apples, berries, broccoli, brussels sprouts, cabbage, endive, green beans, kale, lettuce, leeks, olives, onions, peas, red wine, tea, and tomatoes (Costain, 2001; Selma et al., 2009).

Flavan-3-ols

Examples of monomeric flavan-3-ols (3,4-dihydro-2H-chromen-3-ol structure) include catechin, epicatechin, and gallocatechin. These are found in apples, apricots, blackberries, cacao, coffee, cranberries, dark chocolate, green and black teas, pears, red and white wine, and spinach (Costain, 2001; Selma et al., 2009).

Isoflavones

Examples of isoflavones (3-phenylchromen-4-one structure) include daidzen, equol, genestein, and glycitein (aka phytoestrogens), all of them found in soy products and legumes. Isoflavones have one of the highest rates of absorption compared to other flavonoid classes (Costain, 2001; Selma et al., 2009).

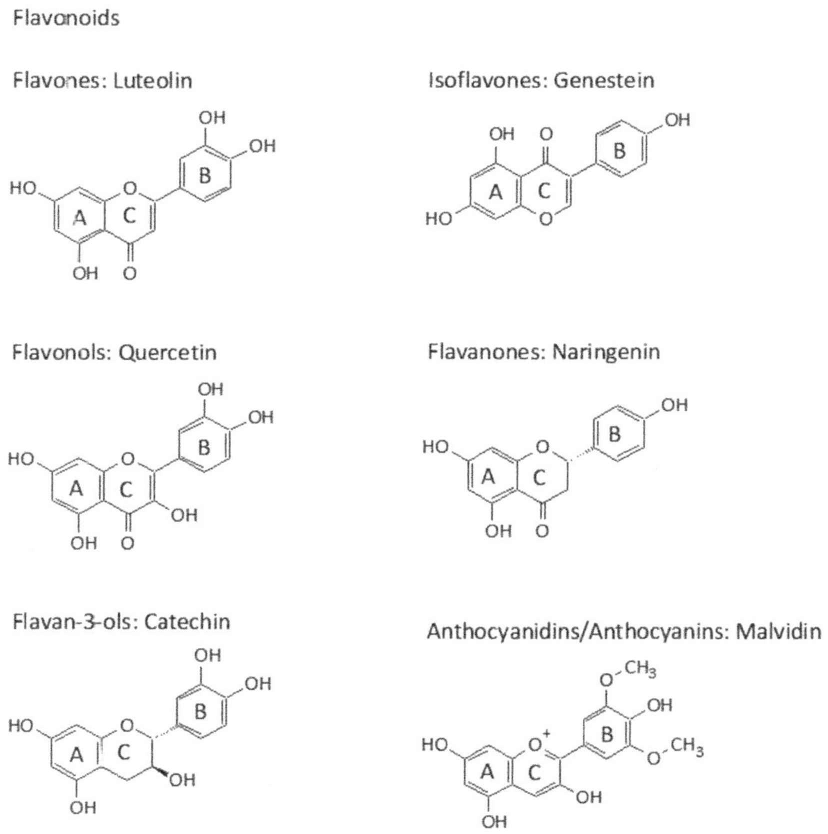

FIGURE 18.3 Structures of flavonoids.

Flavanones

Examples of flavanones (2,3-dihydro-2-phenylchromen-4-one structure) include naringenin in grapefruit (and juice) and hesperidin in cashew nuts, citrus fruits (and juice), and prunes (Costain, 2001; Selma et al., 2009).

Anthocyanidins and Anthocyanins

Anthocyanins are the glycosides of anthocyanidins. As with other flavonoids, classification is based on their R-group binding to H, OH, or OCH_3 as associated with the C6, C3, or C6 structures. Anthocyanins are responsible for the red, blue, purple, and violet colors of fruit. There are at least 300 different kinds of anthocyanins in plants, particularly those that are *Vaccinium* species (Selma et al., 2009). Examples of anthocyanidins (2-phenylchromenylium aglycones of anthocyanins) include cyanidin, delphinidin, malvidin, pelargondidin, peonidin, and petunidin. They are found in pigments in red fruits (e.g., apples, berries, cherries, currants, grapes, peaches, and plums), black and red currants, eggplant, radishes, red cabbage, and onions (Costain, 2001; Selma et al., 2009). Anthocyanins are poorly absorbed (i.e., approximately 0.5% or less compared to other flavonoids; Selma et al., 2009), so they reach the colon where they are metabolized by gut microbes or excreted. Anthocyanin metabolites found in the GI tract include the hydroxycinnamic acids gallic (3,4,5-trihydroxybenzoic acid), protocatechuic (3,4-dihydroxybenzoic acid), syringic (4-hydroxy-3,5-dimethyoxybenzoic acid), and vanillic acids (4-methyl-3-methoxybenzoic acid).

Other Phenolics

Stilbenes

Stilbenes have classical C6–C2–C6 structures with two hydroxyl groups on the A ring and one on the B ring (Fig. 18.4). They exist in plants as aglycones or glycosides, providing protection against bacterial, mold, or fungal

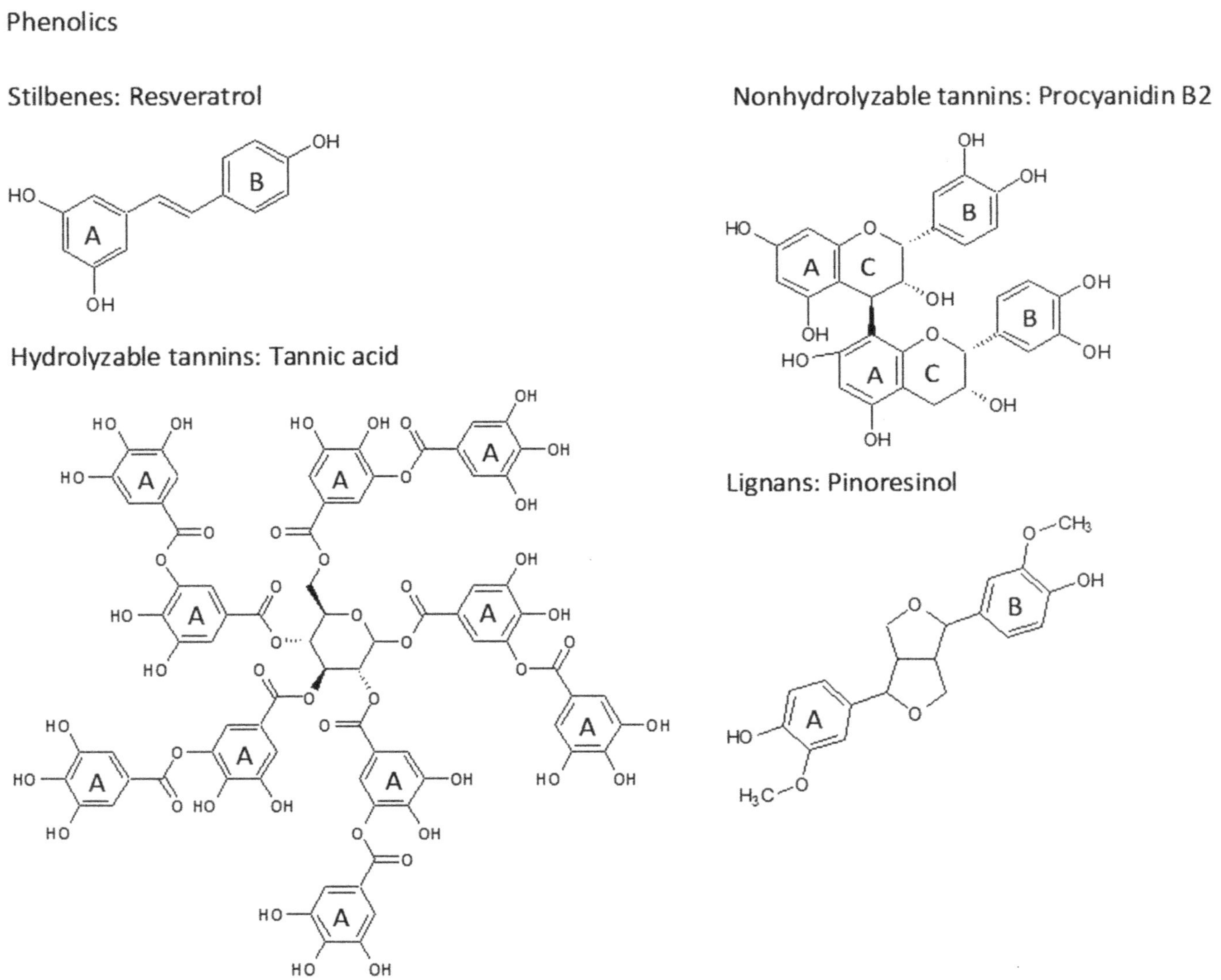

FIGURE 18.4 Structures of other phenolics.

invasion. Examples of stilbenes are the phytoalexins resveratrol and piceatannol, a resveratrol metabolite. They are found in grapes (skin), mulberries, peanuts, and red wine (Selma et al., 2009).

Tannins

There are at least two major classes of tannins: (1) hydrolyzable and nonhydrolyzable (also known as *condensed*) tannins and (2) proanthocyanidins and procyanidins. Structurally, hydrolyzable and nonhydrolyzable tannins are richly hydroxlyated oligomers or polymers of hydroxybenzoic acids such as gallic acid or flavan-3-ols such as catechin, respectively (Fig. 18.4). High-molecular-weight condensed tannins may contain 50 or more flavan-3-ols subunits attached by carbon–carbon bonds (Selma et al., 2009). They are highly astringent and noticeable in unripe fruits and certain wines.

Hydrolyzable Tannins

Examples of hydrolyzable tannins include gallo- and ellagitannins and tannic acid. Berries, grapes, persimmons, and pomegranate contain gallotannins. Berries, coffee, fruits, nuts, tea, and wine from fermented in oak barrels all contain ellagitannins (Costain, 2001; Selma et al., 2009).

Nonhydrolyzable or Condensed Tannins and Proanthocyanidins and Procyanidins

Examples of nonhydrolyzable or condensed tannins and proanthocyanidins and procyanidins include procyanidin A2 and B2, which consist of oligomers or polymers of the flavan-3-ols catechin, epicatechin, and gallocatechin. They are commonly found in chocolate, cocoa, coffee, cranberries, fruits (e.g., pears and apples), legumes (e.g., lentils, black-eyed peas, chickpeas, and red kidney beans), nuts, red and green grapes (and their juice and wine), and tea (Costain, 2001; Selma et al., 2009).

Lignans

Lignans are phenylpropanoids and are made from C6–C3 structures synthesized from phenylalanine, resulting in C6–C3–C3–C6 structures (Selma et al., 2009; Fig. 18.4). Examples include enterodiol, enterolactone, lariciresinol, matairesinol, pinoresinol, secoisolariciresinol, and sesamol found primarily in vegetables (e.g., broccoli, carrots, corn, and onions) and fruit (e.g., apples, cranberries, and pears), as well as in legumes and potatoes (Touillaud et al., 2007; Selma et al., 2009). Alcoholic beverages, coffee, grains (e.g., wheat, rye, and barley), and tea also contain lignans, with lesser amounts in linseed and olive oils and sesame seeds.

ANTIOXIDANT AND ANTIINFLAMMATORY PROPERTIES OF POLYPHENOLS

Antioxidant Properties of Polyphenols

Electrophiles or free radicals are generated from pollution, ozone, UV light, radiation, cigarette and cigar smoke, chemicals, drugs, pesticides, enzymes (e.g., nicotinamide adenine dinucleotide phosphate (NADPH) oxidase, xanthine oxidase, P450s, immune cells (e.g., phagocytes)), and cellular respiration. Examples of free radicals include superoxide ($O_2^\bullet$), hydroxyl ($^\bullet OH$), peroxyl ($LOO^\bullet$), alkoxyl ($LO^\bullet$), hydroperoxyl ($HO_2^\bullet$), nitric oxide ($^\bullet NO$), nitric dioxide ($^\bullet NO_2$), peroxynitrite ($ONOO^\bullet$), and nonlipid ($ROO^\bullet$, $R^\bullet$) radicals (Gropper and Smith, 2013). Free radicals can directly or indirectly cause oxidative damage to DNA, proteins, and polyunsaturated fatty acids, leading to cell mutations, toxicity, and inflammation with dire physiological consequences, including death.

Polyphenols neutralize or scavenge free radicals by electron transfer due to the hydroxyl group(s) associated with their phenol ring structure (C6) (Pietta, 2000). As the number of hydroxyl groups increases, so does the antioxidant potential of the polyphenol (Cao et al., 1997). Polyphenols also decrease free radical concentrations by inducing genes encoding antioxidant enzymes such as heme oxygenase-1, glutathione peroxidase, superoxide dismutase–1/2, catalase, and γ-glutamate-cysteine ligase catalytic subunit by activating the transcription factor nuclear factor–erythroid 2 (NF–E2)-related factor 2 (Nrf2) (Chuang and McIntosh, 2011). Collectively, these antioxidant actions of polyphenols provide a means of preventing oxidative damage mediated by free radicals, a notorious contributor to chronic disease risk.

Antiinflammatory Properties of Polyphenols

Free radicals activate enzymes such as NAPDH oxidase and NO synthase that generate reactive oxygen species and nitric oxide species, respectively. These radicals, in turn, trigger the inflammatory mitogen-activated protein kinases (MAPKs), apoptosis signal-related kinase-1, c-Jun N-terminal kinase, p38, and extracellular signal-related kinase, and the transcription factors nuclear factor kappa B (NFκB), and activator protein-1 (AP-1) that induce inflammatory gene expression. Increased inflammatory gene expression, in turn, leads to the synthesis and release of inflammatory cytokines and chemokines that activate or recruit immune cells to target tissues, which results in tissue inflammation (Chuang and McIntosh, 2011). Proinflammatory species also trigger the synthesis of proinflammatory eicosanoids via activation of phospholipases, cyclooxygenases, lipooxygenases, or P450 enzymes.

Polyphenols have been reported to activate specific transcription factors that antagonize NFκB or AP-1 (Chuang and McIntosh, 2011). For example, enhancing peroxisome proliferator activator receptor-γ (PPARγ) activation antagonizes NFκB and AP-1-mediated inflammatory gene expression, thereby reducing inflammation (Ricote and Glass, 2007). In addition, antiinflammatory, alternatively activated macrophages (i.e., M2s) require PPARγ for their activation (Bouhiel et al., 2007; Odegaard et al., 2007). Furthermore, feeding polyphenol-rich grapes to rats (1) increased cardiac PPARγ and δ mRNA levels and DNA binding activity, (2) decreased cardiac NFκB activity, and (3) decreased systemic markers of inflammation (Seymour et al., 2010). Supplementing high-fat-fed Zucker rats with grape seed procyanidins decreased white adipose tissue (WAT) mRNA levels of tumor necrosis factor alpha (TNF-α), interleukin 6 (IL-6), and C-reactive protein (CRP) and attenuated plasma levels of CRP (Terra et al., 2009).

Consistent with these data, we demonstrated that a polyphenol-rich grape extract or quercetin supplementation of primary cultures of human adipocytes treated with TNF-α (1) increased the activity of PPARγ, (2) increased the mRNA levels of several PPARγ target genes, or (3) decreased inflammatory signaling and insulin resistance (Chuang et al., 2010a,b). We also showed that a polyphenol-rich grape extract or quercetin-attenuated inflammatory signaling in human macrophages and in human primary adipocytes treated with conditioned media obtained from human macrophages (Overman et al., 2010, 2011). Similarly, quercetin and kaempferol increased PPARγ activity and decreased NO levels mediated by lipopolysaccharide (LPS) and insulin resistance in murine 3T3-L1 (pre)adipocytes (Fang et al., 2008). We further demonstrated that polyphenol-rich grape powder improved glucose tolerance acutely and decreased markers of inflammation in blood and WAT chronically in high-fat-fed mice (Chuang et al., 2012). Finally, we demonstrated that the xanthone α-mangostin, a polyphenol derived from *Garcinia mangostana* in Southeast Asia and used as a traditional medicine for skin infections, wounds, and diarrhea, prevented LPS-mediated inflammation or insulin resistance in human adipocytes and macrophages (Bumrungpert et al., 2009, 2010).

Notably, quercetin and *trans*-resveratrol activated the histone deacetylase sirtuin 1 (SIRT-1), causing NFκB deacetylation and thereby attenuating NFκB activity and inflammatory signaling (Howitz et al., 2003). Similarly, resveratrol reduced inflammatory signaling and improved insulin sensitivity in an SIRT-1–dependent manner by deacetylating NFκB (Fischer-Posovszky et al., 2010; Olholm et al., 2010; Yang et al., 2010; Zhu et al., 2008) and PGC1α (Lagouge et al., 2006; Sun et al., 2007), thereby enhancing mitochondrial biogenesis, oxidative phosphorylation, and aerobic capacity (Lagouge et al., 2006). Taken together, these antioxidant and antiinflammatory actions of polyphenols (Chuang and McIntosh, 2011) provide a means of preventing inflammation, a notorious risk factor for chronic disease.

Before discussing the intestinal health benefits of polyphenols, the next sections will examine (1) the influence of polyphenols on nutrient bioavailability, (2) how polyphenols are digested and absorbed, and (3) their interactions with gut microbes.

INFLUENCE OF POLYPHENOLS ON MACRO- AND MICRONUTRIENT BIOAVAILABILITY

Polyphenols may decrease carbohydrate absorption and glycemia by antagonizing amylase activity (Thompson et al., 1984; Forester et al., 2012). Such an effect provides carbohydrates for microbial growth in the GI tract, particularly saccharolytic bacteria such as *Bacteroides, Bifidobacterium, Clostridium, Eubacterium, Lactobacillus*, and *Ruminococcus* (Maukonen and Saarela, 2015). This could enhance microbial fermentation, thereby increasing SCFA synthesis and decreasing intestinal pH. In this way, polyphenols could influence bacterial diversity, gut peptide synthesis, energy harvest, food intake, and insulin sensitivity. Similarly, polyphenols may interact with intestinal lipases or proteases, decreasing fat and protein digestion, respectively, and consequently enhancing their likelihood of being fermented by gut microbes (Jakobek, 2015).

Dietary polyphenols may prevent macro- and micronutrient oxidation given their antioxidant capabilities, thereby maintaining their quality. On the other hand, polyphenols can interfere with mineral absorption. For instance, gallic acid, chlorogenic acids, monomeric flavonoids, and polyphenolic polymerization products inhibit nonheme iron absorption by as much as 50% (Monsen, 1988; Smith et al., 2005). In addition, tannins and gallic acid have been reported to bind to zinc, thereby impairing its absorption (Monsen, 1988). In summary, polyphenols have the capacity to enhance or impair nutrient absorption, depending on the type of polyphenol and nutrient involved. The next section will examine the bioavailability of polyphenols during the digestion, absorption, and utilization.

POLYPHENOL DIGESTION, ABSORPTION, AND UTILIZATION

Polyphenol Bioaccessibility and Bioavailability

The amount of polyphenol available for absorption (i.e., bioaccessibility) and the rate and extent of absorption and availability for metabolism (i.e., bioavailability) are impacted by their structure, degree of polymerization, types of interactions with food matrices, dietary status, diet composition, intestinal pH, and abundance of digestive enzymes (Lila et al., 2012; Bohn, 2014; Neilson and Ferruzzi, 2013). For example, conjugated polyphenols require deconjugation in order to diffuse into the enterocyte (Rein et al., 2013). The brush border of the small intestine contains membrane bound β-glucosidases that hydrolyze gluconated polyphenols into more readily absorbable aglycones (Van

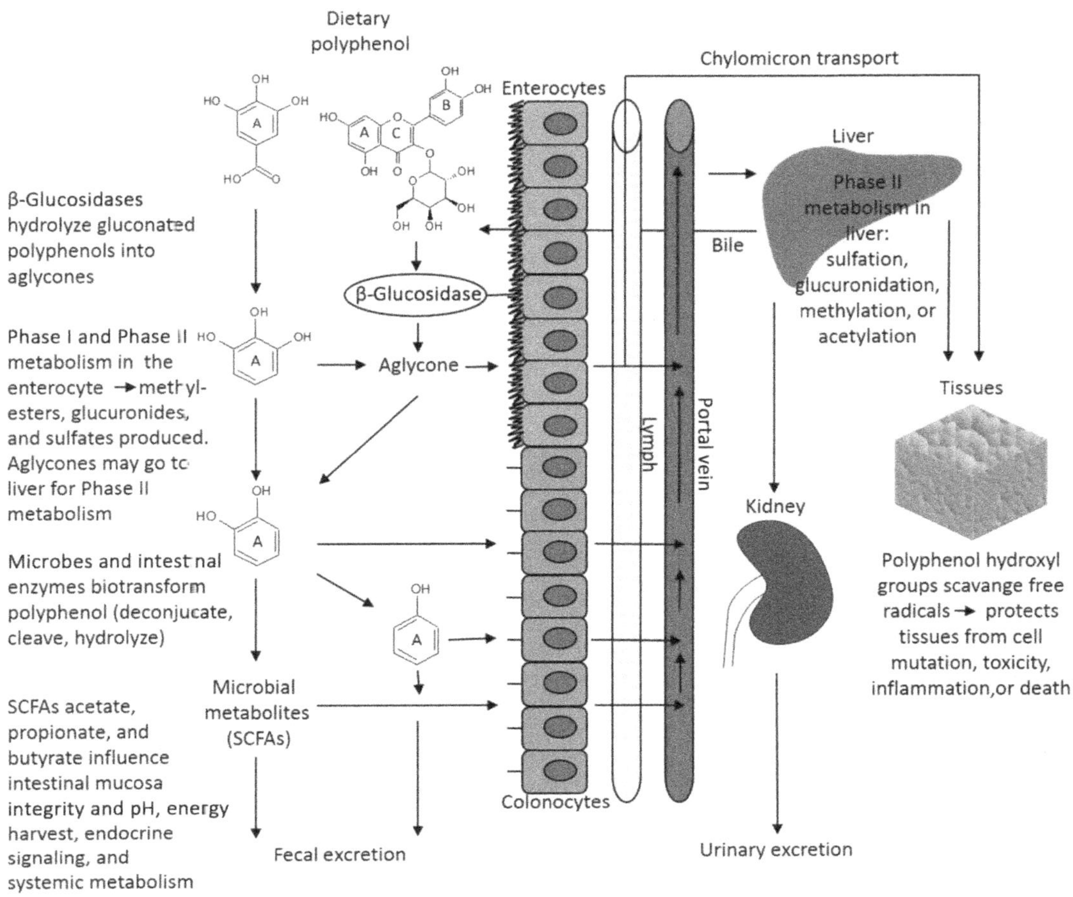

FIGURE 18.5 Metabolism and the fates of dietary polyphenols.

Duynhoven et al., 2011) (Fig. 18.5). Subsequently, the aglycone will undergo Phase I (e.g., reduction, oxidation, or hydrolysis) or Phase II (e.g., conjugation) metabolism in the enterocyte, converting it into a methyl ester, a glucuronide, or sulfate or be transported as an aglycone to the liver for similar metabolism (Chiou et al., 2014). Conjugating aglycones reduces their potential microbial toxicity and makes them easier to transport as biotransformed polyphenols. Furthermore, dietary macronutrients can alter the composition of intestinal microbes, which in turn influences polyphenol biotransformation in the GI tract (Fava et al., 2012). For instance, a high-fat meal increases the bioaccessibility of anthocyanins, whereas protein-rich matrices protect anthocyanins from degradation in the small intestine, thus making them available for colonic microbial biotransformation (Ribnicky et al., 2014).

Bacterial Metabolism of Polyphenols

Dietary polyphenols that reach the colon are metabolized by microbes and intestinal enzymes (Fig. 18.5). Biotransformation of polyphenols (e.g., deconjugated, cleaved, or hydrolyzed) to more or less bioaccessible and bioactive metabolites influences microbial growth and metabolism (Selma et al., 2009; Kemperman et al., 2010). Alternatively, biotransformed polyphenols (e.g., aglycones, monomeric proanthocyanidins, and phenolic acids) may be absorbed into the mucosa or bloodstream, where they can activate local or systemic receptors or transporters, respectively, that impact metabolism (Neilson and Ferruzzi, 2013). For the most part, microbial enzymes (e.g., dehydroxylases, decarboxylases, demethylases, esterases, glucosidases, glucuronidasases, hydrogenases, and isomerases) convert a diverse group of dietary polyphenols into a relatively small group of aromatic metabolites (Selma et al., 2009; Van Duynhoven et al., 2011). For example, benzoic, hippuric, and vanillic acids are the main microbial metabolites of green tea polyphenols (Fang et al., 2008). Those that are absorbed into the portal blood and reach the liver undergo sulfation, glucuronidation, methylation, or acetylation by Phase II enzymes (Neilson and Ferruzzi, 2013). These hepatic polyphenol metabolites, in turn, enter the bloodstream or bile acid pool.

POLYPHENOL–MICROBE INTERACTIONS

Microbial Fermentation Products That Influence Intestinal Health

Polyphenols alter the production of the microbial SCFAs acetate, propionate, and butyrate, which are normally at molar ratios of 60:23:17 (Blaut, 2014). SCFAs contribute approximately 10% of the total daily kcal intake (Bergman, 1990) and can regulate energy harvest. For example, (1) propionate is a precursor for hepatic gluconeogenesis, (2) propionate and acetate are precursors of cholesterol synthesis, and (3) acetate and butyrate are substrates for hepatic and WAT triglyceride (TG) synthesis. In addition, butyrate is the preferred energy substrate for colonocyte growth and differentiation (Roediger, 1980). Butyrate reduces the growth of colorectal cancer cells via upregulation of Wnt–beta-catenin signaling (Lazarova et al., 2014). Butyrate also increases the localization of tight junction proteins on the apical surface of epithelial cells, improving gut barrier function and preventing translocation of endotoxins into the systemic circulation (Cox and Blaser, 2013). Butyrate-inhibits NFκB signaling, thereby reducing inflammatory cytokine synthesis associated with GI inflammatory disease (Segain et al., 2000; Lührs et al., 2002). The acidic nature of SCFAs reduces luminal pH throughout the colon, preventing the growth of certain pathogenic bacteria (e.g., Enterobacteriaceae) (Roe et al., 2002; Hirshfield et al., 2003). This effect on pH may also be a determining factor on which class of fermenters predominates. At more neutral pH (6.5), acetate producers predominate; in contrast, in a more acidic environment (pH 5.5), butyrate producers predominate (Walker et al., 2005).

Activation of Endocrine Cell Signals

Polyphenols, their metabolites, or SCFAs activate G protein receptors (GPRs) on gut endocrine cells (e.g., GPR 41, 43, or 119) that secrete peptides that influence the host. For instance, butyrate increased GLP-1 secretion (Samuel et al., 2008), and GRP-mediated secretion of GLP-1 and -2 inhibited gastric emptying, elevated insulin secretion and sensitivity, and stimulated satiety (Holst, 2007; Wichmann et al., 2013). Similarly, GPR-mediated PYY secretion prevented obesity by increasing satiety, energy expenditure, or sympathetic-mediated thermogenesis in adipose tissue (Mestdagh et al., 2012). Therefore, polyphenol-mediated changes in fermentation products influence intestinal and systemic metabolisms.

INTESTINAL HEALTH BENEFITS OF POLYPHENOLS

Altering the Gut Microbiome and Improving Barrier Function

Dietary polyphenols increase the abundance and diversity of microbial populations (Tuohy et al., 2012). For example, a decreased ratio of Firmicutes to Bacteroidetes and increased *Lactobacilli*, *Bifidobacteria*, *Akkermansia muciniphila*, *Roseburia* spp., *Bacteroides*, and *Prevotella* spp. attenuates gut dysbiosis and accompanying metabolic complications (Selma et al., 2009; Roopchand et al., 2013; Neyrinck et al., 2013; Anhe et al., 2014). High-fat-fed mice consuming Concord grape polyphenols had a robust increase in fecal *A. muciniphila* abundance, which is associated with improved gut barrier function (Roopchand et al., 2015). Mice fed high levels of fat and sugar but supplemented with proanthocyanidin-rich cranberry extract had an increased abundance of fecal *A. muciniphila* (Anhe et al., 2014), a commensal, mucin-degrading bacteria that play a key role in enhancing gut barrier function and reducing inflammation, insulin resistance, and adiposity (Everard et al., 2013).

Polyphenol-rich grape juice increased the growth of the probiotics *L. acidophilus* and *Lactobacillus delbruekii*, and decreased the growth of *Escherichia coli* in vivo (Agte et al., 2010). Resveratrol supplementation of rats treated with dextran sulfate sodium (DSS) saw increased the levels of *Lactobacilli* and *Bifidobacteria* and improved colon mucosa architecture and inflammatory profile compared to controls (Larrosa et al., 2009b). Quercetin supplementation increased the growth of the probiotics *L. acidophilus* and *L. plantarum* (Yadav et al., 2011). Malvindin-3-glucoside increased the growth of *Bifidobacterium* and bacteria from the genuses *Lactobacillus* and *Enterococcus* (Hidalgo et al., 2012). Rats consuming polyphenol-rich grape fiber had increased cecum levels of *Lactobacillus* spp. (Pozuelo et al., 2012). Rats fed polyphenol-rich grape pomace juice had increased abundance of *Lactobacillus* and *Bifidobacterium* and decreased levels of secondary bile acids in their feces (Sembries et al., 2006). A reduction in secondary bile acids is positively associated with a reduced risk of GI cancers. Similarly, rats consuming red wine polyphenols had lower levels of *Clostridium* spp. and higher levels of *Lactobacillus* spp. (Dolara et al., 2005). In addition, adults consuming red wine had an increased abundance of *Enterococcus*, *Prevotella*, *Bacteroides*, *Bifidobacterium*, *Bacteroides uniformis*, *Eggerthella lenta*, *Blautia coccoides*, and *Eubacterium rectale* groups compared to a baseline. The wine consumers had lower blood pressure, blood cholesterol, and CRP levels, which were positively correlated with *Bifidobacteria* (Queipo-Ortuño et al., 2012). Wine polyphenols increased the growth of the probiotic *L. plantarum* (Barrosa et al., 2014). Adult males given a proanthocyanin-rich extract had reduced fecal microbial populations of *Bacteriodes, Clostridium,* and *Propionibacterium* genuses and higher levels of the probiotics *Bacteriodes, Lactobacillus,* and *Bifidobacterium* (Cardona et al., 2013).

High-fat diets cause gut dysbiosis, including increasing the abundance of deleterious sulfidogenic bacteria (Zhang et al., 2010; Shen et al., 2013, 2014) that produce hydrogen sulfide, a toxic gas that damages intestinal cells (Carbonero et al., 2012; Devkota et al., 2012). We demonstrated in butter-fed mice that table grape powder reduced adiposity, improved hepatic TG levels, modestly reduced WAT inflammatory gene expression, and lowered the cecum levels of deleterious sulfidogenic bacteria while tending to increase the abundance of *A. muciniphila* and *Allobaculum* in the proximal colon and cecum (Baldwin et al., 2016). In a follow-up study, we examined the impact of a polyphenol-rich, extractable fraction from table grape powder in mice fed a high-fat, American-type diet. The extractable fraction was rich in polyphenols, particularly anthocyanins and proanthocyanidins. The polyphenol-rich fraction attenuated diet-induced obesity, insulin resistance, steatosis, and chronic inflammation in WAT while improving gut barrier function and altering the bacterial structure of the cecum mucosa (Collins et al., 2016).

Quercetin or *trans*-resveratrol supplementation of mice consuming a high-fat, high-sugar diet decreased body weights and insulin resistance compared to control mice (Etxeberria et al., 2015). Notably, quercetin-mediated improvements in systemic health were positively correlated with a decreased ratio of Firmicutes and Bacteroidetes and an abundance of deleterious bacteria (e.g., Erysipelotrichaceae, *Bacillus*, and *Enubacterium cylindroides*), thereby reducing diet-induced dysbiosis. Quercetin-mediated increases in the Bacteroidetes phylum were accompanied by increases in the Bacteriodaceae and Prevotellaceae families (Etxeberria et al., 2015), which have been previously reported to be decreased in high-fat-fed mice (Hildebrandt et al., 2009). *Trans*-resveratrol–fed mice had suppressed intestinal markers of inflammation and enhanced markers of barrier function but only alterations in gut microbial profiles.

Antimicrobial Properties

Polyphenols have bacteriostatic, bactericidal, or adhesion-preventing properties against disease-causing bacteria (Selma et al., 2009). They have also been shown to inhibit quorum sensing (Gonzalez and Keshavan 2006), disrupt lipid membrane integrity (Kemperman et al., 2010), and DNA polymerase activity of bacteria (Cushnie and Lamb, 2005). For instance, anthocyanin-rich extracts from varieties of vegetables, juices, and tea inhibited the growth of infectious strains of bacteria (Lee et al., 2003, 2006). Polyphenols from tea attenuated the growth of *Candida albicans* (Evensen and Braun, 2009). Microbial metabolites of berries decreased the growth of salmonella (Alakomi et al., 2007). Gallic acid reduced the growth of potential respiratory pathogens, particularly the gram-negative bacteria *Moraxella catarrhalis* and the gram-positive *Staphylococcus aureus* (Cueva et al., 2012). Flavon-3-ol diminished the growth of the *Staphylococcus* genus and several *E. coli* strains in human fecal samples (Cueva et al., 2015). Finally, resveratrol mitigated the growth of drug-resistant strains of *Myobacterium smegmatis* (Lechner et al., 2008).

Suppressing Immune Cell Infiltration or Inflammatory Signaling in the GI Tract

Several intestinally derived polyphenol metabolites (i.e., dihydro-oxyphenylacetic, hydrocaffeic, and hydroferulic acids) suppressed inflammatory prostaglandin production in colon cancer cells and in rodents (Larrosa et al., 2009a). Hydrocaffeic acid reduced inflammation and DNA damage in a DSS-induced model of ulcerative colitis (Larrosa et al., 2009a). Similarly, a microbial metabolite of curcumin (i.e., ferualdehyde) reduced inflammation and extended life span in endotoxin-treated rodents (Radnai et al., 2009). Cranberry products reduced intestinal disease activity indices and markers of inflammation in experimentally induced colitis in mice (Xiao et al., 2015; Popov et al., 2010). Cranberry-derived flavonoids, and procyanidin dimers and oligomers were responsible for preventing lipid peroxidation and inflammatory signaling in intestinal Caco-2 cells treated with prooxidants or LPS (Denis et al., 2015). Rutin, quercetin glycosides, and resveratrol attenuated intestinal inflammation in rodents (Galvez et al., 1997; Kwon et al., 2005; Martin et al., 2004, 2006; Ergun et al., 2007). Polyphenol-rich grape seed extract reduced IBD markers, increased goblet cell number, and decreased myeloperoxidase activity, a constituently expressed enzyme in neutrophils that is positively associated with GI inflammation, in IL-10–deficient mice (Suwannaphet et al., 2010). Consistent with these data, resveratrol decreased nitric oxide synthase activity and mucosal damage in an enterocolitis rat model (Ergun et al., 2007). Intestinal colitis in Wistar rats was suppressed by grape juice flavonoids (Paiotti et al., 2013). Collectively, these data demonstrated the antiinflammatory properties of polyphenols.

Preventing or Treating Peptic Ulcers and Colitis

Two recent reviews describe literature supporting a positive role for dietary polyphenols found in *Piper betel,* apples, curcumin, green tea, grapes, pomegranate, bilberry, olive oil, and citrus fruits for the management of peptic ulcers (Farzaei et al., 2015a) and IBDs (Farzaei et al., 2015b). Mechanisms cited in these reviews for the beneficial effects of these polyphenols include (1) decreasing proinflammatory signaling cascades or enzymes, (2) increasing antioxidant compounds or enzymes, (3) increasing angiogenesis and growth factors, and (4) increasing populations of commensal and decreasing populations of disease-causing gut microbes. For example, apple polyphenols protected against aspirin-induced gastric ulcer (Paturi et al., 2014; D'Argenio et al., 2008; Graziani et al., 2005) in part by increasing the antioxidant status of the gastric mucosa and upregulating genes encoding proteins that defend gastric mucosa from insult. Apple polyphenols also reduced the incidence of colitis in a DSS mouse model of colitis via downregulating MAPKs and the induction of downstream inflammatory genes they regulate (Skyberg et al., 2011). Resveratrol decreased the activity of intestinal myeloperoxidase and improved the antioxidant status and degree of damage of the gastric mucosa in a murine model of acetic acid–induced gastric ulcers (Solmaz et al., 2009). Resveratrol also decreased DSS-mediated injury to colonic mucosa, which was associated with diminished NFκB and MAPK signaling in a mouse model of colitis (Youn et al., 2009). Ellagic acid, a pomegranate metabolite from intestinal bacteria, protected rats against gastric ulcer development in part by suppressing the activation of inflammatory cytokine production and increasing antioxidant activities (Beserra et al., 2011). Ellagic acid decreased trinitrobenzenesulfonic acid–mediated colitis in rats, which was associated with decreased activation of cyclooxygenase-2, iNOS, MAPK, and NFκB pathways that trigger inflammatory gene expression and the recruitment of immune cells into the GI mucosa (Rosillo et al., 2011). Tea polyphenols decreased the abundance of *Helicobacter pylori*, a GI bacterium associated with gastritis, by decreasing LPS-mediated activation of toll-like receptor 4 (Ankolekar et al., 2011). Tea polyphenols also decreased DSS-mediated colitis in mice by attenuating inflammatory gene expression and increasing antioxidant status (Oz et al., 2013).

Reducing GI Cancer Risk

Dietary phytochemicals and other natural products have anticancer properties (Singh et al., 2016a) that target cancer stem cells (Singh et al., 2016b) or the arachidonic acid pathway (Yarla et al., 2016). For instance, rats fed wine polyphenols for 16 weeks had a reduced incidence of colon carcinogenesis, which was positively associated with lower intestinal indicators of oxidative stress and populations of *Bacteriodes, Clostridium*, and *Propionibacterium* spp. (Dolara et al., 2005). Rats treated with the colon carcinogen 1,2-dimethylhydrazine (DMH) and supplemented with resveratrol had a lower colonic tumor burden, which was positively correlated with decreases in microbial biotransforming enzymes (e.g., β-glucuronidase, β-glucosidase, β-galactosidase, mucinase, nitroreductase, and sulfatase) linked with the development of cancer (Sengottuvelan and Nalini, 2006). Consistent with these data, DMH-treated rats consuming resveratrol had reduced colonic DNA damage that was positively associated with increased activities of superoxide dismutase, catalase, and glutathione peroxidase, reductase, and *S*-transferase and higher levels of glutathione, vitamins and E, and beta-carotene. The resveratrol-mediated enhancement of antioxidant status was accompanied by decreased markers of lipid peroxidation compared to nonresveratrol-supplemented mice (Sengottuvelan and Nalini, 2009).

CONCLUSIONS AND IMPLICATIONS

Intestinal dysbiosis is associated with intestinal and systemic diseases. Altering the gut microbiome with prebiotics, probiotics, antibiotics, or fecal microbial transplantation can mitigate dysbiosis and improve intestinal and systemic health. Plants are particularly rich in polyphenols that have significant health benefits when consumed. The three main classes of polyphenols are (1) phenolic acids, (2) flavonoids, and (3) other phenolics. They are abundant in specific types of fruits, beverages made from fruits, vegetables, spices, herbs, nuts, legumes, and plant oils. Plant polyphenols have potent antioxidant and antiinflammatory properties. They have positive and negative influences on nutrient digestion and absorption, depending on the macro- or micronutrient content of the diet. The digestion, absorption, and utilization of polyphenols is determined based on their structure, degree of polymerization, types of interactions with food matrices, dietary status, diet composition, intestinal pH, and abundance of digestive enzymes. Dietary polyphenols are poorly absorbed in the small intestine, so a large percentage of polyphenols (e.g., 90–95%) are metabolized by colonic microbial and intestinal enzymes. In general, microbial enzymes convert a diverse

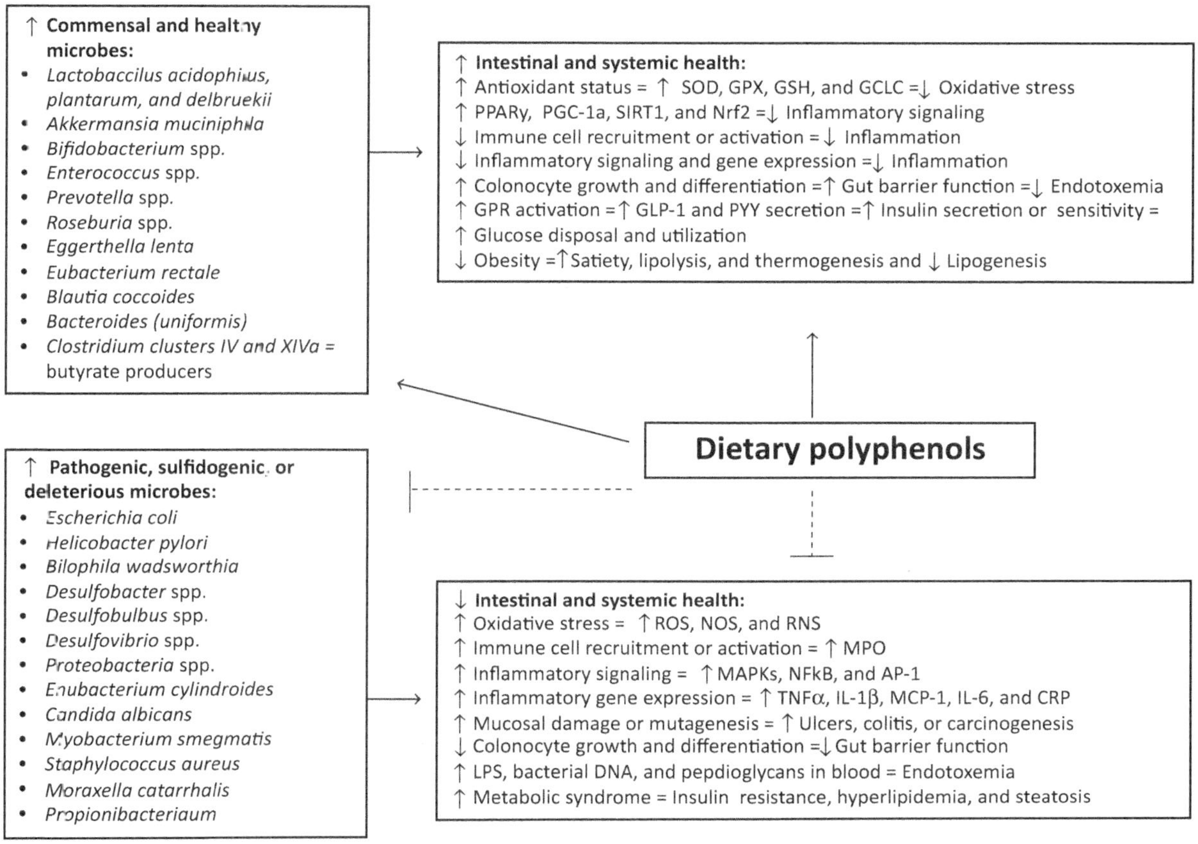

FIGURE 18.6 Summary of the reported effects on dietary polyphenols on intestinal microbes and intestinal and systemic health. *SOD*, superoxide dismutase; *GPX*, glutathione peroxidase; *GSH*, glutathione; *GCLC*, γ-glutamate-cysteine ligase catalytic subunit; *PPAR*, peroxisome proliferator activated receptor; *PGC*, PPARγ coactivator; *SIRT*, sirtuin; *Nrf2*, nuclear factor-erythroid 2 (NF-E2)-related factor 2; *GLP*, glucagon-like peptide; *PYY*, polypeptide YY; *ROS*, reactive oxygen species; *NOS*, nitric oxide species; *RNS*, reactive nitrogen species; *MPO*, myeloperoxidase; *MAPK*, mitogen-activated protein kinase; *NFκB*, nuclear factor kappa B; *AP-1*, activator protein-1; *TNF*, tumor necrosis factor; *IL*, interleukin; *CRP*, C-reactive protein; *LPS*, lipopolysaccharide.

group of dietary polyphenols into a relatively small group of aromatic metabolites that are either absorbed into the portal blood and sent to the liver or excreted in the feces. Those that reach the liver undergo sulfation, glucuronidation, methylation, or acetylation by Phase II enzymes. These hepatic polyphenol metabolites, in turn, enter the (1) bloodstream for uptake by target tissues, (2) the bladder for urinary excretion, or (3) the bile acid pool for remixing with intestinal digesta. Polyphenols alter the production of the microbial SCFAs acetate, propionate, and butyrate, which influences intestinal mucosa integrity and pH, energy harvest, endocrine signaling, and systemic metabolism. Dietary polyphenols increase the abundance and diversity of microbial populations that directly or indirectly impact gut barrier function, pathogenic bacterial growth, immune cell infiltration, and inflammatory status (Fig. 18.6). Such alterations may reduce the risk of intestinal disease, including peptic ulcers, colitis, Crohn's disease, and colon cancer. Collectively, these data support recommendations for consuming phytochemical-rich foods and beverages, including fruits, vegetables, herbs, beverages made from fruits and vegetables, nuts, and certain plant oils.

References

Agte, V., Khetmalis, N., Nilegaonkar, S., Karkamkar, S., Yadav, S., 2010. Prebiotic potential of 'juice grape' varieties and some hybrids. J. Sci. Ind. Res. 69, 850–854.

Alakomi, H.L., Puupponen-Pimia, R., Aura, A.M., Helander, I., Nohynek, L., Oksman-Caldentey, K., et al., 2007. Weakening of salmonella with selected microbial metabolites of berry-derived phenolic compounds and organic acids. J. Agric. Food Chem. 55, 3905–3912.

Alisi, A., Bedogni, G., Baviera, G., Giorgio, V., Porro, E., Paris, C., et al., 2014. Randomised clinical trial: the beneficial effects of VSL#3 in obese children with non-alcoholic steatohepatitis. Aliment. Pharmacol. Ther. 39, 1276–1285.

Anhe, F., Roy, D., Pilon, G., Dudonne, S., Matamoros, S., Varin, T., et al., 2014. A polyphenol-rich cranberry extract protects from diet-induced obesity, insulin resistance, and intestinal inflammation in association with increased *Akkermansia spp.* population in the gut microbiota of mice. Gut 64 (6), 872–880.

Anhe, F., Varin, T., Le Barz, M., Desjardins, Y., Levy, E., Roy, D., et al., 2015. Gut microbiota dysbiosis in obesity-linked metabolic diseases and prebiotic potential of polyphenol-rich extracts. Curr. Obes. Rep. 4, 389–400.

Ankolekar, C., Johnson, D., Pinto Mda, S., Johnson, K., Labbe, R., Shetty, K., 2011. Inhibitory potential of tea polyphenolics and influence of extraction time against Helicobacter pylori and lack of inhibition of beneficial lactic acid bacteria. J. Med. Food 14, 1321–1329.

Bakken, J.S., 2009. Fecal bacteriotherapy for recurrent *Clostridium difficile* infection. Anaerobe 15 (6), 285–289.

Bakken, J.S., Borody, T., Brandt, L.J., Brill, J., Demarco, D., Franzos, M., et al., 2011. Treating *Clostridium difficile* infection with fecal microbiota transplant. Clin. Gastroenterol. Hepatol. 9, 1044–1049.

Baldwin, J., Collins, B., Wolf, P., Shen, W., Martinez, K., Chuang, C.-C., et al., 2016. Table grape consumption reduces adiposity and markers of lipogenesis and alters gut microbiota in butter fat-fed mice. J. Nutr. Biochem. 27, 123–135.

Barrosa, E., Van de Wiele, T., Jimenez-Giron, A., Munoz-Gonzalez, I., Martin-Alvarez, P., Moreno-Arribas, M., et al., 2014. *Lactobacillus plantarum* IFPL935 impacts colonic metabolism in a simulator of the human gut microbiota during feeding with red wine polyphenols. Appl. Microbiol. Biotechnol. 98, 6805–6815.

Bergman, Z.R., 1990. Energy contributions for volatile fatty acids from the gastrointestinal tract in various species. Physiol. Rev. 70, 567–590.

Berry, D., Kuzyk, O., Rauch, I., Heider, S., Schwab, C., Hainzl, E., et al., 2015. Intestinal microbiota signatures associated with inflammation history in mice experiencing recurring colitis. Front. Micro. 6, 1408.

Beserra, A., Calegari, P., Souza, Mdo, C., Dos Santos, R., Lima, J., Silva, R., et al., 2011. Gastroprotective and ulcer-healing mechanisms of ellagic acid in experimental rats. J. Agric. Food Chem. 59, 6957–6965.

Blaut, M., 2014. Gut microbiota and energy balance: role in obesity. Proc. Nutr. Soc. 74 (3), 227–234.

Bohn, T., 2014. Dietary factors affecting polyphenol bioavailability. Nutr. Rev. 72 (7), 429–452.

Borody, T.J., Khoruts, A., 2012. Fecal microbiota transplantation and emerging applications. Nat. Rev. Gastroenterol. Hepatol. 9, 88–96.

Bouhiel, M., Derudas, B., Rigamonti, E., Dievart, R., Brozek, J., Haulon, S., et al., 2007. PPARγ activation primes human monocytes into alternatively activated M2 macrophages with anti-inflammatory properties. Cell Metab. 6, 137–143.

Brandt, L.J., Aroniadis, O.C., 2013. An overview of fecal microbiota transplantation: techniques, indications, and outcomes. Gastrointest. Endosc. 78 (2), 240–249.

Bumrungpert, A., Kalpravidh, R., Chitchumroonchokchai, C., Chuang, C., West, T., Kennedy, A., et al., 2009. Xanthones from mangosteen prevent lipopolysaccharide-mediated inflammation and insulin resistance in primary cultures of human adipocytes. J. Nutr. 139, 1185–1191.

Bumrungpert, A., Kalpravidh, R., Chuang, C., Overman, A., Martinez, K., West, T., et al., 2010. Xanthones from mangosteen inhibit inflammation of human macrophages and in human adipocytes exposed to macrophage-conditioned media. J. Nutr. 140, 842–847.

Cao, G., Sofic, E., Prior, R., 1997. Antioxidant and prooxidant behavior of flavonoids: structure-activity relationships. Free Radic. Biol. Med. 22, 749–760.

Carbonero, F., Benefiel, A., Alizadeh-Ghamsari, A., Gaskins, H., 2012. Microbial pathways in colonic sulfur metabolism and links with health and disease. Front. Physiol. 3, 448.

Cardona, F., Adrés-Lacueva, C., Tulipani, S., Tinahones, F.J., Queipo-Ortuño, M.I., 2013. Benefits of polyphenols on gut microbiota and implications in human health. J. Nutr. Biochem. 24, 1415–1422.

Chiou, Y.S., Wu, J.C., Huang, Q., Shahidi, F., Wang, Y.J., Ho, C.T., et al., 2014. Metabolic and colonic microbiota transformation may enhance the bioactivities of dietary polyphenols. J. Funct. Foods 7, 3–25.

Chuang, C.C., McIntosh, M., 2011. Potential mechanisms by which polyphenol-rich grapes prevent obesity-mediated inflammation and metabolic diseases. Annu. Rev. Nutr. 31, 155–176.

Chuang, C.C., Bumrungpert, A., Kennedy, A., West, T., Dawson, B., McIntosh, M., 2010a. Grape powder extract attenuates tumor necrosis factor α-mediated inflammation and insulin resistance in primary cultures of human adipocytes. J. Nutr. Biochem. 22, 89–94.

Chuang, C.C., Martinez, K., Xie, G., Kennedy, A., Bumrungpert, A., Overman, A., et al., 2010b. Quercetin is equally or more effective than resveratrol in attenuating tumor necrosis factor-{alpha}-mediated inflammation and insulin resistance in primary human adipocytes. Am. J. Clin. Nutr. 92, 1511–1521.

Chuang, C.C., Shen, W., Chen, H., Xie, G., Jia, W., Chung, S., et al., 2012. Differential effects of grape powder and its extract on glucose tolerance and chronic inflammation in high fat-fed obese mice. J. Agric. Food Chem. 60, 12458–12468.

Collins, B., Hoffman, J., Martinez, K., Grace, M., Lila, M.A., Cockrell, C., et al., 2016. A polyphenol-rich fraction obtained from table grapes decreases adiposity, insulin resistance, and markers of inflammation and impacts gut microbiota in high-fat fed mice. J. Nutr. Biochem. 31, 150–165. http://dx.doi.org/10.1016/j.jnutbio.2015.12.021.

Costain, L., 2001. Super Nutrients Handbook. Dorling Kindersley Books, New York, NY.

Cox, L., Blaser, M., 2013. Pathways of microbe-induced obesity. Cell Metab. 17, 883–894.

Cueva, C., Mingo, S., Munoz-Gonzalez, I., Bustos, I., Reguena, T., del Campo, R., et al., 2012. Antibacterial activity of wine phenolic compounds and oenological extracts against potential respiratory pathogens. Lett. Appl. Microbiol. 54, 557–563.

Cueva, C., Bartolome, B., Moreno-Arribas, M., Bustos, I., Reguena, T., Gonzalez-Manzano, S., et al., 2015. Susceptibility and tolerance of human gut culturable aerobic microbiota to wine polyphenols. Microb. Drug Resist. 21, 17–24.

Cushnie, T.P., Lamb, A.J., 2005. Antimicrobial activity of flavonoids. Int. J. Antimicrob. Agents 26, 343–356.

D'Argenio, G., Mazzone, G., Tuccillo, C., Grandone, I., Gravina, A., Graziani, G., et al., 2008. Apple polyphenol extracts prevent aspirin-induced damage to rat gastric mucosa. Br. J. Nutr. 100, 1228–1236.

David, L.A., Maurice, C.F., Carmody, R.N., Gootenberg, D.B., Button, J.E., Wolfe, B.E., et al., 2014. Diet rapidly and reproducibly alters the human gut microbiome. Nature 505, 559–563.

Denis, M.C., Desjardins, Y., Furtos, A., Marcil, V., Dudonne, S., Montoudis, A., et al., 2015. Prevention of oxidative stress, inflammation and mitochondrial dysfunction in the intestine by different cranberry phenolic fractions. Clin. Sci. 128, 197–212.

Devkota, S., Wang, Y., Musch, M., Leone, V., Fehlneer-Peach, H., Nadimpalli, A., et al., 2012. Dietary fat-induced taurocholic acid promotes pathobiont expansion and colitis in IL10$^{-/-}$ mice. Nature 487, 104–108.

Dhiman, R.K., Rana, B., Agrawal, S., Garg, A., Chopra, M., Thumburu, K., et al., 2014. Probiotic VSL#3 reduces liver disease severity and hospitalization in patients with cirrhosis: a randomized, controlled trial. Gastroenterology 147 (6), 1327–1337 e3.

Dolara, P., Luceri, C., De Filippo, C., Giovannelli, L., Caderni, G., Cecchini, C., et al., 2005. Red wine polyphenols influence carcinogenesis, intestinal microflora, oxidative damage, and gene expression profiles of colinc mucosa in F344 rats. Mutat. Res. 591, 237–246.

Eckburg, P.B., Bik, E.M., Bernstein, C.N., Purdom, E., Dethlesfsen, L., Sargent, M., et al., 2005. Diversity of the human intestinal microbial flora. Science 308, 1635–1638.

Ettinger, G., MacDonald, K., Reid, G., Burton, J.P., 2014. The influence of the human microbiome and probiotics on cardiovascular health. Gut Microbes 5 (6), 19–28.

Etxeberria, U., Arias, N., Boque, N., Macarulla, M., Portillo, M., Martinez, J., et al., 2015. Reshaping faecal gut microbiota composition by the intake of trans-resveratrol and quercetin in high-fat sucrose diet-fed mice. J. Nutr. Biochem. 26, 651–660.

Evensen, N., Braun, P., 2009. The effects of tea polyphenols on *Candida albicans*: inhibition of biofilm formation and proteasome inactivation. Can. J. Microbiol. 55, 1033–1039.

Everard, A., Belzer, C., Geurts, L., Ouwerkerk, J.P., Druart, C., Bindels, L.B., et al., 2013. Cross-talk between *Akkermansia muciniphila* and intestinal epithelium controls diet-induced obesity. Proc. Natl. Acad. Sci. USA 110, 9066–9071.

Ergun, O., Ergun, G., Oktem, G., Sevi, N., Dogan, H., Tuncyurek, M., et al., 2007. Enteral resveratrol supplementation attenuates intestinal epithelial inducible nitric oxide synthase activity andmucosal damage in experimental necrotizing enterocolitis. J. Pediatr. Surg. 42, 1687–1694.

Fang, X.K., Gao, J., Zhu, D.N., 2008. Kaempferol and quercetin isolated from *Euonymus alatus* improve glucose uptake of 3T3-L1 cells without adipogenesis activity. Life Sci. 82, 615–622.

Farzaei, M., Abdollahi, M., Rahimi, R., 2015a. Role of dietary polyphenols in the management of peptic ulcer. World J. Gastroenterol. 21, 6499–6517.

Farzaei, M., Rahimi, R., Abdollahi, M., 2015b. The role of dietary polyphenols in the management of inflammatory bowel disease. Curr. Pharm. Biotechnol. 16, 196–210.

Fava, F., Bitau, R., Griffin, B., Gibson, G., Tuohy, K., Lovegrove, J., 2012. The type and quantity of dietary fat and carbohydrate alter faecal micrbiome and short chain fatty acid excretion in a metabolic syndrome at risk population. Int. J. Obesity 37 (2), 216–233.

Fischer-Posovszky, P., Kukulus, V., Tews, D., Unterkircher, T., Debatin, K.M., Fulda, S., et al., 2010. Resveratrol regulates human adipocyte number and function in a Sirt1-dependent manner. Am. J. Clin. Nutr. 92, 5–15.

Flegal, K., Carroll, M., Ogden, C., Curtin, L., 2010. Prevalence and trends in obesity among U.S. adults, 1999–2008. J. Am. Med. Assoc. 303 (3), 235–241.

Forester, S.C., Gu, Y., Lambert, J.D., 2012. Inhibition of starch digestion by the green teapolyphenol, (−)-epigallocatechin-3-gallate. Mol. Nutr. Food Res. 56, 1647–1655.

Galvez, J., Cruz, T., Crespo, E., Ocete, M.A., Lorente, M.D., Sanchez deMedina, F., et al., 1997. Rutoside as mucosal protective in acetic acid induced rat colitis. Planta Med. 63, 409–414.

Gonzalez, J., Keshavan, N., 2006. Messing with bacterial quorum sensing. Microbiol. Mol. Biol. Rev. 70, 859–875.

Ghouri, Y.A., Richards, D.M., Rahimi, E.F., Krill, J.T., Jelinek, K.A., DuPont, A.W., 2014. Systematic review of randomized controlled trials of probiotics, prebiotics, and synbiotics in inflammatory bowel disease. Clin. Exp. Gastroenterol. 7, 473–487.

Graziani, G., D'Argenio, G., Tuccillo, C., Loguercio, C., Ritieni, A., Morisco, F., et al., 2005. Apple polyphenol extracts prevent DNA damage to human gastric epithelial cells in vitro and to rat gastric mucosa in vivo. Gut 54, 193–200.

Gropper, S., Smith, J., 2013. Perspective-antioxidant nutrients, reactive species, and disease Advanced Nutrition and Human Metabolism, sixth ed. Wadsworth, Belmont, CA416–424, Cengage Learning, Independence, KY.

Hartstra, A.V., Bouter, K., Backhed, F., Nieuwdorp, M., 2015. Insights into the role of the microbiome in obesity and type 2 diabetes. Diabetes Care 38, 159–165.

Hidalgo, M., Oruna-Concha, M.J., Kolida, S., Walton, G.E., Kallithraka, S., Spencer, J.P., et al., 2012. Metabolism of anthocyanins by human gut microflora and their influence on gut bacterial growth. J. Agric. Food Chem. 60, 3882–3890.

Hildebrandt, M., Hoffman, C., Sherrill-Mix, S., Keilbaught, S., Hamady, M., Chen, Y., et al., 2009. High-fat diet determines the composition of the murine microbiome independently of obesity. Gastroenterology 137, 1716–1724.

Hirshfield, I.N., Terzulli, S., O'Byrne, C., 2003. Weak organic acids: panoply of effects on bacteria. Sci. Prog. 86, 245–269.

Holst, J., 2007. The physiology of glucagon-like peptide 1. Physiol. Rev. 87, 1409–1439.

Howitz, K.T., Bitterman, K.J., Cohen, H.Y., Lamming, D.W., Lavu, S., Wood, J.G., et al., 2003. Small molecule activators of sirtuins extend *Saccharomyces cerevisiae* lifespan. Nature 425, 191–206.

Jakobek, L., 2015. Interactions of polyphenols with carbohydrates, lipids and proteins. Food Chem. 175, 556–567.

Kaur, N., Chen, C.C., Luther, J., Kao, J.Y., 2011. Intestinal dysbiosis in inflammatory bowel disease. Gut Microbes 2 (4), 211–216.

Kemperman, R., Bolca, S., Roger, L., Vaughan, E., 2010. Novel approaches for analyzing gut microbes and dietary polyphenols; challenges and opportunities. Microbiology 156, 3224–3231.

Kwon, K.H., Murakami, A., Tanaka, T., Ohigashi, H., 2005. Dietary rutin, but not its aglycone quercetin, ameliorates dextran sulfate sodium induced experimental colitis in mice: attenuation of pro-inflammatory gene expression. Biochem. Pharmacol. 69, 395–406.

Lagier, J.C., Million, M., Hugon, P., Armougom, F., Raoult, D., 2012. Human gut microbiota: repertoire and variations. Front. Cell Infect. Microbiol. 2, 136.

Lagouge, M., Argmann, C., Gerhart-Hines, Z., Meziane, H., Lerin, C., Daussin, F., et al., 2006. Resveratrol improves mitochondrial function and protects against metabolic disease by activating SIRT1 and PGC-1alpha. Cell 127, 1109–1122.

Larrosa, M., Luceri, C., Vivoli, E., Pagliuca, C., Lodovici, M., Moneti, G., et al., 2009a. Polyphenol metabolites from colonic microbiota exert anti-inflammatory activity on different inflammation models. Mol. Nutr. Food Res. 53, 1044–1054.

Larrosa, M., Yañéz-Gascón, M.J., Selma, M.V., González-Sarrías, A., Toti, S., Cerón, J.J., et al., 2009b. Effect of a low dose of dietary resveratrol on colon microbiota, inflammation and tissue damage in a DSS-induced colitis rat model. J. Agric. Food Chem. 57, 2211–2220.

Lazarova, D., Lee, A., Wong, T., Marian, B., Chiaro, C., Rainey, C., et al., 2014. Modulation of Wnt activity and cell physiology by butyrate in LT97 microadenoma cells. J. Cancer 5, 203–213.
Lechner, D., Gibbons, S., Bucar, F., 2008. Plant phenols compounds as ethidium bromide efflux inhibitors of *Mycobacterium smegmatis*. J. Antimicrob. Chemother. 62, 345–348.
Lee, H., Jenner, A., Lowa, C., Lee, Y., 2006. Effects of tea phenolics and their aromatic fecal bacterial metabolites on intestinal microbiota. Res. Microbiol. 157, 876–884.
Lee, Y., Cesario, T., Wang, Y., Shanbrom, E., Thrupp, L., 2003. Antibacterial activity of vegetables and juices. Nutrition 19, 994–996.
Ley, R.E., Backhed, F., Turnbaugh, P., Lozupone, C.A., Knight, R.D., Gordon, J.I., 2005. Obesity alters gut microbial ecology. Proc. Natl. Acad. Sci. USA 102 (31), 11070–11075.
Ley, R.E., Turnbaugh, P.J., Klein, S., Gordon, J.I., 2006. Microbial ecology: human gut microbes associated with obesity. Nature 444, 1022–1023.
Lila, M.A., Ribnicky, D., Rojo, L., Rojas-Silva, P., Oren, A., Havenaar, R., et al., 2012. Complementary approaches to gauge the bioavailability and distribution of ingested berry polyphenolics. J. Agric. Food Chem. 60, 5763–5771.
Liou, A.P., Paziuk, M., Luevano Jr., J.M., Machineni, S., Turnbaugh, P.J., Kaplan, L.M., 2013. Conserved shifts in the gut microbiota due to gastric bypass reduce host weight and adiposity. Sci. Transl. Med. 5 (178), 178ra41.
Lührs, H., Gerke, T., Müller, J.G., Melcher, R., Schauber, J., Boxberge, F., et al., 2002. Butyrate inhibits NF-κ B activation in lamina propria macrophages of patients with ulcerative colitis. Scand. J. Gastroenterol. 37, 458–466.
Martin, A.R., Villegas, I., LaCasa, C., de la Lastra, C.A., 2004. Resveratrol, a polyphenol found in grapes, suppresses oxidative damage and stimulates apoptosis during early colonic inflammation in rats. Biochem. Pharmacol. 67, 1399–1410.
Martin, A.R., Villegas, I., Sanchez-Hidalgo, M., de la Lastra, C.A., 2006. The effects of resveratrol, a phytoalexin derived from red wines, on chronic inflammation induced in an experimentally induced colitis model. Br. J. Pharmacol. 147, 873–885.
Martinez, R.C., Bedani, R., Saad, S.M., 2015. Scientific evidence for health effects attributed to the consumption of probiotics and prebiotics: an update for current perspectives and future challenges. Br. J. Nutr. 114 (12), 1993–2015.
Maukonen, J., Saarela, M., 2015. Human gut microbiota: does diet matter? Proc. Nutr. Soc. 74, 23–36.
Mestdagh, R., Dumas, M.E., Rezzi, S., Kochhar, S., Holmes, E., Claus, S., et al., 2012. Gut microbiota modulate the metabolism of brown adipose tissue in mice. J. Proteome Res. 11, 620–630.
Moayyedi, P., Surette, M.G., Kim, P.T., Libertucci, J., Wolfe, M., Onischi, C., et al., 2015. Fecal microbiota transplantation induces remission in patients with active ulcerative colitis in a randomized controlled trial. Gastroenterology 149 (1), 102–109.
Monsen, E., 1988. Iron nutrition and absorption: dietary factors which impact iron availability. J. Am. Diet Assoc. 88, 786–790.
Neilson, A.P., Ferruzzi, M., 2013. Bioavailability and metabolism of bioactive compounds from foods Nutrition in the Prevention and Treatment of Disease, third ed Elsevier Science, Amsterdam.407–423
Neyrinck, A., Van Hee, V., Bindels, L., Possemiers, S., De Backer, F., Cani, P., et al., 2013. Polyphenol-rich extract of pomegranate peel alleviates tissue inflammation and hypercholesterolemia in high-fat-induced obese mice: potential implication of the gut microbiota. Br. J. Nutr. 109, 802–809.
Ng, S.C., Plamondon, S., Kamm, M.A., Hart, A.L., Al-Hassi, H.O., Guenther, T., et al., 2010. Immunosuppressive effects via human intestinal dendritic cells of probiotic bacteria and steroids in the treatment of acute ulcerative colitis. Inflamm. Bowel Dis. 16, 1286–1298.
Odegaard, J., Ricardo-Gonzalez, R., Goforth, M., Morel, C., Subramanian, V., Mukendan, L., et al., 2007. Macrophage-specific PPARγ controls alternative activation and improves insulin resistance. Nature 447, 1116–1120.
Ojeda, P., Bobe, A., Dolan, K., Leone, V., Martinez, K., 2016. Nutritional modulation of gut microbiota-the impact on metabolic disease pathophysiology. J. Nutr. Biochem. 28, 191–200.
Olholm, J., Paulsen, S.K., Cullberg, K.B., Richelsen, B., Pedersen, S.B., 2010. Anti-inflammatory effect of resveratrol on adipokine expression and secretion in human adipose tissue explants. Int. J. Obesity 34, 1546–1553.
Overman, A., Bumrungpert, K., Kennedy, A., Martinez, K., Chuang, C., West, T., et al., 2010. Polyphenol-rich grape extract attenuates inflammation in human macrophages and in human adipocytes exposed to macrophage-conditioned media. Int. J. Obesity 34, 800–808.
Overman, A., Chuang, C.C., McIntosh, M., 2011. Quercetin attenuates inflammation in human macrophages and in human adipocytes exposed to macrophage-conditioned media. Int. J. Obesity 35, 1165–1172.
Oz, H., Chen, T., De Villiers, W., 2013. Green tea polyphenols and sulfasalazine have parallel anti-inflammatory properties in colitis models. Front. Immunol. 4 Article 132 http://dx.doi.org/10.3389/fimmu.2013.00132.
Paiotti, A.P., Neto, R.A., Marchi, P., Silva, R.M., Pazine, V.L., Noguti, J., et al., 2013. The anti-inflammatory potential of phenolic compounds in grape juice concentrate (G8000™) on 2,4,6-trinitrobenzene sulphonic acid-induced colitis. Br. J. Nutr. 110, 973–980.
Paturi, G., Butts, C., Bentley-Hewitt, K., McGhie, T., Saleh, Z., McLeod, A., 2014. Apple polyphenol extracts protect against aspirin-induced gastric mucosal damage in rats. Phytother. Res. 28, 1846–1854.
Pietta, P.G., 2000. Flavonoids as antioxidants. J. Nat. Prod. 63, 1035–1042.
Popov, S.V., Markov, P.A., Nikitina, I.R., Petrishev, S., Smirnov, V., Ovodov, Y.S., 2010. Preventive effect of a pectic polysaccharide of the common cranberry *Vaccinium oxycoccos* L. on acetic acid-induced colitis in mice. World J. Gastroenterol. 12, 6646–6651.
Pozuelo, M.J., Torres, A.A., Hernandez, D.H., Lopez-Olivia, M.E., Martinez, E.M., Rotger, R., et al., 2012. Grape antioxidant dietary fiber stimulates lactobacillus growth in rat cecum. J. Food Sci. 77, H59–H62.
Queipo-Ortuño, M.I., Boto-Ordóñez, M., Murri, M., Gomez-Zumaquero, J.M., Clemente-Postigo, M., Estruch, R., et al., 2012. Influence of red wine polyphenols and ethanol on the gut microbiota ecology and biochemical biomarkers. Am. J. Clin. Nutr. 95, 1323–1334.
Radnai, B., Tucsek, Z., Bognar, Z., Antus, C., Mark, L., Berente, Z., et al., 2009. Ferulaldehyde, a water-soluble degradation product of polyphenols, inhibits the lipopolysaccharide induced inflammatory response in mice. J. Nutr. 139, 291–297.
Rein, M.J., Renouf, M., Cruz-Hernandez, C., Ctis-Goretta, L., Thakkar, S.K., Da Silva, P.M., 2013. Bioavailability of bioactive food compounds: a challenging journey to bioefficacy. Br. J. Clin. Pharmacol. 75, 588–602.
Ribnicky, D., Roopchand, D., Oren, A., Grace, M., Pouleve, A., Lila, M.A., et al., 2014. Effects of a high fat meal matrix and protein complexation on the bioaccessibility of blueberry anthocyanins using TNO gastrointestinal model (TIM-1). Food Chem. 142, 349–357.

Ricote, M., Glass, C., 2007. PPARs and molecular mechanisms of transrepression. Biochim. Biophys. Acta 1771, 926–935.

Roe, A.J., O'Byrne, C., McLaggan, D., Booth, I.R., 2002. Inhibition of *Escherichia coli* growth by acetic acid: a problem with methionine biosynthesis and homocysteine toxicity. Microbiology 148, 2215–2222.

Roediger, W., 1980. Role of anaerobic bacteria in the metabolic welfare of the colonic mucosa in man. Gut 21, 793–798.

Roopchand, D., Kuhn, P., Krueger, C., Moskal, K., Lila, M.A., Raskin, I., 2013. Concord grape pomace polyphenols complexed to soy protein isolate are stable and hypoglycemic in diabetic mice. J. Agric. Food Chem. 61, 11428–11433.

Roopchand, D., Carmody, R., Kuhn, P., Moskal, K., Rojas-Silva, P., Turnbaugh, P., et al., 2015. Dietary polyphenols promote growth of the gut bacterium *Akkermansia muciniphila* and attenuate diet-induced metabolic syndrome. Diabetes 64, 2847–2858.

Rosillo, M., Sanchez-Hildalgo, M., Cardeno, A., Alacon Del La Lastra, C., 2011. Protective effect of ellagic acid, a natural polyphenolic compound in a murine model of Crohn's disease. Biochem. Pharmacol. 82, 737–745.

Samuel, B., Shaito, A., Motoike, T., Rey, F., Backhed, F., Manchester, J., et al., 2008. Effects of gut microbiota on host adiposity are modulated by the short chain fatty-acid binding protein G protein-coupled receptor, Gpr41. Proc. Natl. Acad. Sci. USA 105, 16767–16772.

Sartor, R.B., 2016. Review article: the potential mechanisms of action of rifaximin in the management of inflammatory bowel diseases. Aliment. Pharmacol. Ther. 43 (Suppl. 1), 27–36.

Schaubeck, M., Haller, D., 2015. Reciprocal interaction of diet and microbiome in inflammatory bowel diseases. Curr. Opin. Gastroenterol. 31 (6), 64–70.

Segain, J.P., Raingeard de la Blétière, D., Bourreille, A., Leray, V., Gervois, N., Rosales, C., et al., 2000. Butyrate inhibits inflammatory responses through NFκB inhibition: implications for Crohn's disease. Gut 47, 397–403.

Selma, M.V., Espín, J.C., Tomás-Barberán, F.A., 2009. Interaction between phenolics and gut microbiota: role in human health. J. Agric. Food Chem. 57, 6485–6501.

Sembries, S., Dongowski, G., Mehrlander, K., Will, F., Dietrich, H., 2006. Physiological effects of extraction juices from apple, grape, and red beet pomaces in rats. J. Agric. Food Chem. 54, 10269–10280.

Sengottuvelan, M., Nalini, N., 2006. Dietary supplementation of resveratrol suppresses colonic tumour incidence in 1,2 dimethylhydrazine-treated rats by modulating biotransforming enzymes and aberrant crypt foci development. Br. J. Nutr. 96, 145–154.

Sengottuvelan, M., Nalini, N., 2009. Dietary supplementation with resveratrol suppresses colonic tumour incidence in 1.2-dimethylhydrazine treated rats by modulating biotransforming enzymes and aberrant crypt foci development. Chem. Biol. Interact. 181, 193–201.

Seymour, E.M., Bennink, M.R., Watts, S.W., Bolling, S.F., 2010. Whole grape intake impacts cardiac peroxisome proliferator-activated receptor and nuclear factor κB activity and cytokine expression in rats with diastolic dysfunction. Hypertension 55, 1179–1185.

Shen, W., Gaskins, H., McIntosh, M., 2013. Influence of dietary fat on intestinal microbes, inflammation, barrier function, and metabolic outcomes. J. Nutr. Biochem. 25, 270–280.

Shen, W., Wolf, P., Carbonaro, F., Zhong, W., Reid, T., Gaskins, H., et al., 2014. Intestinal and systemic inflammatory responses are positively associated with sulfidogenic bacteria abundance in high-fat-fed male C57BL/6J mice. J. Nutr. 144, 1181–1197.

Singh, A., Siddiqui, I., Mukhtar, H., Ahmad, N., 2016a. Combination chemoprevention with grape antioxidants. Mol. Nutr. Food Res. 60 (6), 1406–1415. http://dx.doi.org/10.1002/mnfr.201500945.

Singh, A., Sharma, N., Ghosh, M., Park, Y., Jeong, D., 2016b. Emerging importance of dietary phytochemicals in fight against cancer: role in targeting cancer stem cells. Crit. Rev. Food Sci. Nutr. Feb. 6:0 PMID: 26853447.

Skyberg, J., Robison, A., Golden, S., Rollins, M., Callis, G., Huarte, E., et al., 2011. Apple polyphenols require T cells to ameliorate dextran suflfat-sodium-induced colitits and dampen proinflammatory cytokine expression. J. Leukoc. Biol. 90, 1043–1054.

Smith, A., Zoetendal, E., Mackie, R., 2005. Bacterial mechanisms to overcome inhibitory effects of dietary tannins. Microb. Ecol. 50, 197–205.

Solmaz, A., Sener, G., Cetinel, S., Yuksel, M., Yegen, C., Yegen, C., 2009. Protective and therapeutic effects of resveratrol on actetic-acid induced gastric ulcer. Free Radic. Res. 43, 594–603.

Sun, C., Zhang, F., Ge, X., Yan, T., Chen, X., Shi, X., et al., 2007. SIRT1 improves insulin sensitivity under insulin-resistant conditions by repressing PTP1B. Cell Metab. 6, 307–319.

Suwannaphet, W, Meeprom, A., Yibchok-Anun, S., Adisakwattana, S., 2010. Preventive effect of grape seed extract against high-fructose diet-induced insulin resistance and oxidative stress in rats. Food Chem. Toxicol. 48, 1853–1857.

Terra, G., Montagut, M., Bustos, N., Llopiz, A., Ardèvol, C., Bladé, D., et al., 2009. Grape-seed procyanidins prevent low-grade inflammation by modulating cytokine expression in rats fed a high-fat diet. J. Nutr. Biochem. 20, 201–218.

Thompson, L.U., Yoon, J.H., Jenkins, D.J., Wolever, T.M., Jenkins, A.L., 1984. Relationship between polyphenol intake and blood glucose response of normal and diabetic individuals. Am. J. Clin. Nutr. 39, 745–751.

Touillaud, M., Thiebaut, A., Fournier, A., Niravong, M., Boutron-Ruault, M., Chavel-Chapelon, F., 2007. Dietary lignin intake and postmenopausal breast cancer risk by estrogen and progesterone receptor status. J. Natl. Cancer Inst. 99, 475–486.

Tuohy, K.M., Conterno, L., Gasperotti, M., Viola, R., 2012. Up-regulating the human intestinal microbiome using whole plant foods, polyphenols, and/or fiber. J. Agric. Food Chem. 60, 8776–8782.

Turnbaugh, P.J., Backhed, F., Fulton, L., Gordon, J.I., 2008. Diet-induced obesity is linked to marked but reversible alterations in the mouse distal gut microbiome. Cell Host Microbe 3 (4), 213–223.

Van Duynhoven, J., Vaughan, E.E., Jacobs, D.M., Kemperman, R.A., van Velzen, E.J., Gross, G., et al., 2011. Metabolic fate of polyphenols in the human superorganism. Proc. Natl. Acad. Sci. 108 (Suppl. 1), 4531–4538.

Viladomiu, M., Hontecillas, R., Yuan, L., Lu, P., Bassanganya-Riera, J., 2013. Nutritional protective mechanisms against gut inflammation. J. Nutr. Biochem. 24, 929–939.

Vrieze, A., Van Nood, E., Holleman, F., Salojarvi, J., Kootte, R.S., Bartelsman, J.F., et al., 2012. Transfer of intestinal microbiota from lean donors increases insulin sensitivity in individuals with metabolic syndrome. Gastroenterology 143 (4), 913–916 e7.

Walker, A.W., Duncan, S.H., McWilliam Leitch, E.C., Child, M.W., Flint, H.J., 2005. pH and peptide supply can radically alter bacterial populations and short-chain fatty acid ratios within microbial communities from the human colon. Appl. Environ. Microbiol. 71, 3692–3700.

Wichmann, A., Allahyar, A., Greiner, T.U., Plovier, H., Lundén, G.Ö., Larsson, T., et al., 2013. Microbial modulation of energy availability in the colon regulates intestinal transit. Cell Host Microbe 14, 582–590.

Wu, G.D., Chen, J., Hoffmann, C., Bittinger, K., Chen, Y.Y., Keilbaugh, S.A., et al., 2011. Linking long-term dietary patterns with gut microbial enterotypes. Science 334, 105–108.

Xiao, X., Kim, J., Sun, Q., Kim, D., Park, C.S., Lu, T.S., et al., 2015. Preventive effects of cranberry products on experimental colitis induced by dextran sulphate sodium in mice. Food Chem. 167, 438–446.

Yadav, S., Gite, S., Nilegaonkar, S., Agte, V., 2011. Effect of supplementation of micronutrients and phytochemicals to fructooligosaccharides on growth response of probiotics and *E. coli*. Biofactors 37, 58–64.

Yang, Z., Kahn, B.B., Shi, H., Xue, B.Z., 2010. Macrophage alpha1 AMP-activated protein kinase (alpha1AMPK) antagonizes fatty acid-induced inflammation through SIRT1. J. Biol. Chem. 285, 19051–19059.

Yarla, N., Bishayee, A., Sethi, G., Reddanna, P., Kalle, A., Dhananjaya, B., et al., 2016. Targeting arachidonic acid pathway by natural products for cancer prevention and therapy. Semin. Cancer Biol. Feb. 4 http://dx.doi.org/10.1016/j.semcancer.2016.02.001.

Youn, J., Lee, J., Na, H., Kundu, J., Surh, Y., 2009. Resveratrol and piccatannol inhibit iNOS expression and NF-κB activation in dextran sulfate sodium-induced mouse colitis. Nutr. Cancer 61, 847–854.

Zhang, C., Zhang, M., Wang, S., Han, R., Cao, Y., Hua, W., et al., 2010. Interactions between gut microbiota, host genetics, and diet relevant to development of metabolic syndromes in mice. ISME J. 4, 232–241.

Zhu, J., Yong, W., Wu, X., Yu, Y., Lv, J., Liu, C., et al., 2008. Anti-inflammatory effect of resveratrol on TNF-alpha-induced MCP-1 expression in adipocytes. Biochem. Biophys. Res. Commun. 369, 471–477.

CHAPTER

19

Nootropics, Functional Foods, and Dietary Patterns for Prevention of Cognitive Decline

Francesco Bonetti, Gloria Brombo and Giovanni Zuliani

University of Ferrara, Ferrara, Italy

INTRODUCTION

Over the last century we have assisted the aging of the world population, the resulting changes in epidemiology are modifying the problems perceived as fundamental by governments, clinicians, and the general population. In this context of global aging and prolonged life span, the prevalence of dementia has risen to hardly sustainable levels and is expected to triple in a few decades, with severe impacts on communities and health systems (WHO, 2012). Moreover, since achievements in health and medicine are granting more of the population more years (especially in industrialized countries), the concept of spending old age with a good quality of life is gaining popularity, and "normal" (or should we say "common"?) brain aging is becoming less acceptable in a society in which elderly people can live active, satisfying lives while remaining highly productive and socially integrated. Because it is difficult to define normality in terms of cognitive performances among the elderly, it is hard to select the target to aim for in pursuit of satisfactory cognition in this part of the population. If the target is the preservation of a good capability of daily life and activity, then an early intervention with neuroprotective intent could be sufficient. If, on the other hand, we are aiming to restore the function of a central nervous system (CNS) that has already undergone major detrimental modifications, we have to shift from neuroprotection to cognitive enhancement, knowing that current results for the latter approach have been far from excellent.

Based on actual knowledge, it is impossible not to approach cognitive modification during the life span as a holistic problem; the simple and reassuring anatomical subdivision of organs and systems is simply outdated. Nowadays clinicians have to face the fact that the phenotypical manifestation of single system modification (the symptom) is often the result of systemic processes influencing a local condition; the crosstalk among organic systems has to be considered when approaching such complex subjects as CNS function. A demonstration of the latter consideration is the strong association between metabolic derangements or systemic inflammation and cognitive decline (Duarte, 2015; Verdile et al., 2015). Insulin resistance and the consequent metabolic cascade seems to play a major role in cognitive dysfunction (Kim and Feldman, 2015; Verdile et al., 2015). An even more direct correlation can be made between vascular disease and decline in CNS performance, because it markedly influences brain structure and causes easily detectable morphological alterations. So, to plan an efficient program of healthy cognitive aging along with specific neuronal directed care, cardiovascular and metabolic prevention must be considered. Moreover, it is necessary to understand that the human body is not a closed system, so interactions with the environment could have strong repercussions on many physiological and pathological conditions. Nutrition is one major channel of interaction with the environment, largely because of its singular characteristic of frequency and duration in our life. It therefore offers unique possibilities to modulate organic functions both in preventing risky conditions and

Nutrition and Functional Foods for Healthy Aging.
DOI: http://dx.doi.org/10.1016/B978-0-12-805376-8.00019-8

curing established diseases. Epidemiological data support the possible adoption of specific dietary patterns that seem beneficial in preventing or deferring the onset of cognitive decline and dementia (Gillette Guyonnet et al., 2007; Swaminathan and Jicha, 2014; Canevelli et al., 2016). We will now discuss the main evidences about dietary recommendations with possible impacts on cognitive functions, classes of nutrients hypothesized to be beneficial for cognition and the prevention of dementia, and groups of substances that could act as cognitive enhancers.

DIETARY PATTERNS AND COMPLETE NUTRITIONAL PLANS WITH COGNITIVE IMPLICATIONS

The main body of evidence on the effects of diet on cognition has been deduced by retrospective observations. Different cultures have specific dietary habits and because the knowledge that diet has noteworthy repercussions on health is solid and growing, epidemiological research has focused on identifying possible a posteriori protective factors in large cohorts of individuals. In the last two decades, the Mediterranean diet (MeD) has emerged as promising not only for cardiovascular protection but also for preventing cognitive decline (Smith and Blumenthal, 2016). Even if the MeD is largely the most well known nutritional approach to a healthy life, other examples of nutritional habits associated with a successful aging are reaching the attention of the scientific community (Willcox et al., 2014).

Mediterranean Diet

The MeD is representative of a healthy cultural approach to food adopted in many countries in southern Europe. Considered the strong regional characterization of eating habits in countries like Italy, Spain, France, and Greece, united to the geographical modifications in typical recipes that occur even inside the same region at impressive short-distance, it would be naive to think that a monomorphic eating style exists in these countries. The diet regimens historically adopted in states bordering the Mediterranean Sea have a few things in common: a wide base of plant-derived flavonoid-rich products (with seasonal production-oriented rotations that ensure a variety of vegetables, fruits, and spices available for consumption), a daily moderate wine consumption (preferably red), an extensive use of olive oil instead of animal fats, and a preference for low-fat dairy products and limited meat intake substituted by more healthy fish consumption. The actual dietary patterns of Mediterranean countries are the result of repeated and massive beneficial cross-contaminations of cultural heritages (Altomare et al., 2013). The MeD itself has been recognized by the United Nations Educational, Scientific, and Cultural Organization. On the other hand, it is true that nowadays the real mean intake of nutritional component is far from MeD standards in southern Europe (Karamanos et al., 2002), although this highly beneficial nutritional pattern survives in small contexts that maintain high longevity and successful aging phenotypes. The MeD is perfectly in agreement with European Food Safety Authority (EFSA) recommendations on macronutrient composition of a healthy diet (EFSA, 2010a,b, 2012) considering that it should be characterized by a high intake of carbohydrates (approximately 65%—and EFSA recommends 45–65%) with large amounts of vegetables (wild edible herbs included), legumes, fruits and (whole) cereals, moderate consumption of fats (approximately 30%, mostly unsaturated—and EFSA recommends 20–35%) of prevalent origin from plants (olive oil and nuts), low-fat dairy products and fish, and just minor contribution of red meat and animal fat, and lesser amounts of proteins (approximately 15%—and EFSA recommends 10–20%). The typical low-dose alcohol intake should come preferably from red wine (high polyphenol content, resveratrol included), but theoretically it could also come through other forms of fermentation-derived beverages (which often happens because of economic and cultural factors) that could have beneficial effects even if of slightly smaller magnitude (e.g., good-quality beer with low alcohol concentration and high yeast, polyphenols, B vitamins, and silicon, an antagonist of aluminum absorption, content) (Kondo, 2004; González-Muñoz et al., 2008; Arranz et al., 2012).

Only in the last decades has MeD been widely recognized as an effective lifestyle modification that is useful in preventing age-related cognitive decline and dementia (Solfrizzi and Panza, 2014; Valls-Pedret et al., 2015). While the notion of the whole-diet effect was growing, single components—macronutrients and micronutrients—arose as possible functional foods having protective roles (Frisardi et al., 2010; Panza et al., 2004), especially mono- and polyunsaturated fatty acids (MUFAs and PUFAs) with particular regard to omega-3 (O3) and omega-6 (O6), light to moderate alcohol consumption, and fruit and vegetables intake (mainly because of their high vitamin, flavonoid, and antioxidant contents) (Frisardi et al., 2010; Mecocci et al., 2014; Polidori et al., 2009; Solfrizzi et al., 2011). Some authors suggest that the reduced risk of obesity, diabetes, and cardiovascular events in individuals adhering to MeD could at least partially justify the postulated effect of cognitive decline prevention (Solfrizzi et al., 2011), especially considering the impact of brain vascular damage on cognitive vulnerability in the elderly and on the progression of dementia of any etiology, including Alzheimer's disease (AD) (Solfrizzi et al., 2011; Polidori et al., 2012). Moreover, insulin resistance, obesity-related inflammatory state, and obviously overt diabetes are strongly associated with cognitive decline (Biessels and Reagan, 2015; Duarte, 2015; Verdile et al., 2015). Anyway, due to recent scientific acquisitions in terms of synergy among nutraceuticals with neuroprotective effects (Mecocci et al., 2014), it is reasonable to differentiate the vascular protection from the other possible beneficial effects of these substances on CNS.

Dietary Approaches Other Than the Mediterranean Diet

MeD is not the only dietary pattern epidemiologically correlated with successful aging (and cognitive function sparing). In southern Japan, e.g., the Ryukyu Islands (Okinawa prefecture) represent a model of lifestyle compatible with long life and healthy aging (Willcox and Willcox, 2014). The Okinawan traditional diet is a low-caloric nutritionally dense dietary pattern that has been associated with a low incidence of age-related chronic diseases (cardiovascular diseases, cancer, and dementia) (Willcox and Willcox, 2014). Being similar to the MeD, it is characterized by high consumption of vegetables (flavonoid- and antioxidant-rich products) and legumes (mainly soy); moderate consumption of alcohol, fish, and carbohydrates with low glycemic index; and low animal protein and fat intake (the main part of fats are represented by O3 and monounsaturated fats). Willcox and colleagues emphasize the extensive use of functional foods as staple dietary elements that are rich in fiber, antioxidants, and vitamins such as the Okinawan sweet potato (*Ipomoea batatas*), a good source of calories with a really low glycemic index (reportedly as low as 55). Furthermore, Okinawans highlight the habit of mixing herbs and spices (turmeric, pepper, artemisia, seaweeds) to the dishes to enrich them with functional micronutrients and the use of soy-based products and mushrooms as low fat sources of protein (associated in these foods with minerals, vitamins, and flavonoids as isoflavones of the soy). One interesting extract of white-skinned sweet potato peel (caiapo) used in traditional medicine seems to have insulin sensitizer properties (Ludvik et al., 2003); when added to the diet of patients affected by type 2 diabetes, it seems able to reduce adiponectin and surrogate markers of systemic inflammation and ameliorate lipid profile (Ludvik et al., 2004).

The eating plans just described are derived from observations of "naturally occurring dietary patterns", recently also structured complete nutritional plans expressly created for specific health targets are discussed for their possible neuroprotective properties. The Dietary Approaches to Stop Hypertension (DASH), e.g., has shown that it may be able to prevent cognitive decline (Smith and Blumenthal, 2016). DASH has a high-fiber and plant-derived food content and a moderate protein content, with extremely low fat and sodium intake. In this dietary pattern, probably the huge reduction of cardiovascular risk is one of the major contributors of the reported brain health gained by individuals adopting this eating style (Tangney, 2014). DASH is strikingly capable of reducing blood pressure in a short time of adherence (Conlin et al., 2000), and has demonstrated good efficacy in reducing cardiovascular events and deaths (Fung et al., 2008; Salehi-Abargouei et al., 2013; Wengreen et al., 2013). While there is evidence that the DASH eating plan is associated with reduced age-related cognitive decline (Tangney, 2014; Tangney et al., 2014), a specific retrospective analysis of participants in the Memory and Aging Project seems to show evidence that a combination of this pattern with MeD could be more beneficial in terms of cognitive prevention. This approach has been relabeled as the Mediterranean–DASH Diet Intervention for Neurodegenerative Delay (MIND) (Morris et al., 2015).

Other dietary patterns based on different recommendations have been investigated in relation to neurodegeneration: e.g., the Healthy Diet Indicator, Healthy Eating Index, Programme National Nutrition Santé, and Recommended Food Score (van de Rest et al., 2015). Globally, the most common characteristics could be summarized as high consumption of legumes, nuts, and whole grains (Wengreen et al., 2013); low consumption of red meat and saturated fats (Granic et al., 2016) in deference to more fish and unsaturated fats of plant origin (Panza et al., 2004); and the presence of low-caloric, nutrient-dense functional foods such as vegetables, herbs, and spices (Mecocci and Polidori, 2012; Willcox and Willcox, 2014).

MICRONUTRIENTS WITH POSSIBLE EFFECTS ON COGNITION

Currently, it is not easy to find an official definition of *nutraceutical* (a portmanteau of the words *nutrient* and *pharmaceutical*), but Mecocci and colleagues (2014) synthesized a common meaning that defines *nutraceuticals* as foods or food components with properties potentially beneficial in terms of health maintenance or disease treatment. For didactic purposes, in this chapter we will describe first the micronutrients hypothesized to be biologically active to better understand the complexity of the foods defined as "functional." It is important to understand that preclinical studies investigating the activity of a single micronutrient are far away from providing a clear idea of what happens when a particular food is eaten, especially if it is of plant origin, which usually contains a multitude of micronutrients whose interactions in terms of bioavailability, pharmacokinetics, and pharmacodynamics are hardly predictable. So, even if a substance has demonstrated high beneficial activity in vitro or in animal models, high-quality trials conducted on real-life subjects are necessary to demonstrate a clear repercussion on health and disease. Unfortunately, this level of evidence is lacking for many nutraceuticals at the moment. For similar reasons, the biological activity of a food component is not surely inferable from retrospective analyses of the intake of foods containing high concentrations of the substance under consideration, and the same substance cannot be considered a full substitute for the functional food in which it is a single component. That said, some observations coming from both laboratory and dietary analyses are a good starting point for programming future investigations and hypothesizing effective interventions.

Monounsaturated and Polyunsaturated Fatty Acids

The CNS is characterized by a relatively low regenerative reserve when compared with most other organs, but a residual neurogenesis has been demonstrated in at least two brain regions; in fact, axonal and dendritic plasticity are part of normal brain functioning (Lazarov et al., 2010) and even adult neurons and all glial cells require continuous structural maintenance to guarantee the efficiency and integrity of the system. These remodeling processes are modulated by the availability of substances fundamental to the cell machinery (Angulo-Guerrero and Oliart, 1998). Neuronal cell membrane is of primary importance in modulating the genesis and conduction of the nerve signal and in transmitting it from cell to cell via the specialized membrane that characterizes the synaptic junctions. Lipid membrane components and their quantitative ratios directly influence the density and activity of membrane proteins (ion channels, enzymes, and receptors) that are responsible for efficacious neurotransmission (Kamphuis and Wurtman, 2009). Over a wide range of dietary variations in lipid intake, membranes remain relatively constant in their saturated and monounsaturated fatty acid levels; on the other hand, *n*-6 and *n*-3 PUFA levels in the diet influence sensibly quantity and type of phospholipids in neuron membranes, which seem to be most sensitive to O3 and the O3–O6 PUFA ratio. These differences probably are justified by lack of de novo O3 and O6 PUFA synthesis by higher animals (Hulbert et al., 2005). Membrane phospholipids require PUFA, choline, and uridine monophosphate for their synthesis. When all three compounds are administered together to animals, they increase levels of phosphatides, synaptic proteins, dendritic spines, and cholinergic tone in the CNS (Kamphuis and Wurtman, 2009). Among PUFAs present in the human brain, arachidonic acid (AA) and docosahexaenoic acid (DHA) are reported to contribute to about 6% of dry cerebral cortex weight (Svennerholm, 1968). These PUFAs can be obtained by dietary intake (fish and plant oils) or be synthesized from precursors: AA can be produced from linoleic acid (an O6 PUFA present in plant oils, nuts, and legumes) and DHA from α-linolenic acid (an O3 PUFA found in fish and flax seeds) with an intermediate passage through eicosapentaenoic acid and docosapentaenoic acid. In addition to direct metabolic activity on the SNC, these long-chain O3 PUFAs exert various degrees of antiinflammatory effects (Dyall, 2015), a fact that renders them hypothetically useful in mitigating brain aging and many neurodegenerative processes (Janssen and Kiliaan, 2014). PUFA supplementation has shown promising results in experimental studies, and O3 intake over a substantial part of rodent life showed reduced neuronal damage (in terms of hippocampal atrophy and the deposition of amyloid beta, Aβ) and slowing cognitive decline (Cederholm et al., 2013). In humans, our knowledge is derived primarily from epidemiological studies in which fish intake or DHA plasma concentrations correlated with the delay of cognitive decline, better performances at neurological testing, and less brain atrophy (Cederholm et al., 2013); limited good quality trials are available, however. Even if it seems that O3 PUFA supplementation could be beneficial in healthy adults with mild memory complaints, similar positive effects in patients with dementia seem to be restricted to those that are ApoE4 allele negative (Salem et al., 2015), actually there is no conclusive evidence of efficient prevention of incident dementia or significant cognitive advantages in healthy subjects or dementia patients (Sydenham et al., 2012; Burckhardt et al., 2016).

Polyphenols

Polyphenols are constituents of foods of plant origin characterized by one or more hydroxyl groups on an aromatic ring (phenol group). The number of phenol rings and structural elements that bind them are used to classify them. The main groups are flavonoids, phenolic acids, phenolic alcohols, stilbenes, and lignans (D'Archivio et al., 2007). Neuroprotection mediated by polyphenols is mainly due to their antioxidant, antiinflammatory, and antiamyloidogenic effects (Pérez-Hernández et al., 2016). Experimental data strongly support a possible activity of polyphenols in neuroprotection, and epidemiological data indirectly agree with such evidence even though randomized trials are scant and controversial.

Flavonoids

Flavonoids are a group of polyphenolic substances commonly found in several types of food of plant origin. They are easily found in high concentration in vegetables, fruits, cereals (Gupta and Prakash, 2014), herbs, and spices (Mecocci et al., 2014) and sometimes contributing significantly to color, flavor or taste of foods. Flavonoids are a large family of substances (more than 4000, of which several hundred are found in edible plants) and have multiple roles in plants—from attracting pollinating insects to protecting plants from environmental stressors (Kumar and Pandey, 2013). A chemical classification can be adopted to divide them into six categories: flavanols, flavonols, flavones, isoflavones, flavanones, and anthocyanidins (Kumar and Pandey, 2013; Mecocci et al., 2014). Their hypothesized properties, however, can belong to different but often overlapping chemical classes. Flavonoids are reported to interact with neuronal and glial cellular signaling pathways (Moosavi et al., 2015) to perform several functions: promote peripheral and locoregional vasodilation modulating cerebral blood flow (Spencer et al., 2009; Nehlig, 2013; Rendeiro et al., 2015), exert antioxidant and antiinflammatory activity in biological systems that mitigates neuronal and endothelial damage (González et al., 2011; Magalingam et al., 2015), contain pathological damage in neurodegenerative diseases (Magalingam et al., 2015; Moosavi et al., 2015), and act as hormone mimetics that induce possible beneficial modifications (Mecocci et al., 2014; Kridawati et al., 2016). Considering the cognitive impact of these molecules, probably the most interesting proposal has been a possible role for flavonoids in modulating neuroplasticity in terms of both neurogenesis (Spencer et al., 2009) and synaptogenesis (Rendeiro et al., 2015). All of these activities render flavonoids a promising option in attempting to slow age-related declines in cognitive performances and possibly treat neurodegenerative diseases (Spencer et al., 2009). Estimated dietary intakes from multiple databases in the United States seem to suggest that individuals aged 19 years and older consume approximately 200–250 mg/day of flavonoids: mostly flavanols (about 80%) followed by minor quantities of flavonols, flavanones, and anthocyanidins, and less than 1% of isoflavones and flavones (Sebastian et al., 2015; Kim et al., 2016).

Due to the chemical differences of the various compounds belonging to the flavonoid family and the different characteristics of plants that hosts them, their bioavailability varies broadly among subtypes. β-glycosidic bonds of flavonoids are a critical limit to absorption (Nemeth et al., 2003), and aglycan forms (e.g., catechins) are usually considered to be more readily absorbed. Glycosylated forms are more available after degradation by bacterial flora (such as soy isoflavones during fermentation or others in colonic microambient with the side effect of partial degradation of the flavonoids themselves) or small intestine brush border enzymes. An exception that must be mentioned is the active absorption in the small intestine of some hydrophilic flavonoid glycosides (such as quercetin) by membrane transporters that could enhance the bioavailability of these molecules and possibly render it even better than that of their aglycan forms (Hollman et al., 1999; Manach et al., 2004; Makino et al., 2009). It is intuitive that, along with the potency of their biological effects, the bioavailability of flavonoids is a crucial element considering the possible clinical efficacy of a nutritional intervention.

Flavanols

Flavanols, specifically monomeric flavanols (catechin, epicatechin, epigallocatechin, gallocatechin, and their gallate derivatives) and their polymerization products (proanthocyanidine), are present in noteworthy concentrations in cocoa powder and chocolate (Nehlig, 2013), teas, and grapes (Mecocci et al., 2014). In black teas, teaflavin and tearubigin also can be found in significant concentrations. Catechins are the most readily absorbable flavonoids because they are the only form not bound to sugars (flavonoids glicosides are more easily absorbed after transformation in aglycan form) (Kumar and Pandey, 2013). It is debatable whether this class of substances should be grouped with flavonoids since they have a slightly different chemical structure, but they will be discussed here because they share with other compounds of this class a high antioxidant activity, common food sources, and possible beneficial biological functions. Grape and grape juice (rich in catechin and epicatechin) seem capable of reducing glutamate excitotoxicity and exert powerful antioxidant activity and thus ameliorate endothelial function and reduce platelet aggregation and low-density lipoprotein (LDL) oxidation (Mecocci et al., 2014). These effects are a good basis from which to approach reducing the risk of onset or progression of cerebrovascular damage, even if they come from indirect evidence (grape juice and not a single micronutrient administration). Results from preclinical and human studies on flavanol- rich cocoa administration (in which epicatechin is the most represented flavanol) have shown that it could result in the reduction of age-related cognitive decline, the risk of AD, and depression. Moreover, as previously described for the flavonoid class, this substance seems capable of improving cerebral blood flow, synaptic plasticity, and mitochondrial function (Nehlig, 2013). A high-flavanol dietary supplement administered to elder adults was found to enhance activity in brain regions involved in age-related cognitive decline (dentate gyrus, assessed by functional MRI) and to improve performance at cognitive testing (Brickman et al., 2014). Epigallocatechin gallate, the most abundant flavanol in green and black tea, has shown promising preclinical results in reducing AD and cognitive decline induced by vascular damage (Mecocci et al., 2014).

Flavonols

Among flavonols, quercetin is probably the most studied. Along with kaempferol and myricetin, quercetin is probably the most represented flavonol in edible foods (onions, apples, green teas, and capers are good dietary sources of flavonols). Quercetin has shown promising antioxidant (Kelsey et al., 2010) and antiinflammatory capabilities (Bischoff, 2008; Bureau et al., 2008; Mecocci et al., 2014) in preclinical models of neuronal damage, and it is especially known for its ability to chelate and stabilize the generation of iron-reducing radicals (Kumar and Pandey, 2013). The combined antioxidant and antiinflammatory activity could be partially responsible for improvements seen in models of cerebrovascular damage after flavonols administration (Dajas et al., 2003). Moreover, due to its impact on multiple mechanisms related to neurodegenerative diseases, quercetin has been proposed also as a complementary treatment for AD. Preclinical investigations seem to support a favorable interaction with Aβ42, reducing its direct neurotoxicity (Ansari et al., 2009; Tchantchou et al., 2009) and even providing a potential role in improving memory (possibly due to its anticholinesterase activity) (Orhan et al., 2007), hippocampal synaptic plasticity (as observed in models of neuronal damage induced by exposure to lead) (Mecocci et al., 2014), and neurogenesis (Tchantchou et al., 2009). Similar to quercetin, kaempferol has demonstrated an ability to contain oxidative damage in cellular cultures and to improve memory and learning in mice models (Mecocci et al., 2014). Spencer and colleagues report that flavonol intake (including quercetin, kaempferol, and myricetin) has favorable effects on learning and memory (Spencer et al., 2009). The proposed mechanisms of neuroprotection, other than direct interaction with Aβ42 oligomers (Tchantchou et al., 2009), are increased activation of cyclic-AMP response element binding protein and subsequent release of neurotrophins that are important in memory processes (Spencer et al., 2009; Tchantchou et al., 2009). Recently, fisetin also received attention due to its strong antioxidant activity (Ishige et al., 2001), and subsequent studies identified it as a promising neuroprotective compound since it showed antiinflammatory, neurotrophic, and antiamyloid properties and has been proposed to be able to improve memory, probably by facilitating long-term potentiation in hippocampal neuron cells (Currais et al., 2014). Due to its many beneficial properties, fisetin has been proposed as a possible integration in the treatment of AD and Parkinson's disease (PD) (Navabi et al., 2016).

Isoflavones

Isoflavones (genistein, daidzein, glycitin) can be found in high concentrations in soybeans; their supposed beneficial activity seems to be attributable to estrogenic agonism via beta receptors present in the brain (Mecocci et al., 2014). Estrogen-replacement therapy for prevention of cognitive decline and normal brain function maintenance is a debated subject; the supposed increased cholinergic activity and possible neuroprotective effects support a use of this approach (Engler-Chiurazzi et al., 2016) even if the last Cochrane review on the matter found insufficient evidence to support this indication (Hogervorst et al., 2009). Preclinical exploration on administration of soy isoflavones obtained discrete results in terms of improvement of memory and cognition (Kridawati et al., 2016), but epidemiological data on soy consumption are controversial (Gleason et al., 2009), and evidence of active dietary integration in humans is scant (Mecocci et al., 2014). Meta-analyses and interventional trials on this subject showed little or no statistically significant benefits of integration in postmenopausal women (Hogervorst et al., 2009; Henderson et al., 2012; Cheng et al., 2015) as well as in older people of both genders with and without dementia (Gleason et al., 2009, 2015). Some authors suggest that a possible explanation of failures of integration could be found in timing (Cheng et al., 2015) or in the capacity to metabolize the isoflavones (Gleason et al., 2015) (S-equol, a potent agonist of beta estrogen receptors is produced through daizdein elaboration by gut microbiota of some but not all individuals) (Setchell and Clerici, 2010). Nowadays, conclusive evidence on cognitive benefits of soy isoflavones intake is lacking, and their relationship with possible health issues is debated: some authors suggest a possible role in cancer prevention in healthy individuals (Varinska et al., 2015), while others recommend caution especially in administering pure isoflavones to individuals who can be harmed by estrogen replacement (Allred et al., 2004).

Flavones

Several flavones have been explored for neuroprotection in preclinical models. Luteolin, a flavonoid found in parsley, celery, and rosemary (Mecocci et al., 2014), has demonstrated a clear neuroprotective effect in streptozotocin-induced AD rat model ameliorating spatial learning and memory impairment (Wang et al., 2016). Luteolin effects are at least partially explainable by inhibition of microglia-induced inflammation (Jang et al., 2010; Navabi et al., 2015a). In humans, luteolin has shown promising effects on so-called brain fog—impaired cognition, concentration, and multitasking abilities—i.e., sometimes associated with reductions in short- and long-term memory occurring in a wide range of neuropsychiatric disorders and as cognitive complications of systemic syndromes with notable inflammatory components (Theoharides et al., 2015). A liposomal luteolin formulation in olive fruit extract improved attention in children affected by autism spectrum disorders and brain fog in patients affected by systemic diseases with mild cognitive implications (Theoharides et al., 2015). Apigenin, another common flavone, has shown similar prevention activity on neuroinflammation as reported by Millington and colleagues: apigenin-treated mice improved memory and learning abilities reducing fibrillar amyloid deposits via beta-secretase 1 modulation (Millington et al., 2014). Moreover, this flavone seems capable of restoring the cortical *extracellular signal-regulated kinase–cAMP-response element binding protein–brain-derived neurotrophic factor* pathway typically compromised in AD patients and exerts neurovascular protective effects. Finally, in animal models of inflammatory response, it acted to reduce inflammatory cytokines (Millington et al., 2014), and in rat models of diabetes it was able to attenuate diabetes-associated cognitive decline by modulating apoptotic signals and nitric oxide production (Mao et al., 2015). Similar to apigenin, other flavones also have been studied in relation to their neuroprotective capabilities. Chrysin, a flavone present in various fruits, vegetables, and mushrooms, has been proposed as antiinflammatory, antiamyloidogenic, and neurotrophic for nervous cells (Navabi et al., 2015b). Baicalein, oroxylin A, and wogonin (all isolated from *Scutellaria baicalensis* root) enhanced cognitive and mnestic functions in animal models of aging brains and neurodegeneration and demonstrated neuroprotective potential in models of oxidative stress–induced, Aβ and alpha-synuclein–induced neuronal damage (Gasiorowski et al., 2011).

Flavanones

Among flavanones, pinocembrin (present in honey, propolis, ginger roots, wild marjoram, piper leaves, oregano, licorice aerial parts) (Rasul et al., 2013; Lan et al., 2016) is emerging for its neuroprotective characteristics. In animal models of cerebral ischemic damage, pinocembrin ameliorated cognitive impairment and energy metabolism (Guang and Du 2006; Meng et al., 2014) and demonstrated the ability to counteract Aβ toxicity (Liu et al., 2012). In elderly adults, an 8-week consumption of flavanone-rich orange juice was associated with cognitive benefits (Kean et al., 2015).

Anthocyanins

Anthocyanins and their aglycone forms (antocyanidins—malvidin, cyanidin, peonidin, and delphinidin) are flavonoids present in noteworthy concentrations in berries (blueberries, bilberries, cranberries, elderberries, raspberry seeds, and strawberries) (Mecocci et al., 2014). Their intense red, blue, and purple colors render these substances attractive for industries as food coloring additives. Their activity may involve control of inflammation, amelioration of global metabolic profile and mitochondrial energy metabolism, scavenging of reactive oxygen species, and promotion of neuronal plasticity (Domitrovic 2011; de Pascual-Teresa, 2014; Mecocci et al., 2014). It is interesting that anthocyanins can be found in rat brain when fed with blueberries (cerebellum, cortex, hippocampus, or striatum), and their concentration correlates with the rat performance in the Morris water maze, suggesting a possible direct activity on memory and learning (Andres-Lacueva et al., 2005). Anthocyanins demonstrated beneficial effects in both AD (Badshah et al., 2015) and PD (Strathearn et al., 2014) cellular models of neurodegeneration.

Other Polyphenols

Flavonoids are not the only naturally occurring bioactive phenolic compounds to show neuroprotective activity. Among the growing mass of polyphenols subject to investigation as neuroprotectors, resveratrol and curcumin surely reached the attention of the scientific world due to their potential for multiple health implications. Resveratrol is present in high concentrations in grapes and wine, while curcumin is easily isolable by turmeric and other plants of the Zingiberaceae family (ginger family). Both substances have been described as enhancing cerebral blood flow (Awasthi et al., 2010; Kennedy et al., 2010) and acting as antidepressants (plausibly modulating the monoaminergic system) (Kulkarni et al., 2008; Ogle et al., 2013; Al-Karawi et al., 2016); some of these effects are enhanced by piperine (an alkaloid present in the piper family) (Shoba et al., 1998; Bhutani et al., 2009; Huang et al., 2013; Wightman et al., 2014). Sadly, the measured increments in cerebral blood flow did not produce detectable cognitive enhancement (Wightman et al., 2015), and there is the possibility that the augmented bioavailability obtained with coadministration of piperine could decapitate the bioactivity of polyphenols (Arcaro et al., 2014). Resveratrol and curcumin act on a variety of biological processes involved with chronic diseases (Ghosh et al., 2015; Diaz-Gerevini et al., 2016; Pulido-Moran et al., 2016) and have been proposed as anti-AD medications due to their antioxidant, antiinflammatory and antiamyloidogenic properties (Villaflores et al., 2012). In a group of healthy elderly volunteers, acute administration of solid lipid curcumin formulation enhanced attention and working memory tasks when compared with placebo, while chronic supplement has shown benefits to working memory and mood along with reduced total and LDL cholesterol (Cox et al., 2015). The available human trials on dementia patients are few and undersized, and they did not show significant and clinically relevant amelioration of cognition measured with neuropsychological tests or in functional reserve or neuropsychiatric symptomatology (Brondino et al., 2014). Resveratrol, on the other hand, has shown controversial results in AD patients that are difficult to interpret, especially in light of previous experimental evidence: resveratrol altered Aβ40 in cerebrospinal fluid (CSF) and in the plasma of AD patients, resulting in a lesser reduction of the marker over time. Aβ42 has shown a similar trend, but it is not statistically significant; resveratrol-treated patients had increased volume loss as measured with MRI (Turner et al., 2015). These results show that it is probable that oral resveratrol administration would exert effects on the CNS, reaching and modifying the CSF environment. However, because the cited study found no clinical difference between AD patients treated with resveratrol and placebo, it is still not possible to determine if the observed changes reflect a change in the pathological course of the illness or if this eventual change consists in amelioration or worsening of the baseline condition. Aβ42 in CSF has been observed to be reduced by more than 50% in AD patients versus healthy controls (Buchhave et al., 2009), so the trend to lesser reduction in time in the resveratrol group could still emerge as a sign of good interaction between resveratrol and the amyloid-burdened CNS. It is more difficult to interpret the brain volume loss, usually a marker of worse prognosis, as a sign of better CNS functioning; in studies of human immunization against Aβ and in trials on bapinezumab (a murine antibody against Aβ), brain volume loss has been observed in the absence of significant clinical implications (Turner et al., 2015). Until new evidence sheds light on the relationship between resveratrol and dementia, caution should be used in administering high doses of resveratrol supplements to patients affected by AD. Similar caution is advised for high-dose supplementation in healthy subjects because experimental findings on animal models suggest possible inhibition of neural progenitor cell duplication (Park et al., 2012). Further studies are needed to better understand this phenomenon.

Vitamins and Related Substances

Vitamin deficiencies often affect the CNS. The role of different vitamins for prevention and treatment of cognitive decline has been investigated in experimental models, epidemiological studies, and interventional trials. In this field, the possible role of B group vitamins and choline (although the latter is not strictly a vitamin) as either a direct metabolic effect or as a homocysteine-lowering therapy, has been treated elsewhere in this book (see Chapter 15 on the role of B group vitamins and choline in cognition and brain aging). Other vitamins recently investigated for the same purpose are vitamins A (Obulesu et al., 2011), C (Harrison, 2012), D (van der Schaft et al., 2013; Schlögl and Holick, 2014), and E (La Fata et al., 2014).

Vitamin A, Retinoids, and Carotenoids

Vitamin A is a generic name that describes substances with activities similar to retinol (Hinds et al., 1997). Retinoids are substances of natural (mainly animal) or synthetic origin, some of which exert biological activity, but not all the members of this group of substances have the same properties. For example, retinol is a precursor of visual pigments while retinoic acid has no visual functions but is a strong modulator of cellular growth and differentiation (Hinds et al., 1997). Carotenoids, on the other hand, are pigments of plant origin with antioxidant properties, some of which can be converted into retinol or retinyl esters (Hinds et al., 1997). Of the hundreds of different members of the carotenoid family, more than 40 have been found in the human body, among them β-carotene, lycopene, and lutein, which have been investigated in search of neuroprotective properties (Mecocci et al., 2014). Common food sources of vitamin A analogs and precursors are liver, eggs, milk, and some vegetables, especially the orange-yellow ones. Vitamin A has a known role in CNS development and differentiation; in the adult brain, its role is poorly understood, but it plausibly maintains regulatory capacities on genic expression and synaptic plasticity, seriously impacting memory and learning. That suggests a possible role in neurodegenerative diseases (Tafti and Ghyselinck, 2007). Plasma and cerebrospinal concentrations of vitamin A have been reported to be lower in AD patients than in controls, and in vitro evidence supports antiamyloidogenic activities for vitamin A and its precursor, β-carotene (Ono and Yamada, 2012). Although suggested as an addition to therapeutic protocols for a wide range of pathologies (skin, blood, retinal, and pulmonary diseases), vitamin A has a narrow therapeutic index that often limits its use. The CNS activity seems to be no exception: animal models indicate that the beneficial neurotrophic activity of retinoic acid can be disrupted by both deficiency and excess intake of this vitamer, resulting in reduced cell proliferation and synaptic activity in the hippocampus (Olson and Mello, 2010). Being provitamins, carotenoids have a better tolerability profile and exert a significant antioxidant effect different from liposoluble retinoids; concerns of teratogenicity and possible cancer promotion for high-dose supplementation in certain populations suggest caution in choosing dosages of supplementation (Russell, 2004). Among carotenoids lycopene and β-carotene have been found to be associated with better cognitive performance in cognitively healthy individuals (Mecocci et al., 2014).

Further studies are necessary to determine the possible role of bioactive compounds with vitamin A activity on normal brain aging and neurodegenerative diseases.

Vitamins C and E

Both vitamins C (ascorbic acid) and E (a family of compounds of which alpha-tocopherol is probably one of the most studied in the field of neurodegeneration) are potent antioxidants. In patients affected by AD, lower plasma levels of vitamin C and E have been reported (Lopes da Silva et al., 2014), and dietary intake of both vitamins seems to be protective in terms of AD onset (Li et al., 2012). Different results have been observed when supplementation was adopted. From interventional studies, it emerged that vitamin E could be beneficial in treating patients affected by dementia (Sano et al., 1997; Dysken, 2014). Evidence is not conclusive on the effect of vitamin E supplementation (mainly in the form of alpha-tocopherol) to treat mild cognitive impairment and dementia, and a recent meta-analysis did not show any solid effect (Farina et al., 2012). Similar results emerged from vitamin C supplementation studies (Boothby and Doering, 2005). While vitamin C administration has virtually no side effect, prolonged administration of high dosages of vitamin E (twice or more the recommended tolerable upper intake limit of 1100 international units/day) is discouraged due to suspicions of a possible relationship with increased mortality (Miller et al., 2005), possibly due to reduced vitamin K bioavailability and increased hemorrhagic risk.

Vitamin D

Vitamin D comprises a group of a few natural and synthetic vitamers with similar biological activities (Cashman, 2012). Adequate sunlight exposure on the skin in the presence of normal kidney and liver function is usually sufficient to meet the requirements of young and adult individuals; dietary intake has a minor role in these individuals (Cashman, 2012). Older individuals have a high prevalence of deficiency; in these subjects, dietary intake is often fundamental, especially in terms of supplements (Souberbielle, 2016). Cod oil, eggs, and dairy products are food with sensible concentrations of vitamin D (Stephen, 1975; Cortese et al., 2015). In recent years, vitamin D deficiency has been related to cognitive impairment and reduced hippocampal volume (Annweiler et al., 2013; Karakis et al., 2016). Supplementation with exogenous vitamin D has shown to ameliorate the observed impairment, but the level of performance obtained by supplementation was not statistically different from that of the control group (Annweiler et al., 2013). It is not clear if supplementation of healthy individuals could ameliorate cognitive function.

Methylxanthines

Methylxanthines are alkaloids that can be found in high concentrations in tea, coffee, and chocolate. Theophilline, theobromine, and caffeine are the most popular. They can be found in different concentrations in coffee, chocolate, and tea. Caffeine is the main methilxanthine of coffee; theobromine is abundant in chocolate in which the theobromine–caffeine ratio varies widely, but it is typically higher than 1; and theophilline is the primary methylxanthine in tea (Franco et al., 2013). The common experience is that coffee increases attention; in effect, caffeine and other methylxanthines have been described as being able to act as mild psychostimulants (Lorist and Tops, 2003; Nehlig, 2010; Mitchell et al., 2011; Franco et al., 2013). Epidemiological studies related caffeine consumption in healthy subjects with prevention of neurodegenerative diseases (Nehlig, 2010); in particular it seems that consumption of caffeinated coffee could prevent or defer the onset of AD and PD (Maia and de Mendonca, 2002; Eskelinen et al., 2009; Costa et al., 2010). Methylxanthine mechanisms of action at the CNS level include antagonism of adenosine receptors, regulation of intracellular calcium levels, phosphodiesterase inhibition, and modulation of GABA receptor action (Franco et al., 2013). Moderate consumption of methylxanthine from food sources is safe, but high doses (e.g., caffeine supplements) could produce anxiety and increase heart rate and gastric acid secretion (Franco et al., 2013).

Terpenes

Carnosic and rosmarinic acids, two phenolic acids that can be found in rosemary, seem to act as neuroprotectors in vitro and in animal models (Mecocci et al., 2014). Their mechanism of action is far from being completely understood, and more evidence, especially on human subjects, is needed to express a preliminary opinion on the matter. Surely, as with many other compounds cited in this chapter, terpenes have the requisites to be considered seriously for future research.

FOODS, HERBS, SPICES, AND DIETARY COMPLEMENTS WITH FUNCTIONAL PROPERTIES IN TERMS OF NEUROPROTECTION AND POSSIBLE COGNITIVE ENHANCEMENT

So far we have described the full dietary patterns that are actually identified from retrospective analyses as the healthiest for achieving a successful cognitive aging. We also have examined more extensively the micronutrients assumed to be among the causes of the aforementioned epidemiological data. Now we can focus on complex dietary elements (containing more than one beneficial micronutrient) that have the characteristics to be described as functional foods for cognition with a better comprehension of the possible underlying mechanisms. The majority of them exert mainly neuroprotective effects, while others can be defined *nootropics* (from the Greek root *noos* for mind and *tropein* for toward) (Lanni et al., 2008)—in other words, substances that are able to ameliorate cognitive performances as either acute or chronic effects.

Berries

With the name *berries*, we group fruits belonging to different plant families (e.g., strawberry, raspberry, and blackberry belong to Rosacee, and blueberry and cranberry to Ericaceae) that have in common a high content of polyphenolic compounds (Skrovankova et al., 2015), vitamins (A, C, E, and B group vitamins with the exception of vitamin B_{12}) in various concentrations. All of them have strong antioxidant capacities (Pribis and Shukitt-Hale, 2014). Currently, several experiments have demonstrated the capacity of berry consumption to slow age-related cognitive decline, enhance neuroplasticity, and ameliorate cognitive functions in animal models of dementia (Balk et al., 2006; Subash et al., 2014). On the basis of experimental evidence, several longitudinal studies are ongoing to ascertain if berries consumption can achieve results in human that are similar to the ones observed for laboratory animals (Pribis and Shukitt-Hale, 2014). Recently, a long-term longitudinal observation conducted on participants in the Nurses' Health Study has shown lesser cognitive decline in patients with greater intakes of blueberries and strawberries (Devore et al., 2012).

Nuts

Nuts exhibit a singular mix of neuroprotective compounds. They are particularly rich in fats (mainly MUFAs and PUFAs) and soluble fibers, high-quality vegetal proteins, vitamins (folate, riboflavin, and tocopherols), phytosterols and polyphenols, and minerals and trace elements (Ros, 2010; Pribis and Shukitt-Hale, 2014). The most consumed tree nuts are cashews, macadamias, pistachios, hazelnuts, almonds, and walnuts (the latter two are probably the ones among nuts with more evidence of possible effects on cognition). Peanuts, although botanically grouped as legumes, have nutritional characteristics similar to tree nuts and can be grouped with them for the purpose of this chapter (Pribis and Shukitt-Hale, 2014). Numerous experimental and epidemiological studies have correlated nut consumption with better cognitive performance. Antioxidant, anticholinesterase, procholinergic, and cholesterol-reducing activities have been suggested as possible mechanisms of action (Pribis and Shukitt-Hale, 2014). Recently, in a cohort of cognitively healthy adult and elderly Spanish volunteers, the addition of nut intake (30 g/daily of mixed nuts) to a Mediterranean dietary pattern showed improved cognitive function versus a control group fed only with a low-fat diet (Valls-Pedret et al., 2015). Although the latter evidence is biased by the coadoption of MeD (known to exert beneficial effects on cognition), these data should be considered as a solid base for future investigation on the matter.

Olive Oil

Virgin olive oil is a cornerstone of MeD. Although it is a fat, olive oil contains a unique pattern of MUFAs and PUFAs united to a variety of polyphenols (mainly oleuropein aglycone and oleocanthal) that have shown promising results in experimental AD models (Rigacci, 2015). It seems that the polyphenols associated with this plant-derived product could also ameliorate patient lipid profile by reducing LDL and increasing HDL cholesterol and preventing atherosclerosis, maybe due to their capacity to contain lipoprotein oxidation (Hernáez et al., 2014, 2015). Few randomized controlled trials correlate virgin olive oil intake with improved cognitive function (Martínez-Lapiscina et al., 2013; Valls-Pedret et al., 2015), but evidence is still insufficient to determine the real impact of virgin olive oil supplementation.

Fish

Fish is an important source of long-chain *n*-3 PUFAs, high quality animal proteins, trace elements, and vitamins A, D, and B group (Gil and Gil, 2015). A meta-analysis of 21 cohort studies suggests that consumption of fishery products is associated with reduced incidence of cognitive impairment and dementia (Zhang et al., 2016). This effect on cognitive performance preservation seems to be appreciable even in cohorts of elderly people (Nurk et al., 2007). Actually, there are no sufficient data from randomized controlled trials to establish a sure direct causal effect between fish consumption and cognition, and often researchers focus mainly on O3 rather than on fish itself. However, there is no question that the strong correlation between fish intake and neuroprotection is solid evidence that could itself justify the recommendation to regularly consume fish products. The only concerns emerge from the widespread finding of pollutants in fish, especially those higher in the food chain. Methylmercury is one of the most common pollutants found in fish, but other compounds also have neurotoxic and cancerogenic potential (heavy metals and organic compounds such as organochlorine pesticides, polycyclic aromatic hydrocarbons, polychlorinated biphenyls, dioxins, and dibenzofurans) (Gil and Gil, 2015). Actually, there is no reason to contain an a priori fish intake (Gil and Gil, 2015); the only recommendation is to choose safe and controlled products—as with all other foods.

Allium sativum

Garlic (*Allium sativum*) has been extensively investigated for its multiple potential health benefits. The documented antioxidant, antiatherogenic, antiapoptotic, and antiamyloidogenic activities of various types of garlic extracts are promising features that define this vegetable generally used for seasoning as a possible functional food for neuroprotection at least in terms of preventing AD and neurovascular damage (Mathew and Biju, 2008). Both aged garlic extract (a specific garlic preparation) (Ray et al., 2011) and fresh garlic (Haider et al., 2008) administration seem to be able to improve memory and cognitive functions in laboratory animals. In the last decades, many bioactive compounds have been extracted from garlic. Allicin seems able to slow down atherosclerotic processes in humans (Mahdavi-Roshan et al., 2013) and prevent oxidative stress–induced apoptosis in cellular models (Chen et al., 2014), thiacremonone exhibited antiinflammatory and antioxidant effects and ameliorated cognitive performance in mouse AD models (Yun et al., 2016), and S-allyl-L-cysteine ameliorated cognitive impairment in mouse AD models, probably like the aforementioned compounds that reduce oxidative stress (Javed et al., 2011) and modulate the intracellular pathways related to synaptic degeneration and neuroinflammation (Ray et al., 2011). Moreover, in addition to cognitive improvement, studies examining the whole extract and not the single components have shown reduced mitochondrial impairment, insulin resistance, plasma cholesterol, visceral fat, and body weight in obese insulin-resistant rats fed with a high-fat diet (Pintana et al., 2014) and increased serotoninergic activity in adult rats (Haider et al., 2008).

Another proposed possible mechanism of action for both neuro- and cardioprotective effects of garlic is enhancement of hydrogen sulfide synthesis (Gupta et al., 2010; Kashfi and Olson, 2013), which was recently identified as a gasotransmitter with beneficial effects on endothelial cells and neuromodulatory properties (facilitating long-term potentiation in hippocampal cells via activation of *N*-methyl-D-aspartate receptors, which promotes calcium influx in astrocytes and modulates several intracellular signaling cascades related to neurodegeneration) (Kimura, 2013). The only concern about garlic extract administration could be the impaired hippocampal neurogenesis observed after diallyl disulfide administration (Ji et al., 2013). Better characterization of the compounds contained in garlic extract could assist understanding of the effects on the CNS and improve cognitive outcomes. Considering the similarities observed in sulfur-containing bioactive principles in garlic and onion (*Allium cepa*) (Lanzotti, 2006), it would be interesting also to explore the possible activity on the CNS of this latter vegetable extract.

Cruciferous Vegetables

Epidemiological results from the Hordaland Health Study correlated the consumption of cruciferous vegetables (cauliflower, cabbage, garden cress, bok choy, broccoli, and brussels sprouts, among many others) with better cognitive performance in elderly subjects (Nurk et al., 2010). A possible bioactive molecule responsible for the effects observed in relation to cruciferous vegetable consumption could be sulforaphane, an organosulfur compound (Lee et al., 2014). Sulforaphane reduces cognitive impairment in animal models, seems involved in improving cholinergic neurotransmission (Lee et al., 2014), exerts anxiolytic and antidepressant effects (plausibly inhibiting the hypothalamic–pituitary–adrenal axis and the stress-induced inflammatory response) (Wu et al., 2016), attenuates microglial detrimental interactions with neurons modulating inflammatory response and oxidative stress (Townsend and

Johnson, 2016), and improves mitochondrial function (Carrasco-Pozo et al., 2015). Moreover, it has shown significant action on reducing blood–brain barrier disruption when administered acutely in animal models of brain traumatic injury (Dash et al., 2009) and focal cerebral ischemia (Ma et al., 2015). Prospective studies on humans are required to understand the real impact of this family of vegetables on brain aging and the prevention and treatment of neurodegenerative diseases.

Wine, Grape Juice, and Alcohol

Alcohol is a psychotropic substance known to be neurotoxic in a dose-dependent manner, both in acute intoxication and chronic abuse (Costardi et al., 2015). Similar to what has been observed for coronary heart disease (Roerecke and Rehm, 2014), however, light to moderate alcohol intake seems to be protective for the development of cognitive decline and dementia (Peters et al., 2008; Anstey et al., 2009). Some authors observed a J-shaped relationship between alcohol consumption and progression from mild cognitive impairment to dementia (Xu et al., 2009), confirming the strong suspect that the advantage gained by light alcohol consumption is rapidly lost in heavy drinkers. Wine could represent a good form of alcoholic beverage to be consumed in small quantities daily to prevent cognitive decline due to its modest alcohol concentration and concomitant high polyphenols content (Basli et al., 2012) (for resveratrol hypothesized mechanisms of neuroprotection, see the previous section title "Other Polyphenols"). To support this hypothesis, concord grape juice alone (not fermented) has also shown the ability to enhance memory functions even in the absence of alcohol (Krikorian et al., 2010). The possibility of enriching the diet plan of an individual with limited wine intake should balance the possible benefits and risks (biological and psychological) based on the subject's characteristics and eventual conditions or comorbidities.

Zingiberaceae

Plants belonging to the Zingiberaceae family are rich in polyphenols. Turmeric (*Curcuma longa*) has been proposed as a neuroprotector. The hypothetical effects of its active metabolite curcumin were previously discussed. In one randomized controlled trial, curcumin ameliorated working memory and attention (Cox et al., 2015), but more evidence is required to understand the possible clinical effect of *C. longa* on cognition. *Zingiber officinalis* (ginger) also belongs to the Zingiberaceae family and contains substances similar to the ones found in turmeric; dry ginger extract (Mathew and Subramanian, 2014) and 6-shoganol (Moon et al., 2014) demonstrated neuroprotective activity in vitro. Human evidence is lacking. The only concern is for patients treated with anticoagulants because Zingeiberaceae intake in large quantities could modify their bleeding risk.

Piper nigrum

Black pepper (*Piper nigrum*) is a spice used widely in many traditional cuisines. Recently, the alkamides present in piper have been studied for their antioxidant and anticholinesterase activities (Tu et al., 2015). Among the alkamides isolated from *P. nigrum* extract, piperine, piperettine, and piperettyline exhibited inhibitory activities against both acetylcholinesterase and butyrylcholinesterase, while feruperine was a potent inhibitor only of butyrylcholinesterase (Tu et al., 2015). *Piper nigrum* and piperine improved cognitive functions and exerted antiamyloidogenic activities in animal models of AD (Subedee et al., 2015). Pharmacological research is now aiming to improve piperine bioavailability to develop possible treatments for AD, and there are reports of formulations that have effects similar to donepezil in animal models (Yusuf et al., 2012; Elnaggar et al., 2015). Human studies are lacking, and the utility of piperine still has to be demonstrated in AD patients. Actually, piperine has a recognized role in amplifying the effect of other substances such as curcumin (which increases the bioavailability up to 20-fold when coadministered with piperine) (Patil et al., 2016).

Plants With Anticholinesterase Activity

It has been proposed that AD and age-related cognitive decline could be sustained by an extensive loss of cholinergic activity (Terry and Buccafusco, 2003), which is why AD therapy is now based mainly on cholinesterase inhibitors. Other drugs that improve the cholinergic system activity are considered possible cognitive enhancers. Several plant-derived compounds exhibit anticholinesterase activity in preclinical studies (Konrath et al., 2013; Pinho et al., 2013), but for most molecules human studies are needed to clarify whether these experimental results could be confirmed in vivo. Among actual approved therapies for AD, galanthamine, an alkaloid of natural origin derived from plants belonging to the Amaryllidaceae family, is derived from traditional Chinese medicine and exerts selective action on the enzyme acetylcholinesterase (Ortiz et al., 2012). In addition to cholinergic neurotransmission potentiation, galanthamine has also been described as easing oxidative stress, modulating *N*-methyl-D-aspartate receptor activity, and upregulating antiapoptotic protein expression (Wu et al., 2011). Trials on humans have shown that galanthamine could be beneficial in ameliorating cognitive deficits in AD patients (Tan et al., 2014) and perhaps also in individuals who suffer vascular-induced cognitive impairment even if to a lesser extent (Birks and Craig, 2006). Other herbal remedies used in Chinese and Ayurvedic medicine have been described as having cholinesterase inhibition properties, among them *Huperzia serrata*, *Salvia officinalis*, and *Bacopa monnieri* have also been studied on humans. Huperzine A is an alkaloid extracted from the plant *H. serrata*, which was identified in the 1980s as a potent acetylcholinesterase inhibitor. More recently, a meta-analysis of 20 randomized clinical trials found huperzine to be capable of improving cognitive function, daily living activities, and global clinical assessment in AD patients (Yang et al., 2013). Cognitive effects have also been described for vascular dementia (Xu et al., 2012). A small low-quality study reported mnesic benefits in young healthy subjects (Sun et al., 1999). Some authors report an effect comparable to approved treatments for AD like galanthamine and donepezil (Yang et al., 2013). Leafy parts of plants belonging to *Salvia* species are used in Chinese medicine as herbal remedies for cognitive impairments. At least two sage species (*S. officinalis* and *Salvia lavandulaefolia*) have been studied for their hypothetical nootropic properties (Miroddi et al., 2014). *S. officinalis* extract has antioxidant properties and inhibits acetylcholinesterase in vitro (Wu et al., 2011). A randomized controlled trial in which *S. officinalis* extract was matched against a placebo in mild to moderate AD patients has shown a better cognitive outcome in the treated group (Akhondzadeh et al., 2003). Essential oil and monoterpenoid extract from *S. lavandulaefolia* exhibited cognitive-enhancing properties on small groups of healthy adults (Tildesley et al., 2005; Kennedy et al., 2011). A possible bioactive compound responsible for the cognitive effects of sage has been identified as ursolic acid, a pentacyclic triterpenoid carboxylic acid (Wu et al., 2011). *B. monnieri*, also known as Indian pennywort, is a perennial creeping plant used in Ayurvedic medicine that seems able to improve cognitive performance in neuropsychological tests that require divided attention and programming, reducing choice reaction time (Kongkeaw et al., 2014). The putative bioactive compound responsible for cognitive effects of *B. monnieri* has been named *Bacoside A* (a mix of saponins) (Ramasamy et al., 2015). The hypothesized nootropic mechanisms are acetylcholinesterase inhibition, choline acetyltransferase activation, Aβ reduction, increased cerebral blood flow, and monoamine (dopamine and serotonin) potentiation (Aguiar and Borowski, 2013; Ramasamy et al., 2015).

Tea, Coffee, and Cocoa

Tea, coffee, and cocoa share similar micronutrients. The main bioactive compounds found in these foods with possible cognitive implications are polyphenols (flavonoids) and methylxanthines. The hypothesized effects of these substances have been extensively explored in this chapter. Cocoa has shown neuroprotective properties (Nehlig, 2013), and in the Cocoa, Cognition, and Aging Study, the administration of cocoa drinks containing variable concentrations of flavanols in 90 elderly individuals affected by mild cognitive impairment showed a reduction in blood pressure and insulin resistance and an improvement in cognitive functions measured with neuropsychological tests after just 8 weeks of treatment (Desideri et al., 2012); the effect was proportional to flavanol concentration in the treatment. The consumption of tea, coffee, or caffeine has been often related in epidemiological studies to reduce the incidence of cognitive decline and dementia (Arab et al., 2013), but the variability of the populations studied, the small sample size of cohorts, and the short- to mid-term observations do not ensure that these results could not be biased by confounders (Panza et al., 2015); larger and better designed trials are needed to confirm the beneficial effects of tea and coffee on dementia prevention. Acute administration of caffeine, on the other hand, increases alertness and seems to improve performance in memory tasks, but not all individuals respond equally (several studies have shown that extroverts perform better than introverts after caffeine intake) (Liguori et al., 1999; Smith, 2013), and it is possible that caffeine biological mechanisms modulate neural networks strongly affected by mood and behavior.

Gingko biloba

Ginkgo biloba is an ancient plant and has been found in fossils dating to more than 200 million years ago. *Ginkgo biloba* leaf extract—mainly identified with a mixture of flavonoids, terpenes, and organic acids labeled Egb761—possesses several beneficial properties. In experimental studies, it has been related to improved mitochondrial impairment, antagonism of *N*-methyl-D-aspartate receptors, scavenging of free radicals, inflammation containment, neuroprotection, and reduction of platelet aggregation (Wu et al., 2011). Meta-analyses on *G. biloba*'s nootropic and neuroprotective effects have brought controversial results. In 2009, a Cochrane review concluded that no conclusive evidence supported the use of *G. biloba* for cognitive decline (Birks and Grimley Evans, 2009). More recently, two different meta-analyses agreed on the beneficial effect of *Ginkgo* extract versus placebo (Weinmann et al., 2010; Tan et al., 2015). This plant extract seems to be safe (the only concern is the augmented risk of hemorrhage, especially in patients who use anticoagulants) (Jiang et al., 2005; Birks and Grimley Evans, 2009). Good-quality trials with adequate statistical power will be required to confirm and quantify the effects of *G. biloba* leaf extract.

Crocus sativus

Extracts of *Crocus sativus*, a plant belonging to the Iridaceas family, have shown promising neuroprotective activities in experimental studies. Saffron, a spice derived from the flower of *C. sativus*, contains three bioactive compounds—crocin, crocetin, and saffranal—that exert antioxidant and antiinflammatory effects on the CNS (Khazdair et al., 2015). Due to interactions with dopaminergic, cholinergic, and glutamatergic systems, it has been proposed as an integration in the treatment of various neurodegenerative disorders, especially AD and PD (Khazdair et al., 2015). In AD patients, saffron supplementation has obtained short-term improvement of cognition measured with neuropsychological testing (Akhondzadeh et al., 2010). To date, there is still not sufficient evidence to confirm the efficacy of saffron's bioactive components on cognitive decline prevention or dementia treatment, but preclinical and preliminary clinical data are encouraging.

MEDICAL FOODS

The definition of medical food in the US Orphan Drug Act (21 U.S.C. 360ee (b) (3)) is "a food which is formulated to be consumed or administered enterally under the supervision of a physician and which is intended for the specific dietary management of a disease or condition for which distinctive nutritional requirements, based on recognized scientific principles, are established by medical evaluation" (FDA, 2014). Several medical foods have been developed for treatment of cognitive decline (mainly AD), but we focus here on products that have some evidence of effects on humans (Thaipisuttikul and Galvin, 2012).

Souvenaid®

Souvenaid® is a drink low in calories that has been enriched with a combination of substances (known as Fortasyn Connect) that is supposed to enhance synaptogenesis as observed in animal models (Wurtman, 2014). It contains uridine monophosphate, phospholipids, choline, O3 fatty acids, vitamins, and antioxidants (Thaipisuttikul and Galvin, 2012). Many of these substances can be found in food, but it is difficult to reach the dosages supposed to improve dendritic spine outgrowth with just dietary intake; moreover, uridine in foods usually has a very low bioavailability (Wurtman, 2014). Theoretically improved synaptogenesis should slow or revert cognitive impairment in AD patients, where the disruption of neural networks is a key event in the progression of cognitive decline (de Waal et al., 2014). Few randomized controlled trials are available on human subjects. This medical food appears to be safe, at least for midterm use (48 weeks) (Olde Rikkert et al., 2015). Early instrumental findings in a 24-week trial on drug-naive patients with mild AD treated with Souvenaid® (Souvenir II study) seems to confirm the capability of this medical food of maintaining brain network organization versus a placebo (de Waal et al., 2014). Results from a direct comparison of neuropsychological performances in the Souvenir II study group has shown an improvement in the memory subscale of the neuropsychological test battery used to measure cognitive trajectories, but not in the whole battery score, which presented a not statistically significant trend toward better results in the treated group (Scheltens et al., 2012). New data on long-term administration of this drink will be necessary to properly assess possible effects on AD patients.

Axona®

Axona® is a medical food that contains a medium-chain triglyceride, caprylic acid, that acts as a ketogenic compound and is supposed to bypass the energy metabolism impairment observed in AD patients (Thaipisuttikul and Galvin, 2012). AD patients seem to suffer from decreased glucose use in the CNS, especially the carriers of ApoE4 allele (Ohnuma et al., 2016). Ketogenic diets have shown to be able to improve cognitive performances in AD patients, and these findings have been the basis for the development of a ketogenic medical food. Axona® has shown an ability to ameliorate cognitive functions in ApoE4-negative patients with mild to moderate AD when compared to placebo (Henderson, 2008; Henderson et al., 2009; Roman, 2010; Henderson and Poirier, 2011; Ohnuma et al., 2016) This medical food appears to be safe; the main adverse effects are mild gastrointestinal symptoms and diarrhea (Ohnuma et al., 2016). Further studies are needed to select the patients that can benefit most from this medical food, which still must be assessed to determine whether the effects are only symptomatic or if even a transient amelioration of the energy metabolism resolves in an enhanced neuron survival.

CONCLUSIONS

It is incontrovertible that dietary impact on cognitive function is massive. Actually, since effective therapeutic choices are lacking, preventing cognitive decline is the better strategy for facing the expected rise in dementia prevalence. A dietary plan that contemplates low-caloric dishes rich in micronutrients; is low in refined sugars, salt, and fats (especially of animal origin); and has a predominance of plant-derived products and a minor contribution of high-quality animal foods (fish, eggs, low-fat dairy products) is a good approach to pursuing healthy cognitive aging. Particular attention should be paid to reaching an adequate vitamin status, especially late in life when vitamin deficiencies are more common and requirements could be altered by concomitant diseases. In the presence of specific diseases and polypharmacy, a personalized approach (preferably guided by a medical consultant) is certainly more effective than the simple adherence to global guidelines and is safer when speaking of intervention with dietary complements (a product of "natural origin" is not synonymous with "harmless," especially when rich in bioactive compounds). In the presence of cognitive decline, several foods and spice-derived complements could be helpful before or alongside a pharmaceutical approach. In the face of mounting epidemiological data, few high-quality randomized controlled trials are available to confirm and quantify the effect of the multitude of food-derived substances with possible cognitive effects. Medical foods composed of wide-spectrum bioactive compounds have the possibility of multilevel intervention, which represents a great advantage when compared to the high selectivity of tightly targeted drugs. Actually, only two structured medical foods present evidence of a possible effective approach to cases of severe cognitive impairment. Hopefully, in the next decades a better understanding of the biological mechanisms that underlie neurodegeneration and neuroplasticity will grant us a wider choice of effective therapeutic approaches.

References

Aguiar, S., Borowski, T., 2013. Neuropharmacological review of the nootropic herb *Bacopa monnieri*. J. Rejuvenation Res. 16 (4), 313–326.

Akhondzadeh, S., Noroozian, M., Mohammadi, M., Ohadinia, S., Jamshidi, A.H., Khani, M., 2003. *Salvia officinalis* extract in the treatment of patients with mild to moderate Alzheimer's disease: a double blind, randomized and placebo-controlled trial. J. Clin. Pharm. Ther. 28 (1), 53–59.

Akhondzadeh, S., Sabet, M.S., Harirchian, M.H., Togha, M., Cheraghmakani, H., Razeghi, S., et al., 2010. Saffron in the treatment of patients with mild to moderate Alzheimer's disease: a 16-week, randomized and placebo-controlled trial. J. Clin. Pharm. Ther. 35 (5), 581–588.

Al-Karawi, D., Al Mamoori, D.A., Tayyar, Y., 2015. The role of curcumin administration in patients with major depressive disorder: mini meta-analysis of clinical trials. Phytother. Res. 30 (2), 175–183.

Allred, C.D., Allred, K.F., Ju, Y.H., Goeppinger, T.S., Doerge, D.R., Helferich, W.G., 2004. Soy processing influences growth of estrogen-dependent breast cancer tumors. Carcinogenesis 25 (9), 1649–1657.

Altomare, R., Cacciabaudo, F., Damiano, G., Palumbo, V.D., Gioviale, M.C., Bellavia, M., et al., 2013. The Mediterranean diet: a history of health. Iran J. Public Health 42 (5), 449–457.

Andres-Lacueva, C., Shukitt-Hale, B., Galli, R., Jauregui, O., Lamuela-Raventos, R.M., Joseph, J.A., 2005. Anthocyanins in aged blueberry-fed rats are found centrally and may enhance memory. Nutr. Neurosci. 8 (2), 111–120.

Angulo-Guerrero, O., Oliart, R.R., 1998. Effects of dietary polyunsaturated fatty acids on rat brain plasma membrane fatty acid composition. Arch. Latinoam. Nutr. 48 (4), 287–292.

Annweiler, C., Montero-Odasso, M., Llewellyn, D.J., Richard-Devantoy, S., Duque, G., Beauchet, O., 2013. Meta-analysis of memory and executive dysfunctions in relation to vitamin D. J. Alzheimers Dis. 37 (1), 147–171.

Ansari, M.A., Abdul, H.M., Joshi, G., Opii, W.O., Butterfield, D.A., 2009. Protective effect of quercetin in primary neurons against Abeta(1–42): relevance to Alzheimer's disease. J. Nutr. Biochem. 20, 269–275.

Anstey, K.J., Mack, H.A., Cherbuin, N., 2009. Alcohol consumption as a risk factor for dementia and cognitive decline: meta-analysis of prospective studies. Am. J. Geriatr. Psychiatry 17 (7), 542–555.

Arab, L., Khan, F., Lam, H., 2013. Epidemiologic evidence of a relationship between tea, coffee, or caffeine consumption and cognitive decline. Adv. Nutr. 4 (1), 115–122.

Arcaro, C.A., Gutierres, V.O., Assis, R.P., Moreira, T.F., Costa, P.I., Baviera, A.M., et al., 2014. Piperine, a natural bioenhancer, nullifies the antidiabetic and antioxidant activities of curcumin in streptozotocin-diabetic rats. PLoS One 9 (12), e113993.

Arranz, S., Chiva-Blanch, G., Valderas-Martínez, P., Medina-Remón, A., Lamuela-Raventós, R.M., Estruch, R., 2012. Wine, beer, alcohol and polyphenols on cardiovascular disease and cancer. Nutrients 4 (7), 759–781.

Awasthi, H., Tota, S., Hanif, K., Nath, C., Shukla, R., 2010. Protective effect of curcumin against intracerebral streptozotocin induced impairment in memory and cerebral blood flow. Life Sci. 86 (3–4), 87–94.

Badshah, H., Kim, H., Kim, M.O., 2015. Protective effects of anthocyanins against amyloid beta-induced neurotoxicity in vivo and in vitro. Neurochem. Int. 80, 51–59.

Balk, E., Chung, M., Raman, G., Tatsioni, A., Chew, P., Ip, S., et al., 2006. B vitamins and berries and age-related neurodegenerative disorders. Evid. Rep. Technol. Assess. (Full Rep.) 134, 1–161.

Basli, A., Soulet, S., Chaher, N., Mérillon, J.M., Chibane, M., Monti, J.P., et al., 2012. Wine polyphenols: potential agents in neuroprotection. Oxid. Med. Cell. Longev. 2012, 805762.

Bhutani, M.K., Bishnoi, M., Kulkarni, S.K., 2009. Anti-depressant like effect of curcumin and its combination with piperine in unpredictable chronic stress-induced behavioral, biochemical and neurochemical changes. Pharmacol. Biochem. Behav. 92 (1), 39–43.

Biessels, G.J., Reagan, L.P., 2015. Hippocampal insulin resistance and cognitive dysfunction. Nat. Rev. Neurosci. 16 (11), 660–671.

Birks, J., Craig, D., 2006. Galantamine for vascular cognitive impairment. Cochrane Database Syst. Rev. 4, CD004746.

Birks, J., Grimley Evans, J., 2009. Ginkgo biloba for cognitive impairment and dementia. Cochrane Database Syst. Rev. (1), CD003120.

Bischoff, S.C., 2008. Quercetin: potentials in the prevention and therapy of disease. Curr. Opin. Clin. Nutr. Metab. Care 11, 733–740.

Boothby, L.A., Doering, P.L., 2005. Vitamin C and vitamin E for Alzheimer's disease. Ann. Pharmacother. 39 (12), 2073–2080.

Brickman, A.M., Khan, U.A., Provenzano, F.A., Yeung, L.K., Suzuki, W., Schroeter, H., et al., 2014. Enhancing dentate gyrus function with dietary flavanols improves cognition in older adults. Nat. Neurosci. 17 (12), 1798–1803.

Brondino, N., Re, S., Boldrini, A., Cuccomarino, A., Lanati, N., Barale, F., et al., 2014. Curcumin as a therapeutic agent in dementia: a mini systematic review of human studies. ScientificWorldJournal 2014, 174282.

Buchhave, P., Blennow, K., Zetterberg, H., Stomrud, E., Londos, E., Andreasen, N., et al., 2009. Longitudinal study of CSF biomarkers in patients with Alzheimer's disease. PLoS One 4 (7), e6294.

Burckhardt, M., Herke, M., Wustmann, T., Watzke, S., Langer, G., Fink, A., 2016. Omega-3 fatty acids for the treatment of dementia. Cochrane Database Syst. Rev. 4, CD009002. [Epub ahead of print].

Bureau, G., Longpre, F., Martinoli, M.G., 2008. Resveratrol and quercetin, two natural polyphenols, reduce apoptotic neuronal cell death induced by neuroinflammation. J. Neurosci. Res. 86, 403–410.

Canevelli, M., Lucchini, F., Quarata, F., Bruno, G., Cesari, M., 2016. Nutrition and dementia: evidence for preventive approaches? Nutrients 8 (3) pii: E144.

Carrasco-Pozo, C., Tan, K.N., Borges, K., 2015. Sulforaphane is anticonvulsant and improves mitochondrial function. Neurochemistry 135 (5), 932–942.

Cashman, K.D., 2012. The role of vitamers and dietary-based metabolites of vitamin D in prevention of vitamin D deficiency. Food Nutr. Res. 56

Cederholm, T., Salem Jr, N., Palmblad, J., 2013. ω-3 fatty acids in the prevention of cognitive decline in humans. Adv. Nutr. 4 (6), 672–676.

Chen, S., Tang, Y., Qian, Y., Chen, R., Zhang, L., Wo, L., et al., 2014. Allicin prevents H_2O_2-induced apoptosis of HUVECs by inhibiting an oxidative stress pathway. BMC Complement Altern. Med. 14, 321.

Cheng, P.F., Chen, J.J., Zhou, X.Y., Ren, Y.F., Huang, W., Zhou, J.J., et al., 2015. Do soy isoflavones improve cognitive function in postmenopausal women? A meta-analysis. Menopause 22 (2), 198–206.

Conlin, P.R., Chow, D., Miller 3rd, E.R., Svetkey, L.P., Lin, P.H., Harsha, D.W., et al., 2000. The effect of dietary patterns on blood pressure control in hypertensive patients: results from the Dietary Approaches to Stop Hypertension (DASH) trial. Am. J. Hypertens. 13 (9), 949–955.

Cortese, M., Riise, T., Bjørnevik, K., Holmøy, T., Kampman, M.T., Magalhaes, S., et al., 2015. Timing of use of cod liver oil, a vitamin D source, and multiple sclerosis risk: the EnvIMS study. Mult. Scler. 21 (14), 1856–1864.

Costa, J., Lunet, N., Santos, C., Santos, J., Vaz-Carneiro, A., 2010. Caffeine exposure and the risk of Parkinson's disease: a systematic review and meta-analysis of observational studies. J. Alzheimer's Dis. 20, S221–S238.

Costardi, J.V., Nampo, R.A., Silva, G.L., Ribeiro, M.A., Stella, H.J., Stella, M.B., et al., 2015. A review on alcohol: from the central action mechanism to chemical dependency. Rev. Assoc. Med. Bras. 61 (4), 381–387.

Cox, K.H., Pipingas, A., Scholey, A.B., 2015. Investigation of the effects of solid lipid curcumin on cognition and mood in a healthy older population. J. Psychopharmacol. 29 (5), 642–651.

Currais, A., Prior, M., Dargusch, R., Armando, A., Ehren, J., Schubert, D., et al., 2014. Modulation of p25 and inflammatory pathways by fisetin maintains cognitive function in Alzheimer's disease transgenic mice. Aging Cell 13 (2), 379–390.

D'Archivio, M., Filesi, C., Di Benedetto, R., Gargiulo, R., Giovannini, C., Masella, R., 2007. Polyphenols, dietary sources and bioavailability. Ann. Ist. Super. Sanita. 43 (4), 348–361.

Dajas, F., Rivera-Megret, F., Blasina, F., Arredondo, F., Abin-Carriquiry, J.A., Costa, G., et al., 2003. Neuroprotection by flavonoids. Braz. J. Med. Biol. Res. 36, 1613–1620.

Dash, P.K., Zhao, J., Orsi, S.A., Zhang, M., Moore, A.N., 2009. Sulforaphane improves cognitive function administered following traumatic brain injury. Neurosci. Lett. 460 (2), 103–107.

de Pascual-Teresa, S., 2014. Molecular mechanisms involved in the cardiovascular and neuroprotective effects of anthocyanins. Arch. Biochem. Biophys. 559, 68–74.

Desideri, G., Kwik-Uribe, C., Grassi, D., Necozione, S., Ghiadoni, L., Mastroiacovo, D., et al., 2012. Benefits in cognitive function, blood pressure, and insulin resistance through cocoa flavanol consumption in elderly subjects with mild cognitive impairment: the Cocoa, Cognition, and Aging (CoCoA) study. Hypertension 60 (3), 794–801.

Devore, E.E., Kang, J.H., Breteler, M.M., Grodstein, F., 2012. Dietary intakes of berries and flavonoids in relation to cognitive decline. Ann. Neurol. 72 (1), 135–143.

Diaz-Gerevini, G.T., Repossi, G., Dain, A., Tarres, M.C., Das, U.N., Eynard, A.R., 2016. Beneficial action of resveratrol: How and why? Nutrition 32 (2), 174–178.

Domitrovic, R., 2011. The molecular basis for the pharmacological activity of anthocyans. Curr. Med. Chem. 18 (29), 4454–4469.

Duarte, J.M., 2015. Metabolic alterations associated to brain dysfunction in diabetes. Aging Dis. 6 (5), 304–321.

Dyall, S.C., 2015. Long-chain omega-3 fatty acids and the brain: a review of the independent and shared effects of EPA, DPA and DHA. Front. Aging Neurosci. 7, 52.

Dysken, M.W., Sano, M., Asthana, S., Vertrees, J.E., Pallaki, M., Llorente, M., et al., 2014. Effect of vitamin E and memantine on functional decline in Alzheimer disease: the TEAM-AD VA cooperative randomized trial. JAMA 311 (1), 33–44.

EFSA Panel on Dietetic Products, Nutrition, and Allergies (NDA), 2010a. Scientific Opinion on Dietary Reference Values for carbohydrates and dietary fibre. EFSA J. 8 (3), 1462.

EFSA Panel on Dietetic Products, Nutrition, and Allergies (NDA), 2010b. Scientific Opinion on Dietary Reference Values for fats, including saturated fatty acids, polyunsaturated fatty acids, monounsaturated fatty acids, trans fatty acids, and cholesterol. EFSA J. 8 (3), 1461.

EFSA Panel on Dietetic Products, Nutrition, and Allergies (NDA), 2012. Scientific Opinion on Dietary Reference Values for protein. EFSA J. 10 (2), 2557.

Elnaggar, Y.S., Etman, S.M., Abdelmonsif, D.A., Abdallah, O.Y., 2015. Novel piperine-loaded Tween-integrated monoolein cubosomes as brain-targeted oral nanomedicine in Alzheimer's disease: pharmaceutical, biological, and toxicological studies. Int. J. Nanomedicine 10, 5459–5473.

Engler-Chiurazzi, E.B., Singh, M., Simpkins, J.W., 2016. From the 90's to now: a brief historical perspective on more than two decades of estrogen neuroprotection. Brain Res. 633, 96–100.

Eskelinen, M.H., Ngandu, T., Tuomilehto, J., Soininen, H., Kivipelto, M., 2009. Midlife coffee and tea drinking and the risk of late-life dementia: a population-based CAIDE study. J. Alzheimer's Dis. 16, 85–91.

Farina, N., Isaac, M.G., Clark, A.R., Rusted, J., Tabet, N., 2012. Vitamin E for Alzheimer's dementia and mild cognitive impairment. Cochrane Database Syst. Rev. 11, CD002854.

FDA, 2014. Medical Foods Guidance Documents & Regulatory Information. Available online at: <http://www.fda.gov/Food/GuidanceRegulation/GuidanceDocumentsRegulatoryInformation/MedicalFoods/> (accessed 28.04.16.).

Franco, R., Oñatibia-Astibia, A., Martínez-Pinilla, E., 2013. Health benefits of methylxanthines in cacao and chocolate. Nutrients 5 (10), 4159–4173.

Frisardi, V., Panza, F., Seripa, D., Imbimbo, B.P., Vendemiale, G., Pilotto, A., et al., 2010. Nutraceutical properties of Mediterranean diet and cognitive decline: possible underlying mechanisms. J. Alzheimers Dis. 22 (3), 715–740.

Fung, T.T., Chiuve, S.E., McCullough, M.L., Rexrode, K.M., Logroscino, G., Hu, F.B., 2008. Adherence to a DASH-style diet and risk of coronary heart disease and stroke in women. Arch. Intern. Med. 168 (7), 713–720.

Gasiorowski, K., Lamer-Zarawska, E., Leszek, J., Parvathaneni, K., Yendluri, B.B., Błach-Olszewska, Z., et al., 2011. Flavones from root of *Scutellaria baicalensis* Georgi: drugs of the future in neurodegeneration? CNS Neurol. Disord. Drug Targets 10 (2), 184–191.

Ghosh, S., Banerjee, S., Sil, P.C., 2015. The beneficial role of curcumin on inflammation, diabetes and neurodegenerative disease: a recent update. Food Chem. Toxicol. 83, 111–124.

Gil, A., Gil, F., 2015. Fish, a Mediterranean source of n-3 PUFA: benefits do not justify limiting consumption. Br. J. Nutr. 113 (Suppl. 2), S58–S67.

Gillette Guyonnet, S., Abellan Van Kan, G., Andrieu, S., Barberger Gateau, P., Berr, C., Bonnefoy, M., et al., 2007. IANA task force on nutrition and cognitive decline with aging. J. Nutr. Health Aging 11 (2), 132–152.

Gleason, C.E., Carlsson, C.M., Barnet, J.H., Meade, S.A., Setchell, K.D., Atwood, C.S., et al., 2009. A preliminary study of the safety, feasibility and cognitive efficacy of soy isoflavone supplements in older men and women. Age Ageing 38 (1), 86–93.

Gleason, C.E., Fischer, B.L., Dowling, N.M., Setchell, K.D., Atwood, C.S., Carlsson, C.M., et al., 2015. Cognitive effects of soy isoflavones in patients with Alzheimer's disease. J. Alzheimers Dis. 47 (4), 1009–1019.

González-Muñoz, M.J., Peña, A., Meseguer, I., 2008. Role of beer as a possible protective factor in preventing Alzheimer's disease. Food Chem. Toxicol. 46 (1), 49–56.

González, R., Ballester, I., López-Posadas, R., Suárez, M.D., Zarzuelo, A., Martínez-Augustin, O., et al., 2011. Effects of flavonoids and other polyphenols on inflammation. Crit. Rev. Food Sci. Nutr. 51 (4), 331–362.

Granic, A., Davies, K., Adamson, A., Kirkwood, T., Hill, T.R., Siervo, M., et al., 2016. Dietary patterns high in red meat, potato, gravy, and butter are associated with poor cognitive functioning but not with rate of cognitive decline in very old adults. J. Nutr. 146 (2), 265–274.

Guang, H.M., Du, G.H., 2006. Protections of pinocembrin on brain mitochondria contribute to cognitive improvement in chronic cerebral hypoperfused rats. Eur. J. Pharmacol. 542 (1–3), 77–83.

Gupta, C., Prakash, D., 2014. Nutraceuticals for geriatrics. J. Tradit. Complement. Med. 5 (1), 5–14.

Gupta, Y.K., Dahiya, A.K., Reeta, K.H., 2010. Gaso-transmitter hydrogen sulphide: potential new target in pharmacotherapy. Indian J. Exp. Biol. 48 (11), 1069–1077.

Haider, S., Naz, N., Khaliq, S., Perveen, T., Haleem, D.J., 2008. Repeated administration of fresh garlic increases memory retention in rats. J. Med. Food 11 (4), 675–679.

Harrison, F.E., 2012. A critical review of vitamin C for the prevention of age-related cognitive decline and Alzheimer's disease. J. Alzheimers Dis. 29 (4), 711–726.

Henderson, S.T., 2008. Ketone bodies as a therapeutic for Alzheimer's disease. Neurotherapeutics 5 (3), 470–480.

Henderson, S.T., Poirier, J., 2011. Pharmacogenetic analysis of the effects of polymorphisms in APOE, IDE and IL1B on a ketone body based therapeutic on cognition in mild to moderate Alzheimer's disease; a randomized, double-blind, placebo-controlled study. BMC Med. Genet. 12, 137.

Henderson, S.T., Vogel, J.L., Barr, L.J., Garvin, F., Jones, J.J., Costantini, L.C., 2009. Study of the ketogenic agent AC-1202 in mild to moderate Alzheimer's disease: a randomized, double-blind, placebo-controlled, multicenter trial. Nutr. Metab. (Lond.) 6, 31.

Henderson, V.W., St John, J.A., Hodis, H.N., Kono, N., McCleary, C.A., Franke, A.A., et al., 2012. Long-term soy isoflavone supplementation and cognition in women: a randomized, controlled trial. Neurology 78 (23), 1841–1848.

Hernáez, Á., Fernández-Castillejo, S., Farràs, M., Catalán, Ú., Subirana, I., Montes, R., et al., 2014. Olive oil polyphenols enhance high-density lipoprotein function in humans: a randomized controlled trial. Arterioscler. Thromb. Vasc. Biol. 34 (9), 2115–2119.

Hernáez, Á., Remaley, A.T., Farràs, M., Fernández-Castillejo, S., Subirana, I., Schröder, H., et al., 2015. Olive oil polyphenols decrease LDL concentrations and LDL atherogenicity in men in a randomized controlled trial. J. Nutr. 145 (8), 1692–1697.

Hinds, T.S., West, W.L., Knight, E.M., 1997. Carotenoids and retinoids: a review of research, clinical, and public health applications. J. Clin. Pharmacol. 37 (7), 551–558.

Hogervorst, E., Yaffe, K., Richards, M., Huppert, F.A., 2009. Hormone replacement therapy to maintain cognitive function in women with dementia. Cochrane Database Syst. Rev. 21 (1), CD003799.
Hollman, P.C.H., Buijsman, M.N.C.P., van Gameren, Y., Cnossen, P.J., de Vries, J.H.M., Katan, M.B., 1999. The sugar moiety is a major determinant of the absorption of dietary flavonoid glycosides in man. Free Radic. Res. 31 (6), 569–573.
Huang, W., Chen, Z., Wang, Q., Lin, M., Wu, S., Yan, Q., et al., 2013. Piperine potentiates the antidepressant-like effect of trans-resveratrol: involvement of monoaminergic system. Metab. Brain Dis. 28 (4), 585–595.
Hulbert, A.J., Turner, N., Storlien, L.H., Else, P.L., 2005. Dietary fats and membrane function: implications for metabolism and disease. Biol. Rev. Camb. Philos. Soc. 80 (1), 155–169.
Ishige, K., Schubert, D., Sagara, Y., 2001. Flavonoids protect neuronal cells from oxidative stress by three distinct mechanisms. Free Radic. Biol. Med 30, 433–446.
Jang, S., Dilger, R.N., Johnson, R.W., 2010. Luteolin inhibits microglia and alters hippocampal-dependent spatial working memory in aged mice. J. Nutr. 140 (10), 1892–1898.
Janssen, C.I., Kiliaan, A.J., 2014. Long-chain polyunsaturated fatty acids (LCPUFA) from genesis to senescence: the influence of LCPUFA on neural development, aging, and neurodegeneration. Prog. Lipid Res. 53, 1–17.
Javed, H., Khan, M.M., Khan, A., Vaibhav, K., Ahmad, A., Khuwaja, G., et al., 2011. S-allyl cysteine attenuates oxidative stress associated cognitive impairment and neurodegeneration in mouse model of streptozotocin-induced experimental dementia of Alzheimer's type. Brain Res. 1389, 133–142.
Ji, S.T., Kim, M.S., Park, H.R., Lee, E., Lee, Y., Jang, Y.J., et al., 2013. Diallyl disulfide impairs hippocampal neurogenesis in the young adult brain. Toxicol. Lett. 221 (1), 31–38.
Jiang, X., Williams, K.M., Liauw, W.S., Ammit, A.J., Roufogalis, B.D., Duke, C.C., et al., 2005. Effect of ginkgo and ginger on the pharmacokinetics and pharmacodynamics of warfarin in healthy subjects. Br. J. Clin. Pharmacol. 59 (4), 425–432.
Kamphuis, P.J., Wurtman, R.J., 2009. Nutrition and Alzheimer's disease: pre-clinical concepts. Eur. J. Neurol. 16 (Suppl. 1), 12–18.
Karakis, I., Pase, M.P., Beiser, A., Booth, S.L., Jacques, P.F., Rogers, G., et al., 2016. Association of serum vitamin D with the risk of incident dementia and subclinical indices of brain aging: The Framingham Heart Study. J. Alzheimers Dis. 51 (2), 451–461.
Karamanos, B., Thanopoulou, A., Angelico, F., Assaad-Khalil, S., Barbato, A., Del Ben, M., et al., 2002. Nutritional habits in the Mediterranean Basin. The macronutrient composition of diet and its relation with the traditional Mediterranean diet. Multi-centre study of the Mediterranean Group for the Study of Diabetes (MGSD). Eur. J. Clin. Nutr. 56 (10), 983–991.
Kashfi, K., Olson, K.R., 2013. Biology and therapeutic potential of hydrogen sulfide and hydrogen sulfide-releasing chimeras. Biochem. Pharmacol. 85 (5), 689–703.
Kean, R.J., Lamport, D.J., Dodd, G.F., Freeman, J.E., Williams, C.M., Ellis, J.A., et al., 2015. Chronic consumption of flavanone-rich orange juice is associated with cognitive benefits: an 8-wk, randomized, double-blind, placebo-controlled trial in healthy older adults. Am. J. Clin. Nutr. 101 (3), 506–514.
Kelsey, N.A., Wilkins, H.M., Linseman, D.A., 2010. Nutraceutical antioxidants as novel neuroprotective agents. Molecules 15 (11), 7792–7814.
Kennedy, D.O., Wightman, E.L., Reay, J.L., Lietz, G., Okello, E.J., Wilde, A., et al., 2010. Effects of resveratrol on cerebral blood flow variables and cognitive performance in humans: a double-blind, placebo-controlled, crossover investigation. Am. J. Clin. Nutr. 91 (6), 1590–1597.
Kennedy, D.O., Dodd, F.L., Robertson, B.C., Okello, E.J., Reay, J.L., Scholey, A.B., et al., 2011. Monoterpenoid extract of sage (*Salvia lavandulaefolia*) with cholinesterase inhibiting properties improves cognitive performance and mood in healthy adults. J. Psychopharmacol. 25 (8), 1088–1100.
Khazdair, M.R., Boskabady, M.H., Hosseini, M., Rezaee, R.M., Tsatsakis, A., 2015. The effects of *Crocus sativus* (saffron) and its constituents on nervous system: a review. Avicenna J. Phytomed. 5 (5), 376–391.
Kim, B., Feldman, E.L., 2015. Insulin resistance as a key link for the increased risk of cognitive impairment in the metabolic syndrome. Exp. Mol. Med. 47, e149.
Kim, K., Vance, T.M., Chun, O.K., 2016. Estimated intake and major food sources of flavonoids among US adults: changes between 1999-2002 and 2007-2010 in NHANES. Eur. J. Nutr. 55 (2), 833–843.
Kimura, H., 2013. Physiological role of hydrogen sulfide and polysulfide in the central nervous system. Neurochem. Int. 63 (5), 492–497.
Kondo, K., 2004. Beer and health: preventive effects of beer components on lifestyle-related diseases. Biofactors 22 (1–4), 303–310.
Kongkeaw, C., Dilokthornsakul, P., Thanarangsarit, P., Limpeanchob, N., Norman Scholfield, C., 2014. Meta-analysis of randomized controlled trials on cognitive effects of *Bacopa monnieri* extract. J Ethnopharmacol 151 (1), 528–535.
Konrath, E.L., Passos, C., dos, S., Klein Jr, L.C., Henriques, A.T., 2013. Alkaloids as a source of potential anticholinesterase inhibitors for the treatment of Alzheimer's disease. J. Pharm. Pharmacol. 65 (12), 1701–1725.
Kridawati, A., Hardinsyah, Sulaeman, A., Damanik, R., Winarto, A., Rahardjo, T.B., et al., 2016. Tempereversed effects of ovariectomy on brain function in rats: effects of age and type of soy product. J. Steroid Biochem. Mol. Biol. 160, 37–42.
Krikorian, R., Nash, T.A., Shidler, M.D., Shukitt-Hale, B., Joseph, J.A., 2010. Concord grape juice supplementation improves memory function in older adults with mildcognitive impairment. Br. J. Nutr. 103, 730–734.
Kulkarni, S.K., Bhutani, M.K., Bishnoi, M., 2008. Antidepressant activity of curcumin: involvement of serotonin and dopamine system. Psychopharmacology (Berl.) 201 (3), 435–442.
Kumar, S., Pandey, A.K., 2013. Chemistry and biological activities of flavonoids: an overview. ScientificWorldJournal 2013, 162750.
La Fata, G., Weber, P., Mohajeri, M.H., 2014. Effects of vitamin E on cognitive performance during ageing and in Alzheimer's disease. Nutrients 6 (12), 5453–5472.
Lan, X., Wang, W., Li, Q., Wang, J., 2016. The natural flavonoid pinocembrin: molecular targets and potential therapeutic applications. Mol. Neurobiol. 53 (3), 1794–1801.
Lanni, C., Lenzken, S.C., Pascale, A., Del Vecchio, I., Racchi, M., Pistoia, F., et al., 2008. Cognition enhancers between treating and doping the mind. Pharmacol. Res. 57 (3), 196–213.
Lanzotti, V., 2006. The analysis of onion and garlic. J. Chromatogr. A 1112 (1–2), 3–22.
Lazarov, O., Mattson, M.P., Peterson, D.A., Pimplikar, S.W., van Praag, H., 2010. When neurogenesis encounters aging and disease. Trends Neurosci. 33 (12), 569–579.

Lee, S., Kim, J., Seo, S.G., Choi, B.R., Han, J.S., Lee, K.W., et al., 2014. Sulforaphane alleviates scopolamine-induced memory impairment in mice. Pharmacol. Res. 85, 23–32.

Li, F.J., Shen, L., Ji, H.F., 2012. Dietary intakes of vitamin E, vitamin C, and β-carotene and risk of Alzheimer's disease: a meta-analysis. J. Alzheimers Dis. 31 (2), 253–258.

Liguori, A., Grass, J.A., Hughes, J.R., 1999. Subjective effects of caffeine among introverts and extraverts in the morning and evening. Exp. Clin. Psychopharmacol. 7 (3), 244–249.

Liu, R., Wu, C.X., Zhou, D., Yang, F., Tian, S., Zhang, L., et al., 2012. Pinocembrin protects against β-amyloid-induced toxicity in neurons through inhibiting receptor for advanced glycation end products (RAGE)-independent signaling pathways and regulating mitochondrion-mediated apoptosis. BMC Med. 10, 105.

Lopes da Silva, S., Vellas, B., Elemans, S., Luchsinger, J., Kamphuis, P., Yaffe, K., et al., 2014. Plasma nutrient status of patients with Alzheimer's disease: systematic review and meta-analysis. Alzheimers Dement. 10 (4), 485–502.

Lorist, M.M., Tops, M., 2003. Caffeine, fatigue, and cognition. Brain Cogn. 53, 82–94.

Ludvik, B., Waldhäusl, W., Prager, R., Kautzky-Willer, A., Pacini, G., 2003. Mode of action of *Ipomoea batatas* (Caiapo) in type 2 diabetic patients. Metabolism 52 (7), 875–880.

Ludvik, B., Neuffer, B., Pacini, G., 2004. Efficacy of *Ipomoea batatas* (Caiapo) on diabetes control in type 2 diabetic subjects treated with diet. Diabetes Care 27 (2), 436–440.

Ma, L.L., Xing, G.P., Yu, Y., Liang, H., Yu, T.X., Zheng, W.H., et al., 2015. Sulforaphane exerts neuroprotective effects via suppression of the inflammatory response in a rat model of focal cerebral ischemia. Int. J. Clin. Exp. Med. 8 (10), 17811–17817.

Magalingam, K.B., Radhakrishnan, A.K., Haleagrahara, N., 2015. Protective mechanisms of flavonoids in Parkinson's disease. Oxid. Med. Cell. Longev. 2015, 314560.

Mahdavi-Roshan, M., Zahedmehr, A., Mohammad-Zadeh, A., Sanati, H.R., Shakerian, F., Firouzi, A., et al., 2013. Effect of garlic powder tablet on carotid intima-media thickness in patients with coronary artery disease: a preliminary randomized controlled trial. Nutr. Health 22 (2), 143–155.

Maia, L., de Mendonca, A., 2002. Does caffeine intake protect from Alzheimer's disease? Eur. J. Neurol. 9, 377–382.

Makino, T., Shimizu, R., Kanemaru, M., Suzuki, Y., Moriwaki, M., Mizukami, H., 2009. Enzymatically modified isoquercitrin, alpha-oligoglucosyl quercetin 3-O-glucoside, is absorbed more easily than other quercetin glycosides or aglycone after oral administration in rats. Biol. Pharm. Bull. 32 (12), 2034–2040.

Manach, C., Scalbert, A., Morand, C., Rémésy, C., Jiménez, L., 2004. Polyphenols: food sources and bioavailability. Am. J. Clin. Nutr. 79 (5), 727–747.

Mao, X.Y., Yu, J., Liu, Z.Q., Zhou, H.H., 2015. Apigenin attenuates diabetes-associated cognitive decline in rats via suppressing oxidative stress and nitric oxide synthase pathway. Int. J. Clin. Exp. Med. 8 (9), 15506–15513.

Martínez-Lapiscina, E.H., Clavero, P., Toledo, E., San Julián, B., Sanchez-Tainta, A., Corella, D., et al., 2013. Virgin olive oil supplementation and long-term cognition: the PREDIMED-NAVARRA randomized, trial. J. Nutr. Health Aging 17 (6), 544–552.

Mathew, B., Biju, R., 2008. Neuroprotective effects of garlic a review. Libyan J. Med. 3 (1), 23–33.

Mathew, M., Subramanian, S., 2014. In vitro evaluation of anti-Alzheimer effects of dry ginger (*Zingiber officinale* Roscoe) extract. Indian J. Exp. Biol. 52 (6), 606–612.

Mecocci, P., Polidori, M.C., 2012. Antioxidant clinical trials in mild cognitive impairment and Alzheimer's disease. Biochim. Biophys. Acta. 1822 (5), 631–638.

Mecocci, P., Tinarelli, C., Schulz, R.J., Polidori, M.C., 2014. Nutraceuticals in cognitive impairment and Alzheimer's disease. Front. Pharmacol. 5, 147.

Meng, F., Wang, Y., Liu, R., Gao, M., DU, G., 2014. Pinocembrin alleviates memory impairment in transient global cerebral ischemic rats. Exp. Ther. Med. 8 (4), 1285–1290.

Miller 3rd, E.R., Pastor-Barriuso, R., Dalal, D., Riemersma, R.A., Appel, L.J., Guallar, E., 2005. Meta-analysis: high-dosage vitamin E supplementation may increase all-cause mortality. Ann. Intern. Med. 142 (1), 37–46.

Millington, C., Sonego, S., Karunaweera, N., Range, A., Aldrich-Wright, J.R., Campbell, I.L., et al., 2014. Chronic neuroinflammation in Alzheimer's disease: new perspectives on animal models and promising candidate drugs. Biomed. Res. Int. 2014, 309129.

Miroddi, M., Navarra, M., Quattropani, M.C., Calapai, F., Gangemi, S., Calapai, G., 2014. Systematic review of clinical trials assessing pharmacological properties of Salvia species on memory, cognitive impairment and Alzheimer's disease. CNS Neurosci. Ther. 20 (6), 485–495.

Mitchell, E.S., Slettenaar, M., vd Meer, N., Transler, C., Jans, L., Quadt, F., et al., 2011. Differential contributions of theobromine and caffeine on mood, psychomotor performance and blood pressure. Physiol. Behav. 104 (5), 816–822.

Moon, M., Kim, H.G., Choi, J.G., Oh, H., Lee, P.K., Ha, S.K., et al., 2014. 6-Shogaol, an active constituent of ginger, attenuates neuroinflammation and cognitive deficits in animal models of dementia. Biochem. Biophys. Res. Commun. 449 (1), 8–13.

Moosavi, F., Hosseini, R., Saso, L., Firuzi, O., 2015. Modulation of neurotrophic signaling pathways by polyphenols. Drug Des. Devel. Ther. 10, 23–42.

Morris, M.C., Tangney, C.C., Wang, Y., Sacks, F.M., Barnes, L.L., Bennett, D.A., et al., 2015. MIND diet slows cognitive decline with aging. Alzheimers Dement. 11 (9), 1015–1022.

Nabavi, S.F., Braidy, N., Gortzi, O., Sobarzo-Sanchez, E., Daglia, M., Skalicka-Woźniak, K., et al., 2015a. Luteolin as an anti-inflammatory and neuroprotective agent: a brief review. Brain Res. Bull. 119 (Pt A), 1–11.

Nabavi, S.F., Braidy, N., Habtemariam, S., Orhan, I.E., Daglia, M., Manayi, A., et al., 2015b. Neuroprotective effects of chrysin: from chemistry to medicine. Neurochem. Int. 90, 224–231.

Nabavi, S.F., Braidy, N., Habtemariam, S., Sureda, A., Manayi, A., Nabavi, S.M., 2016. Neuroprotective effects of Fisetin in Alzheimer's and Parkinson's diseases: from chemistry to medicine. Curr. Top. Med. Chem. 16 (17), 1910–1915.

Nehlig, A., 2010. Is caffeine a cognitive enhancer? J. Alzheimers Dis. 20 (Suppl. 1), S85–S94.

Nehlig, A., 2013. The neuroprotective effects of cocoa flavanol and its influence on cognitive performance. Br. J. Clin. Pharmacol. 75 (3), 716–727.

Nemeth, K., Plumb, G.W., Berrin, J.G., Juge, N., Jacob, R., Naim, H.Y., et al., 2003. Deglycosylation by small intestinal epithelial cell β-glucosidases is a critical step in the absorption and metabolism of dietary flavonoid glycosides in humans. Eur. J. Nutr. 42 (1), 29–42.

Nurk, E., Drevon, C.A., Refsum, H., Solvoll, K., Vollset, S.E., Nygård, O., et al., 2007. Cognitive performance among the elderly and dietary fish intake: the Hordaland Health Study. Am. J. Clin. Nutr. 86 (5), 1470–1478.

Nurk, E., Refsum, H., Drevon, C.A., Tell, G.S., Nygaard, H.A., Engedal, K., et al., 2010. Cognitive performance among the elderly in relation to the intake of plant foods. The Hordaland Health Study. Br. J. Nutr. 104 (8), 1190–1201.

Obulesu, M., Dowlathabad, M.R., Bramhachari, P.V., 2011. Carotenoids and Alzheimer's disease: an insight into therapeutic role of retinoids in animal models. Neurochem. Int. 59 (5), 535–541.

Ogle, W.O., Speisman, R.B., Ormerod, B.K., 2013. Potential of treating age-related depression and cognitive decline with nutraceutical approaches: a mini-review. Gerontology 59 (1), 23–31.

Ohnuma, T., Toda, A., Kimoto, A., Takebayashi, Y., Higashiyama, R., Tagata, Y., et al., 2016. Benefits of use, and tolerance of, medium-chain triglyceride medical food in the management of Japanese patients with Alzheimer's disease: a prospective, open-label pilot study. Clin. Interv. Aging 11, 29–36.

Olde Rikkert, M.G., Verhey, F.R., Blesa, R., von Arnim, C.A., Bongers, A., Harrison, J., et al., 2015. Tolerability and safety of Souvenaid in patients with mild Alzheimer's disease: results of multi-center, 24-week, open-label extension study. J. Alzheimers Dis. 44 (2), 471–480.

Olson, C.R., Mello, C.V., 2010. Significance of vitamin A to brain function, behavior and learning. Mol. Nutr. Food Res. 54 (4), 489–495.

Ono, K., Yamada, M., 2012. Vitamin A and Alzheimer's disease. Geriatr. Gerontol. Int. 12 (2), 180–188.

Orhan, I., Kartal, M., Tosun, F., Sener, B., 2007. Screening of various phenolic acids and flavonoid derivatives for their anticholinesterase potential. Z. Naturforsch. C 62 (11–12), 829–832.

Ortiz, J.E., Berkov, S., Pigni, N.B., Theoduloz, C., Roitman, G., Tapia, A., et al., 2012. Wild Argentinian Amaryllidaceae, a new renewable source of the acetylcholinesterase inhibitor galanthamine and other alkaloids. Molecules 17 (11), 13473–13482.

Panza, F., Solfrizzi, V., Colacicco, A.M., D'Introno, A., Capurso, C., Torres, F., et al., 2004. Mediterranean diet and cognitive decline. Public Health Nutr. 7 (7), 959–963.

Panza, F., Solfrizzi, V., Barulli, M.R., Bonfiglio, C., Guerra, V., Osella, A., et al., 2015. Coffee, tea, and caffeine consumption and prevention of late-life cognitive decline and dementia: a systematic review. J. Nutr. Health Aging 19 (3), 313–328.

Park, H.R., Kong, K.H., Yu, B.P., Mattson, M.P., Lee, J., 2012. Resveratrol inhibits the proliferation of neural progenitor cells and hippocampal neurogenesis. J. Biol. Chem. 287 (51), 42588–42600.

Patil, V.M., Das, S., Balasubramanian, K., 2016. Quantum chemical and docking insights into bioavailability enhancement of curcumin by piperine in pepper. J. Phys. Chem. A 120 (20), 3643–3653.

Pérez-Hernández, J., Zaldívar-Machorro, V.J., Villanueva-Porras, D., Vega-Ávila, E., Chavarría, A., 2016. A potential alternative against neurodegenerative diseases: phytodrugs. Oxid. Med. Cell. Longev. 2016, 8378613.

Peters, R., Peters, J., Warner, J., Beckett, N., Bulpitt, C., 2008. Alcohol, dementia and cognitive decline in the elderly: a systematic review. Age Ageing 37 (5), 505–512.

Pinho, B.R., Ferreres, F., Valentão, P., Andrade, P.B., 2013. Nature as a source of metabolites with cholinesterase-inhibitory activity: an approach to Alzheimer's disease treatment. J. Pharm. Pharmacol. 65 (12), 1681–1700.

Pintana, H., Sripetchwandee, J., Supakul, L., Apaijai, N., Chattipakorn, N., Chattipakorn, S., 2014. Garlic extract attenuates brain mitochondrial dysfunction and cognitive deficit in obese-insulin resistant rats. Appl. Physiol. Nutr. Metab. 39 (12), 1373–1379.

Polidori, M.C., Praticó, D., Mangialasche, F., Mariani, E., Aust, O., Anlasik, T., et al., 2009. High fruit and vegetable intake is positively correlated with antioxidant status and cognitive performance in healthy subjects. J. Alzheimers Dis. 17, 921–927.

Polidori, M.C., Pientka, L., Mecocci, P., 2012. A review of the major vascular risk factors related to Alzheimer's disease. J. Alzheimers Dis. 32, 521–530.

Pribis, P., Shukitt-Hale, B., 2014. Cognition: the new frontier for nuts and berries. Am. J. Clin. Nutr. 100 (Suppl. 1), 347S–352S.

Pulido-Moran, M., Moreno-Fernandez, J., Ramirez-Tortosa, C., Ramirez-Tortosa, M., 2016. Curcumin and Health. Molecules 21 (3) pii: E264.

Ramasamy, S., Chin, S.P., Sukumaran, S.D., Buckle, M.J., Kiew, L.V., Chung, L.Y., 2015. In silico and in vitro analysis of bacoside A aglycones and its derivatives as the constituents responsible for the cognitive effects of *Bacopa monnieri*. PLoS One 10 (5), e0126565.

Rasul, A., Millimouno, F.M., Ali Eltayb, W., Ali, M., Li, J., Li, X., 2013. Pinocembrin: a novel natural compound with versatile pharmacological and biological activities. Biomed. Res. Int. 2013, 379850.

Ray, B., Chauhan, N.B., Lahiri, D.K., 2011. The "aged garlic extract:" (AGE) and one of its active ingredients S-allyl-L-cysteine (SAC) as potential preventive and therapeutic agents for Alzheimer's disease (AD). Curr. Med. Chem. 18 (22), 3306–3313.

Rendeiro, C., Rhodes, J.S., Spencer, J.P., 2015. The mechanisms of action of flavonoids in the brain: direct versus indirect effects. Neurochem. Int. 89, 126–139.

Rigacci, S., 2015. Olive oil phenols as promising multi-targeting agents against Alzheimer's disease. Adv. Exp. Med. Biol. 863, 1–20.

Roerecke, M., Rehm, J., 2014. Alcohol consumption, drinking patterns, and ischemic heart disease: a narrative review of meta-analyses and a systematic review and meta-analysis of the impact of heavy drinking occasions on risk for moderate drinkers. BMC Med. 12, 182.

Roman, M.W., 2010. Axona (Accera, Inc): a new medical food therapy for persons with Alzheimer's disease. Issues Ment. Health Nurs. 31 (6), 435–436.

Ros, E., 2010. Health benefits of nut consumption. Nutrients 2 (7), 652–682.

Russell, R.M., 2004. The enigma of beta-carotene in carcinogenesis: what can be learned from animal studies. J. Nutr. 134 (1), 262S–268S.

Salehi-Abargouei, A., Maghsoudi, Z., Shirani, F., Azadbakht, L., 2013. Effects of Dietary Approaches to Stop Hypertension (DASH)-style diet on fatal or nonfatal cardiovascular diseases—incidence: a systematic review and meta-analysis on observational prospective studies. Nutrition 29 (4), 611–618.

Salem Jr, N., Vandal, M., Calon, F., 2015. The benefit of docosahexaenoic acid for the adult brain in aging and dementia. Prostaglandins Leukot Essent Fatty Acids 92, 15–22.

Sano, M., Ernesto, C., Thomas, R.G., Klauber, M.R., Schafer, K., Grundman, M., et al., 1997. A controlled trial of selegiline, alpha-tocopherol, or both as treatment for Alzheimer's disease. The Alzheimer's Disease Cooperative Study. N. Engl. J. Med. 336 (17), 1216.

Scheltens, P., Twisk, J.W., Blesa, R., Scarpini, E., von Arnim, C.A., Bongers, A., et al., 2012. Efficacy of Souvenaid in mild Alzheimer's disease: results from a randomized, controlled trial. J. Alzheimers Dis. 31 (1), 225–236.

Schlögl, M., Holick, M.F., 2014. Vitamin D and neurocognitive function. Clin. Interv. Aging 9, 559–568.

Sebastian, R.S., Wilkinson Enns, C., Goldman, J.D., Martin, C.L., Steinfeldt, L.C., Murayi, T., et al., 2015. A new database facilitates characterization of flavonoid intake, sources, and positive associations with diet quality among US Adults. J. Nutr. 145 (6), 1239–1248.

Setchell, K.D., Clerici, C., 2010. Equol: history, chemistry, and formation. J. Nutr. 140 (7), 1355S–1362S.

Shoba, G., Joy, D., Joseph, T., Majeed, M., Rajendran, R., Srinivas, P.S., 1998. Influence of piperine on the pharmacokinetics of curcumin in animals and human volunteers. Planta Med. 64 (4), 353–356.

Skrovankova, S., Sumczynski, D., Mlcek, J., Jurikova, T., Sochor, J., 2015. Bioactive Compounds and Antioxidant Activity in Different Types of Berries. Int. J. Mol. Sci. 16 (10), 24673–24706.

Smith, A.P., 2013. Caffeine, extraversion and working memory. J. Psychopharmacol. 27 (1), 71–76.

Smith, P.J., Blumenthal, J.A., 2016. Dietary Factors and Cognitive Decline. J. Prev. Alzheimers Dis. 3 (1), 53–64.

Solfrizzi, V., Panza, F., 2014. Mediterranean diet and cognitive decline. A lesson from the whole-diet approach: what challenges lie ahead? J. Alzheimers Dis. 39 (2), 283–286.

Solfrizzi, V., Frisardi, V., Seripa, D., Logroscino, G., Imbimbo, B.P., D'Onofrio, G., et al., 2011. Mediterranean diet in predementia and dementia syndromes. Curr. Alzheimer Res 8 (5), 520–542.

Souberbielle, J.C., 2016. Epidemiology of vitamin-D deficiency. Geriatr. Psychol. Neuropsychiatr. Vieil. 14 (1), 7–15.

Spencer, J.P., Vauzour, D., Rendeiro, C., 2009. Flavonoids and cognition: the molecular mechanisms underlying their behavioural effects. Arch. Biochem. Biophys. 492 (1-2), 1–9.

Stephen, J.M., 1975. Epidemiological and dietary aspects of rickets and osteomalacia. Proc. Nutr. Soc. 34 (2), 131–138.

Strathearn, K.E., Yousef, G.G., Grace, M.H., Roy, S.L., Tambe, M.A., Ferruzzi, M.G., et al., 2014. Neuroprotective effects of anthocyanin- and proanthocyanidin-rich extracts in cellular models of Parkinson's disease. Brain Res. 1555, 60–77.

Subash, S., Essa, M.M., Al-Adawi, S., Memon, M.A., Manivasagam, T., Akbar, M., 2014. Neuroprotective effects of berry fruits on neurodegenerative diseases. Neural. Regen. Res. 9 (16), 1557–1566.

Subedee, L., Suresh, R.N., Mk, J., Hl, K., Am, S., Vh, P., 2015. Preventive role of Indian black pepper in animal models of Alzheimer's disease. J. Clin. Diagn. Res. 9 (4), FF01–FF04.

Sun, Q.Q., Xu, S.S., Pan, J.L., Guo, H.M., Cao, W.Q., 1999. Huperzine-A capsules enhance memory and learning performance in 34 pairs of matched adolescent students. Zhongguo Yao Li Xue Bao 20 (7), 601–603.

Svennerholm, L., 1968. Distribution and fatty acid composition of phosphoglycerides in normal human brain. J. Lipid Res. 9 (5), 570–579.

Swaminathan, A., Jicha, G.A., 2014. Nutrition and prevention of Alzheimer's dementia. Front. Aging Neurosci. 6, 282.

Sydenham, E., Dangour, A.D., Lim, W.S., 2012. Omega 3 fatty acid for the prevention of cognitive decline and dementia. Cochrane Database Syst. Rev. 6, CD005379.

Tafti, M., Ghyselinck, N.B., 2007. Functional implication of the vitamin A signaling pathway in the brain. Arch. Neurol. 64 (12), 1706–1711.

Tan, C.C., Yu, J.T., Wang, H.F., Tan, M.S., Meng, X.F., Wang, C., et al., 2014. Efficacy and safety of donepezil, galantamine, rivastigmine, and memantine for the treatment of Alzheimer's disease: a systematic review and meta-analysis. J. Alzheimers Dis. 41 (2), 615–631.

Tan, M.S., Yu, J.T., Tan, C.C., Wang, H.F., Meng, X.F., Wang, C., et al., 2015. Efficacy and adverse effects of ginkgo biloba for cognitive impairment and dementia: a systematic review and meta-analysis. J. Alzheimers Dis. 43 (2), 589–603.

Tangney, C.C., 2014. DASH and Mediterranean-type Dietary Patterns to Maintain Cognitive Health. Curr. Nutr. Rep. 3 (1), 51–61.

Tangney, C.C., Li, H., Wang, Y., Barnes, L., Schneider, J.A., Bennett, D.A., et al., 2014. Relation of DASH- and Mediterranean-like dietary patterns to cognitive decline in older persons. Neurology 83 (16), 1410–1416.

Tchantchou, F., Lacor, P.N., Cao, Z., Lao, L., Hou, Y., Cui, C., et al., 2009. Stimulation of neurogenesis and synaptogenesis by bilobalide and quercetin via common final pathway in hippocampal neurons. J. Alzheimers Dis. 18 (4), 787–798.

Terry Jr, A.V., Buccafusco, J.J., 2003. The cholinergic hypothesis of age and Alzheimer's disease-related cognitive deficits: recent challenges and their implications for novel drug development. J. Pharmacol. Exp. Ther. 306 (3), 821–827.

Thaipisuttikul, P., Galvin, J.E., 2012. Use of medical foods and nutritional approaches in the treatment of Alzheimer's disease. Clin. Pract (Lond) 9 (2), 199–209.

Theoharides, T.C., Stewart, J.M., Hatziagelaki, E., Kolaitis, G., 2015. Brain "fog," inflammation and obesity: key aspects of neuropsychiatric disorders improved by luteolin. Front. Neurosci. 9, 225.

Tildesley, N.T., Kennedy, D.O., Perry, E.K., Ballard, C.G., Wesnes, K.A., Scholey, A.B., 2005. Positive modulation of mood and cognitive performance following administration of acute doses of Salvia lavandulaefolia essential oil to healthy young volunteers. Physiol. Behav. 83 (5), 699–709.

Townsend, B.E., Johnson, R.W., 2016. Sulforaphane induces Nrf2 target genes and attenuates inflammatory gene expression in microglia from brain of young adult and aged mice. Exp. Gerontol. 73, 42–48.

Tu, Y., Zhong, Y., Du, H., Luo, W., Wen, Y., Li, Q., et al., 2016. Anticholinesterases and antioxidant alkamides from *Piper nigrum* fruits. Nat. Prod. Res. 30 (17) 1945–1949.

Turner, R.S., Thomas, R.G., Craft, S., van Dyck, C.H., Mintzer, J., Reynolds, B.A., et al., 2015. Alzheimer's Disease Cooperative Study.A randomized, double-blind, placebo-controlled trial of resveratrol for Alzheimer disease. Neurology 85 (16), 1383–1391.

Valls-Pedret, C., Sala-Vila, A., Serra-Mir, M., Corella, D., de la Torre, R., Martínez-González, M.Á., et al., 2015. Mediterranean Diet and age-related cognitive decline: a randomized clinical trial. JAMA Intern. Med. 175 (7), 1094–1103.

van de Rest, O., Berendsen, A.A., Haveman-Nies, A., de Groot, L.C., 2015. Dietary patterns, cognitive decline, and dementia: a systematic review. Adv. Nutr. 6 (2), 154–168.

van der Schaft, J., Koek, H.L., Dijkstra, E., Verhaar, H.J., van der Schouw, Y.T., Emmelot-Vonk, M.H., 2013. The association between vitamin D and cognition: a systematic review. Ageing Res. Rev. 12 (4), 1013–1023.

Varinska, L., Gal, P., Mojzisova, G., Mirossay, L., Mojzis, J., 2015. Soy and breast cancer: focus on angiogenesis. Int. J. Mol. Sci. 16 (5), 11728–11749.

Verdile, G., Keane, K.N., Cruzat, V.F., Medic, S., Sabale, M., Rowles, J., et al., 2015. Inflammation and Oxidative Stress: The Molecular Connectivity between Insulin Resistance, Obesity, and Alzheimer's Disease. Mediators Inflamm. 2015, 105828.

Villaflores, O.B., Chen, Y.J., Chen, C.P., Yeh, J.M., Wu, T.Y., 2012. Curcuminoids and resveratrol as anti-Alzheimer agents. Taiwan J. Obstet. Gynecol. 51 (4), 515–525.

de Waal, H., Stam, C.J., Lansbergen, M.M., Wieggers, R.L., Kamphuis, P.J., Scheltens, P., et al., 2014. The effect of souvenaid on functional brain network organisation in patients with mild Alzheimer's disease: a randomised controlled study. PLoS One 9 (1), e86558.

Wang, H., Wang, H., Cheng, H., Che, Z., 2016. Ameliorating effect of luteolin on memory impairment in an Alzheimer's disease model. Mol. Med. Rep. 13 (5), 4215–4220.

Weinmann, S., Roll, S., Schwarzbach, C., Vauth, C., Willich, S.N., 2010. Effects of Ginkgo biloba in dementia: systematic review and meta-analysis. BMC Geriatr. 10, 14.

Wengreen, H., Munger, R.G., Cutler, A., Quach, A., Bowles, A., Corcoran, C., et al., 2013. Prospective study of Dietary Approaches to Stop Hypertension- and Mediterranean-style dietary patterns and age-related cognitive change: the Cache County Study on Memory, Health and Aging. Am. J. Clin. Nutr. 98 (5), 1263–1271.

WHO (World Health Organization) and Alzheimer's Disease International, 2012. Dementia: a public health priority. Available online at: http://www.who.int/mental_health/publications/dementia_report_2012/en/

Wightman, E.L., Reay, J.L., Haskell, C.F., Williamson, G., Dew, T.P., Kennedy, D.O., 2014. Effects of resveratrol alone or in combination with piperine on cerebral blood flow parameters and cognitive performance in human subjects: a randomised, double-blind, placebo-controlled, cross-over investigation. Br. J. Nutr. 112 (2), 203–213.

Wightman, E.L., Haskell-Ramsay, C.F., Reay, J.L., Williamson, G., Dew, T., Zhang, W., et al., 2015. The effects of chronic trans-resveratrol supplementation on aspects of cognitive function, mood, sleep, health and cerebral blood flow in healthy, young humans. Br. J. Nutr. 114 (9), 1427–1437.

Willcox, B.J., Willcox, D.C., 2014. Caloric restriction, caloric restriction mimetics, and healthy aging in Okinawa: controversies and clinical implications. Curr. Opin. Clin. Nutr. Metab. Care 17 (1), 51–58.

Willcox, D.C., Scapagnini, G., Willcox, B.J., 2014. Healthy aging diets other than the Mediterranean: a focus on the Okinawan diet. Mech. Ageing Dev. 136-137, 148–162.

Wu, T.Y., Chen, C.P., Jinn, T.R., 2011. Traditional Chinese medicines and Alzheimer's disease. Taiwan J. Obstet. Gynecol. 50 (2), 131–135.

Wu, S., Gao, Q., Zhao, P., Gao, Y., Xi, Y., Wang, X., et al., 2016. Sulforaphane produces antidepressant- and anxiolytic-like effects in adult mice. Behav. Brain Res. 301, 55–62.

Wurtman, R.J., 2014. A nutrient combination that can affect synapse formation. Nutrients 6 (4), 1701–1710.

Xu, G., Liu, X., Yin, Q., Zhu, W., Zhang, R., Fan, X., 2009. Alcohol consumption and transition of mild cognitive impairment to dementia. Psychiatry Clin. Neurosci. 63 (1), 43–49.

Xu, Z.Q., Liang, X.M., Juan-Wu, Zhang, Y.F., Zhu, C.X., Jiang, X.J., 2012. Treatment with Huperzine A improves cognition in vascular dementia patients. Cell Biochem. Biophys. 62 (1), 55–58.

Yang, G., Wang, Y., Tian, J., Liu, J.P., 2013. Huperzine A for Alzheimer's disease: a systematic review and meta-analysis of randomized clinical trials. PLoS One 8 (9), e74916.

Yun, H.M., Jin, P., Park, K.R., Hwang, J., Jeong, H.S., Kim, E.C., et al., 2016. Thiacremonone potentiates anti-oxidant effects to improve memory dysfunction in an APP/PS1 transgenic mice model. Mol. Neurobiol. 53 (4), 2409–2420.

Yusuf, M., Khan, M., Khan, R.A., Ahmed, B., 2012. Preparation, characterization, in vivo and biochemical evaluation of brain targeted Piperine solid lipid nanoparticles in an experimentally induced Alzheimer's disease model. J. Drug Target [Epub ahead of print].

Zhang, Y., Chen, J., Qiu, J., Li, Y., Wang, J., Jiao, J., 2016. Intakes of fish and polyunsaturated fatty acids and mild-to-severe cognitive impairment risks: a dose-response meta-analysis of 21 cohort studies. Am. J. Clin. Nutr 103 (2), 330–340.

CHAPTER

20

Chalcones Target the Tumor Necrosis Factor–Related Apoptosis-Inducing Ligand (TRAIL) Signaling Pathway for Cancer Chemoprevention

Małgorzata Kłósek[1], *Andrzej Karol Kuropatnicki*[2], *Ewelina Szliszka*[1], *Ilona Korzonek-Szlacheta*[1] *and Wojciech Król*[1]

[1]Medical University of Silesia, Katowice, Poland [2]Pedagogical University of Krakow, Krakow, Poland

INTRODUCTION

Chalcones are natural biocides and considered as intermediate in the biosynthesis of flavonoids. They are commonly found in edible plants. Their name derives from a Greek word χαλκός meaning copper or brass (Nickon and Silversmith, 1987). Chalcones and their derivatives constitute an interesting class of compounds due to their synthetic versatility. They have been shown to possess numerous effective biological activities such as antiinflammatory, anticancer, antihypertensive, antibacterial, antiretroviral, antimalarial, antioxidant, antifungal, antispasmodic, antiparasitic, antidiabetic, antihistamine, antiangiogenic, antiarrhythmic, antinociceptive, antiplasmodial, and anti-obesity as well as hypnotic, cardioprotective, immunosuppressant, and cytotoxic (Singh et al., 2014).

The first dihydrochalcone, phlorizin (phloridzin), a naturally occurring flavonoid, was initially described by Philipp Lorentz Geiger in 1834. The German pharmacist and professor of pharmacy at the University of Heidelberg isolated it from apple root bark. One year later, in 1835, Laurent-Guillaume de Koninck, a Belgian chemist, characterized phlorizin and named it using the Greek words φλόος for "bark" and ῥίζα for "root" (Definitions.net "phlorizin"; Koninck et al., 1835). Phlorizin occurs in minute and slightly pinkish crystals and is sparingly soluble in cold water, alcohol, and ether (Krotoszyner and Stevens, 1917). The first chalcone described as a naturally occurring compound was carthamine, a natural red pigment from safflower (*Carthamus tinctorius*), a dye plant used in India (Bhardwaj and Jain, 1982). Carthamine was used as a dye not only in ancient times (Candolle, 1885) but also later in the European wool-dyeing industry as well as in Japan for making cosmetics for use by geishas and kabuki artists (Definitions.net "carthamin").

Stanisław Kostanecki, a Polish organic chemist who worked at the University in Bern, Switzerland, pioneered in vegetable dye chemistry. In 1893, he found out that the phenol derivative of benzopirene is a matrix substance of chrysine, which was named by him *flavonoid* after Latin term *flavus* for yellow (Kuropatnicki et al., 2014). Kostanecki together with Josef Tambor was the first who coined the term *chalcone* (Kostanecki and Tambor, 1899). In 1925, H. F. Dean and M. Nierenstein described the isomeric relationship involving the ring opening of flavanones to yield chalcones (Dean and Nierenstein, 1925).

Polyphenols are secondary plant metabolites present especially in fruit, vegetables, spices, green tea, olive oil, red wine, and beer—they have become integral parts of the human diet. More than 8000 different phenolic compounds

Nutrition and Functional Foods for Healthy Aging.
DOI: http://dx.doi.org/10.1016/B978-0-12-805376-8.00020-4

have been identified in the plant kingdom (Dai and Mumper, 2010; Pietta, 2000) and can be divided into flavonoids, phenolic acids, stilbenes, and lignans (Pandey and Rizvi, 2009). Flavonoids are further subdivided into nine classes, including flavonols, flavones, flavanones, flavan-3-ols, anthocyanidins, isoflavones, proanthocyanidins, aurones, and chalcones (Mahapatra et al., 2015). The basic chemical structure of flavonoids is the flavan backbone in which two phenolic rings, A and B, are linked by a heterocyclic ring, C (Busch et al., 2015; Pietta, 2000; Vue et al., 2015).

Chalcones, an important group of the flavonoids, have interesting biological properties. So far, they have received increasing attention due to their potent antioxidant properties and anticancer effects (Orlikova et al., 2011). Much attention has been given to chemoprevention as an alternative approach to cancer control.

Cancer development is a multistage process that starts with initial mutations that are followed by promotion and progression and ultimately some form of malignancy. At the beginning of the 21st century, cancer was the second leading cause of death after heart disease in the European Union and the United States (Kang et al., 2011). Chemoprevention is one of the most promising approaches used against many cancer cells to arrest or reverse the process of carcinogenesis through dietary compounds or synthetic pharmacological agents or both (Sporn et al., 1976). In the last 20 years, numerous preclinical and epidemiological studies have shown that natural dietary products play role in the prevention of cancers (Sirerol et al., 2016).

Chalcones can inhibit cancerogenesis from the its earliest stages, including tumor initiation, promotion, and progression. One important event for cancer chemoprevention is the induction of apoptosis. In some cancer cells, one pathway—the tumor necrosis factor–related apoptosis-inducing ligand (TRAIL)—mediates apoptosis by making tumors attractive targets for the chemopreventive activities of specific dietary agents. Chalcones can target the TRAIL-induced apoptotic pathway and sensitize cancer cells. However, some tumor cells are resistant to apoptosis as mediated by TRAIL. New strategies to overcome this resistance are critically important to cancer chemoprevention. This chapter shows the mechanisms of sensitization of TRAIL resistance cancer cells by chalcones.

CHARACTERISTICS OF TRAIL AND APOPTOSIS INDUCED BY TRAIL

TRAIL is a 20-kilodalton protein encoded by a gene located on chromosome 3. It was discovered by two independent groups as a novel pro-apoptotic member of the tumor necrosis factor superfamily with the highest homology to CD95L (FasL/APO-1L) (Pitti et al., 1996; Wiley et al., 1995). TRAIL is a type II transmembrane protein but can be cleaved by metalloproteases to yield a soluble form (Secchiero et al., 2010). This ligand is expressed on the surface of immune effector cells such as dendritic cells, macrophages, natural killer cells, and cytotoxic T cells (Holoch and Griffith, 2009). It has the ability to selectively induce apoptosis in cancer cells without having toxic effects for normal cells. Several TRAIL receptors have been discovered to date, including TRAIL-R1 (DR4), TRAIL-R2 (DR5), TRAIL-R3 (DcR1), TRAIL-R4 (DcR2), and soluble osteoprotegerin (OPG) (Emery et al., 1998; MacFarlane et al., 1997). TRAIL-R1 and TRAIL-R2 are called *death receptors* because they have ability to transduce signals to apoptosis (Mahmood and Shukla, 2010). TRAIL-R3 and TRAIL-4 are called *decoy receptors* because they lack a functional death domain and are unable to activate apoptotic signaling. TRAIL-R3 lacks an intracellular domain and has a glycosylphosphatidylinositol membrane anchor instead. TRAIL-R4 has a truncated death domain and is missing 52 of the 76 amino acids found in the death domains (DDs) of death receptors (Amarante-Mendes and Griffith, 2015). OPGs may also function as decoy receptors, although their relevance is unclear (Amarante-Mendes and Griffith, 2015; Emery et al., 1998). The physiological role of osteoprotegerin is to inhibit the RANKL–RANK interaction in bone morphogenesis (Boyce and Xing, 2007). The types of TRAIL receptors are shown in Fig. 20.1.

Two pathways of TRAIL-induced apoptosis have been identified: the extrinsic (receptor-mediated) and the intrinsic (mitochondrial) (Fig. 20.2) (MacFarlane, 2003; Sayers, 2011). TRAIL induces apoptosis in cancer cells via a receptor-mediated pathway. It binds to the death receptor TRAIL-R1 (DR4) or TRAIL-R2 (DR5) (or both) and leads to the trimerization of receptors. This results in the recruitment of the adaptor molecule, Fas-associated death domain (FADD), to form the death-inducing signaling complex (DISC) (Pennarun et al., 2010). The death effectors domain (DED) of Fas-associated protein has been recognized by the DED of caspase-8, leading to its autoactivation. In type I cells, activation of caspase-8 is sufficient for subsequent activation of effector caspase-3 or caspase-7, leading to apoptosis. In type II cells, signal amplification via the intrinsic pathway is necessary for apoptosis (Ozören and El-Deiry, 2002). In this type of cell, caspase-8 cleaves Bid to truncated Bid (tBid), which migrates to the mitochondrial membrane and stimulates the oligomerization of Bak and Bax to form pores in the outer mitochondrial membrane. This allows for the release of mitochondria proteins such as cytochrome c, apoptosis-inducing factor,

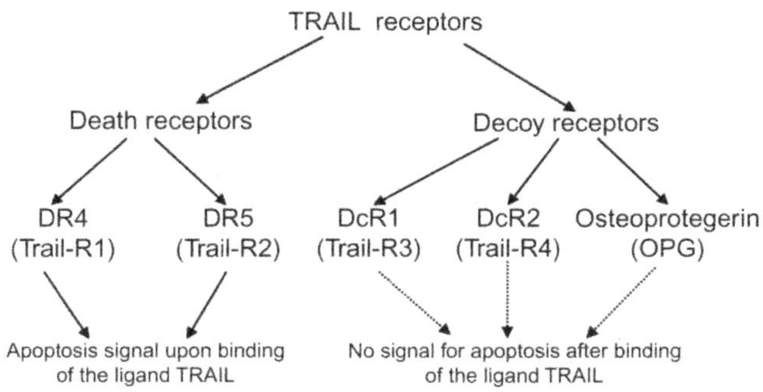

FIGURE 20.1 TRAIL receptors and the ability to induce apoptosis mediated by TRAIL.

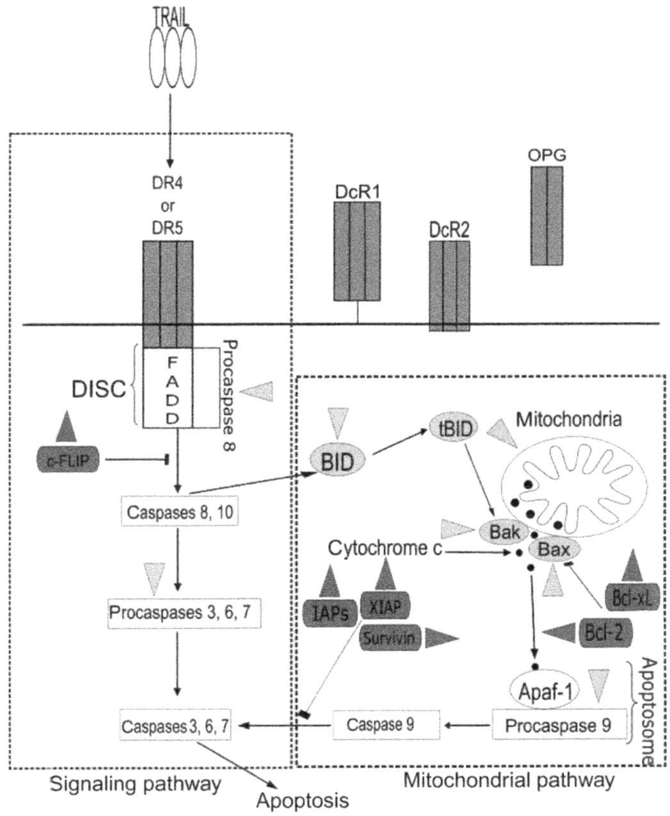

FIGURE 20.2 The pathways of TRAIL-induced apoptosis and molecular targets of chalcones. *Bluemarks* TRAIL's receptors, *yellow arrowheads* mark activation, and *red arrowheads* mark inhibition.

and Smac/DIABLO into the cytosol. Cytochrome c binds apoptotic peptidase activating factor 1 (Apaf-1), dATP, and caspase-9 to form apoptosome. Caspase-9 is activated and cleaves caspase-3 to initiate apoptosis (Holland, 2013; Mellier et al., 2010; Russo et al., 2010; Schulze-Osthoff et al., 1998).

Some cancer cells are resistant to TRAIL-mediated cell death through a variety of survival mechanisms. One reason is deletion in TRAIL-R1 observed in nasopharyngeal cancer and mutations in TRAIL-R2 in breast cancer, lung cancer, and head and neck cancer (Lim et al., 2015; Zhang and Fang, 2005). In turn, a lack of expression of TRAIL-R1 due to epigenetic silencing has been observed in ovarian cancer cells (Horak et al., 2005a). On the other hand, high mRNA expression of DcR1 and DcR2 found in human osteoblast cells also correlates with resistance to TRAIL-mediated apoptosis (Lim et al., 2015). High levels of c-FLIP that inhibit activation of caspase-8 at the DISC have been correlated with resistance to TRAIL observed in several cancer types, including lung and breast cancers, colon cancers, ovarian cancers, and B-cell chronic lymphocytic leukemia (Guseva et al., 2008; Horak et al., 2005b; Wang et al., 2008). Overexpression of antiapoptotic proteins Bcl-2 in breast cancer cells and Bcl-xL in pancreatic cancer cells have reportedly resulted in TRAIL resistance (Fulda et al., 2002; Hinz et al., 2000). High levels of anti-apoptotic proteins XIAP, cIAP-1, cIAP-2, and survivins lead to TRAIL resistance in prostate cancer cells (McEleny et al., 2002). High XIAP expression has been postulated as a mechanism of resistance to TRAIL in colon cancer and pancreatic cancer (Li et al., 2013; Ndozangue-Touriguine et al., 2008; Ozören and El-Deiry, 2002). Mutation in the pro-apoptotic protein Bax has been shown to contribute to TRAIL resistance in human colon carcinoma cells (LeBlanc et al., 2002). Understanding mechanisms of TRAIL resistance in cancer cells can help researchers find more suitable strategies to overcome TRAIL resistance and obtain better therapeutic outcomes.

CHARACTERISTICS OF CHALCONES

Chalcones or 1,3-diaryl-2-propen-1-ones are a group of polyphenolic compounds belonging to the flavonoids family. They are the precursors of flavonoids and isoflavonoids (Sahu et al., 2012). Chemically, they consist of open-chain flavonoids in which the two aromatic rings are joined together by three carbons in an α,-unsaturated system (Nowakowska, 2007) (Fig. 20.3).

The structure of chalcones is diverse due to the number and position of various substituents, including hydroxy or methoxy groups on the A or B rings. Chalcones are also C-prenylated and. more rarely, O-prenylated. The most frequent type of prenylation is 3,3-dimethylallyl substitution (prenyl group). Besides this, they also have isopentenyl, furano, dimethylchromano, geranyl, and farnesyl groups (Zsuzsanna Rozmer, 2014). Most prenylated chalcones have been isolated from the Moraceae (broussochalcone A) and Leguminosae families, and several compounds were isolated from *Humulus lupulus* (xanthohumol, desmethylxanthohumol) (Botta et al., 2005; Zsuzsanna Rozmer, 2014). Dihydrochalcones belong to a small group of flavonoids in which a three-carbon bridge double bond has been reduced as in asebogenin or phloridzin.

The chromone—1-benzopyran-4-one—is the core in several flavonoids. One of the first methods for synthesizing chromones was introduced by the aforementioned Stanisław Kostanecki; hence, this reaction is now known as the *Kostanecki acylation*. Chalcones are synthesized by Claisen-Schmidt condensation of an aromatic aldehyde and ketone in a polar solvent. Chalcones can easily be cyclized to flavanones by a Michael addition at the β position of the carbonyl (Claisen and Claparède, 1881; Orlikova et al., 2011; Zhang et al., 2013). Reaction of 2′-hydroxyacetophenone with benzaldehyde in the 0.1 M NaOH gives 2′-hydroksychalcone (Fig. 20.4) (Avupati and Yejella, 2014).

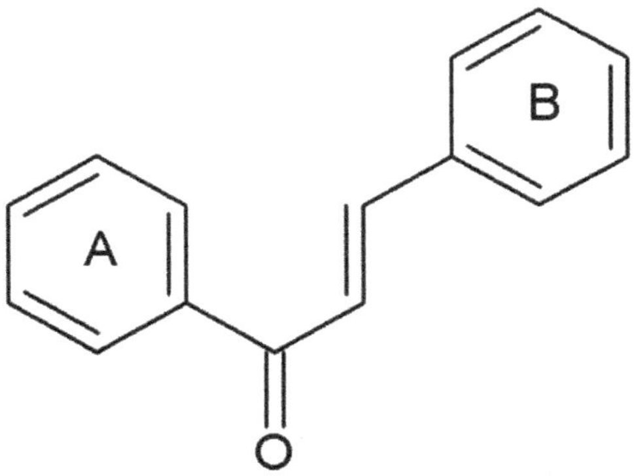

FIGURE 20.3 The core of chalcone structure.

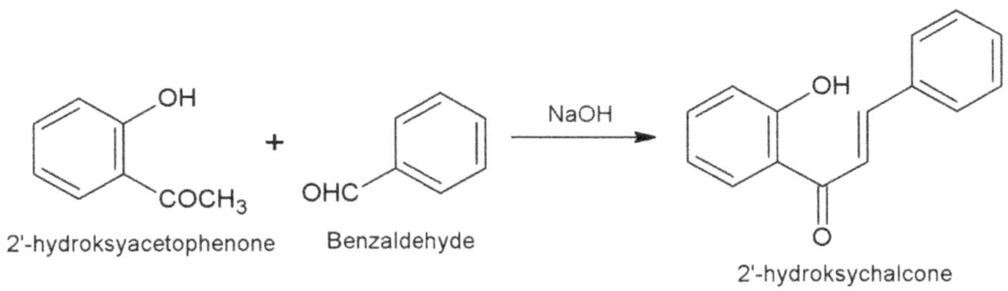

FIGURE 20.4 Synthesis of 2′-hydroksychalcone in Claisen-Schmidt condensation between 2′-hydroxyacetophenone and benzaldehyde.

Condensation between acetophenone and benzaldehyde by sonochemical and thermally activated reactions over a zeolite as catalyst to give chalcone is presented in Fig. 20.5 (Avupati and Yejella, 2014).

Other methods for obtaining chalcone use Suzuki, Friedel-Crafts, or Julia-Kocienski reactions. Synthesis of chalcones in a Suzuki reaction occurs between activated cinnamic acids and phenylboronic acids (Fig. 20.6) or between activated benzoic acids and phenylvinylboronic acids (Eddarir et al., 2003).

A different method of chalcones synthesis is the reaction of arylboronic acids with benzoic anhydride in the presence of $PdCl_2$ and Na_2CO_3 in H_2O/acetone (Fig. 20.7) (Selepe and Van Heerden, 2013).

The biosynthesis of chalcones in plants is initiated by chalcone synthase, which leads to condensation of three acetate units starting from malonyl-CoA with *p*-coumaroyl-CoA to 4,2′,4′,6′-tetrahydroxychalcone, also known as *naringenin chalcone* (Fig. 20.8) (Schijlen et al., 2004).

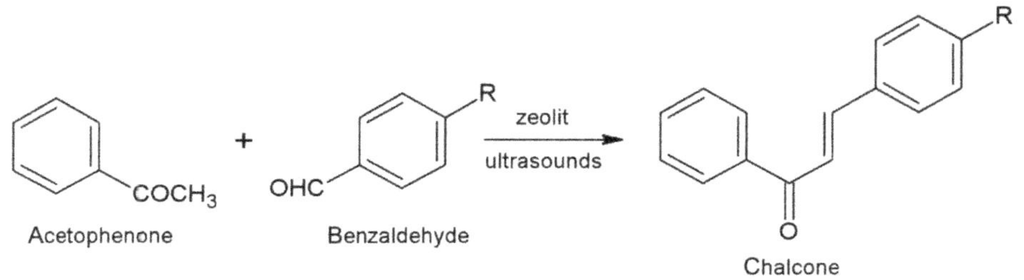

FIGURE 20.5 Synthesis of chalcone in Claisen-Schmidt condensation between acetophenone and benzaldehyde.

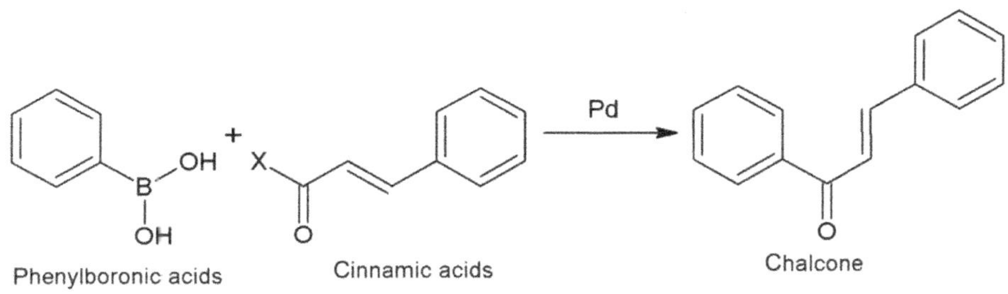

FIGURE 20.6 Synthesis of chalcone in Suzuki reaction between phenylvinylboronic acids and cinnamic acids.

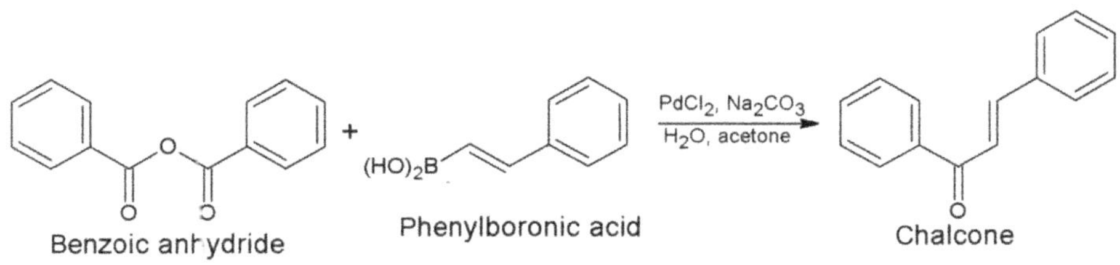

FIGURE 20.7 Synthesis of chalcone between benzoic anhydride and arylboronic acids.

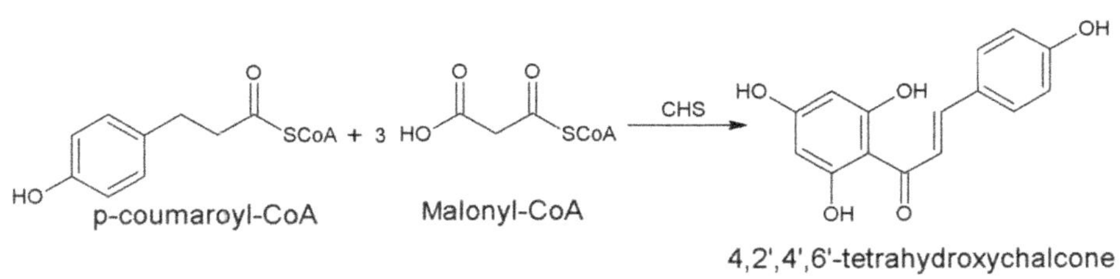

FIGURE 20.8 Synthesis of chalcone in plants.

Many plants do not accumulate chalcones, and this reaction is the first step in the synthesis of the remaining class of flavonoids such as flavanones, dihydroflavonols, and anthocyanins. In turn, isoflavones, flavones, flavonols, aurones, or proanthocyanidins represent side branches of the flavonoid pathway. Chalcones can be found in many plants (Table 20.1).

Chalcones represent an important class of natural flavonoids useful in medicine and pharmacology. Many patents describe the isolation of chalcones from plant extracts and use them as additives in cosmetics and other preparations. Isoliquiritigenin used in the treatment and prevention of cardiovascular diseases was patented for the prevention of skin aging by cosmetics companies. Licochalcone A was patented as cosmetic toner, antiacne, and skin-whitening agent. Isobavachalcone was patented as an agent for treating inflammatory nerve diseases (Matos et al., 2015). As previously mentioned, chalcones have a broad spectrum of biological properties such as antioxidant, antimicrobial, and antiinflammatory activities (Sahu et al., 2012). Over the past 10 years, about 90 compounds of chalcones with

TABLE 20.1 Examples of chalcones naturally occurring in plants

Chalcone	Major Sources	References
Asebogenin (dihydrochalcone)	*Piper aduncum* leaves, *Piper longicaudatum*, *Pieris japonica* leaves	Joshi et al., 2001; Orjala et al., 1994; Yao et al., 2005
Aurentiacin	*Syzygium samarangense*	Kim et al., 2012
Broussochalcone A (prenylated chalcone)	*Broussonetia papyrifera*	Sohn et al., 2004
Butein	Stembark of cashews, *Semecarpus anacardium*, the heartwood of *Dalbergia odorifera*, traditional Chinese and Tibetan medicinal herbs, *Caragana jubata*, and *Rhus verniciflua* Stokes	Cheng et al., 1998; Yadav et al., 2011
Cardamonin	Herbal tea *Catimbium speciosum*, pulp and seeds of the fruits of *Syzygium samarangense*	Ohtsuki et al., 2009; Simirgiotis et al., 2008
Derricin	*Lonchocarpus neuroscapha*	Gonçalves de Lima et al., 1975
Desmethylxanthohumol (prenylated chalcone)	Female flowers of hops (*Humulus lupulus*)	De Keukeleire et al., 2003
Flawokawain B	*Piper methysticum* (Kava)	Lebot et al., 2014; Tang et al., 2010
Flavokawain C	*Piper methysticum* (Kava)	Tang et al., 2010
Isobavachalcone (prenylated chalcone)	*Psoralea corylifolia*, *Psoralea longum*, *Angelica keiskei*, *Maclura tinctoria*	ElSohly et al., 2001; Yan et al., 2015
Isocordoin	*Aeschynomene fascicularis*	Caamal-Fuentes et al., 2015
Isoliquiritin	*Glycyrrhiza* sp.	Wu and Meng, et al., 2013
Isoliquiritigenin	*Dalbergia odorifera*, roots of *Glycyrrhiza uralensis*, *Glycyrrhiza glabra*, *Mongolian glycyrrhiza*	Li et al., 2010; Peng et al., 2015; Zhao et al., 2011
Licochalcone A	Root of *Glycyrrhiza inflata*, *Glycyrrhiza glabra*	Fu et al., 2004; Furusawa et al., 2009
Licochalcone E	Roots of *Glycyrrhiza inflata*	Kwon et al., 2013
Millepachine	*Millettia pachycarpa*	Wu and Ye, et al., 2013
Myrigalone B	*Myrica gale*	Mathiesen et al., 1997
Panduratin A	*Kaempferia pandurata*	Lee et al., 2010
Phloretin (dihydrochalcone)	Leaves of *Malus* (crabapple), leaves of *Pieris japonica*	Qin et al., 2015; Yao et al., 2005
Phlorizin (phloridzin) (dihydrochalcone)	leaves of *Malus* (crabapple), leaves of *Pieris japonica*	Qin et al., 2015; Yao et al., 2005
Pinocembrin chalcone	*Helichrysum trilineatum*	Bremner and Meyer, 1998
Stercurensin	Pulp and seeds of fruits of *Syzygium samarangense*	Simirgiotis et al., 2008
Viscolin	*Viscum coloratum*	Hwang et al., 2006
Xanthoangelol (prenylated chalcone)	*Angelica keiskei*	Ohnogi et al., 2012; Tabata et al., 2005
Xanthohumol (prenylated chalcone)	Female flowers of hops (*Humulus lupulus*)	Lee et al., 2012; Liu et al., 2014

antitumor activities have been found (Zhang et al., 2013). Chalcones show cytotoxicity against a wide range of cancer cell lines, including prostate cancer, breast cancer, leukemia, hepatoma, stomach cancer, and colorectal cancer. The IC50 values of the majority of compounds were found to be below 50 μM (Zhang et al., 2013). Calcones induce apoptosis in cancer cells through a death receptor–mediated pathway, a mitochondrial-mediated pathway, or a nuclear factor kappa B pathway.

CHALCONE POTENTIAL FOR ENHANCING TRAIL-MEDIATED APOPTOSIS IN CANCER CELLS

TRAIL resistance in some cancer cells can be overcome by flavonoids. The preclinical studies have shown that chalcones in combination with TRAIL can sensitize TRAIL-resistant cancer cells to apoptosis induced by TRAIL. Chalcones such as butein, cardamonin, chalcone, xanthohumol, isobavachalcone, isoliquiritigenin, licochalcone A, and flavokawain B augment anticancer activities through different mechanisms in the apoptotic pathway. The molecular targets for chalcones in many cancer cells are presented in Table 20.2 and Fig. 20.2.

Butein is a 3,4,2′,4′-tetrahydroxychalcone isolated from *Toxicodendron verniciﬂuum* (*Rhus verniciflua*), *Butea monosperma*, *Semecarpus anacardium*, or *Dalbergia odorifera* (Padmavathi et al., 2015). Szliszka et al. have shown that butein at concentrations of 20 and 50 μM in combination with TRAIL at concentrations of 20–100 ng/mL increased the percentage of cell death in LNCaP prostate cancer cells from 36.82 ± 0.87% to 81.97 ± 0.84% (Szliszka et al., 2009). Leukemia cell lines U937, Jurkat, and K562 were pretreated with butein for 12 h at concentrations of 5 and 7.5 μg/mL and further incubated with TRAIL for 24 hours at concentrations of 50–200 ng/mL. The tested compound showed enhanced sensitivity to TRAIL-mediated cell death (Kim, 2008). Kim showed that butein in combination with TRAIL significantly induces apoptosis in TRAIL-resistant leukemia U937 cells by increased caspase-3 and caspase-8 activation (Kim, 2008). The sequence of a promoter region in TRAIL-R2 is different from that in TRAIL-R1, and the regulation of each TRAIL receptor is different from that of other receptors (Yoshida and Sakai, 2004). TRAIL-R2 mRNA expression was upregulated in the leukemia U937 cells and leukemia Jurkat cells after 12 h treatment with butein compared to those untreated cells. The expression of TRAIL-R1 was not significantly increased by butein (Kim, 2008). In solid tumor cells such as those in renal cancer, prostate cancer, lung cancer, and bladder cancer, the initiation of the apoptotic process is carried out mainly by the TRAIL-R2 receptor (Wu et al., 2007). Moon et al. have demonstrated that butein enhances TRAIL-induced apoptosis in hepatoma HepG2 and Hep3B cancer cells, HCT116 colon cancer cells, PC3 prostate cancer cells, and leukemia U937 cancer cells through upregulation of TRAIL-R2 (Moon et al., 2010). A combined treatment with butein and TRAIL increased caspase-3 activation in leukemia U937 cancer cells (Kim, 2008). A combination of butein and TRAIL leads to cleavage of caspase-3, -8, -9, Bid, and poly(ADP-ribose) polymerase (PARP) as well as the release of cytochrome c from the mitochondria into the cytosol in hepatoma HepG2 cancer cells (little or no change was observed in cells treated with a single agent). The combined treatment decreased the expression of Bcl-2, XIAP, IAP-1, and IAP- 2 in hepatoma cancer cells (Moon et al., 2010). The molecular target of chalcones is presented in Fig. 20.2.

Cardamonin can be found in cardamom spice and many other plant species, including *Alpinia* sp., *Boesenbergia pandurate*, *Catimbium speciosum*, *Elettaria cardamomum*, and *Syzygium samarangense* (Gonçalves et al., 2014; Ohtsuki et al., 2009; Simirgiotis et al., 2008). Cardamonin sensitizes TRAIL-resistant human gastric adenocarcinoma cells (AGS) gastric carcinoma cells to TRAIL through the induction of TRAIL-R1 and TRAIL-R2. Cardamonin upregulates TRAIL-R1, TRAIL-R2, and downregulates DcR1 in leukemia KMB-5, multiple myeloma U266, pancreatic cancer MiaPaCa, and prostate cancer DU145 and PC3. The tested compound induced CCAAT/enhancer-binding protein homologous protein (CHOP) expression, a transcriptional factor that regulates TRAIL-R2 expression (Ohtsuki et al., 2009). Cardamonin combined treatment with TRAIL increased caspase-3, -8, and -9 activity in a dose-dependent manner in DLD1/TR colon cancer cells, AGS gastric cancer cells, and HCT116 colon cancer cells (Ohtsuki et al., 2009; Yadav et al., 2012). Treatment of TRAIL-resistant colorectal adenocarcinoma cell line (DLD1/TR) colon cancer cells with cardamonin decreased mRNA and protein levels of antiapoptotic Bcl-xL protein.

A prenylated chalcone xantohumol is the main prenylated flavonoid present in hops (*H. lupulus*) (Botta et al., 2005; Stevens and Page, 2004), and isobavachalcone is found in medicinal plants such as *Angelica keiskei*, *Broussonetia papyrifera*, *Psoralea corylifolia*, and *Maclura tinctoria* (ElSohly et al., 2001; Yan et al., 2015). Szliszka et al. (2009) have shown that xanthohumol and isobavachalcone markedly augmented TRAIL-mediated apoptosis and cytotoxicity in LNCaP prostate cancer cells. Similar results were obtained for butein, licochalcone A, and chalkon. Szliszka et al. also demonstrated that chalcone, isobavachalcone, licochalcone A, and xanthohumol at concentrations of 25 μM significantly increased TRAIL-R2 protein levels of HeLa cervical cancer cells after 24-h (Szliszka et al., 2012). The studies were continued by Kłósek, who showed that xanthohumol sensitizes cancer cells to TRAIL-mediated

TABLE 20.2 Examples of chalcones that enhance TRAIL-induced apoptosis in cancer cells

Naturally Occurring Chalcone	Chemical Structure	Targets	Cell Lines	References
Butein	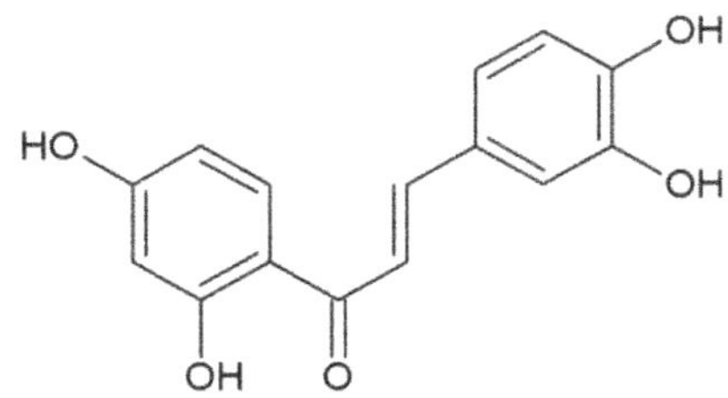	Increase: DR5, caspase-3, caspase-8, caspase-9, PARP, cytochrome c release; activation Bid to tBid Decrease: Bcl-2, XIAP, IAP-1, IAP-2	Prostate cancer LNCaP, prostate cancer PC3,Leukemia U937, leukemia Jurkat, leukemia K562, hepatocellular cancer Hep3B and HepG2, colon cancer HCT116	Kim, 2008; Moon et al., 2010; Szliszka et al., 2009
Cardamonin	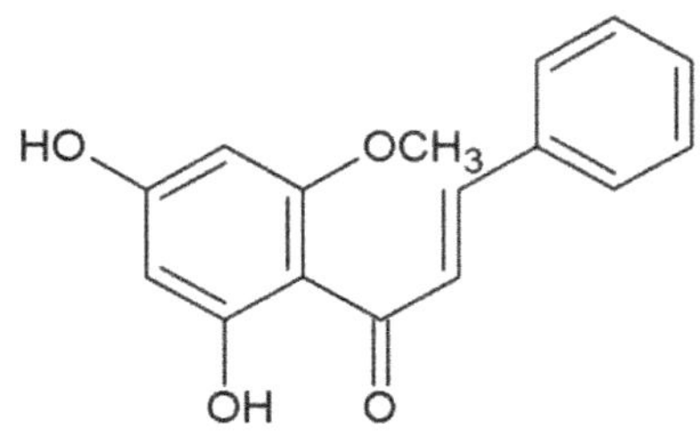	Increase: DR4, DR5, caspase-3, caspase-8, caspase-9 Decrease: Bcl-xL	Colon cancer DLD-1, colon cancer HCT116, gastric carcinoma AGS, leukemia KMB-5, ultiple myeloma U266, pancreatic cancer MiaPaCa, prostate cancer DU145, prostate cancer PC3	Kim et al., 2012; Ohtsuki et al., 2009; Yadav et al., 2012
Chalcone	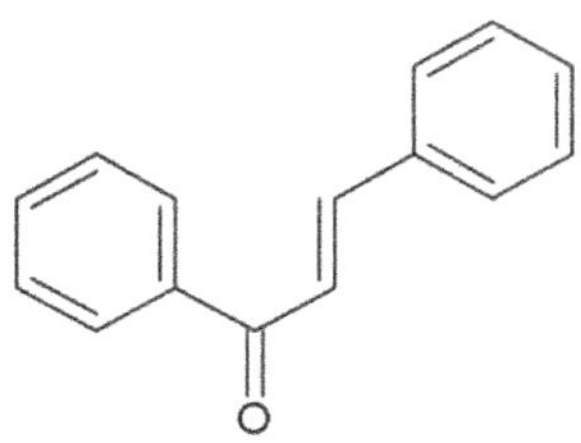	Increase: DR5	Prostate cancer LNCaP, cervical cancer HeLa	Szliszka et al., 2010; Szliszka et al., 2009; Szliszka et al., 2012
Xanthohumol	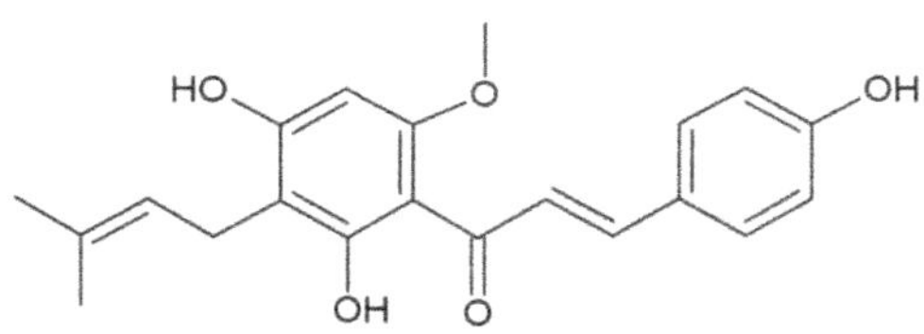	Increase: DR5	Prostate cancer LNCaP, cervical cancer HeLa	Szliszka et al., 2009; Szliszka et al., 2012
Isobavachalcone	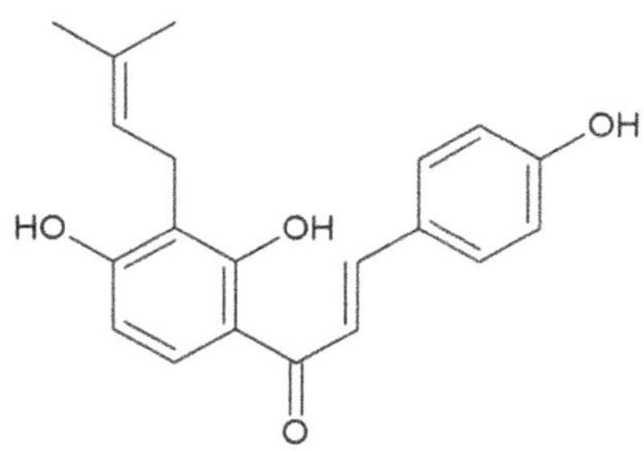	Increase: DR5	Prostate cancer LNCaP, cervical cancer HeLa	Szliszka et al., 2009; Szliszka et al., 2012
Isoliquiritigenin	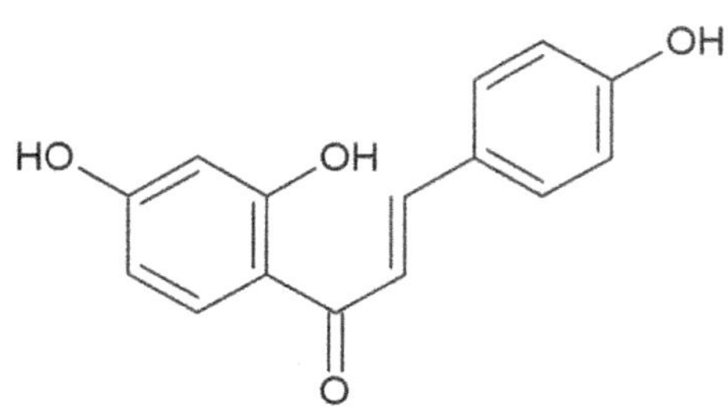	Increase: DR5, caspase-3, caspase-8, caspase-9, caspase-10	Colon cancer HT29	Yoshida et al., 2008

(*Continued*)

TABLE 20.2 Examples of chalcones that enhance TRAIL-induced apoptosis in cancer cells (Continued)

Naturally Occurring Chalcone	Chemical Structure	Targets	Cell Lines	References
Licochalcone A	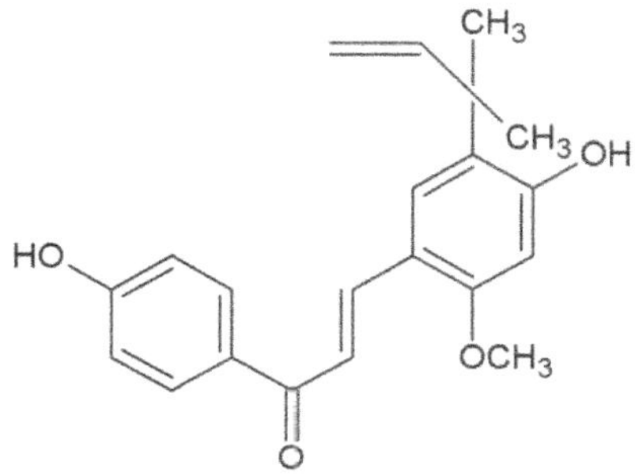	Increase: DR5	Prostate cancer LNCaP, cervical cancer HeLa	Szliszka et al., 2009; Szliszka et al., 2012
Flavokawain B	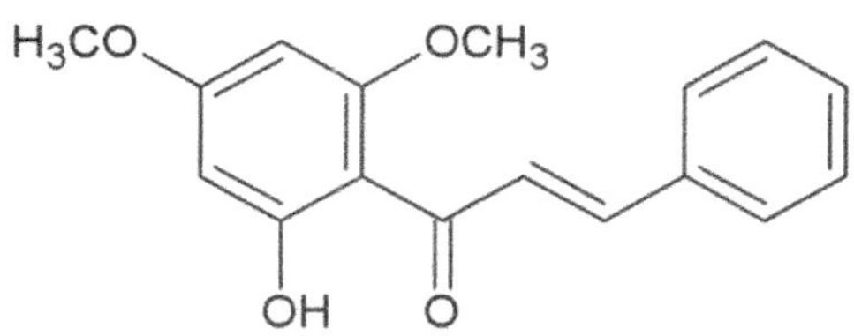	Increase: DR5, caspase-3, caspase-8, caspase-9, Bax, Bim, Puma Decrease: XIAP, survivin	Prostate cancer PC-3	Tang et al., 2010

apoptosis through activation of caspases-3, -8, and -9 and activation of Bid increase the expression of Bax, decrease of the expression of Bcl-xL, and decrease the mitochondrial membrane potential. No change was observed in the expression of death receptors on the surface of LNCaP cancer cells (Kłósek, 2014).

Isoliquiritigenin isolated from the roots of plants belonging to *Glycyrrhiza uralensis, Glycyrrhiza glabra*, and *Mongolian glycyrrhiza* have many biological properties (Peng et al., 2015). Yoshida et al. have shown that isoliquiritigenin increases the level of TRAIL-R2 but not TRAIL-R1 through activation of caspase-8, -10, -9, and -3 in HT29 colon cancer cells (Yoshida et al., 2008). The tested compound did not significantly increase the levels of the pro-apoptotic protein Bax and antiapoptotic proteins Bcl-2 and Bcl-xL.

Flavokawain A, B, and C constitute about 0.46%, 0.015%, and 0.012% of kava extracts (Dharmaratne et al., 2002). Flavokawain B found in *Piper methysticum* (Kava) has anticarcinogenic properties (Lebot et al., 2014). Tang et al. demonstrated that flavokawain B induces apoptosis in DU145 and PC3 prostate cancer cells via activation of caspases-3, -8, and -9 (Tang et al., 2010). The tested compound increases the mRNA expression of TRAIL-R2 in PC3 cancer cells and enhances TRAIL-induced apoptosis. Tang et al. have also shown that flavokawain B activates the pro-apoptotic protein Bax and mitochondrially mediated apoptotic pathway by upregulation of Bim and Puma. The tested compound also decreased expression of inhibitors of apoptosis proteins XIAP and survivin in PC3 and DU145 prostate cancer cells (Tang et al., 2010).

In summary, chalcones in combination with TRAIL increase the expression of death receptors and pro-apoptotic proteins and also decrease the expression of antiapoptotic proteins in many cancer cells. Molecular targets of chalcones in the TRAIL signaling pathway lead to sensitization of cancer cells to TRAIL-mediated apoptosis. Chalcones have potential chemopreventive effects and may be a therapeutic strategy for malignant diseases.

References

Amarante-Mendes, G.P., Griffith, T.S., 2015. Therapeutic applications of TRAIL receptor agonists in cancer and beyond. Pharmacol. Ther. 155, 117–131.

Avupati, V.R., Yejella, R.P., 2014. Chalcones: a mini review, 1713–1742.

Bhardwaj, H.C., Jain, K.K., 1982. Indian Dyes and Dyeing Industry during 18–19th Century. Indian J. Hist. Sci. 17, 70–81.

Botta, B., Vitali, A., Menendez, P., Misiti, D., Delle Monache, G., 2005. Prenylated flavonoids: pharmacology and biotechnology. Curr. Med. Chem. 12, 717–739.

Boyce, B.F., Xing, L., 2007. Biology of RANK, RANKL, and osteoprotegerin. Arthritis Res. Ther. 9 (Suppl 1), S1.

Bremner, P.D., Meyer, J.J., 1998. Pinocembrin chalcone: an antibacterial compound from *Helichrysum trilineatum*. Planta Med. 64, 777.

Busch, C., Burkard, M., Leischner, C., Lauer, U.M., Frank, J., Venturelli, S., 2015. Epigenetic activities of flavonoids in the prevention and treatment of cancer. Clin. Epigenetics 7, 64.

Caamal-Fuentes, E.E., Peraza-Sánchez, S.R., Torres-Tapia, L.W., Moo-Puc, R.E., 2015. Isolation and identification of cytotoxic compounds from *Aeschynomene fascicularis*, a Mayan medicinal plant. Molecules 20, 13563–13574.

Candolle, A., 1885. Origin of Cultivated Plants. D. Appleton & Co, New York. 164.

carthamin, definitions.net, STANDS4 LLC, 2016. "*carthamin*." Accessed February 22, 2016. <http://www.definitions.net/definition/carthamin>.

Cheng, Z.J., Kuo, S.C., Chan, S.C., Ko, F.N., Teng, C.M., 1998. Antioxidant properties of butein isolated from *Dalbergia odorifera*. Biochim. Biophys. Acta 1392, 291–299.

Claisen, L., Claparède, A., 1881. Condensationen von Ketonen mit Aldehyden. Chem. Ber 14, 2460–2468.

Dai, J., Mumper, R.J., 2010. Plant phenolics: extraction, analysis and their antioxidant and anticancer properties. Molecules 15, 7313–7352.

De Keukeleire, J., Ooms, G., Heyerick, A., Roldan-Ruiz, I., Van Bockstaele, E., De Keukeleire, D., 2003. Formation and accumulation of alpha-acids, beta-acids, desmethylxanthohumol, and xanthohumol during flowering of hops (*Humulus lupulus* L.). J. Agric. Food Chem. 51, 4436–4441.

Dean, H.F., Nierenstein, M., 1925. Attempts to synthesize myricetin. J. Am. Chem. Soc. 47, 1676–1684.

Definitions.net, STANDS4 LLC, 2016. "*phlorizin*". Accessed March 3, 2016. <http://www.definitions.net/definition/phlorizin>.

Dharmaratne, H.R., Nanayakkara, N.P., Khan, I.A., 2002. Kavalactones from Piper methysticum, and their 13C NMR spectroscopic analyses. Phytochemistry 59, 429–433.

Eddarir, S., Cotelle, N., Bakkoura, Y., Rolandoa, C., 2003. An efficient synthesis of chalcones based on the Suzuki reaction. Tetrahedron Lett. 44, 5359–5363.

ElSohly, H.N., Joshi, A.S., Nimrod, A.C., Walker, L.A., Clark, A.M., 2001. Antifungal chalcones from *Maclura tinctoria*. Planta Med. 67, 87–89.

Emery, J.G., McDonnell, P., Burke, M.B., Deen, K.C., Lyn, S., Silverman, C., et al., 1998. Osteoprotegerin is a receptor for the cytotoxic ligand TRAIL. J. Biol. Chem. 273, 14363–14367.

Fu, Y., Hsieh, T.C., Guo, J., Kunicki, J., Lee, M.Y., Darzynkiewicz, Z., et al., 2004. Licochalcone-A, a novel flavonoid isolated from licorice root (Glycyrrhiza glabra), causes G2 and late-G1 arrests in androgen-independent PC-3 prostate cancer cells. Biochem. Biophys. Res. Commun. 322, 263–270.

Fulda, S., Meyer, E., Debatin, K.M., 2002. Inhibition of TRAIL-induced apoptosis by Bcl-2 overexpression. Oncogene 21, 2283–2294.

Furusawa, J., Funakoshi-Tago, M., Mashino, T., Tago, K., Inoue, H., Sonoda, Y., et al., 2009. Glycyrrhiza inflata-derived chalcones, Licochalcone A, Licochalcone B and Licochalcone D, inhibit phosphorylation of NF-kappaB p65 in LPS signaling pathway. Int. Immunopharmacol. 9, 499–507.

Gonçalves de Lima, O., de Méllo, J.F., de Barros Coêlho, J.S., de Andrade Lyra, F.D., Machado de Albuquerque, M., Marini-Bettólo, G.B., et al., 1975. New prenylated chalcones from Lonchocarpus neuroscapha Benth. (Cordoa piaca). Farmaco Sci. 30, 326–342.

Gonçalves, L.M., Valente, I.M., Rodrigues, J.A., 2014. An overview on cardamonin. J. Med. Food 17, 633–640.

Guseva, N.V., Rokhlin, O.W., Taghiyev, A.F., Cohen, M.B., 2008. Unique resistance of breast carcinoma cell line T47D to TRAIL but not anti-Fas is linked to p43cFLIP(L). Breast Cancer Res. Treat. 107, 349–357.

Hinz, S., Trauzold, A., Boenicke, L., Sandberg, C., Beckmann, S., Bayer, E., et al., 2000. Bcl-XL protects pancreatic adenocarcinoma cells against CD95- and TRAIL-receptor-mediated apoptosis. Oncogene 19, 5477–5486.

Holland, P.M., 2013. Targeting Apo2L/TRAIL receptors by soluble Apo2L/TRAIL. Cancer Lett. 332, 156–162.

Holoch, P.A., Griffith, T.S., 2009. TNF-related apoptosis-inducing ligand (TRAIL): a new path to anti-cancer therapies. Eur. J. Pharmacol. 625, 63–72.

Horak, P., Pils, D., Haller, G., Pribill, I., Roessler, M., Tomek, S., et al., 2005a. Contribution of epigenetic silencing of tumor necrosis factor-related apoptosis inducing ligand receptor 1 (DR4) to TRAIL resistance and ovarian cancer. Mol. Cancer Res. 3, 335–343.

Horak, P., Pils, D., Kaider, A., Pinter, A., Elandt, K., Sax, C., et al., 2005b. Perturbation of the tumor necrosis factor-related apoptosis-inducing ligand cascade in ovarian cancer: overexpression of FLIPL and deregulation of the functional receptors DR4 and DR5. Clin. Cancer Res. 11, 8585–8591.

Hwang, T.L., Leu, Y.L., Kao, S.H., Tang, M.C., Chang, H.L., 2006. Viscolin, a new chalcone from Viscum coloratum, inhibits human neutrophil superoxide anion and elastase release via a cAMP-dependent pathway. Free Radic. Biol. Med. 41, 1433–1441.

Joshi, A.S., Li, X.C., Nimrod, A.C., elSohly, H.N., Walker, L.A., Clark, A.M., 2001. Dihydrochalcones from Piper longicaudatum. Planta Med. 67, 186–188.

Kang, N.J., Shin, S.H., Lee, H.J., Lee, K.W., 2011. Polyphenols as small molecular inhibitors of signaling cascades in carcinogenesis. Pharmacol. Ther. 130, 310–324.

Kim, N., 2008. Butein sensitizes human leukemia cells to apoptosis induced by tumor necrosis factor-related apoptosis inducing ligand (TRAIL). Arch. Pharm. Res. 31, 1179–1186.

Kim, Y.J., Kim, H.C., Ko, H., Amor, E.C., Lee, J.W., Yang, H.O., 2012. Inhibitory effects of aurentiacin from *Syzygium samarangense* on lipopolysaccharide-induced inflammatory response in mouse macrophages. Food Chem. Toxicol. 50, 1027–1035.

Kłósek, M., 2014. TRAIL-indukowana apoptoza komórek raka gruczołu krokowego po zastosowaniu ksantohumolu [TRAIL-induced apoptosis of prostate cancer cells after treatment of xanthohumol]. Unpublished PhD dissertation. Medical University of Silesia.

Koninck, L., 1835. Ueber das Phloridzin (Phlorrizin). Annales Pharmaceutiques 15, 75–77.de Koninck, L., 1835. Weitere Notiz über das Phloridzin. Annales Pharmaceutiques 15, 238–263.

Kostanecki, S., Tambor, J., 1899. Über die sechs isomeren Monooxybenzal-acetophenone. Berichte der Deutschen Chemischen Gesellschaft 32, 1921.

Krotoszyner, M., Stevens, W.E., 1917. The Intravenous Phlorizin Test. JAMA LXIX (22), 1865–1873. http://dx.doi.org/10.1001/jama.1917.02590490029006.

Kuropatnicki, A., Kłósek, M., Król, W., 2014. Uczniowie prof. Stanisława Kostaneckiego. In: Kopacz, M., Pusz, J., Kalembkiewicz, J. (Eds.), Flawonoidy i ich zastosowanie. Oficyna Wydawnicza Politechniki Rzeszowskiej, Rzeszów, pp. 11–20. [in Polish].

Kwon, S.J., Park, S.Y., Kwon, G.T., Lee, K.W., Kang, Y.H., Choi, M.S., et al., 2013. Licochalcone E present in licorice suppresses lung metastasis in the 4T1 mammary orthotopic cancer model. Cancer Prev. Res. (Phila) 6, 603–613.

LeBlanc, H., Lawrence, D., Varfolomeev, E., Totpal, K., Morlan, J., Schow, P., et al., 2002. Tumor-cell resistance to death receptor-induced apoptosis through mutational inactivation of the proapoptotic Bcl-2 homolog Bax. Nat. Med. 8, 274–281.

Lebot, V., Do, T.K., Legendre, L., 2014. Detection of flavokavins (A, B, C) in cultivars of kava (Piper methysticum) using high performance thin layer chromatography (HPTLC). Food Chem. 151, 554–560.

Lee, C.W., Kim, H.S., Kim, H.K., Kim, J.W., Yoon, J.H., Cho, Y., et al., 2010. Inhibitory effect of panduratin A isolated from Kaempferia panduarata Roxb. on melanin biosynthesis. Phytother. Res. 24, 1600–1604.

Lee, Y.M., Hsieh, K.H., Lu, W.J., Chou, H.C., Chou, D.S., Lien, L.M., et al., 2012. Xanthohumol, a prenylated flavonoid from hops (*Humulus lupulus*), prevents platelet activation in human platelets. Evid. Based Complement Alternat. Med. 2012, 852362.

Li, S., Li, W., Wang, Y., Asada, Y., Koike, K., 2010. Prenylflavonoids from *Glycyrrhiza uralensis* and their protein tyrosine phosphatase-1B inhibitory activities. Bioorg. Med. Chem. Lett. 20, 5398–5401.

Li, S., Sun, J., Yang, J., Zhang, L., Wang, L., Wang, X., et al., 2013. XIAP expression is associated with pancreatic carcinoma outcome. Mol. Clin. Oncol. 1, 305–308.

Lim, B., Allen, J.E., Prabhu, V.V., Talekar, M.K., Finnberg, N.K., El-Deiry, W.S., 2015. Targeting TRAIL in the treatment of cancer: new developments. Expert Opin. Ther. Targets 19, 1171–1185.

Liu, M., Yin, H., Liu, G., Dong, J., Qian, Z., Miao, J., 2014. Xanthohumol, a prenylated chalcone from beer hops, acts as an α-glucosidase inhibitor in vitro. J. Agric. Food Chem. 62, 5548–5554.

MacFarlane, M., 2003. TRAIL-induced signalling and apoptosis. Toxicol. Lett. 139, 89–97.

MacFarlane, M., Ahmad, M., Srinivasula, S.M., Fernandes-Alnemri, T., Cohen, G.M., Alnemri, E.S., 1997. Identification and molecular cloning of two novel receptors for the cytotoxic ligand TRAIL. J. Biol. Chem. 272, 25417–25420.

Mahapatra, D.K., Bharti, S.K., Asati, V., 2015. Anti-cancer chalcones: structural and molecular target perspectives. Eur. J. Med. Chem. 98, 69–114.

Mahmood, Z., Shukla, Y., 2010. Death receptors: targets for cancer therapy. Exp. Cell Res. 316, 887–899.

Mathiesen, L., Malterud, K.E., Sund, R.B., 1997. Hydrogen bond formation as basis for radical scavenging activity: a structure-activity study of C-methylated dihydrochalcones from Myrica gale and structurally related acetophenones. Free Radic. Biol. Med. 22, 307–311.

Matos, M.J., Vazquez-Rodriguez, S., Uriarte, E., Santana, L., 2015. Potential pharmacological uses of chalcones: a patent review (from June 2011 - 2014). Expert Opin. Ther. Pat. 25, 351–366.

McEleny, K.R., Watson, R.W., Coffey, R.N., O'Neill, A.J., Fitzpatrick, J.M., 2002. Inhibitors of apoptosis proteins in prostate cancer cell lines. Prostate 51, 133–140.

Mellier, G., Huang, S., Shenoy, K., Pervaiz, S., 2010. TRAILing death in cancer. Mol. Aspects Med. 31, 93–112.

Moon, D.O., Kim, M.O., Choi, Y.H., Kim, G.Y., 2010. Butein sensitizes human hepatoma cells to TRAIL-induced apoptosis via extracellular signal-regulated kinase/Sp1-dependent DR5 upregulation and NF-kappaB inactivation. Mol. Cancer Theraphy 9, 1583–1595.

Ndozangue-Touriguine, O., Sebbagh, M., Mérino, D., Micheau, O., Bertoglio, J., Bréard, J., 2008. A mitochondrial block and expression of XIAP lead to resistance to TRAIL-induced apoptosis during progression to metastasis of a colon carcinoma. Oncogene 27, 6012–6022.

Nickon, A., Silversmith, E.F., 1987. Organic Chemistry. The Name Game. Modern Coined Words and their Origins. Pergamon Press, Bungay.307.

Nowakowska, Z., 2007. A review of anti-infective and anti-inflammatory chalcones. Eur. J. Med. Chem. 42, 125–137.

Ohnogi, H., Kudo, Y., Tahara, K., Sugiyama, K., Enoki, T., Hayami, S., et al., 2012. Six new chalcones from *Angelica keiskei* inducing adiponectin production in 3T3-L1 adipocytes. Biosci. Biotechnol. Biochem. 76, 961–966.

Ohtsuki, T., Kikuchi, H., Koyano, T., Kowithayakorn, T., Sakai, T., Ishibashi, M., 2009. Death receptor 5 promoter-enhancing compounds isolated from Catimbium speciosum and their enhancement effect on TRAIL-induced apoptosis. Bioorg. Med. Chem. 17, 6748–6754.

Orjala, J., Wright, A.D., Behrends, H., Folkers, G., Sticher, O., Rüegger, H., et al., 1994. Cytotoxic and antibacterial dihydrochalcones from *Piper aduncum*. J. Nat. Prod. 57, 18–26.

Orlikova, B., Tasdemir, D., Golais, F., Dicato, M., Diederich, M., 2011. Dietary chalcones with chemopreventive and chemotherapeutic potential. Genes Nutr. 6, 125–147.

Ozören, N., El-Deiry, W.S., 2002. Defining characteristics of Types I and II apoptotic cells in response to TRAIL. Neoplasia 4, 551–557.

Padmavathi, G., Rathnakaram, S.R., Monisha, J., Bordoloi, D., Roy, N.K., Kunnumakkara, A.B., 2015. Potential of butein, a tetrahydroxychalcone to obliterate cancer. Phytomedicine 22, 1163–1171.

Pandey, K.B., Rizvi, S.I., 2009. Plant polyphenols as dietary antioxidants in human health and disease.. Oxid Med Cell Longev 2, 270–278.

Peng, F., Du, Q., Peng, C., Wang, N., Tang, H., Xie, X., et al., 2015. A review: the pharmacology of isoliquiritigenin. Phytother. Res. 29, 969–977.

Pennarun, B., Meijer, A., de Vries, E.G., Kleibeuker, J.H., Kruyt, F., de Jong, S., 2010. Playing the DISC: turning on TRAIL death receptor-mediated apoptosis in cancer. Biochim. Biophys. Acta 1805, 123–140.

Pietta, P.G., 2000. Flavonoids as antioxidants. J. Nat. Prod. 63, 1035–1042.

Pitti, R.M., Marsters, S.A., Ruppert, S., Donahue, C.J., Moore, A., Ashkenazi, A., 1996. Induction of apoptosis by Apo-2 ligand, a new member of the tumor necrosis factor cytokine family. J. Biol. Chem. 271, 12687–12690.

Qin, X., Xing, Y.F., Zhou, Z., Yao, Y., 2015. Dihydrochalcone compounds isolated from crabapple leaves showed anticancer effects on human cancer cell lines. Molecules 20, 21193–21203.

Russo, M., Mupo, A., Spagnuolo, C., Russo, G.L., 2010. Exploring death receptor pathways as selective targets in cancer therapy. Biochem. Pharmacol. 80, 674–682.

Sahu, N.K., Balbhadra, S.S., Choudhary, J., Kohli, D.V., 2012. Exploring pharmacological significance of chalcone scaffold: a review. Curr. Med. Chem. 19, 209–225.

Sayers, T.J., 2011. Targeting the extrinsic apoptosis signaling pathway for cancer therapy. Cancer Immunol. Immunother. 60, 1173–1180.

Schijlen, E.G., Ric de Vos, C.H., van Tunen, A.J., Bovy, A.G., 2004. Modification of flavonoid biosynthesis in crop plants. Phytochemistry 65, 2631–2648.

Schulze-Osthoff, K., Ferrari, D., Los, M., Wesselborg, S., Peter, M.E., 1998. Apoptosis signaling by death receptors. Eur. J. Biochem. 254, 439–459.

Secchiero, P., Gonelli, A., Corallini, F., Ceconi, C., Ferrari, R., Zauli, G., 2010. Metalloproteinase 2 cleaves in vitro recombinant TRAIL: potential implications for the decreased serum levels of TRAIL after acute myocardial infarction. Atherosclerosis 211, 333–336.

Selepe, M.A., Van Heerden, F.R., 2013. Application of the Suzuki–Miyaura reaction in the synthesis of flavonoids. Molecules 18, 4739–4765.

Simirgiotis, M.J., Adachi, S., Satoshi, To, Yang, H., Reynertson, K.A., Basile, M.J., et al., 2008. Cytotoxic chalcones and antioxidants from the fruits of a *Syzygium samarangense* (Wax Jambu). Food Chem. 107, 813–819.

Singh, P., Anand, A., Kumar, V., 2014. Recent developments in biological activities of chalcones: A mini review. Eur. J. Med. Chem. 85, 758–777.
Sirerol, J.A., Rodríguez, M.L., Mena, S., Asensi, M.A., Estrela, J.M., Ortega, A.L., 2016. Role of natural stilbenes in the prevention of cancer. Oxid. Med. Cell Longev. 2016, 3128951.
Sohn, H.Y., Son, K.H., Kwon, C.S., Kwon, G.S., Kang, S.S., 2004. Antimicrobial and cytotoxic activity of 18 prenylated flavonoids isolated from medicinal plants: *Morus alba* L., *Morus mongolica* Schneider, *Broussnetia papyrifera* (L.) Vent, Sophora flavescens Ait and *Echinosophora koreensis* Nakai. Phytomedicine 11, 666–672.
Sporn, M.B., Dunlop, N.M., Newton, D.L., Smith, J.M., 1976. Prevention of chemical carcinogenesis by vitamin A and its synthetic analogs (retinoids). Fed. Proc. 35, 1332–1338.
Stevens, J.F., Page, J.E., 2004. Xanthohumol and related prenylflavonoids from hops and beer: to your good health!. Phytochemistry 65, 1317–1330.
Szliszka, E., Czuba, Z.P., Mazur, B., Paradysz, A., Krol, W., 2010. Chalcones and dihydrochalcones augment TRAIL-mediated apoptosis in prostate cancer cells. Molecules 15, 5336–5353.
Szliszka, E., Czuba, Z.P., Mazur, B., Sedek, L., Paradysz, A., Krol, W., 2009. Chalcones enhance TRAIL-induced apoptosis in prostate cancer cells. Int. J. Mol. Sci. 11, 1–13.
Szliszka, E., Jaworska, D., Ksek, M., Czuba, Z.P., Król, W., 2012. Targeting death receptor TRAIL-R2 by chalcones for TRAIL-induced apoptosis in cancer cells. Int. J. Mol. Sci. 13, 15343–15359.
Tabata, K., Motani, K., Takayanagi, N., Nishimura, R., Asami, S., Kimura, Y., et al., 2005. Xanthoangelol, a major chalcone constituent of *Angelica keiskei*, induces apoptosis in neuroblastoma and leukemia cells. Biol. Pharm. Bull. 28, 1404–1407.
Tang, Y., Li, X., Liu, Z., Simoneau, A.R., Xie, J., Zi, X., 2010. Flavokawain B, a kava chalcone, induces apoptosis via up-regulation of death-receptor 5 and Bim expression in androgen receptor negative, hormonal refractory prostate cancer cell lines and reduces tumor growth. Int. J. Cancer 127, 1758–1768.
Vue, B., Zhang, S., Chen, Q.H., 2015. Flavonoids with therapeutic potential in prostate cancer. Anticancer Agents Med. Chem 16, 1205–1209.
Wang, X., Chen, W., Zeng, W., Bai, L., Tesfaigzi, Y., Belinsky, S.A., et al., 2008. Akt-mediated eminent expression of c-FLIP and Mcl-1 confers acquired resistance to TRAIL-induced cytotoxicity to lung cancer cells. Mol. Cancer Theraphy 7, 1156–1163.
Wiley, S.R., Schooley, K., Smolak, P.J., Din, W.S., Huang, C.P., Nicholl, J.K., et al., 1995. Identification and characterization of a new member of the TNF family that induces apoptosis. Immunity 3, 673–682.
Wu, W., Ye, H., Wan, L., Han, X., Wang, G., Hu, J., et al., 2013. Millepachine, a novel chalcone, induces G2/M arrest by inhibiting CDK1 activity and causing apoptosis via ROS-mitochondrial apoptotic pathway in human hepatocarcinoma cells in vitro and in vivo. Carcinogenesis 34, 1636–1643.
Wu, X.X., Jin, X.H., Zeng, Y., El Hamed, A.M., Kakehi, Y., 2007. Low concentrations of doxorubicin sensitizes human solid cancer cells to tumor necrosis factor-related apoptosis-inducing ligand (TRAIL)-receptor (R) 2-mediated apoptosis by inducing TRAIL-R2 expression. Cancer Sci. 98, 1969–1976.
Wu, Y.P., Meng, X.S., Bao, Y.R., Wang, S., 2013. Pharmacokinetic study of four flavones of Glycyrrhiza in rat plasma using HPLC-MS. J. Ethnopharmacol. 148, 266–270.
Yadav, V.R., Prasad, S., Aggarwal, B.B., 2012. Cardamonin sensitizes tumour cells to TRAIL through ROS- and CHOP-mediated up-regulation of death receptors and down-regulation of survival proteins. Br. J. Pharmacol. 165, 741–753.
Yadav, V.R., Prasad, S., Sung, B., Aggarwal, B.B., 2011. The role of chalcones in suppression of NF-κB-mediated inflammation and cancer. Int. Immunopharmacol. 11, 295–309.
Yan, C., Wu, Y., Weng, Z., Gao, Q., Yang, G., Chen, Z., et al., 2015. Development of an HPLC method for absolute quantification and QAMS of flavonoids components in *Psoralea corylifolia* L. J. Anal. Methods Chem. 2015, 792637.
Yao, G.M., Ding, Y., Zuo, J.P., Wang, H.B., Wang, Y.B., Ding, B.Y., et al., 2005. Dihydrochalcones from the leaves of *Pieris japonica*. J. Nat. Prod. 68, 392–396.
Yoshida, T., Horinaka, M., Takara, M., Tsuchihashi, M., Mukai, N., Wakada, M., et al., 2008. Combination of isoliquiritigenin and tumor necrosis factor-related apoptosis-inducing ligand induces apoptosis in colon cancer HT29 cells. Environ. Health Prev. Med. 13, 281–287.
Yoshida, T., Sakai, T., 2004. Promoter of TRAIL-R2 gene. Vitam. Horm. 67, 35–49.
Zhang, E.H., Wang, R.F., Guo, S.Z., Liu, B., 2013. An update on antitumor activity of naturally occurring chalcones. Evid. Based Complement. Alternat. Med. 2013, 815621.
Zhang, L., Fang, B., 2005. Mechanisms of resistance to TRAIL-induced apoptosis in cancer. Cancer Gene Theraphy 12, 228–237.
Zhao, X., Mei, W., Gong, M., Zuo, W., Bai, H., Dai, H., 2011. Antibacterial activity of the flavonoids from *Dalbergia odorifera* on *Ralstonia solanacearum*. Molecules 16, 9775–9782.
Zsuzsanna Rozmer, P.P., 2014. Naturally occurring chalcones and their biological activities. Phytochem. Rev. 15, 87–120.

C H A P T E R

21

Anti-inflammatory Dietary Ingredients, Medicinal Plants, and Herbs Exert Beneficial Health Effects in Aging

Kiran S. Panickar and Dennis E. Jewell

Hill's Pet Nutrition Center, Topeka, KS, United States

INTRODUCTION

One hallmark of aging is chronic low-grade inflammation (Brüünsgaard and Pedersen, 2003; Candore et al., 2010) that is accompanied by an increase in circulating pro-inflammatory cytokines (Roubenoff et al., 1998; Bruunsgaard, 2002, Michaud et al., 2013). A pro-inflammatory state contributes to various aging-associated dysfunctions at the cellular and molecular levels.

The immune system is a key component of inflammation and is body's natural response to injury or infection. Immune function involves several cell types that regulate both innate and adaptive responses as well as interactions among them while responding to an antigen. Innate immune response is nonspecific and relatively immediate whereas adaptive immune response is antigen-specific and delayed. Inflammation is generally classified as acute or chronic. While many features of the acute inflammatory response may also manifest themselves in chronic inflammation, there are distinguishing features. For instance, acute inflammation, as its name indicates, is a quick response to an infection or injury and is often resolved quickly; chronic inflammation may develop in days and can be progressive. While neutrophils play an important role in acute inflammation, monocytes, macrophages, and lymphocytes play a major role in chronic inflammation. One form of early response to infection or injury is the acute phase response (APR). The APR is characterized by the production of plasma protein-derived proteins such as C-reactive protein (CRP) and serum amyloids A and P, and they complement proteins by the liver generally in response to cell-derived mediators such as prostaglandins, nitric oxide, leukotrienes, and cytokines. The goal of the early response includes (1) destroying or inhibiting the activity of foreign bodies in particular microbes, (2) exerting protective effects that may limit infection, (3) removing necrotic tissue, and (4) initiating cell repair. This response is distinct from a state of mild inflammation, which is associated with chronically elevated levels of inflammatory markers, including C-reactive protein as well as cytokines such as interleukin-6 (IL-6) and tumor necrosis factor-α (TNF-α).

Immunosenescence is the gradual decline of the immune system with age (Franceschi et al., 2000). Both innate and adaptive responses are dampened with aging, and there is also a decline in the diversity of the antigen repertoire and an accumulation of functionally impaired memory lymphocytes that can affect the ability to fight infection or recover from injury. While there is consensus that the immune responses decline with aging, the specific changes in the repertoire of specific cell types leading to a compromised immune system are not clear. For instance, there might be a decrease in the levels of cluster of differentiation (CD) cells CD27 and CD28 and the generation of immature B cells but an increase in CD244 and memory B cells (see Alam and Pawelec, 2012 for review). This signifies the complexity of the immune system in aging. CD244, for instance, is a cell surface receptor on natural killer (NK) cells, which might imply increased NK-mediated cytolytic activity. In addition, this receptor can also be expressed

Nutrition and Functional Foods for Healthy Aging.
DOI: http://dx.doi.org/10.1016/B978-0-12-805376-8.00021-6

on nonlymphocytes such as eosinophils, mast cells, and dendritic cells. Whereas taking this one example in isolation would indicate an increased immune function in aging, a generalized dampened immune function in aging is likely the resultant composite function of the immune system as a whole. In canines, there does not appear to be clear consensus on the types of leukocytes that decline with aging although a general decline in immune function with aging is observed. Kearns et al. (1999) reported an age-associated decline in the proliferative capacity of lymphocytes in fox terriers and Labrador retrievers, indicating a reduced immune activity. Fleming et al. (2011) reported that older dogs died of neoplastic, traumatic, and infectious disorders, which indicates a possibly reduced immune function and ability to fight infection. Nevertheless, in older canines an ability to mount a primary humoral response to novel antigens is generally retained but the magnitude of the response is likely reduced relative to titers achieved in younger animals (Day, 2010). Aged beagle dogs have decreased neutrophil phagocytosis when compared to young ones as assessed by their ability to phagocytize *Lactococcus lactis* ex vivo (Hall et al., 2010). In the same study, younger dogs had significantly higher levels of messenger RNA (mRNA) for IL8R, L-selectin, and interleukin-1β-converting enzyme. While this indicates a generally depressed innate immune response in older dogs, the ability to fight infections was not assessed in the study.

Dietary modifications also can influence the immune system in elderly humans (Lesourd, 1997; Lesourd and Mazari, 1999). However, several ingredients have not had the desired beneficial immune effects although their effects in animal studies have been generally beneficial. In humans, dietary inclusions of certain ingredients including β-carotene (Santos et al., 1997) or black-currant seed oil rich in both gamma-linolenic (18:3n-6) and alpha-linolenic (18:3n-3) acids (Wu et al., 1999) have not been reported to have significant effects on the immune system in the elderly. In contrast, vitamin E (800 mg dl-α-tocopheryl acetate) appeared to enhance cell-mediated immunity in healthy elders (Meydani et al., 1990). Immunosenescence in canines can be modulated by caloric restriction (Greeley et al., 2006), and there is an important role for nutrition in regulating immune function (Sheffy and Williams, 1981). Hall et al. (2011) reported that a diet fortified with vitamins C and E and added fish oil reduced the pro-inflammatory markers, including nuclear factor kappa B (NFκB), toll-like receptors 2 and 4 (TLR-2 and TLR-4), cyclooxygenase-2, and myeloperoxidase (MPO) in the neutrophils isolated from adult and aged dogs. Consumption of high concentrations of α-tocopheryl acetate in elderly healthy dogs resulted in higher percentages of CD8+ cells when compared to those consuming low concentrations (Hall et al., 2003). These studies indicate an important role of nutrition in regulating the immune function in aging.

RENAL FUNCTION

A reduction in age-associated kidney function in humans has been well established (see Abdel-Rahman and Okusa, 2014, for review). In addition to a reduction in renal mass during aging (Mulder and Hillen, 2001), morphological changes in the glomeruli are associated with kidney dysfunction, including decreases in glomerular filtration rate (GFR) and renal blood flow (Anderson and Brenner, 1986; Weinstein and Anderson, 2010). Similarly, a reduction in renal function with age has also been reported in cats (Hall et al., 2014) and dogs (Hall et al., 2015). In canines, chronic renal failure (CRF) is the most common form of renal disease; while CRF may occur at all ages, its incidence increases with age (Rubin, 1997). Inflammation is associated with a decline in renal function. Costa et al. (2013) reported impaired renal function in older rats (18 months old) and significantly higher urea and creatinine as well as interferon gamma (INFγ) when compared to young rats (two months). Increased pro-inflammatory cytokines and chemokines (CCLs), including CCL3, CCL4, CCL5, CD80, TNF-α, and IL-12b are upregulated in aging rat kidney when compared to young (Xi et al., 2014). Other pro-inflammatory mediators in kidney dysfunction in aging include NFκB (Moreno et al., 2011). In canines, there was an increased expression of the cytokines IL-1α, IL-1β, transforming growth factor beta (TGF-β), and the enzyme 5-lipoxygenase (5-LO) in the venous whole blood of dogs with renal disease (Nentwig et al., 2016). There was a significant relation between serum CRP concentrations and kidney function, which indicates an important role for CRP in the pathogenesis of naturally occurring canine renal disease (Raila et al., 2011). Median CRP concentration of miniature schnauzer dogs was slightly higher than that of other breeds of dogs (Wong et al., 2011), indicating that breed specificity may also be an important factor to consider when assessing inflammation in dogs. In cats, chronic kidney disease (CKD) is the most common metabolic disease of aged domesticated cats (>12 years of age; Brown et al. (2016). Inflammation contributes to the progression of renal fibrosis in CKD in cats; when urine cytokine levels in both healthy and CKD cats were compared, significantly higher levels of IL-8 and transforming growth factor-β1 (TGF-β1) concomitant with lower vascular endothelial growth factor (VEGF) levels were reported (Habenicht et al., 2013).

A common aging effect shared by cats, dogs, and humans is declining renal function (see Panickar and Jewell, 2015 for review; Hall et al.; Hall et al., 2016a; Hall et al., 2016b). There are multiple observational studies in humans that show diets rich in fruits and vegetables reduce the risk of chronic kidney disease (Jain and Reilly, 2014). There is also a reduction in renal function when foods high in pro-inflammatory ingredients are compared to foods with high anti-inflammatory dietary ingredients; the pro-inflammatory regimen was also associated with increased systemic inflammation (Xu et al., 2015). Therefore, it is reasonable to conclude that inflammation is one pathway through which kidney function is influenced and foods that reduce inflammation may be beneficial in reducing age-associated declines in kidney function.

Nutritional intervention to reduce kidney dysfunction is important in maintaining kidney health. In evaluating the effect of anti-inflammatory ingredients and botanicals on early intervention to change age-associated declines in renal function, a food rich in antioxidants (alpha-lipoic acid, vitamins E and C), fish oil, and botanicals (fruits and vegetables) were fed to dogs for a period of six months. Dogs that did not receive the renal protective food (RPF) but were maintained on their owner's choice food had numerically increased blood urea nitrogen (BUN) and symmetric dimethyl arginine (SDMA), while those that received the RPF decreased BUN and SDMA. The control dogs did not change blood creatinine concentration, whereas the RPF fed dogs declined in circulating creatinine concentration. These improvements in markers of renal function in geriatric dogs show the benefit of anti-inflammatory ingredients and botanicals (Hall et al., 2016b). A major role of the kidneys is to also maintain phosphorus homeostasis in the body. In general, in dogs with chronic renal failure the combination of low protein and low phosphorus in the diet appears to be beneficial. In addition, several ingredients have been demonstrated to attenuate stress associated with kidney function in aging as well as in nonaging-related kidney dysfunction. Table 21.1 provides a list of anti-inflammatory botanical extracts that may prove beneficial as nephroprotective agents when included in the diet. In cats, similar to what was observed in dogs, an RPF enriched with antioxidants (vitamins E and C), fish oil, L-carnitine, and botanicals (vegetables) had an improvement in renal function when compared to cats that did not receive nutritional intervention with the RPF. In this study, the control cats had no change in BUN and increased SDMA concentration while urine specific gravity decreased. In contrast, cats fed the RPF saw reduced concentrations of BUN, creatinine, and SDMA. Like the dog, these improvements in markers of renal function in the geriatric cats show the benefits of anti-inflammatory ingredients and botanicals (Hall et al., 2016a). Anorexia or hyporexia is a common problem in cats with CKD and may lead to cats being fed suboptimal diets for their disease (Markovich et al., 2015), indicating an importance of nutrition in cats with kidney disease.

The nephroprotective effects of bioactive components from dietary ingredients, including botanical extracts, in rodent studies have been reported. In rats made obese with a high-fat diet, lycopene, a major component of tomato, reduced TNF-α levels in the kidney when supplemented in the high-fat diet (Pierine et al., 2014). Anti-inflammatory effects of lycopene have been reported in the kidney of obese rats (Pierine et al., 2014), in diabetic nephropathy in mice (Guo et al., 2015), and in contrast-induced nephropathy in rats (Buyuklu et al., 2015). Inclusion of polyphenols, which generally have anti-inflammatory effects, has also been shown to have a nephroprotective effect. In a mouse model of diabetes, the low-molecular-weight polyphenol oligonol, derived from lychee fruit, reduced diabetes-induced increase in advanced glycation end product (AGE) formation and apoptosis in the kidneys (Park et al., 2014). A polyphenol-rich extract from amla (*Emblica officinalis Gaertn*) reduced the expression of renal nuclear factor kappa B (NFκB), inhibitory κB in cytoplasm, inducible nitric oxide synthase (iNOS), and cyclooxygenase 2 (COX-2) protein levels that were elevated in aged rats (Yokozawa et al., 2007).

In summary, it is apparent that a diet that includes anti-inflammatory and specific botanically active ingredients can reduce or reverse the decline in kidney function associated with aging. This effectiveness is likely due in part to the known beneficial effect of the anti-inflammatory ingredients but may also be the result of a specific action of individual botanical compounds on the kidney.

COGNITIVE FUNCTION

Cognitive function declines with aging, but it is not uniform; some people experience very little cognitive decline whereas others suffer from mild to moderate to severe decline in some components of cognitive function. The causes or mechanisms of this decline are not clear, but there is evidence to indicate a role for inflammation in reducing cognitive ability. In aged rats that received a single injection of lipopolysaccharide (LPS), there was an impaired reversal of learning and attentional shifts but not effect on discrimination learning (Culley et al., 2014). Further, in this study, although an increase in monocyte chemoattractant protein 1 (MCP-1) was found elevated 2h after LPS administration, the levels returned to normal at the time of testing. Whether the increase and subsequent decrease in TNF and CCL2 following LPS injection in the rats had initiated a cascade of events that affected subsequent cognitive function is not clear but is a possibility. Increased levels of TNFα and IL1β were reported in the 24-month group (older

TABLE 21.1 Anti-inflammatory and Immune-Modulating Effects of Some Herbal and Plant Extracts in Both In Vivo and In Vitro Models of Inflammatory Conditions

Bioactive Component or Extract	Class of Compound	Efficacy in Health Conditions	Potential Anti-Inflammatory Mechanism	References
β-caryophyllene (clove oil, rosemary, hops, basil)	Sesquiterpene	Neuroprotective, nephroprotective, immune modulation	Inhibits pathways due to activation of toll-like receptor complex CD14/TLR4/MD2; reduces pro-inflammatory cytokines, including IL-1β, TNF-α, IL-6; exhibits synergy with μ-opioid receptor–dependent pathways; activates peroxisome proliferator-activated receptor gamma (PPARγ) pathway	Bento et al., 2011; Horváth et al., 2012; Guo et al., 2014; Sharma et al., 2016
Eugenol (clove)	Phenylpropene	Inflammation, nephroprotective	Inhibits IL-1β, IL-6, and matrix metalloproteinase 9 (MMP-9); inhibits mouse paw edema induced by carrageenan; anti-inflammatory effect on gentamycin-induced nephrotoxicity in rat kidney	Valacchi et al., 2009; Said 2011; Taher et al., 2015
Zingerone, shogaols, and gingerols (ginger extract)	Guaiacol (zingerone)	Aging, nephroprotective	Zingerone partially prevented age-related decline in PPAR expression and suppressed pro-inflammatory NFκB activity in rats; gingerol induces nephroprotective effect on gentamycin-mediated nephropathy and reduces IL-2, TNF-α, and IFN-γ.	Chung et al., 2009; Kim et al., 2010; Rodrigues et al., 2014
Proanthocyanidins (grape seed extract, cinnamon extract)	Polyphenol	Cognition, nephroprotective	Grape seed extract ameliorates renal injury in type 2 diabetic rats; proanthocyanidins from persimmon peel reduced inflammation in streptozotocin-induced diabetic rats; proanthocyanidin-rich fraction obtained from the bark of *Croton celtidifolius* Baill has anti-inflammatory as well as beneficial effects on cognitive functions in rats	Lee et al., 2007; Moreira et al., 2010; Panickar, 2014; Bao et al., 2015
			Suppressed NFkB and activator protein 1 pathways; prostaglandin E2 (PGE2), COX-2; reduction in cMyc, H-ras, and p53-related genes; inhibited signal transducer and activator of transcription 4 (STAT-4), mitogen-activated protein kinases (MAPKs); reduces TNF-α, IL-2, IL-4, IFN-γ, and chemokines (CXCL8, CCL2, CCL3, CCL4)	
Ellagitannin, gallocatechin, delphinidin (pomegranate extract)	Polyphenol	Nephroprotective, cognition	Urolithins, gut microbiota–derived metabolites of ellagitannins, inhibit LPS-induced inflammation in RAW 264.7 murine macrophages; punicalagin, a bioactive ellagitannin, inhibits LPS-induced inflammation in a macrophage cell line; consumption of pomegranate juice decreased inflammation and strengthened innate immunity in hemodialysis patients; improves cognitive performance in diabetic rats as well as in a mouse model of Alzheimer's disease.	Cambay et al. 2011; Shema-Didi et al., 2012; Xu et al., 2014; Piwowarski et al., 2015; Subash et al., 2015
Piperine (black pepper extract)	Alkaloid	Aging, nephroprotective	Inhibits STAT-1; reduces NFκB activation, suppresses Akt, ERKs; reduces IL-2, IL-4, IL-5, iNOS, COX-2, INF-γ	Kim and Lee, 2009; Bae et al., 2012
			Reduces eosinophil infiltration; decreases MMP-3, MMP-13 responses	
Rutin (buckwheat and citrus fruit rinds)	Polyphenol	Cognition	Improves cognition and reduces neuroinflammation in a mouse model of Alzheimer's disease; Improves long-term and short-term episodic memory deficits in Wistar rats	Kwon et al., 2005; Koda et al., 2009; Javed et al., 2012; Ramalingayya et al., 2016
			Reduces tissue levels of IFN-γ, IL-1β, IL-4, IL-5, IL-10, IL-17; IL-31, and IL-32; reduces NFκB activation, COX-2, iNOS, TNF-α; inhibits MMP-3	

Carnosol (rosemary extract, sage extract)	Polyphenol	Cognition	*Rosmarinus officinalis* leaf extract improves memory deficits in a rats; rosemary extract and carnosol both inhibited COX1 and COX2 activity in mice.	Ozarowski et al., 2013; Emami et al., 2013
Oleocanthal, oleuropein, (olive oil)	Polyphenol, phenylethanoid (oleocanthal)	Nephroprotective, cognition	Dietary olive oil reduces inflammation and renal injury in mice; anti-inflammatory effects of oleuropein aglycone in neurodegeneration and peripheral inflammatory disorders	Casamenti et al., 2015; Aparicio Soto et al., 2016
Rhubarb extract,rhubarb (*Rheum rhabarbarum*)	Anthraquinones	Nephroprotective	Nephroprotective and anti-fibrotic activities in patients with chronic kidney disease; anthraquinones from rhubarb reduce $HgCl2$-induced acute renal failure in rats.	Zhang et al., 2015; Gao et al., 2016
Withania somnifera	Tropine and cuscohygrine (alkaloid also found in cocoa), withaferin A (steroidal lactone)	Nephroprotective, cognition	Oral administration of *W. somnifera* significantly protected against bromobenzene-induced nephrotoxicity and renal dysfunction in rats. *W. somnifera* extract improved cognitive and psychomotor performance in healthy male subjects.	Vedi et al., 2014; Pingali et al., 2014
Magnolol (*Magnolia officinalis*)	Lignan	Mobility	Anti-arthritic effects of magnolol reported in a Mycobacterium butyricum-induced arthritis model in rats	Wang et al., 2012
Fenugreek extract,fenugreek (*Trigonella foenum-graecum L*)	Alkaloids, flavonoids	Nephroprotective	Fenugreek oil reduced renal toxicity in alloxan-induced diabetic rats.	Hamden et al., 2010; Yadav & Baquer, 2014
Black cumin (*Nigella sativa*)	Thymoquinone, tannins	Nephroprotective, cognition	*N. sativa* administration antagonized paracetamol-induced kidney pathological damage, improved cognition in healthy adolescent males as well as in elderly human subjects.	Bin Sayeed et al., 2013, 2014; Canayakin et al., 2016
Mangosteen (*Garcinia mangostana*)	Xanthones (gartanin and α-mangostin)	Cognition, nephroprotective, mobility	Mangosteen attenuated the deficit in spatial memory retrieval in a mouse model of Alzheimer's disease. α-mangosteen had a renoprotective effect in a cisplatin-induced model of nephrotoxicity in rats. Isogarcinol, isolated from *Garcinia mangostana*, reduced inflammation in collagen-induced arthritis in animals.	Pérez-Rojas et al., 2009; Huang et al., 2014; Fu et al., 2014
Silibinin (milk thistle: *Silybum marianum*)	Polyphenol	Mobility, cognition, nephroprotective	Silymarin, primarily made of three isomers—silybin, silydianin, and silychristin—exhibited significant anti-inflammatory and antiarthritic activities in the papaya latex–induced model of inflammation in rats; silymarin significantly reversed high-fat diet-induced cognitive deficits in mice; silymarin significant attenuated the nephrotoxic effects in a rat model of kidney stress.	Gupta et al., 2000; Neha et al., 2014; Alcaraz-Contreras et al., 2016
Scutellaria baicalensis and *Oroxylum indicum* (Indian trumpetflower)	Baicalein (flavonoid)	Nephroprotective, cognitive, mobility	Baicalein attenuated kidney injury induced by myocardial ischemia and reperfusion in rats; baicalein inhibited inflammatory process through inactivation of NF-κB and MAPK signal pathways to exert antifibrotic actions in obstructive kidney disease in mice; baicalein prevented spatial learning and memory retention deficits following whole brain irradiation in mice; baicalein attenuated expression of MMPs and ameliorated cartilage damage in rabbit model of osteoarthritis.	Oh et al., 2013; Chen et al., 2015; Wang et al., 2015; Lai et al., 2016

Source: Table modified from Panickar, K.S., 2014. Anti-inflammatory properties of botanical extracts contribute to their protective effects in brain edema in cerebral ischemia. In: Watson, R., Preedy, V. (Eds), Bioactive Nutriceuticals and Dietary Supplements in Neurological and Brain Disease: Prevention and Therapy, Academic Press, New York, pp. 3– 15.

group) when compared to the young group of rats (Gocmez et al., 2016). In another study in aged rats, following laparotomy (abdominal cavity surgery) memory and learning functions were impaired and there was a significant upregulation of TNF-α, interleukin (IL)-1β, IL-4, and IL-6 in the hippocampal tissues. However, intracisternal administration of the TNF-α receptor antagonist R-7050 during surgery attenuated these defects in cognitive function and inhibited the production of the pro-inflammatory cytokines (Ma et al., 2015).

In human subjects, a study reported that a pro-inflammatory diet at midlife might be associated with subsequent lower cognitive functioning (Kesse-Guyot et al., 2016). In the Singapore Longitudinal Aging Study, significant associations of soluble IL-2 receptor alpha chain, soluble tumor necrosis factor receptor 2, and soluble glycoprotein 130 were found along with cognitive impairment in community-dwelling older persons (Gao et al., 2016). In the Berlin Aging Study II, levels of IL-6, IL-10, and CRP were inversely associated with executive function and processing speed, but IL-6 to IL-10 ratio was not predictive for executive function and processing speed (Tegeler et al., 2016). Further, in the same study, no associations were found between inflammatory markers and verbal episodic memory. The underlying mechanisms or the neuroanatomical correlates on why certain inflammatory markers are associated with certain components of memory are not clear. In nondemented subjects aged 70–90 years, higher levels of serum macrophage inhibitory cytokine-1 (MIC-1), also called *growth differentiation factor 15* (GDF15), were associated with lower global cognition (Fuchs et al., 2013). A higher intracellular cytokine production of IL-1β and IL-6 by activated monocytes were predictive of lower cognitive performance in working memory in healthy older individuals aged 55–70 years (Simpson et al., 2013). In a prospective population-based cohort study with data collected over 20 years, it was reported that higher serum CRP and IL-6 were associated with a likelihood of cognitive impairment (Wichmann et al., 2014). Nascimento et al. (2014) reported an association of pro-inflammatory cytokines, including TNF-α and IL6, with mild cognitive impairment in elderly humans. Such elevated levels of the pro-inflammatory cytokines, however, could be reduced with physical exercise, which also correlated with subsequent positive effects on cognition. Taken together, these studies indicate that an increased risk of cognitive decline is associated with age-related inflammatory conditions.

In canines, an age-dependent decline is seen in learning and memory, and neuropathological changes are also observed in canines that are generally similar to those seen in normal human aging or in early Alzheimer's disease (Head, 2011; Vite and Head, 2014; Schütt et al., 2016). Cognitive dysfunction syndrome has also been described in canines and felines (Landsberg et al., 2012; Bosch et al., 2013). Interferon gamma (IFN-γ) expression was increased in the homogenates of dentate gyrus, a region of the limbic system involved in cognition, in aged dogs when compared to adult dogs (Hwang et al., 2008). A battery of cognitive tests were then administered to dogs that were divided into young (1–4 years), middle-aged (5–8 years), cognitively unimpaired aged (≥9 years), and cognitively impaired aged (≥9 years). The younger dogs (<9 years) successfully located the food more quickly in a food-seeking task and with more success than the aged groups (≥9 years) (González-Martínez et al., 2013). In another study with pet dogs. there were no significant effects of age on learning or retention tasks, but older dogs (≥8 years) were significantly impaired on the reversal learning task when compared with younger ones (<8 years). In addition, the trial response latency was significantly increased in aged dogs in both the initial and reversal learning tasks but not on the retention task (Mongillo et al., 2013). These studies indicate that pro-inflammatory markers are associated with a decline in cognitive function, but the facets of cognitive components affected by various inflammatory markers are yet unclear.

Diet-induced improvement in cognitive function has been demonstrated and it appears that more research is warranted. In the Whitehall II prospective cohort study, a dietary pattern with a higher intake of red and processed meat, peas, legumes and fried food, and lower intake of whole grains was associated with higher inflammatory markers and accelerated cognitive decline at older ages (Ozawa et al., 2016). Intervention studies using eicosapentaenoic acid (EPA) and docosahexaenoic acid (DHA), fatty acids which have anti-inflammatory effects, to adults with mild cognitive impairment or age-related cognitive impairment have shown beneficial effects although no differences in cognitive decline between treated and nontreated participants were observed in healthy older adults (Cederholm et al., 2013). In a population-based cohort of nondemented Asian subjects aged 60–93 years, when the authors compared the Mini-Mental State Examination (MMSE) scores for three categories of regular curry (curcumin) consumption they found that those who consumed curry "occasionally" and "often or very often" had significantly better MMSE scores than did subjects who "never or rarely" consumed curry (Ng et al., 2006). The anti-inflammatory effects of curcumin have been well established in several studies (for reviews, see Boyanapalli and Tony Kong, 2015; Ghosh et al., 2015; Sahebkar et al., 2016).

In canines, higher serum vitamin E concentrations from vitamin E supplemented food correlated with improved performance on landmark-discrimination tasks in aged dogs (Ikeda-Douglas et al., 2004). Although vitamin E (generally tocopherols) has been reported to have antioxidant effects, their anti-inflammatory effects have also been reported (Betti et al., 2011; England et al., 2012). Whether the improvement in cognitive tasks was a consequence of their anti-inflammatory actions or a combination of antioxidant and anti-inflammatory actions is not clear but is a possibility. A combination of antioxidant and mitochondrial cofactor improved the performance of aged dogs in a three-choice size-discrimination task (Siwak et al., 2005). Canine puppies fed a diet rich in DHA (and with higher concentrations of vitamin E, taurine, choline, and L-carnitine) performed significantly better on cognitive tasks when compared to moderate and low DHA groups (Zicker et al., 2012). In addition to the anti-inflammatory actions of vitamin E, DHA also has been reported to have anti-inflammatory actions in beagles (Hall et al., 2011). Canines supplemented with medium-chain triglycerides (MCT) showed improved memory in some but not all of the cognitive tasks administered in aged dogs (Pan et al., 2010). The mechanisms underlying the improvement in cognitive functions in the previously mentioned studies is not clear, but certainly ingredients with anti-inflammatory potential may be important in attenuating cognitive decline.

In adult rats, anthocyanins reversed the D-galactose–induced neuroinflammation-mediated cognitive impairment (Rehman et al., 2016). In aged rats, dietary supplementation with the polyphenol-rich açaí pulps (*Euterpe oleracea Mart.* and *Euterpe precatoria Mart.*) improved cognition in aged rats and concomitantly reduced levels of TNF-α were also reported in the serum (Carey et al., 2015). In mice, supplementing a diet with resveratrol reduced the LPS-related neuroinflammation and deficits in working memory in aged mice (Abraham and Johnson, 2009). Similarly, resveratrol was effective in preventing cognitive deficit in aged rats by inhibiting the production of inflammatory cytokines (Gocmez et al., 2016). The inclusion of mushroom (*Agaricus bisporus*), which has anti-inflammatory effects, in the daily diet of aged rats had beneficial effects on age-related deficits in cognitive and motor function (Thangthaeng et al., 2015). Supplementation with blueberry polyphenols attenuated the kainic acid–induced increase in the expression of IL-1β, TNF-α, and NFκB, and expression of insulin-like growth factor 1 (IGF-1) and a concomitant reduction in learning impairments following the neurotoxic insult (Shukitt-Hale et al., 2008). In addition, the effects of polyphenol-rich extracts from grape, strawberry, blackberry, and plum reportedly have beneficial effects in cognition in rodent models (Shukitt-Hale et al., 2006; Shukitt-Hale et al., 2009; Cherniack, 2012). Table 21.1 lists some natural compounds that may provide beneficial health effects by reducing inflammation and may also benefit cognition. In short, the studies mentioned indicate that dietary ingredients, in particular botanical extracts with anti-inflammatory properties, may be useful in improving several components of cognitive function.

CONCLUSION

Aging-associated increases in low-grade systemic inflammation could contribute to the pathogenesis of various chronic conditions in aging, including kidney dysfunction, diminished cognition, and a reduction in an effective immune function. The causal factors for the increased systemic low-grade inflammation are not clear but likely multifactorial. Strategies to effectively combat aging-associated inflammation have included nutrition, drugs, lifestyle changes, and recently stem cell therapies to modulate the immune system. Nutritional intervention is a particularly important strategy to lower systemic inflammation in aging, and evidence for this comes from laboratory animal studies, clinical studies, and epidemiological studies. Dietary factors, including a polyphenol-rich diet from fruits, vegetables, and herbs, as well as a diet rich in ω-3 fatty acids and some vitamins appear to have beneficial effects or the potential to reduce systemic inflammation in aging. In general, there appears to be a health benefit in reducing systemic inflammation in aging. Given the complexity and breadth of the inflammatory profile, in particular in aging, it is imperative that the anti-inflammatory and immune-modulating properties of herbal or plant extracts be investigated further as part of the dietary regimen.

CONFLICT OF INTEREST

The authors are employees at the Science and Technology Center of the Hillspet Nutrition Center, a Colgate-Palmolive company.

References

Abdel-Rahman, E.M., Okusa, M.D., 2014. Effects of aging on renal function and regenerative capacity. Nephron Clin. Pract. 127 (1–4), 15–20.

Abraham, J., Johnson, R.W., 2009. Consuming a diet supplemented with resveratrol reduced infection-related neuroinflammation and deficits in working memory in aged mice. Rejuvenation Res. 12 (6), 445–453.

Alam, I., Pawelec, G., 2012. Aging, nutrition and immunity – their relationship and interaction. Nutr. Aging 1, 151–165.

Alcaraz-Contreras, Y., Mendoza-Lozano, R.P., Martínez-Alcaraz, E.R., Martínez-Alfaro, M., Gallegos-Corona, M.A., Ramírez-Morales, M.A., et al., 2016. Silymarin and dimercaptosuccinic acid ameliorate lead-induced nephrotoxicity and genotoxicity in rats. Hum. Exp. Toxicol 35 (4), 398–403.

Anderson, S., Brenner, B.M., 1986. Effects of aging on the renal glomerulus. Am. J. Med. 80 (3), 435–442.

Aparicio-Soto, M., Sánchez-Hidalgo, M., Cárdeno, A., Rosillo, M.Á., Sánchez-Fidalgo, S., Utrilla, J., et al., 2016. Dietary extra virgin olive oil attenuates kidney injury in pristane-induced SLE model via activation of HO-1/Nrf-2 antioxidant pathway and suppression of JAK/STAT, NF-κB and MAPK activation. J. Nutr. Biochem. 27, 278–288.

Bae, G.S., Kim, J.J., Park, K.C., Koo, B.S., Jo, I.J., Choi, S.B., et al., 2012. Piperine inhibits lipopolysaccharide-induced maturation of bone-marrow-derived dendritic cells through inhibition of ERK and JNK activation. Phytother. Res. 26 (12), 1893–1897.

Bao, L., Zhang, Z., Dai, X., Ding, Y., Jiang, Y., Li, Y., et al., 2015. Effects of grape seed proanthocyanidin extract on renal injury in type 2 diabetic rats. Mol. Med. Rep. 1 (1), 645–652.

Bento, A.F., Marcon, R., Dutra, R.C., Claudino, R.F., Cola, M., Leite, D.F., et al., 2011. β-Caryophyllene inhibits dextran sulfate sodium-induced colitis in mice through CB2 receptor activation and PPARγ pathway. Am. J. Pathol. 178 (3), 1153–1166.

Betti, M., Minelli, A., Ambrogini, P., Ciuffoli, S., Viola, V., Galli, F., et al., 2011. Dietary supplementation with α-tocopherol reduces neuroinflammation and neuronal degeneration in the rat brain after kainic acid-induced status epilepticus. Free Radic. Res. 45 (10), 1136–1142.

Bin Sayeed, M.S., Asaduzzaman, M., Morshed, H., Hossain, M.M., Kadir, M.F., Rahman, M.R., 2013. The effect of *Nigella sativa* Linn. seed on memory, attention and cognition in healthy human volunteers. J. Ethnopharmacol. 148 (3), 780–786.

Bin Sayeed, M.S., Shams, T., Fahim Hossain, S., Rahman, M.R., Mostofa, A., Fahim Kadir, M., et al., 2014. *Nigella sativa* L. seeds modulate mood, anxiety and cognition in healthy adolescent males. J. Ethnopharmacol. 152 (1), 156–162.

Bosch, M.N., Gimeno-Bayón, J., Rodríguez, M.J., Pugliese, M., Mahy, N., 2013. Rapid improvement of canine cognitive dysfunction with immunotherapy designed for Alzheimer's disease. Curr. Alzheimer Res. 10 (5), 482–493.

Boyanapalli, S.S., Tony Kong, A.N., 2015. "Curcumin, the King of Spices": epigenetic regulatory mechanisms in the prevention of cancer, neurological, and inflammatory diseases. Curr. Pharmacol. Rep. 1 (2), 129–139.

Brown, C.A., Elliott, J., Schmiedt, C.W., Brown, S.A., 2016. Chronic kidney disease in aged cats: clinical features, morphology, and proposed pathogeneses. Vet. Pathol. 53 (2), 309–326.

Bruunsgaard, H., 2002. Effects of tumor necrosis factor-alpha and interleukin-6 in elderly populations. Eur. Cytokine Netw. 13 (4), 389–391.

Brüünsgaard, H., Pedersen, B.K., 2003. Age-related inflammatory cytokines and disease. Immunol. Allergy Clin. North Am. 23 (1), 15–39.

Buyuklu, M., Kandemir, F.M., Ozkaraca, M., Set, T., Bakirci, E.M., Topal, E., et al., 2015. Benefical effects of lycopene against contrast medium-induced oxidative stress, inflammation, autophagy, and apoptosis in rat kidney. Hum. Exp. Toxicol. 34 (5), 487–496.

Cambay, Z., Baydas, G., Tuzcu, M., Bal, R., 2011. Pomegranate (*Punica granatum* L.) flower improves learning and memory performances impaired by diabetes mellitus in rats. Acta Physiol. Hung. 98 (4), 409–420.

Canayakin, D., Bayir, Y., Kilic Baygutalp, N., Sezen Karaoglan, E., Atmaca, H.T., Kocak Ozgeris, F.B., et al., 2016. Paracetamol-induced nephrotoxicity and oxidative stress in rats: the protective role of *Nigella sativa*. Pharm. Biol. 9, 1–10.

Candore, G., Caruso, C., Jirillo, E., Magrone, T., Vasto, S., 2010. Low grade inflammation as a common pathogenetic denominator in age-related diseases: novel drug targets for anti-ageing strategies and successful ageing achievement. Curr. Pharm. Des. 16 (6), 584–596.

Carey, A.N., Miller, M.G., Fisher, D.R., Bielinski, D.F., Gilman, C.K., Poulose, S.M., et al., 2015. Dietary supplementation with the polyphenol-rich açaí pulps (Euterpe oleracea Mart. and Euterpe precatoria Mart.) improves cognition in aged rats and attenuates inflammatory signaling in BV-2 microglial cells. Nutr. Neurosci. Nov 30. [Epub ahead of print].

Casamenti, F., Grossi, C., Rigacci, S., Pantano, D., Luccarini, I., Stefani, M., 2015. Oleuropein aglycone: a possible drug against degenerative conditions. in vivo evidence of its effectiveness against Alzheimer's disease. J. Alzheimers Dis. 45 (3), 679–688.

Cederholm, T., Salem, N. Jr, Palmblad, J., 2013. ω-3 fatty acids in the prevention of cognitive decline in humans. Adv. Nutr. 4 (6), 672–676.

Chen, W.P., Xiong, Y., Hu, P.F., Bao, J.P., Wu, L.D., 2015. Baicalein inhibits MMPs expression via a MAPK-dependent mechanism in chondrocytes. Cell Physiol. Biochem. 36 (1), 325–333.

Cherniack, E.P., 2012. A berry thought-provoking idea: the potential role of plant polyphenols in the treatment of age-related cognitive disorders. Br. J. Nutr. 108 (5), 794–800.

Chung, S.W., Kim, M.K., Chung, J.H., Kim, D.H., Choi, J.S., Anton, S., et al., 2009. Peroxisome proliferator-activated receptor activation by a short-term feeding of zingerone in aged rats. J. Med. Food 12 (2), 345–350.

Costa, E., Fernandes, J., Ribeiro, S., Sereno, J., Garrido, P., Rocha-Pereira, P., et al., 2013. Aging is associated with impaired renal function, INF-gamma induced inflammation and with alterations in iron regulatory proteins gene expression. Aging Dis. 5 (6), 356–365.

Culley, D.J., Snayd, M., Baxter, M.G., Xie, Z., Lee, I.H., Rudolph, J., et al., 2014. Systemic inflammation impairs attention and cognitive flexibility but not associative learning in aged rats: possible implications for delirium. Front. Aging Neurosci. 6, 107.

Day, M.J., 2010. Ageing, immunosenescence and inflammageing in the dog and cat. J. Comp. Pathol. 142 (Suppl 1), S60–S69.

Emami, F., Ali-Beig, H., Farahbakhsh, S., Mojabi, N., Rastegar-Moghadam, B., Arbabian, S., et al., 2013. Hydroalcoholic extract of Rosemary (*Rosmarinus officinalis* L.) and its constituent carnosol inhibit formalin-induced pain and inflammation in mice. Pak. J. Biol. Sci. 16 (7), 309–316.

England, A., Valdes, A.M., Slater-Jefferies, J.L., Gill, R., Howell, W.M., Calder, P.C., et al., 2012. Variants in the genes encoding TNF-α, IL-10, and GSTP1 influence the effect of α-tocopherol on inflammatory cell responses in healthy men. Am. J. Clin. Nutr. 95 (6), 1461–1467.

Franceschi, C., Bonafe, M., Valensin, S., 2000. Human immunosenescence: the prevailing of innate immunity, the failing of clonotypic immunity, and the filling of immunological space. Vaccine 18 (16), 1717–1720.

Fleming, J.M., Creevy, K.E., Promislow, D.E., 2011. Mortality in North American dogs from 1984 to 2004: an investigation into age-, size-, and breed-related causes of death. J. Vet. Internal Med. 25, 187–198.

Fu, Y., Zhou, H., Wang, M., Cen, J., Wei, Q., 2014. Immune regulation and anti-inflammatory effects of isogarcinol extracted from *Garcinia mangostana* L. against collagen-induced arthritis. J Agric Food Chem. 62 (18), 4127–4134.

Fuchs, T., Trollor, J.N., Crawford, J., Brown, D.A., Baune, B.T., Samaras, K., et al., 2013. Macrophage inhibitory cytokine-1 is associated with cognitive impairment and predicts cognitive decline-the Sydney Memory and Aging Study. Aging Cell 12 (5), 882–889.

Gao, Q., Camous, X., Lu, Y.X., Lim, M.L., Larbi, A., Ng, T.P., 2016. Novel inflammatory markers associated with cognitive performance: Singapore Longitudinal Ageing Studies. Neurobiol. Aging 39, 140–146.

Gao, D., Zeng, L.N., Zhang, P., Ma, Z.J., Li, R.S., Zhao, Y.L., et al., 2016. Rhubarb anthraquinones protect rats against mercuric chloride ($HgCl_2$)-induced acute renal failure. Molecules 21 (3).

Ghosh, S., Banerjee, S., Sil, P.C., 2015. The beneficial role of curcumin on inflammation, diabetes and neurodegenerative disease: a recent update. Food Chem. Toxicol. 83, 111–124.

Gocmez, S.S., Gacar, N., Utkan, T., Gacar, G., Scarpace, P.J., Tumer, N., 2016. Protective effects of resveratrol on aging-induced cognitive impairment in rats. Neurobiol. Learn. Mem 131, 131–136.

González-Martínez, A., Rosado, B., Pesini, P., García-Belenguer, S., Palacio, J., Villegas, A., et al., 2013. Effect of age and severity of cognitive dysfunction on two simple tasks in pet dogs. Vet. J. 198 (1), 176–181.

Greeley, E.H., Spitznagel, E., Lawler, D.F., Kealy, R.D., Segre, M., 2006. Modulation of canine immunosenescence by life-long caloric restriction. Vet. Immunol. Immunopathol. 111 (3–4), 287–299.

Guo, K., Mou, X., Huang, J., Xiong, N., Li, H., 2014. Trans-caryophyllene suppresses hypoxia-induced neuroinflammatory responses by inhibiting NF-κB activation in microglia. J. Mol. Neurosci. 54 (1), 41–48.

Guo, Y., Liu, Y., Wang, Y., 2015. Beneficial effect of lycopene on anti-diabetic nephropathy through diminishing inflammatory response and oxidative stress. Food Funct. 6 (4), 1150–1156.

Gupta, O.P., Sing, S., Bani, S., Sharma, N., Malhotra, S., Gupta, B.D., et al., 2000. Anti-inflammatory and anti-arthritic activities of silymarin acting through inhibition of 5-lipoxygenase. Phytomedicine 7 (1), 21–24.

Habenicht, L.M., Webb, T.L., Clauss, L.A., Dow, S.W., Quimby, J.M., 2013. Urinary cytokine levels in apparently healthy cats and cats with chronic kidney disease. J. Feline Med. Surg. 15 (2), 99–104.

Hall, J.A., Tooley, K.A., Gradin, J.L., Jewell, D.E., Wander, R.C., 2003. Effects of dietary n-6 and n-3 fatty acids and vitamin E on the immune response of healthy geriatric dogs. Am. J. Vet. Res. 64 (6), 762–772.

Hall, J.A., Chinn, R.M., Vorachek, W.R., Gorman, M.E., Jewell, D.E., 2010. Aged Beagle dogs have decreased neutrophil phagocytosis and neutrophil-related gene expression compared to younger dogs. Vet. Immunol. Immunopathol. 137 (1–2), 130–135.

Hall, J.A., Chinn, R.M., Vorachek, W.R., Gorman, M.E., Greitl, J.L., Joshi, D.K., et al., 2011. Influence of dietary antioxidants and fatty acids on neutrophil mediated bacterial killing and gene expression in healthy Beagles. Vet. Immunol. Immunopathol. 139 (2–4), 217–228.

Hall, J.A., Yerramilli, M., Obare, E., Yerramilli, M., Jewell, D.E., 2014. Comparison of serum concentrations of symmetric dimethylarginine and creatinine as kidney function biomarkers in cats with chronic kidney disease. J. Vet. Intern. Med. 28 (6), 1676–1683.

Hall, J.A., Yerramilli, M., Obare, E., Yerramilli, M., Melendez, L.D., Jewell, D.E., 2015. Relationship between lean body mass and serum renal biomarkers in healthy dogs. J. Vet. Intern. Med. 29 (3), 808–814.

Hall, J.A., MacLeay, J., Yerramilli, M., Obare, E., Yerramilli, M., Schiefelbein, H., et al., 2016a. Positive Impact of nutritional interventions on serum symmetric dimethylarginine and creatinine concentrations in client-owned geriatric cats. PLoS One 11 (4), e0153654.

Hall, J.A., MacLeay, J., Yerramilli, M., Obare, E., Yerramilli, M., Schiefelbein, H., et al., 2016b. Positive impact of nutritional interventions on serum symmetric dimethylarginine and creatinine concentrations in client-owned geriatric dogs. PLoS One 11 (4), e0153653.

Hamden, K., Masmoudi, H., Carreau, S., Elfeki, A., 2010. Immunomodulatory, beta-cell, and neuroprotective actions of fenugreek oil from alloxan-induced diabetes. Immunopharmacol. Immunotoxicol. 32 (3), 437–445.

Head, E., 2011. Neurobiology of the aging dog. Age (Dordr) 33 (3), 485–496.

Horváth, B., Mukhopadhyay, P., Kechrid, M., Patel, V., Tanchian, G., Wink, D.A., et al., 2012. β-Caryophyllene ameliorates cisplatin-induced nephrotoxicity in a cannabinoid 2 receptor-dependent manner. Free Radic. Biol. Med. 52 (8), 1325–1333.

Huang, H.J., Chen, W.L., Hsieh, R.H., Hsieh-Li, H.M., 2014. Multifunctional effects of mangosteen pericarp on cognition in C57BL/6J and triple transgenic Alzheimer's mice. Evid Based Complement Alternat Med, 813672.

Hwang, I.K., Lee, C.H., Li, H., Yoo, K.Y., Choi, J.H., Kim, D.W., et al., 2008. Comparison of ionized calcium-binding adapter molecule 1 immunoreactivity of the hippocampal dentate gyrus and CA1 region in adult and aged dogs. Neurochem. Res. 33 (7), 1309–1315.

Ikeda-Douglas, C.J., Zicker, S.C., Estrada, J., Jewell, D.E., Milgram, N.W., 2004. Prior experience, antioxidants, and mitochondrial cofactors improve cognitive function in aged beagles. Vet. Ther. 5 (1), 5–16.

Jain, N., Reilly, R.F., 2014. Effects of dietary interventions on incidence and progression of CKD. Nat. Rev. Nephrol. 10, 712–724.

Javed, H., Khan, M.M., Ahmad, A., Vaibhav, K., Ahmad, M.E., Khan, A., et al., 2012. Rutin prevents cognitive impairments by ameliorating oxidative stress and neuroinflammation in rat model of sporadic dementia of Alzheimer type. Neuroscience 210, 340–352.

Kearns, R.J., Hayek, M.G., Turek, J.J., Meydani, M., Burr, J.R., Greene, R.J., et al., 1999. Effect of age, breed and dietary omega-6 (n-6): omega-3 (n-3) fatty acid ratio on immune function, eicosanoid production, and lipid peroxidation in young and aged dogs. Vet. Immunol. Immunopathol. 69 (2–4), 165–183.

Kesse-Guyot, E., Assmann, K.E., Andreeva, V.A., Touvier, M., Neufcourt, L., Shivappa, N., et al., 2016. Long-term association between the dietary inflammatory index and cognitive functioning: findings from the SU.VI.MAX study. Eur. J. Nutr. Apr 7. [Epub ahead of print].

Kim, M.K., Chung, S.W., Kim, D.H., Kim, J.M., Lee, E.K., Kim, J.Y., et al., 2010. Modulation of age-related NF-kappaB activation by dietary zingerone via MAPK pathway. Exp. Gerontol. 45 (6), 419–426.

Lai, C.C., Huang, P.H., Yang, A.H., Chiang, S.C., Tang, C.Y., Tseng, K.W., et al., 2016. Baicalein, a component of scutellaria baicalensis, attenuates kidney injury induced by myocardial ischemia and reperfusion. Planta Med. 82 (3), 181–189.

Landsberg, G.M., Nichol, J., Araujo, J.A., 2012. Cognitive dysfunction syndrome: a disease of canine and feline brain aging. Vet. Clin. North Am. Small Anim. Pract. 42 (4), 749–768.

Lee, Y.A., Kim, Y.J., Cho, E.J., Yokozawa, T., 2007. Ameliorative effects of proanthocyanidin on oxidative stress and inflammation in streptozotocin-induced diabetic rats. J. Agric. Food Chem. 55 (23), 9395–9400.

Kim, S.H., Lee, Y.C., 2009. Piperine inhibits eosinophil infiltration and airway hyperresponsiveness by suppressing T cell activity and Th2 cytokine production in the ovalbumin-induced asthma model. J. Pharm. Pharmacol. 61 (3), 353–359.

Koda, T., Kuroda, Y., Imai, H., 2009. Rutin supplementation in the diet has protective effects against toxicant-induced hippocampal injury by suppression of microglial activation and pro-inflammatory cytokines: protective effect of rutin against toxicant-induced hippocampal injury. Cell Mol. Neurobiol. 29 (4), 523–531.

Kwon, K.H., Murakami, A., Tanaka, T., Ohigashi, H., 2005. Dietary rutin, but not its aglycone quercetin, ameliorates dextran sulfate sodium-induced experimental colitis in mice: attenuation of proinflammatory gene expression. Biochem. Pharmacol. 69 (3), 395–406.

Lesourd, B.M., 1997. Nutrition and immunity in the elderly: modification of immune responses with nutritional treatments. Am. J. Clin. Nutr. 66 (2), 478S–484S.

Lesourd, B., Mazari, L., 1999. Nutrition and immunity in the elderly. Proc. Nutr. Soc. 58 (3), 685–695.

Markovich, J.E., Freeman, L.M., Labato, M.A., Heinze, C.R., 2015. Survey of dietary and medication practices of owners of cats with chronic kidney disease. J. Feline Med. Surg. 17 (12), 979–983.

Ma, Y., Cheng, Q., Wang, E., Li, L., Zhang, X., 2015. Inhibiting tumor necrosis factor-α signaling attenuates postoperative cognitive dysfunction in aged rats. Mol. Med. Rep. 12 (2), 3095–3100.

Meydani, S.N., Barklund, M.P., Liu, S., Meydani, M., Miller, R.A., Cannon, J.G., et al., 1990. Vitamin E supplementation enhances cell-mediated immunity in healthy elderly subjects. Am. J. Clin. Nutr. 52 (3), 557–563.

Michaud, M., Balardy, L., Moulis, G., Gaudin, C., Peyrot, C., Vellas, B., et al., 2013. Proinflammatory cytokines, aging, and age-related diseases. J. Am. Med. Dir. Assoc. 14 (12), 877–882.

Mongillo, P., Araujo, J.A., Pitteri, E., Carnier, P., Adamelli, S., Regolin, L., et al., 2013. Spatial reversal learning is impaired by age in pet dogs. Age (Dordr) 35 (6), 2273–2282.

Moreira, E.L., Rial, D., Aguiar Jr., A.S., Figueiredo, C.P., Siqueira, J.M., DalBó, S., et al., 2010. Proanthocyanidin-rich fraction from Croton celtidifolius Baill confers neuroprotection in the intranasal 1-methyl-4-phenyl-1,2,3,6-tetrahydropyridine rat model of Parkinson's disease. J. Neural Transm. (Vienna) 117 (12), 337–351.

Moreno, J.A., Izquierdo, M.C., Sanchez-Niño, M.D., Suárez-Alvarez, B., Lopez-Larrea, C., Jakubowski, A., et al., 2011. The inflammatory cytokines TWEAK and TNFα reduce renal klotho expression through NFκB. J. Am. Soc. Nephrol. 22 (7), 1315–1325.

Mulder, W.J., Hillen, H.F.P., 2001. Renal function and renal disease in the elderly. Part I. Eur. J. Intern. Med. 12, 86–97.

Nascimento, C.M., Pereira, J.R., De Andrade, L.P., Garuffi, M., Talib, L.L., Forlenza, O.V., et al., 2014. Physical exercise in MCI elderly promotes reduction of pro-inflammatory cytokines and improvements on cognition and BDNF peripheral levels. Curr. Alzheimer Res. 11 (8), 799–805.

Neha, Kumar, A., Jaggi, A.S., Sodhi, R.K., Singh, N., 2014. Silymarin ameliorates memory deficits and neuropathological changes in mouse model of high-fat-diet-induced experimental dementia. Naunyn Schmiedebergs Arch. Pharmacol. 387 (8), 777–787.

Nentwig, A., Schweighauser, A., Maissen-Villiger, C., Bruckmaier, R.M., Zurbriggen, A., Van Dorland, H.A., et al., 2016. Assessment of the expression of biomarkers of uremic inflammation in dogs with renal disease. Am. J. Vet. Res. 77 (2), 218–224.

Ng, T.P., Chiam, P.C., Lee, T., Chua, H.C., Lim, L., Kua, E.H., 2006. Curry consumption and cognitive function in the elderly. Am. J. Epidemiol. 164 (9), 898–906.

Oh, S.B., Park, H.R., Jang, Y.J., Choi, S.Y., Son, T.G., Lee, J., 2013. Baicalein attenuates impaired hippocampal neurogenesis and the neurocognitive deficits induced by γ-ray radiation. Br. J. Pharmacol. 168 (2), 421–431.

Ozarowski, M., Mikolajczak, P.L., Bogacz, A., Gryszczynska, A., Kujawska, M., Jodynis-Liebert, J., et al., 2013. Rosmarinus officinalis L. leaf extract improves memory impairment and affects acetylcholinesterase and butyrylcholinesterase activities in rat brain. Fitoterapia 91, 261–271.

Ozawa, M., Shipley, M., Kivimaki, M., Singh-Manoux, A., Brunner, E.J., 2016. Dietary pattern, inflammation and cognitive decline: The Whitehall II prospective cohort study. Clin. Nutr. S0261-5614(16)00035-2.

Pan, Y., Larson, B., Araujo, J.A., Lau, W., De Rivera, C., Santana, R., et al., 2010. Dietary supplementation with medium-chain TAG has long-lasting cognition-enhancing effects in aged dogs. Br. J. Nutr. 103 (12), 1746–1754.

Panickar, K.S., 2014. Anti-inflammatory properties of botanical extracts contribute to their protective effects in brain edema in cerebral ischemia. In: Watson, R., Preedy, V. (Eds.), Bioactive Nutriceuticals and Dietary Supplements in Neurological and Brain Disease: Prevention and Therapy. Academic Press, New York, pp. 3–15.

Panickar, K.S., Jewell, D.E., 2015. The beneficial role of anti-inflammatory dietary ingredients in attenuating markers of chronic low-grade inflammation in aging. Horm. Mol. Biol. Clin. Investig. 23 (2), 59–70.

Park, C.H., Yokozawa, T., Noh, J.S., 2014. Oligonol, a low-molecular-weight polyphenol derived from lychee fruit, attenuates diabetes-induced renal damage through the advanced glycation end product-related pathway in db/db mice. J. Nutr. 144 (8), 1150–1157.

Pérez-Rojas, J.M., Cruz, C., García-López, P., Sánchez-González, D.J., Martínez-Martínez, C.M., Ceballos, G., et al., 2009. Renoprotection by alpha-Mangostin is related to the attenuation in renal oxidative/nitrosative stress induced by cisplatin nephrotoxicity. Free Radic. Res 43 (11), 1122–1132.

Pierine, D.T., Navarro, M.E., Minatel, I.O., Luvizotto, R.A., Nascimento, A.F., Ferreira, A.L., et al., 2014. Lycopene supplementation reduces TNF-α via RAGE in the kidney of obese rats. Nutr. Diabetes 10 (4), e142.

Pingali, U., Pilli, R., Fatima, N., 2014. Effect of standardized aqueous extract of Withania somnifera on tests of cognitive and psychomotor performance in healthy human participants. Pharmacognosy Res. 6 (1), 12–18.

Piwowarski, J.P., Kiss, A.K., Granica, S., Moeslinger, T., 2015. Urolithins, gut microbiota-derived metabolites of ellagitannins, inhibit LPS-induced inflammation in RAW 264.7 murine macrophages. Mol. Nutr. Food Res. 59 (11), 2168–2177.

Raila, J., Schweigert, F.J., Kohn, B., 2011. C-reactive protein concentrations in serum of dogs with naturally occurring renal disease. J. Vet. Diagn. Investig. 23 (4), 710–715.

Ramalingayya, G.V., Nampoothiri, M., Nayak, P.G., Kishore, A., Shenoy, R.R., Mallikarjuna Rao, C., et al., 2016. Naringin and rutin alleviates episodic memory deficits in two differentially challenged object recognition tasks. Pharmacogn. Mag. 12 (Suppl 1), S63–S70.

Rehman, S.U., Shah, S.A., Ali, T., Chung, J.I., Kim, M.O., 2016. Anthocyanins reversed D-Galactose-induced oxidative stress and neuroinflammation mediated cognitive impairment in adult rats. Mol. Neurobiol. [Epub ahead of print]. PMID: 26738855.

Rodrigues, F.A., Prata, M.M., Oliveira, I.C., Alves, N.T., Freitas, R.E., Monteiro, H.S., et al., 2014. Gingerol fraction from Zingiber officinale protects against gentamicin-induced nephrotoxicity. Antimicrob. Agents Chemother. 58 (4), 1872–1878.

Roubenoff, R., Harris, T.B., Abad, L.W., Wilson, P.W., Dallal, G.E., Dinarello, C.A., 1998. Monocyte cytokine production in an elderly population: effect of age and inflammation. J. Gerontol. A Biol. Sci. Med. Sci. 53 (1), M20–M26.

Rubin, S.I., 1997. Chronic renal failure and its management and nephrolithiasis. Vet. Clin. North Am. Small Anim. Pract. 27 (6), 1331–1354.

Sahebkar, A., Cicero, A.F., Simental-Mendía, L.E., Aggarwal, B.B., Gupta, S.C., 2016. Curcumin downregulates human tumor necrosis factor-α levels: a systematic review and meta-analysis ofrandomized controlled trials. Pharmacol. Res. 107, 234–242.

Santos, M.S., Leka, L.S., Ribaya-Mercado, J.D., Russell, R.M., Meydani, M., Hennekens, C.H., et al., 1997. Short- and long-term beta-carotene supplementation do not influence T cell-mediated immunity in healthy elderly persons. Am. J. Clin. Nutr. 66 (4), 917–924.

Said, M.M., 2011. The protective effect of eugenol against gentamicin-induced nephrotoxicity and oxidative damage in rat kidney. Fundam. Clin. Pharmacol. 25 (6), 708–716.

Schütt, T., Helboe, L., Østergaard Pedersen, L., Waldemar, G., Berendt, M., Pedersen, J.T., 2016. Dogs with cognitive dysfunction as a spontaneous model for early Alzheimer's disease: a translational study of neuropathological and inflammatory markers. J. Alzheimers Dis. [Epub ahead of print].

Sharma, C., Al Kaabi, J., Nurulain, S.M., Goyal, S.N., Kamal, M.A., Ojha, S., 2016. Polypharmacological properties and therapeutic potential of β-caryophyllene: a dietary phytocannabinoid of pharmaceutical promise. Curr. Pharm. Des. [Epub ahead of print].

Sheffy, B.E., Williams, A.J., 1981. Nutrition and the aging animal. Vet. Clin. North Am. Small Anim. Pract. 11 (4), 669–675.

Shema-Didi, L., Sela, S., Ore, L., Shapiro, G., Geron, R., Moshe, G., et al., 2012. One year of pomegranate juice intake decreases oxidative stress, inflammation, and incidence of infections in hemodialysis patients: a randomized placebo-controlled trial. Free Radic. Biol. Med. 53 (2), 297–304.

Shukitt-Hale, B., Carey, A., Simon, L., Mark, D.A., Joseph, J.A., 2006. Effects of Concord grape juice on cognitive and motor deficits in aging. Nutrition 22 (3), 295–302.

Shukitt-Hale, B., Lau, F.C., Carey, A.N., Galli, R.L., Spangler, E.L., Ingram, D.K., et al., 2008. Blueberry polyphenols attenuate kainic acid-induced decrements in cognition and alter inflammatory gene expression in rat hippocampus. Nutr. Neurosci. 11 (4), 172–182.

Shukitt-Hale, B., Cheng, V., Joseph, J.A., 2009. Effects of blackberries on motor and cognitive function in aged rats. Nutr. Neurosci. 12 (3), 135–140.

Simpson, E.E., Hodkinson, C.F., Maylor, E.A., McCormack, J.M., Rae, G., Strain, S., et al., 2013. Intracellular cytokine production and cognition in healthy older adults. Psychoneuroendocrinology 38 (10), 2196–2208.

Siwak, C.T., Tapp, P.D., Head, E., Zicker, S.C., Murphey, H.L., Muggenburg, B.A., et al., 2005. Chronic antioxidant and mitochondrial cofactor administration improves discrimination learning in aged but not young dogs. Prog. Neuropsychopharmacol. Biol. Psychiatry 29 (3), 461–469.

Subash, S., Braidy, N., Essa, M.M., Zayana, A.B., Ragini, V., Al-Adawi, S., et al., 2015. Long-term (15 mo) dietary supplementation with pomegranates from Oman attenuates cognitive and behavioral deficits in a transgenic mice model of Alzheimer's disease. Nutrition 31 (1), 223–229.

Taher, Y.A., Samud, A.M., El-Taher, F.E., Ben-Hussin, G., Elmezogi, J.S., Al-Mehdawi, B.F., et al., 2015. Experimental evaluation of anti-inflammatory, antinociceptive and antipyretic activities of clove oil in mice. Libyan J. Med. 10, 28685.

Tegeler, C., O'Sullivan, J.L., Bucholtz, N., Goldeck, D., Pawelec, G., Steinhagen-Thiessen, E., et al., 2016. The inflammatory markers CRP, IL-6, and IL-10 are associated with cognitive function-data from the Berlin Aging Study II. Neurobiol. Aging 38, 112–117.

Thangthaeng, N., Miller, M.G., Gomes, S.M., Shukitt-Hale, B., 2015. Daily supplementation with mushroom (Agaricus bisporus) improves balance and working memory in aged rats. Nutr. Res. 35 (12), 1079–1084.

Valacchi, G., Pecorelli, A., Mencarelli, M., Maioli, E., Davis, P.A., 2009. β-carotene prevents ozone-induced proinflammatory markers in murine skin. Toxicol. Ind. Health 25 (4–5), 241–247.

Vedi, M., Rasool, M., Sabina, E.P., 2014. Protective effect of administration of Withania somifera against bromobenzene induced nephrotoxicity and mitochondrial oxidative stress in rats. Ren. Fail 36 (7), 1095–1103.

Vite, C.H., Head, E., 2014. Aging in the canine and feline brain. Vet. Clin. North Am. Small Anim. Pract. 44 (6), 1113–1129.

Xi, Y., Shao, F., Bai, X.Y., Cai, G., Lv, Y., Chen, X., 2014. Changes in the expression of the Toll-like receptor system in the aging rat kidneys. PLoS One 9 (5), e96351.

Xu, X., Yin, P., Wan, C., Chong, X., Liu, M., Cheng, P., et al., 2014. Punicalagin inhibits inflammation in LPS-induced RAW264.7 macrophages via the suppression of TLR4-mediated MAPKs and NF-κB activation. Inflammation 37 (3), 956–965.

Xu, H., Sjogren, P., Arnlov, J., Banerjee, T., Cederholm, T., Riserus, U., et al., 2015. A proinflammatory diet is associated with systemic inflammation and reduced kidney function in elderly adults. J. Nutr. 145, 729–735.

Wang, J.H., Shih, K.S., Liou, J.P., Wu, Y.W., Chang, A.S., Wang, K.L., et al., 2012. Anti-arthritic effects of magnolol in human interleukin 1β-stimulated fibroblast-like synoviocytes and in a rat arthritis model. PLoS One 7 (2), e31368.

Wang, W., Zhou, P.H., Xu, C.G., Zhou, X.J., Hu, W., Zhang, J., 2015. Baicalein attenuates renal fibrosis by inhibiting inflammation via down-regulating NF-κB and MAPK signal pathways. J. Mol. Histol. 46 (3), 283–290.

Weinstein, J.R., Anderson, S., 2010. The aging kidney: physiological changes. Adv. Chronic Kidney Dis. 17 (4), 302–307.

Wichmann, M.A., Cruickshanks, K.J., Carlsson, C.M., Chappell, R., Fischer, M.E., Klein, B.E., et al., 2014. Long-term systemic inflammation and cognitive impairment in a population-based cohort. J. Am. Geriatr. Soc. 62 (9), 1683–1691.

Wong, V.M., Kidney, B.A., Snead, E.C., Myers, S.L., Jackson, M.L., 2011. Serum C-reactive protein concentrations in healthy Miniature Schnauzer dogs. Vet. Clin. Pathol. 40 (3), 380–383

Wu, D., Meydani, M., Leka, L.S., Nightingale, Z., Handelman, G.J., Blumberg, J.B., et al., 1999. Effect of dietary supplementation with black currant seed oil on the immune response of healthy elderly subjects. Am. J. Clin. Nutr. 70 (4), 536–543.

Yadav, U.C., Baquer, N.Z., 2014. Pharmacological effects of Trigonella foenum-graecum L. in health and disease. Pharm. Biol. 52 (2), 243–254.

Yokozawa, T., Kim, H.Y., Kim, H.J., Tanaka, T., Sugino, H., Okubo, T., et al., 2007. Amla (Emblica officinalis Gaertn.) attenuates age-related renal dysfunction by oxidative stress. J. Agric. Food Chem. 55 (19), 7744–7752.

Zhang, Z.H., Wei, F., Vaziri, N.D., Cheng, X.L., Bai, X., Lin, R.C., et al., 2015. Metabolomics insights into chronic kidney disease and modulatory effect of rhubarb against tubulointerstitial fibrosis. Sci. Rep. 5, 14472.

Zicker, S.C., Jewell, D.E., Yamka, R.M., Milgram, N.W., 2012. Evaluation of cognitive learning, memory, psychomotor, immunologic, and retinal functions in healthy puppies fed foods fortified with docosahexaenoic acid-rich fish oil from 8 to 52 weeks of age. J. Am. Vet. Med. Assoc. 241 (5), 583–594.

CHAPTER

22

Calorie Restriction Mimetics From Functional Foods: Impact on Promoting a Healthy Life Span

Wai Yan Sun and Yu Wang

The University of Hong Kong, Hong Kong, China

INTRODUCTION: CALORIE RESTRICTION

The life expectancy of humans has dramatically increased over the past few centuries, which is imposing negative impacts on age-associated diseases and the medical cost of health care. Aging is a multifactorial biological process, progressively degenerative in nature and resulting in loss of physical or mental functions (or both) (Dabhade and Kotwal, 2013; Shokolenko et al., 2014). *Primary aging* refers to the currently inevitable process of the functional deterioration of organs as well as slowing movement, fading vision, progressive hearing loss, and increased susceptibility to infection. In contrast, *secondary aging* is preventable and results largely from disease processes, harmful environmental factors, and poor lifestyle decisions such as smoking and a lack of physical activity (Anstey et al., 1993). Numerous signaling pathways that are commonly or specifically involved in age-related diseases—including type 2 diabetes mellitus, cardiovascular disease, and Alzheimer's disease (AD)—have been identified and characterized (Masri, 2015). As a result, the protections against secondary aging lead to a significant increase in the average life span (Fontana et al., 2010). However, our knowledge of the underlying causes for primary aging remain primitive. Accordingly, the maximal longevity of humans remains largely unchanged.

Calorie intake influences the rate of aging and the onset of age-related diseases in animals and humans. Calorie restriction is a dietary regimen to limit the consumption of food without causing malnutrition, which effectively slows the process of primary aging and protects secondary aging in rodents (McCay et al. 1935; Weindruch and Sohal 1997) as well as in nonhuman primates (Lane et al., 1996; Colman et al., 2009). The effects are robust as evident in mice with long-term 55% to 65% calorie restriction leading to a 65% extension of maximal life span when compared to the control group with ad libitum feeding (Weindruch, 1996). Two long-term calorie restriction studies using rhesus monkeys by the Wisconsin National Primate Research Center (WNPRC) and the National Institute on Aging (NIA) produced controversial results. The former was initiated in 1989, and its results were published in 2014 with the conclusion that a long-term approximately 30% restricted diet significantly improved age-related and all-cause survival in rhesus monkeys (Colman et al., 2014). The NIA initiated its study in 1987, and the interim report in 2012 showed that calorie restriction did not increase the median life span of rhesus monkeys (Mattison et al., 2012). Notably, WNPRC study performed 30% dietary restriction that was individualized for each monkey, whereas the monkeys of NIA study were fed with 22% to 24% reduced calories based on the standardized chart of food intake by the National Academy of Science. In addition, all monkeys in the NIA study were supplemented with minerals and vitamins above the adequate amount in order to avoid any compromising factors. However, only the

Nutrition and Functional Foods for Healthy Aging.
DOI: http://dx.doi.org/10.1016/B978-0-12-805376-8.00022-8

calorie-restricted monkeys were supplemented in WNPRC study. The control monkeys at NIA weighed less than those at the WNPRC at all time points, suggesting an inadequate food intake (Tenenbaum, 2014).

Long-term calorie restriction reduces body weight and has beneficial effects on the health span of nonhuman primates by reducing cancer development, neurodegeneration, and metabolic disorders (Mattison et al., 2012; Libert and Guarente, 2013). Intermittent calorie restriction also shows similar benefits in improving the health span in humans, but consistent weight loss is unlikely to be seen (Heilbronn et al., 2005). In mice, calorie restriction not only reduces body weight and fat mass but also decreases insulin-like growth factor 1 (IGF-1), leptin, fasting blood glucose, and insulin levels (Mai et al., 2003; Tatar et al., 2003; Wang et al., 2013). Overall, calorie restriction enhances metabolic and anti-inflammatory profiles. Effects such as lowered blood glucose and insulin occur quickly but also diminish rapidly when calorie restriction stops (Anderson and Herman, 1972; Mitchell et al., 2015). Thus, to be beneficial, intervention must be sustained. Nevertheless, calorie restriction lowers the susceptibility of a wide spectrum of age-associated diseases. For instance, mice on a calorie-restricted diet showed attenuation of age-related neuronal loss seen in Parkinson's disease (Duan and Mattson, 1999) and in AD (Zhu et al., 1999); improvement for the brain's plasticity in learning (Mattson, 2000); prevention of age-associated declines in psychomotor and spatial memory tasks (Ingram et al., 1987); and reductions in autoimmune disease, kidney damage, and diabetes (Fernandes and Good, 1984). Taken together, calorie restriction protects secondary aging in rodents and nonhuman primates.

Long-term population studies of calorie restriction are hard to conduct for primary aging in humans (Holloszy and Fontana, 2007). Physiological and metabolic variables are determined as the biomarkers for secondary aging. The Biosphere 2 study initiated in 1991 with eight healthy humans (four males and four females) sealed inside a 3.15-acre enclosure began with a limited food supply. After six months, the occupants' body weights, blood pressure, serum cholesterol, fasting glucose, and leukocyte counts were significantly reduced without any changes in physical or mental health status (Walford et al., 1992). The Comprehensive Assessment of Long-Term Effects of Reducing Intake of Energy was the first random trial in free-living nonobese men and women investigating the effects of calorie restriction (Stewart et al., 2013; Romashkan et al., 2016). During the two-year study period, individuals on an 11% calorie-restricted diet exhibited 10% weight loss, whereas the body weight of the control counterparts remained unchanged (Ravussin et al., 2015). Calorie restriction significantly reduced the levels of triiodothyronine and tumor necrosis factor alpha (a marker of inflammation) (Ravussin et al., 2015). Memory and learning performance is enhanced, and insulin sensitivity is improved in healthy elderly persons subject to calorie restriction (Witte et al., 2009). Furthermore, diabetic elderly patients on calorie restriction for 12 weeks show improved blood pressure, glucose and lipid profiles, as well as liver functions, all of which contribute to low cardiovascular risks (Choi et al., 2013).

In the 1950s, Okinawan elders were consuming a calorie-restricted diet that was approximately 1800 cal/day and approximately 20% lower than the national average of Japan (Heilbronn and Ravussin, 2003). Public health care and the quality of the diet on Okinawa were sufficiently good to prevent nutritional deficiencies and infectious diseases. Thus, life expectancy was 81.2 years, significantly higher than those of European countries (e.g., 78.3 years in Italy and 78.1 years in Greece) and the United States (76.8 years) (Sohal and Weindruch, 1996). Because of poverty, however, elderly Okinawans growth was significantly stunted. In fact, long-term calorie restriction may not be a desirable dietary method for improving health span as well as longevity in humans. On the one hand, personal motivation to undergo long-term calorie restriction may be lacking. Thus, a 30% to 60% calorie restriction is not achievable by most human subjects, especially the elderly. On the other hand, the side effects of long-term calorie reduction remain unclear, but include reduced bone mineral densities, functional disability, infertility, and slow recovery from injuries (Ingram and Roth, 2011; Romashkan et al., 2016). Moreover, calorie restriction can provoke unpleasant common side effects such as reduced body temperature and libido (Ingram and Roth, 2011).

Recent decades have seen the introduction of *calorie restriction mimetics* (CRMs), which are also known as *energy restriction mimetics*, in which a class of natural or synthetic pharmacological substances are provided as food supplements to mimic the beneficial anti-aging effects of calorie restriction (Chen and Guarente, 2007; Lee and Min, 2013). The genes and pathways involved in the actions of calorie restriction are the targets for discovering and developing CRMs (Ingram et al., 2006). An effective CRM activates the same physiological and metabolic pathways as calorie restriction, triggers stress-response mechanisms for protection against cellular damage, and extends health and life span without the requirement of dietary or energy restriction. In the following sections, the mechanisms of action for CRMs derived from functional foods will be discussed with a focus on their roles in mimicking the metabolic or signaling pathways of calorie restriction.

CRMs IN MEDIATING METABOLIC PATHWAYS OF CALORIE RESTRICTION

A precise understanding of the mechanisms underlying the actions of calorie restriction is needed for identifying and generating CRMs. Starvation of cells or dietary restriction in mammals leads to a rapid reduction of intracellular acetyl coenzyme A (acetyl-CoA), which is coupled to the status of protein acetylation and deacetylation (Bao and Sack, 2010). Decreased acetyl-CoA levels occur before the reduction of adenosine triphosphate (ATP), oxidation of nicotinamide adenine dinucleotide phosphate (NADH), and the depletion of amino acids. The coordinated alterations of these metabolites trigger a number of key cellular defense mechanisms via the activation of nutrient sensors, including adenosine monophosphate (AMP)-activated protein kinase (AMPK) and silent mating type information regulation 2 homologue 1 (SIRT-1), as well as inactivation of mammalian target of rapamycin (Cetrullo et al., 2015).

Targeting Glycolysis and the Citric Acid Cycle to Limit Energy Supply

In cells, glycolysis is a multistep process that utilizes energy (ATP) to break down glucose into pyruvate, which is then decarboxylated into acetyl-CoA (Akram, 2014). Glycolytic inhibition has been suggested as a strategy for developing CRMs (Roth et al., 1999) based on the rationale that reducing energy supply enhances the metabolic responses in cells, a process mimicking calorie restriction (Ingram and Roth. 2011). There are several key enzymes for targeting the glycolytic pathway. In particular, phosphoglucose isomerase, which converts glucose-6-phosphate to fructose-6-phosphate, is the target of 2-deoxy-D-glucose (2DG) (Ingram and Roth, 2011). Low doses of 2DG enhance oxidative stress protection and neuronal resistance by upregulating heat shock protein 70 (HSP-70) and glucose-regulated protein 78, resulting in neuroprotection (Lee et al., 1999). Glycolytic inhibition delays secondary aging and prevents neurodegenerative disorders.

Glyceraldehyde-3-phosphate dehydrogenase is another target of glycolytic inhibition in vitro in which administration of iodoacetate that inhibits this enzyme can upregulate the expression of HSP-70 and HSP-90 in neurons against excitotoxic and oxidative injury (Guo et al., 2001). Other glycolytic inhibitors—including glucosamine, mannoheptulose, and 3-bromopyruvate—are also candidate CRMs. The phosphorylated form of glucosamine, glucosamine-6-phosphate, is an inhibitor of hexokinase, which is involved in the first step of glycolysis (Marshall et al., 2005). Glucosamine activates autophagy, which is an important cellular mechanism for anti-aging and discussed in later (Carames et al., 2013). In antitumor studies, mannoheptulose and 3-bromopyruvate exhibit inhibitory effects on the glycolytic enzyme hexokinase activity, where this early part of the glycolytic reactions is utilized by cancer cells to generate their own energy (Pedersen, 2007; Wang et al., 2016). However, the underlying mechanisms for CRM are not fully known in vivo. When dogs were fed mannoheptulose, their fasting insulin levels were reduced in a dose-dependent manner, but the serum glucose levels did not differ (McKnight et al., 2014; Ingram and Roth, 2015). These agents can be candidates for CRM, but further studies are required to investigate their full mechanisms of action.

The citric acid cycle (also known as the Krebs cycle or tricarboxylic acid cycle) consists of a series of reactions conducted within the mitochondria of eukaryotic cells or in the cytoplasm of prokaryotic cells (Kornberg, 2000; Korla and Mitra, 2014). It is a central driver of cellular respiration and takes acetyl-CoA as the starting material. Oxaloacetate is the end product of one citric acid cycle. Supplementation with oxaloacetate has been shown to increase longevity in *Caenorhabditis elegans* via an increase in the ratio of nicotinamide adenine dinucleotide (NAD) to NADH and activation of the AMPK pathway (Williams et al., 2009). The conversion of oxaloacetate to malate promotes the conversion of NADH to NAD. Unlike 2DG, oxaloacetate supports glycolysis and cellular respiration (Wilkins et al., 2016). In mice, administration of oxaloacetate increases brain bioenergetic function by activating hippocampal neurogenesis and reducing neuroinflammation via the Akt signaling pathway (Wilkins et al., 2014). A recent study has revealed the safety profile of oxaloacetate in humans, but the efficacy in AD or other age-associated diseases has yet to be elucidated (Swerdlow et al., 2016).

Acetyl-CoA Depletion to Induce Cellular Stress Responses

Formation of intracellular acetyl-CoA occurs in both mitochondrial and nucleocytosolic compartments. In mammals, the mitochondrial acetyl-CoA is produced from pyruvate, fatty acid, and branched-chain amino acids via glycolysis, lipolysis, and oxidative decarboxylation (Madeo et al., 2014). Acetyl-CoA in the mitochondrial matrix is condensed with oxaloacetate into citrate, which can be exported into the cytoplasm, where it freely diffuses in and out of nucleus. The extramitochondrial acetyl-CoA is produced from citrate by ATP citrate lyase or from acetate by acetyl-CoA synthase (Choudhary et al., 2014; Marino et al., 2014; Schroeder et al., 2014). Excessive nutrient supply enhances the transportation of acetyl-CoA from mitochondria to cytosol for the synthesis of fatty acids and sterols (Wellen et al., 2009; Cai et al., 2011; Shi and Tu, 2015). Short-term removal of nutrients in human cell culture and overnight fasting of rodents rapidly reduces acetyl-CoA levels (Marino et al., 2014). Notably, when cells commit to proliferate, the intracellular levels of acetyl-CoA are substantially elevated to promote histone acetylation so the gene expression for growth can be switched on (Cai et al., 2011). This mechanism requires energy consumption and is pro-aging. Conversely, reduction of acetyl-CoA levels is observed when arresting cell growth to reserve energy, which favors anti-aging.

A number of natural compounds act as CRMs to reduce acetyl-CoA or inhibit protein acetylation. For example, hydroxycitrate (Hackenschmidt et al., 1972) and epigallocatechin-3-gallate (EGCG), one of the major active compounds in green tea (Santana et al., 2015), stimulate the activity of acetyl-CoA carboxylase, a biotin-dependent enzyme that irreversibly catalyzes the carboxylation of acetyl-CoA to form malonyl-CoA. Anacardic acid (6-pentadecyl-salicylic acid from the nutshell of the cashew, *Anacardium occidentale*), garcinol (from the fruit of the kokum tree, *Garcinia indica*), and spermidine (a polyamine found at particular high concentrations in durian fruit, fermented soybeans, and wheat germs) reduce the overall lysine acetylation of cellular protein via inhibition of acetyltransferases, in turn inducing autophagy (Pietrocola et al., 2015).

Nucleocytosolic acetyl-CoA production is a metabolic repressor of autophagy, a self-cannibalistic pathway to eliminate damaged organelles and toxic protein aggregates, thus mobilizing energy reserves when external resources are limited (Levine and Kroemer, 2008). During this process, the unique organelle known as the *autophagosome* delivers the cellular components to a lysosome for degradation. A number of autophagy-related proteins (Atg) are involved in the formation of autophagosome (Ravikumar et al., 2010). Notably, the biological process of autophagy decreases with age (Cavallini et al., 2007). Deficiency or attenuation of autophagy causes premature aging and leads to various age-dependent diseases (Levine and Kroemer, 2008; Hartleben et al., 2010; Cui et al., 2013). Conversely, activation of autophagy by overexpression of Atg can increase the life span of mice (Pyo et al., 2013).

Calorie restriction is one physiological trigger for autophagy. Depletion of nucleocytosolic acetyl-CoA in yeast and knockdown of acetyl-CoA synthase in *Drosophila melanogaster* attenuates the global acetylation of proteins, activating autophagy to promote longevity (Eisenberg et al., 2014; Schroeder et al., 2014). Starvation-induced autophagy is associated with the reduced acetylation of Atg, tubulin, and microtubule-associated proteins (Lee and Finkel, 2009; Geeraert et al., 2010). Inhibition of endogenous E1A-binding protein p300 (EP300), an acetyl transferase and transcription coactivator, causes induction of forkhead box protein O promotor activity (Senf et al., 2011) and reduces acetylation of Atg5, Atg7, Atg8, and Atg12 (Lee and Finkel, 2009) A variety of agents that inhibit EP300 are used in traditional medicine, including curcumin (from the South Asian spice turmeric, *Curcuma longa*, one of the principal ingredients of curry powder), EGCG, garcinol, and spermidine (Pietrocola et al., 2015).

Spermidine belongs to the family of polyamines that can be found naturally in oranges, soybeans, rice bran, green pepper, broccoli, mushrooms, and green tea (Morselli et al., 2011). At the cellular level, polyamines interact with negatively charged molecules such as DNA, RNA, and lipids and regulate cell growth, proliferation, and death as well as lipid metabolism (Minois et al., 2011). Spermidine increases the life span in yeast *Saccharomyces cerevisiae*, nematode worm *C. elegans*, and fruit flies *D. melanogaster* (Eisenberg et al., 2009; Madeo et al., 2010; Minois et al., 2012). Autophagy has been identified as the main mechanism of action underlying the antiaging effects of spermidine (Minois, 2014). Administration of spermidine at low doses induces full autophagic responses and extends life span in yeast (Morselli et al., 2011). Spermidine-fed flies show enhanced autophagy and are protected from age-induced memory impairment (Gupta et al., 2013). In addition, spermidine inhibits acetyltransferases and affects global protein acetylation status by triggering deacetylation in the cytosol or acetylation in the nucleus (or both) (Eisenberg et al., 2009; Minois et al., 2012). The intracellular concentrations of polyamines decline with age in rodents and humans (Nishimura et al., 2006; Eisenberg et al., 2009). Supplementation with spermidine reduces age-associated pathology and mortality in aged mice (Soda et al., 2009; LaRocca et al., 2013). However, the evidence for spermidine to increase primate and human life spans has yet to be revealed. Recently, the endogenous levels of spermidine have been shown to be positively correlated with left ventricular ejection fraction and heart rate in humans (Meana et al., 2016). Whether supplementation of spermidine has beneficial effects for preventing age-associated diseases, especially cardiovascular diseases, needs further investigation.

Increasing NAD Levels to Reverse Aging

Calorie restriction increases mitochondrial NAD in order to promote survival (Yang et al., 2007). The salvage pathway for NAD biosynthesis begins with either nicotinamide (NAM) or nicotinic acid (NA), collectively known as niacin or vitamin B_3 (Rongvaux et al., 2003). NAM is converted to nicotinamide mononucleotide (NMN) by nicotinamide phosphoribosyltransferase (NAMPT). The production of NAD from NMN and ATP is catalyzed by a family of NMN adenylyltransferases (NMNATs). In lower eukaryotes—including *S. cerevisiae, D. melanogaster*, and *C. elegans*—no NAMPT activity has been found. NAM is converted to NA, which then enters the parallel salvage pathway found in all eukaryotic species. Alternatively, nicotinamide riboside (NR) forms a precursor for NAD synthesis, connecting to the NAM salvage pathway through NMN. While the NAM salvage biosynthesis pathway is considered the main pathway for maintaining NAD levels, the latter can also be de novo synthesized from L-tryptophan (L-Trp). Note that the three major precursors for NAD biosynthesis (NAM, NA, and L-Trp) are all approved drugs or food supplements. NA has been a treatment option for lowering circulating lipid levels for many years (MacKay et al., 2012).

The intermediary metabolites previously mentioned regulate life span in different ways. Supraphysiological concentrations of NAD and NA extend life span in a fashion that depends on SIR-2.1, the nematodal ortholog of SIRT-1 (Hashimoto et al., 2010). By contrast, high concentration of NAM decreases nematodal life span, whereas low physiological doses of NAM or its metabolite, N^1-methylnicotinamide (MNA), extend life span independently of SIR-2.1 (Schmeisser et al., 2013). Supplementation with NAM reduces chronic infection in humans (Bogan and Brenner, 2008), improves cognition in mice (Green et al., 2008; Gong et al., 2013), and increases longevity in yeast (Schmeisser et al., 2013). However, excessive NAM can cause immune intolerance and cancers (Bogan and Brenner, 2008). Nicotinamide N-methyltransferase (NNMT) is the mammalian enzyme that methylates NAM using *S*-adenosylmethionine as a methyl donor to generate MNA. In contrast to the discovery in lower organisms, Kraus et al. (2014) reported that knocking down NNMT protects against diet-induced obesity. Moreover, increased *Nnmt* expression is found in obese compared to nonobese human subjects, and the urinary MNA is elevated in humans and animals with obesity and type 2 diabetes (Salek et al., 2007).

Poly(ADP-ribose) polymerases (PARPs) catalyze the polymerization of ADP–ribose units of the target proteins with donor NAD molecules, which causes the formation of linear or branched polymers (Kim et al., 2005). A strong positive correlation between longevity and the polymer synthesis capacity of PARPs has been shown in mammalian cells (Beneke et al., 2010). Mice with *PARP1* genetically knocked out exhibit faster aging than their wild-type counterparts (Piskunova et al., 2008). Thus, inhibition of PARPs has been proposed to increase NAD availability to elicit the anti-aging activity (El Ramy et al., 2009). Overall, maintaining high levels of NAD can increase the life span of the lower organisms by preventing primary aging, and it promotes the health spans of higher organisms.

TARGETING SIRT-1 FOR CRM DISCOVERY AND DEVELOPMENT

Sirtuins are a family of NAD-dependent protein deacetylases that exert diversified cellular functions by interacting with a wide range of signaling molecules, transcription factors, histones, and enzymes (Wang et al., 2012). *Sir2* (silent information regulator 2), the first gene discovered in this family, was originally shown to extend life span in yeast and promote transcriptional silencing through deacetylation of the epsilon-amino groups of lysine in the amino-terminal domains of histones (Gottlieb and Esposito, 1989; Aparicio et al., 1991). Budding yeast cultured under low glucose conditions (i.e., calorie restriction) exhibits a significant extension of proliferative life span, which is *Sir2*-dependent (Kaeberlein et al., 1999). Depletion or mutation of *Sir2* significantly reduces life span in yeast, worms, and flies (Longo and Kennedy, 2006; Chen and Guarente, 2007).

Over the last decade, sirtuins have attracted major attention due to their potential in expanding life span and protecting against age-associated disorders (Baur et al., 2012). Of all mammalian sirtuins, SIRT-1 is the ortholog most highly related to *Sir2* (Law et al., 2009; Wang et al., 2011; Wang et al., 2012). Both proteins possess NAD-dependent deacetylase and ADP-ribosyltransferase activities and are upregulated by calorie restriction (Hassa et al., 2006; Kanfi et al., 2008). Genetic variations of SIRT-1 are associated with accelerated aging in human populations (Kuningas et al., 2007). Mice lacking SIRT-1 fail to show an increased activity and extended life span in response to calorie restriction (Chen et al., 2005; Boily et al., 2008). Small molecular activators of SIRT-1 replicate signaling pathways triggered by calorie restriction and extend life span in mice (Smith et al., 2009; Mitchell et al., 2014). In vitro overexpression of SIRT-3 shows protective benefit of calorie restriction by increasing NADPH levels against oxidative stress-induced cell death (Someya et al., 2010). Similarly, overexpression of SIRT-6 in male mice increases the maximal life span with reduced levels of IGF-1 in serum (Kanfi et al., 2012). Recent studies have shown that a genetic variant within the SIRT-1 gene promoter is not associated with longevity in elderly Italians (Albani et al., 2015), but single nucleotide polymorphisms of SIRT-3 are involved in the longevity of female elderly within the same population (Albani et al., 2014).

The anti-aging activity of SIRT-1 has been largely attributed to its role in regulating energy metabolism. The requirement of NAD as a cosubstrate implies that SIRT-1 acts as a sensor of cellular energy and reduction–oxidation status (Lin et al., 2004). SIRT-1 not only mediates the metabolic changes associated with calorie restriction but also protects against metabolic damage caused by chronic exposure to a high-fat diet (Pfluger et al., 2008). It is a principal regulator of energy homeostasis and systemic insulin sensitivity (Chang and Guarente, 2014). Mice overexpressing SIRT-1 are leaner and exhibit improved energy homeostasis (Bordone et al., 2007). Genetic variations of SIRT-1 in humans are associated with body mass index and adiposity, especially visceral obesity (Peeters et al., 2008; Shimoyama et al., 2011). Although the molecular basis underlying the antiaging functions of SIRT-1 remains to be elucidated, activators of this longevity element represent a promising class of drugs for the treatment of aging-related diseases (Imai and Guarente, 2014).

Tissue-Specific Activation of SIRT-1 Mediates the Beneficial Effects of Calorie Restriction

Aging is associated with a significant change of body fat composition that is characterized by a gradual decrease in fat free mass (especially skeletal muscle) and a significant increase in fat mass (especially in the abdominal cavity). These changes, referred to as *sarcopenic obesity*, contributes to impaired physical and psychological functions and the development of many aging-related ailments (Batsis et al., 2013). In fact, adiposity, particularly around the abdomen, is positively linked to reduced life expectancy (Bluher, 2008). While various factors such as decreased energy expenditure and alterations of hormone productions influence body fat distribution in aged individuals, as an endocrine and metabolic organ, adipose tissue per se actively participates in the aging process (Tchkonia et al., 2013). For example, accumulation of visceral fat (central obesity) leads to metabolic syndrome and shortens life span, in part by increasing the inflammatory factors and decreasing adiponectin, an insulin-sensitizing and cardiovascular protective hormone (Hanauer, 2005). In addition, fat redistribution is often associated with the dysregulation of fatty acid storage and release. The overflow of fatty acids in the form of diacylglycerols, ceramides, and long-chain acyl-coenzymes A exert adverse effects on systemic energy homeostasis and insulin sensitivity (Jensen, 2008; Jung and Choi, 2014). Since abnormal adipose tissue distribution and function are key components of a vicious cycle accelerating the aging process, adipose tissue engineering may represent an effective anti-aging approach. Indeed, many longevity modulators including calorie restriction and physical excise elicit their beneficial effects via regulating fat distribution and metabolism (Jung and Choi, 2014). Long-term calorie restriction decreases adiposity, elevates gene expression involved in energy metabolism, and reduces the expression of more than 50 proinflammatory genes in white adipose tissues (Higami et al., 2006).

Calorie restriction reduces body weight and fat mass, especially visceral fat, which is an indicator of metabolic disorders in mammals (Li et al., 2003; Ye and Keller, 2010). Calorie restriction-induced reduction of visceral fat leads to an increase in life span and reduced renal diseases in rodents (Muzumdar et al., 2008). Calorie restriction study in overweight men and women has shown that visceral fat is largely reduced in conjugation with other benefits of lowering metabolic rate, core body temperature, and insulin resistance as well as the prevention of cardiovascular diseases (Larson-Meyer et al., 2006; Lefevre et al., 2009). Specific depletion or expansion of the visceral fat depot using genetic or surgical tools in rodents have direct effects on aging-related disease risks (Huffman and Barzilai, 2009). Mice with genetically increased life spans (Ames dwarf, Snell dwarf, insulin growth hormone receptor, pregnancy-associated plasma protein A knockout mice) have substantially reduced visceral fat (Junnila et al., 2013; Menon et al., 2014). Elevated insulin sensitivity, reduced oxidative stress, augmented adiponectin production, significantly improved whole body glucose homeostasis, and lipid metabolism contribute to the increased life span in these mice.

SIRT-1 is a key mediator coordinating the physiological responses to calorie restriction. The expression and activity of SIRT-1 is dynamically regulated in major metabolic organs. Calorie restriction-induced SIRT-1 expression occurs predominantly in adipose tissues but not liver or muscle tissues (Chen et al., 2008). In fact, SIRT-1 exerts its effects on metabolism and insulin sensitivity in a tissue-specific manner (Wang et al., 2012). SIRT-1 in liver may not be the major contributor to systemic glucose homeostasis and insulin sensitivity (Rodgers et al., 2005; Erion et al., 2009; Purushotham et al., 2009) but appears to maintain hepatic lipid homeostasis and control the bile acid metabolism (Garcia-Rodriguez et al., 2014; Li et al., 2014). In skeletal muscle, SIRT-1 expression is decreased under insulin-resistant conditions (Sun et al., 2007). It regulates the differentiation and metabolism of muscle cells (Lee and Min, 2013). However, specific overexpression or knockout of SIRT-1 in skeletal muscle does not affect whole-body energy expenditure in mice on either a standard diet or energy-restricted diets (White et al., 2013).

The role of adipose SIRT-1 as an important regulator of energy metabolism and systemic insulin sensitivity has been suggested by both clinical and animal studies (Picard and Guarente, 2005; Wang et al., 2012). In humans,

SIRT-1 expression is decreased in both obese and type 2 diabetic patients (Pedersen et al., 2008; Song et al., 2013). Extensive weight loss significantly increases SIRT-1 expression in adipose tissues (Moschen et al., 2013). In mice, both expression and activity of SIRT-1 in adipose tissues progressively decrease during aging but are markedly elevated by calorie restriction (Xu et al., 2013; Xu et al., 2015). SIRT-1 acts as a nutrient-dependent modulator to inhibit adipose tissue inflammation (Gillum et al., 2011; Chalkiadaki and Guarente, 2012; Kotas et al., 2013). In 3T3-L1 adipocytes, SIRT-1 promotes fat mobilization by interacting with corepressors NcoR and SMART (Picard et al., 2004). SIRT-1–dependent deacetylation of peroxisome proliferator activator receptor gamma (PPARγ) facilitates the brown remodeling of white adipose tissues (Qiang et al., 2012). Knockdown of SIRT-1 inhibits insulin-stimulated glucose uptake and GLUT4 translocation, whereas treatment of adipocytes with specific SIRT-1 activators leads to an increase in insulin-stimulated glucose uptake (Yoshizaki et al., 2009). SIRT-1 also modulates the expression and secretion of adiponectin (Qiao and Shao, 2006; Qiang et al., 2007). In mice, activation of SIRT-1 selectively in adipose tissue protects mice against metabolic deterioration during aging and facilitates energy homeostasis; these effects resemble those elicited by calorie restriction (Wang et al., 2012; Xu et al., 2013; Wang, 2014; Xu et al., 2015).

Intermediary Metabolites as Modulators of SIRT-1 Function

The expression and activity of SIRT-1 decline during aging and contribute to the development of age-related complications (Yuan et al., 2016). Thus, a forced SIRT-1 activation or induction represents a strategy for identifying and developing CRMs. SIRT-1 is dynamically regulated by intermediary metabolites. Its cofactor, the pyridine nucleotide NAD, metabolically acts as a hydride acceptor to form NADH (donor for oxidoreductases) and as an enzyme substrate. However, NAD usually presents at a much higher level than its *Km* for SIRT-1 activation, precluding this metabolite from being a rate-limiting factor for SIRT-1 functions in vivo (Sauve and Youn, 2012). On the other hand, NAD metabolites may be more dynamically involved in regulating SIRT-1 (Lee et al., 2008).

SIRT-1 activity can be increased by supplementation of NA or NAM for NAD biosynthesis (Yoshino et al., 2011) or by inhibiting the enzyme CD38 or *PARP* to reduce NAD consumption (Aksoy et al., 2006; de Picciotto et al., 2016). Supplementation with purine nucleotide metabolites of NAD, such as NR, enhances oxidative metabolism and protects against high-fat-diet–induced metabolic abnormalities in SIRT-1–dependent manners (Canto et al., 2012). In addition, modulating the activity of enzymes involved in NAD metabolic pathways such as NAMPT (Song et al., 2014), NNMT (Kraus et al., 2014), and PARP (Bai et al., 2011) exerts marked effects on energy metabolism in mice. Recent evidence has further expanded the scope of intermediary metabolites for SIRT-1 regulation, including various acyl-CoA donors (Feldman et al., 2012) and biotin and biotin-5′-AMP (Xu et al., 2013; Wang, 2014).

The initial breakthrough of identification of *Sir2* as a deacetylase with weak ADP–ribosyltransferase activity came along with the identification of the *Salmonella typhimurium* CobB protein as a *Sir2* homolog (Tsang and Escalante-Semerena, 1998). CobB compensates for the lack of CobT mutants during vitamin B_{12} biosynthesis and possesses nicotinate mononucleotide (NaMN)–dependent phosphoribosyltransferase activity. Thus, CobB catalyzes the release of NA from NaMN, whereas *Sir2* and SIRT-1 remove NAM from NAD. This evidence suggests that the biosynthesis or homeostasis of B vitamins [including vitamin B_3 (NA/NAM) and B_7 (biotin)] regulate the enzymatic activities of SIRT-1. Indeed, SIRT-1 can be potently inhibited by biotin and its metabolite biotinyl-5′-AMP (Xu et al., 2013). Chronic biotin supplementation abolishes SIRT-1-mediated health benefits (Wang, 2014). In mice, biotin storage in adipose tissues increases with age, which is accompanied by a progressively decreased SIRT-1 activity (Xu et al., 2013). Calorie restriction activates SIRT-1 partly by preventing the accumulation of biotin in adipose tissue (Xu et al., 2013, 2015). In summary, the dynamic changes of endogenous intermediary metabolites that regulate SIRT-1 activity are potential pathways for rational design and development of CRMs.

SIRT-1–Activating Compounds Derived From Functional Foods

Various functional foods are able to boost SIRT-1′s activity or expression (Park et al., 2016). It is implicated in mitochondrial homeostasis, autophagy regulation, protein deacetylation, and longevity induced by a number of CRMs derived from functional foods (Lee et al., 2008; Mouchiroud et al., 2013; Ou et al., 2014). Resveratrol, known as 3,4′,5-trihydroxystilbene, is a natural polyphenolic compound primarily found in plants (Fremont, 2000). It presents in either *trans-* or *cis-* isomers, where the *trans*-resveratrol has been widely studied and found enriched in grapes and grape products, berries, peanuts, and some herbal plants (Wenzel and Somoza, 2005; Giovinazzo et al., 2012). Many health benefits of *trans*-resveratrol have been reported, ranging from being cardio- and neuroprotective, antioxidant, antiinflammatory, antiatherosclerotic to anti-tumorigenic (Sale et al., 2004; Das and Maulik, 2006; Kwon et al., 2011; Smoliga et al., 2011).

Resveratrol is an activator of SIRT-1 and is able to induce AMPK, both of which are involved in its antiaging functions (Diaz-Ruiz et al., 2015). Resveratrol has been reported to increase DNA stability and extension of life span in yeast (Howitz et al., 2003). However, the effects on life span failed to be observed in higher organisms such as *D. melanogaster* (Bass et al., 2007) and rodents (Pearson et al., 2008; Miller et al., 2011). Nevertheless, resveratrol exerts beneficial effects on secondary aging—that is, the prevention of age-associated diseases and functional loss. Resveratrol-treated mice had lower total cholesterol levels in plasma and reduced incidence of atherosclerotic lesion formation when compared to control counterparts (Do et al., 2008). Treatment with resveratrol in the aged mice activated SIRT-1 expression, where the subsequent apoptotic pathway involving forkhead box protein O3 was inhibited (Lin et al., 2014). It increases glucose uptake in response to insulin stimulation in skeletal muscle, adipocytes, and hepatocytes via activation of SIRT-1 and AMPK (Sun et al., 2007; Breen et al., 2008). Resveratrol can penetrate the blood–brain barrier to reach the central nervous system. In the animal model of Alzheimer's disease, resveratrol-treated mice show a delayed onset as well as a slow progression of impaired memory (Kim et al., 2007; Venigalla et al., 2016) due partly at least to SIRT-1-mediated inhibition of nuclear factor kappa B (NFκB) signaling (Chen et al., 2005). Resveratrol rescued SIRT-1 activity suppressed by betaamyloid peptide 25–35 in a dose-dependent manner, which led to significant attenuation of apoptosis in mouse neurons (Feng et al., 2013; Witte et al., 2014; Zhang et al., 2014; Turner et al., 2015).

Fisetin (3, 7, 3′, 4′-tetrahydroxyflavone) is a flavonol that can be found in vegetables and fruits such as strawberries and apples (Kim et al., 2015). It increases the expression of adiponectin in a dose-dependent manner to protect obesity-related malfunctions and vascular abnormalities (Jin et al., 2014). By suppressing PPARs, it regulates cell metabolism (Kim et al., 2015). Mechanistically, fisetin not only promotes SIRT-1 activity to mediate the deacetylation of PPARγ and FOXO1 but also enhances the association of SIRT-1 with the promoter of PPARγ, which results in attenuation of adipogenesis (Kim et al., 2015). Oligonol contains catechin-type oligomers that are found in lychee fruit and grape seed (Fujii et al., 2007). Mice treated with oligonol exhibit reduced serum lipid concentration, improved kidney function, and attenuated cognitive impairment (Noh et al., 2010; Sakurai et al., 2013). By upregulation of SIRT-1 expression, oligonol attenuates mitochondrial superoxide formation and activates autophagy (Park et al., 2016).

Melatonin (known as N-acetyl 5-methoxy tryptamine) is an indole hormone that is expressed by various plants and animals (Reiter et al., 2013). Plants synthesize melatonin from the essential amino acid L-trytophan, but melatonin in animals is mainly secreted from the pineal gland but is also present in skin, the immune system, the reproductive system, and the gastrointestinal tract (Slominski et al., 2002; Acuna-Castroviejo et al., 2014; Ramis et al., 2015). However, the absorption of melatonin is low in humans because the plasma levels of melatonin after the ingestion of melatonin-rich food are far less than the amount of melatonin ingested (Kennaway, 2015). Melatonin regulates circadian cycle (Hardeland et al., 2012) and elicits antioxidant (Galano et al., 2013) and anti-inflammatory activities (Agil et al., 2013). The circadian rhythm of melatonin is disturbed and deteriorated by aging (Waller et al., 2016). The loss of melatonin rhythm in the elderly not only causes sleep disorders but also leads to desynchronization of gene expression that affects general well-being (Jung-Hynes et al., 2010). Melatonin increases the expression of SIRT-1 protein and decreases the levels of acetylated p53 and NFκB in mice prone to accelerated senescence (Gutierrez-Cuesta et al., 2008). However, melatonin exhibits anti-tumor activity by downregulating SIRT-1 and upregulating acetylated p53 in human osteosarcoma cells (Cheng et al., 2013). Whether or not melatonin-mediated SIRT-1 expressions are specific to certain cell types warrants further study.

CONCLUDING REMARKS AND PERSPECTIVES

The average life expectancy has been creeping upward in most developed countries for many years. While the ultimate goal of science and technology is to extend the life span beyond its current natural limits, the contemporary challenge of anti-aging program is to eliminate or reduce aging-associated medical burdens from the world's leading causes of death, including cancer and cardiovascular, neurodegenerative, musculoskeletal, and metabolic diseases. To focus on molecules that mediate the beneficial effects of caloric restriction represents one of the most straightforward approaches for developing anti-aging remedies. Accordingly, a bunch of CRMs emerge for either depletion of the energy supply or targeting specific signaling pathways such as autophagy. Functional foods represent the most promising source of CRMs. In particular, those that activate the expression or function of SIRT-1 hold great potential to delay the onset of aging and age-related diseases. In this respect, actions specific to adipose tissue by SIRT-1 are directly related to the anti-aging effects of caloric restriction. Adipose tissue is the body's largest endocrine organ that secretes inflammatory and immune mediators. During aging, the most prominent changes in our body are the loss of functional lean (fat-free) mass and the accumulation of fat, especially in the abdominal region (Jackson et al., 2012). From the ages of 40 to 79, visceral fat in men increased by 42.9% and by 65.3% in women, whereas the fat-free mass decreased by 6.6% to 23.3% in both genders (Yamada et al., 2014). This phenomenon, referred as *sarcopenic obesity*, is assuming a prominent role in aging-related diseases (Prado et al., 2012). The important role of adipose tissues in human aging provides a more convenient but focused strategy for discovering SIRT-1–activating compounds in functional foods.

References

Acuna-Castroviejo, D., Escames, G., Venegas, C., Diaz-Casado, M.E., Lima-Cabello, E., Lopez, L.C., et al., 2014. Extrapineal melatonin: sources, regulation, and potential functions. Cell Mol Life Sci. 71 (16), 2997–3025.

Agil, A., Reiter, R.J., Jimenez-Aranda, A., Iban-Arias, R., Navarro-Alarcon, M., Marchal, J.A., et al., 2013. Melatonin ameliorates low-grade inflammation and oxidative stress in young Zucker diabetic fatty rats. J. Pineal Res. 54 (4), 381–388.

Akram, M., 2014. Citric acid cycle and role of its intermediates in metabolism. Cell Biochem. Biophys. 68 (3), 475–478.

Aksoy, P., Escande, C., White, T.A., Thompson, M., Soares, S., Benech, J.C., et al., 2006. Regulation of SIRT 1 mediated NAD dependent deacetylation: a novel role for the multifunctional enzyme CD38. Biochem. Biophys. Res. Commun. 349 (1), 353–359.

Albani, D., Ateri, E., Mazzuco, S., Ghilardi, A., Rodilossi, S., Biella, G., et al., 2014. Modulation of human longevity by SIRT3 single nucleotide polymorphisms in the prospective study "Treviso Longeva (TRELONG)." Age (Dordr) 36 (1), 469–478.

Albani, D., Mazzuco, S., Chierchia, A., Fusco, F., Boeri, L., Martines, R., et al., 2015. The SIRT1 promoter polymorphic site rs12778366 increases IL-6 related human mortality in the prospective study "Treviso Longeva (TRELONG)." Int. J. Mol. Epidemiol. Genet. 6 (1), 20–26.

Anderson, J.W., Herman, R.H., 1972. Effect of fasting, caloric restriction, and refeeding on glucose tolerance of normal men. Am. J. Clin. Nutr. 25 (1), 41–52.

Anstey, K., Stankov, L., Lord, S., 1993. Primary aging, secondary aging, and intelligence. Psychol. Aging 8 (4), 562–570.

Aparicio, O.M., Billington, B.L., Gottschling, D.E., 1991. Modifiers of position effect are shared between telomeric and silent mating-type loci in S. cerevisiae. Cell 66 (6), 1279–1287.

Bai, P., Canto, C., Oudart, H., Brunyanszki, A., Cen, Y., Thomas, C., et al., 2011. PARP-1 inhibition increases mitochondrial metabolism through SIRT1 activation. Cell Metab. 13 (4), 461–468.

Bao, J., Sack, M.N., 2010. Protein deacetylation by sirtuins: delineating a post-translational regulatory program responsive to nutrient and redox stressors. Cell Mol. Life Sci. 67 (18), 3073–3087.

Bass, T.M., Weinkove, D., Houthoofd, K., Gems, D., Partridge, L., 2007. Effects of resveratrol on lifespan in *Drosophila melanogaster* and *Caenorhabditis elegans*. Mech. Ageing Dev. 128 (10), 546–552.

Batsis, J.A., Barre, L.K., Mackenzie, T.A., Pratt, S.I., Lopez-Jimenez, F., Bartels, S.J., 2013. Variation in the prevalence of sarcopenia and sarcopenic obesity in older adults associated with different research definitions: dual-energy X-ray absorptiometry data from the National Health and Nutrition Examination Survey 1999–2004. J. Am. Geriatr. Soc. 61 (6), 974–980.

Baur, J.A., Ungvari, Z., Minor, R.K., Le Couteur, D.G., de Cabo, R., 2012. Are sirtuins viable targets for improving healthspan and lifespan? Nat. Rev. Drug Discov. 11 (6), 443–461.

Beneke, S., Scherr, A.L., Ponath, V., Popp, O., Burkle, A., 2010. Enzyme characteristics of recombinant poly(ADP-ribose) polymerases-1 of rat and human origin mirror the correlation between cellular poly(ADP-ribosyl)ation capacity and species-specific life span. Mech. Ageing Dev. 131 (5), 366–369.

Bluher, M., 2008. Fat tissue and long life. Obes. Facts 1 (4), 176–182.

Bogan, K.L., Brenner, C., 2008. Nicotinic acid, nicotinamide, and nicotinamide riboside: a molecular evaluation of NAD+ precursor vitamins in human nutrition. Annu Rev. Nutr. 28, 115–130.

Boily, G., Seifert, E.L., Bevilacqua, L., He, X.H., Sabourin, G., Estey, C., et al., 2008. SirT1 regulates energy metabolism and response to caloric restriction in mice. PLoS One 3 (3), e1759.

Bordone, L., Cohen, D., Robinson, A., Motta, M.C., van Veen, E., Czopik, A., et al., 2007. SIRT1 transgenic mice show phenotypes resembling calorie restriction. Aging Cell 6 (6), 759–767.

Breen, D.M., Sanli, T., Giacca, A., Tsiani, E., 2008. Stimulation of muscle cell glucose uptake by resveratrol through sirtuins and AMPK. Biochem. Biophys. Res. Commun. 374 (1), 117–122.

Cai, L., Sutter, B.M., Li, B., Tu, B.P., 2011. Acetyl-CoA induces cell growth and proliferation by promoting the acetylation of histones at growth genes. Mol. Cell 42 (4), 426–437.

Canto, C., Houtkooper, R.H., Pirinen, E., Youn, D.Y., Oosterveer, M.H., Cen, Y., et al., 2012. The NAD(+) precursor nicotinamide riboside enhances oxidative metabolism and protects against high-fat diet-induced obesity. Cell Metab. 15 (6), 838–847.

Carames, B., Kiosses, W.B., Akasaki, Y., Brinson, D.C., Eap, W., Koziol, J., et al., 2013. Glucosamine activates autophagy in vitro and in vivo. Arthritis Rheum 65 (7), 1843–1852.

Cavallini, G., Donati, A., Taddei, M., Bergamini, E., 2007. Evidence for selective mitochondrial autophagy and failure in aging. Autophagy 3 (1), 26–27.

Cetrullo, S., D'Adamo, S., Tantini, B., Borzi, R.M., Flamigni, F., 2015. mTOR, AMPK, and Sirt1: key players in metabolic stress management. Crit. Rev. Eukaryot Gene Expr. 25 (1), 59–75.

Chalkiadaki, A., Guarente, L., 2012. High-fat diet triggers inflammation-induced cleavage of SIRT1 in adipose tissue to promote metabolic dysfunction. Cell Metab. 16 (2), 180–188

Chang, H.C., Guarente, L., 2014. SIRT1 and other sirtuins in metabolism. Trends Endocrinol. Metab. 25 (3), 138–145.

Chen, D., Guarente, L., 2007. SIR2: a potential target for calorie restriction mimetics. Trends Mol. Med. 13 (2), 64–71.

Chen, D., Bruno, J., Easlon, E., Lin, S.J., Cheng, H.L., Alt, F.W., et al., 2008. Tissue-specific regulation of SIRT1 by calorie restriction. Genes Dev. 22 (13), 1753–1757.

Chen, J., Zhou, Y., Mueller-Steiner, S., Chen, L.F., Kwon, H., Yi, S., et al., 2005. SIRT1 protects against microglia-dependent amyloid-beta toxicity through inhibiting NF-kappaB signaling. J. Biol. Chem. 280 (48), 40364–40374.

Cheng, Y., Cai, L., Jiang, P., Wang, J., Gao, C., Feng, H., et al., 2013. SIRT1 inhibition by melatonin exerts antitumor activity in human osteosarcoma cells. Eur. J. Pharmacol. 715 (1-3), 219–229.

Choi, K.M., Han, K.A., Ahn, H.J., Lee, S.Y., Hwang, S.Y., Kim, B.H., et al., 2013. The effects of caloric restriction on fetuin-A and cardiovascular risk factors in rats and humans: a randomized controlled trial. Clin. Endocrinol. (Oxf) 79 (3), 356–363.

Choudhary, C., Weinert, B.T., Nishida, Y., Verdin, E., Mann, M., 2014. The growing landscape of lysine acetylation links metabolism and cell signalling. Nat. Rev. Mol. Cell Biol. 15 (8), 536–550.

Colman, R.J., Anderson, R.M., Johnson, S.C., Kastman, E.K., Kosmatka, K.J., Beasley, T.M., et al., 2009. Caloric restriction delays disease onset and mortality in rhesus monkeys. Science 325 (5937), 201–204.

Colman, R.J., Beasley, T.M., Kemnitz, J.W., Johnson, S.C., Weindruch, R., Anderson, R.M., 2014. Caloric restriction reduces age-related and all-cause mortality in rhesus monkeys. Nat. Commun. 5, 3557.

Cui, J., Shi, S., Sun, X., Cai, G., Cui, S., Hong, Q., et al., 2013. Mitochondrial autophagy involving renal injury and aging is modulated by caloric intake in aged rat kidneys. PLoS One 8 (7), e69720.

Dabhade, P., Kotwal, S., 2013. Tackling the aging process with bio-molecules: a possible role for caloric restriction, food-derived nutrients, vitamins, amino acids, peptides, and minerals. J. Nutr. Gerontol. Geriatr. 32 (1), 24–40.

Das, D.K., Maulik, N., 2006. Resveratrol in cardioprotection: a therapeutic promise of alternative medicine. Mol. Interval 6 (1), 36–47.

de Picciotto, N.E., Gano, L.B., Johnson, L.C., Martens, C.R., Sindler, A.L., Mills, K.F., et al., 2016. Nicotinamide mononucleotide supplementation reverses vascular dysfunction and oxidative stress with aging in mice. Aging Cell.

Diaz-Ruiz, C., Rodriguez-Perez, A.I., Beiroa, D., Rodriguez-Pallares, J., Labandeira-Garcia, J.L., 2015. Reciprocal regulation between sirtuin-1 and angiotensin-II in the substantia nigra: implications for aging and neurodegeneration. Oncotarget 6 (29), 26675–26689.

Do, G.M., Kwon, E.Y., Kim, H.J., Jeon, S.M., Ha, T.Y., Park, T., et al., 2008. Long-term effects of resveratrol supplementation on suppression of atherogenic lesion formation and cholesterol synthesis in apo E-deficient mice. Biochem. Biophys. Res. Commun. 374 (1), 55–59.

Duan, W., Mattson, M.P., 1999. Dietary restriction and 2-deoxyglucose administration improve behavioral outcome and reduce degeneration of dopaminergic neurons in models of Parkinson's disease. J. Neurosci. Res. 57 (2), 195–206.

Eisenberg, T., Knauer, H., Schauer, A., Buttner, S., Ruckenstuhl, C., Carmona-Gutierrez, D., et al., 2009. Induction of autophagy by spermidine promotes longevity. Nat. Cell Biol. 11 (11), 1305–1314.

Eisenberg, T., Schroeder, S., Andryushkova, A., Pendl, T., Kuttner, V., Bhukel, A., et al., 2014. Nucleocytosolic depletion of the energy metabolite acetyl-coenzyme a stimulates autophagy and prolongs lifespan. Cell Metab. 19 (3), 431–444.

El Ramy, R., Magroun, N., Messadecq, N., Gauthier, L.R., Boussin, F.D., Kolthur-Seetharam, U., et al., 2009. Functional interplay between Parp-1 and SirT1 in genome integrity and chromatin-based processes. Cell Mol. Life Sci. 66 (19), 3219–3234.

Erion, D.M., Yonemitsu, S., Nie, Y., Nagai, Y., Gillum, M.P., Hsiao, J.J., et al., 2009. SirT1 knockdown in liver decreases basal hepatic glucose production and increases hepatic insulin responsiveness in diabetic rats. Proc. Natl. Acad. Sci. USA 106 (27), 11288–11293.

Feldman, J.L., Dittenhafer-Reed, K.E., Denu, J.M., 2012. Sirtuin catalysis and regulation. J. Biol. Chem 287 (51), 42419–42427.

Feng, X., Liang, N., Zhu, D., Gao, Q., Peng, L., Dong, H., et al., 2013. Resveratrol inhibits beta-amyloid-induced neuronal apoptosis through regulation of SIRT1-ROCK1 signaling pathway. PLoS One 8 (3), e59888.

Fernandes, G., Good, R.A., 1984. Inhibition by restricted-calorie diet of lymphoproliferative disease and renal damage in MRL/lpr mice. Proc. Natl. Acad. Sci. USA 81 (19), 6144–6148.

Fontana, L., Partridge, L., Longo, V.D., 2010. Extending healthy life span-from yeast to humans. Science 328 (5976), 321–326.

Fremont, L., 2000. Biological effects of resveratrol. Life Sci. 66 (8), 663–673.

Fujii, H., Nakagawa, T., Nishioka, H., Sato, E., Hirose, A., Ueno, Y., et al., 2007. Preparation, characterization, and antioxidative effects of oligomeric proanthocyanidin-L-cysteine complexes. J. Agric. Food Chem. 55 (4), 1525–1531.

Galano, A., Tan, D.X., Reiter, R.J., 2013. On the free radical scavenging activities of melatonin's metabolites, AFMK and AMK. J. Pineal Res. 54 (3), 245–257.

Garcia-Rodriguez, J.L., Barbier-Torres, L., Fernandez-Alvarez, S., Gutierrez-de Juan, V., Monte, M.J., Halilbasic, E., et al., 2014. SIRT1 controls liver regeneration by regulating bile acid metabolism through farnesoid X receptor and mammalian target of rapamycin signaling. Hepatology 59 (5), 1972–1983.

Geeraert, C., Ratier, A., Pfisterer, S.G., Perdiz, D., Cantaloube, I., Rouault, A., et al., 2010. Starvation-induced hyperacetylation of tubulin is required for the stimulation of autophagy by nutrient deprivation. J. Biol. Chem. 285 (31), 24184–24194.

Gillum, M.P., Kotas, M.E., Erion, D.M., Kursawe, R., Chatterjee, P., Nead, K.T., et al., 2011. SirT1 regulates adipose tissue inflammation. Diabetes 60 (12), 3235–3245.

Giovinazzo, G., Ingrosso, I., Paradiso, A., De Gara, L., Santino, A., 2012. Resveratrol biosynthesis: plant metabolic engineering for nutritional improvement of food. Plant Foods Hum. Nutr. 67 (3), 191–199.

Gong, B., Pan, Y., Vempati, P., Zhao, W., Knable, L., Ho, L., et al., 2013. Nicotinamide riboside restores cognition through an upregulation of proliferator-activated receptor-gamma coactivator 1alpha regulated beta-secretase 1 degradation and mitochondrial gene expression in Alzheimer's mouse models. Neurobiol. Aging 34 (6), 1581–1588.

Gottlieb, S., Esposito, R.E., 1989. A new role for a yeast transcriptional silencer gene, SIR2, in regulation of recombination in ribosomal DNA. Cell 56 (5), 771–776.

Green, K.N., Steffan, J.S., Martinez-Coria, H., Sun, X., Schreiber, S.S., Thompson, L.M., et al., 2008. Nicotinamide restores cognition in Alzheimer's disease transgenic mice via a mechanism involving sirtuin inhibition and selective reduction of Thr231-phosphotau. J. Neurosci. 28 (45), 11500–11510.

Guo, Z., Lee, J., Lane, M., Mattson, M., 2001. Iodoacetate protects hippocampal neurons against excitotoxic and oxidative injury: involvement of heat-shock proteins and Bcl-2. J. Neurochem. 79 (2), 361–370.

Gupta, V.K., Scheunemann, L., Eisenberg, T., Mertel, S., Bhukel, A., Koemans, T.S., et al., 2013. Restoring polyamines protects from age-induced memory impairment in an autophagy-dependent manner. Nat. Neurosci. 16 (10), 1453–1460.

Gutierrez-Cuesta, J., Tajes, M., Jimenez, A., Coto-Montes, A., Camins, A., Pallas, M., 2008. Evaluation of potential pro-survival pathways regulated by melatonin in a murine senescence model. J. Pineal Res. 45 (4), 497–505.

Hackenschmidt, J., Barth, C., Decker, K., 1972. Stimulation of acetyl-CoA carboxylase by (-)-Hydroxycitrate. FEBS Lett. 27 (1), 131–133.

Hanauer, S.B., 2005. Obesity and visceral fat: a growing inflammatory disease. Nat. Clin. Pract. Gastroenterol. Hepatol. 2 (6), 245.

Hardeland, R., Madrid, J.A., Tan, D X., Reiter, R.J., 2012. Melatonin, the circadian multioscillator system and health: the need for detailed analyses of peripheral melatonin signaling. J. Pineal Res. 52 (2), 139–166.

Hartleben, B., Godel, M., Meyer-Schwesinger, C., Liu, S., Ulrich, T., Kobler, S., et al., 2010. Autophagy influences glomerular disease susceptibility and maintains podocyte homeostasis in aging mice. J. Clin. Investig. 120 (4), 1084–1096.

Hashimoto, T., Horikawa, M., Nomura, T., Sakamoto, K., 2010. Nicotinamide adenine dinucleotide extends the lifespan of Caenorhabditis elegans mediated by sir-2.1 and daf-16. Biogerontology 11 (1), 31–43.

Hassa, P.O., Haenni, S.S., Elser, M., Hottiger, M.O., 2006. Nuclear ADP-ribosylation reactions in mammalian cells: where are we today and where are we going? Microbiol. Mol. Biol. Rev. 70 (3), 789–829.

Heilbronn, L.K., Ravussin, E., 2003. Calorie restriction and aging: review of the literature and implications for studies in humans. Am. J. Clin. Nutr. 78 (3), 361–369.

Heilbronn, L.K., Smith, S.R., Martin, C.K., Anton, S.D., Ravussin, E., 2005. Alternate-day fasting in nonobese subjects: effects on body weight, body composition, and energy metabolism. Am. J. Clin. Nutr. 81 (1), 69–73.

Higami, Y., Barger, J.L., Page, G.P., Allison, D.B., Smith, S.R., Prolla, T.A., et al., 2006. Energy restriction lowers the expression of genes linked to inflammation, the cytoskeleton, the extracellular matrix, and angiogenesis in mouse adipose tissue. J. Nutr. 136 (2), 343–352.

Holloszy, J.O., Fontana, L., 2007. Caloric restriction in humans. Exp. Gerontol. 42 (8), 709–712.

Howitz, K.T., Bitterman, K.J., Cohen, H.Y., Lamming, D.W., Lavu, S., Wood, J.G., et al., 2003. Small molecule activators of sirtuins extend Saccharomyces cerevisiae lifespan. Nature 425 (6954), 191–196.

Huffman, D.M., Barzilai, N., 2009. Role of visceral adipose tissue in aging. Biochim. Biophys. Acta 1790 (10), 1117–1123.

Imai, S., Guarente, L., 2014. NAD+ and sirtuins in aging and disease. Trends Cell Biol. 24 (8), 464–471.

Ingram, D.K., Roth, G.S., 2011. Glycolytic inhibition as a strategy for developing calorie restriction mimetics. Exp. Gerontol. 46 (2-3), 148–154.

Ingram, D.K., Roth, G.S., 2015. Calorie restriction mimetics: can you have your cake and eat it, too? Ageing Res. Rev. 20, 46–62.

Ingram, D.K., Weindruch, R., Spangler, E.L., Freeman, J.R., Walford, R.L., 1987. Dietary restriction benefits learning and motor performance of aged mice. J. Gerontol. 42 (1), 78–81.

Ingram, D.K., Zhu, M., Mamczarz, J., Zou, S., Lane, M.A., Roth, G.S., et al., 2006. Calorie restriction mimetics: an emerging research field. Aging Cell 5 (2), 97–108.

Jackson, M.F., Luong, D., Vang, D.D., Garikipati, D.K., Stanton, J.B., Nelson, O.L., et al., 2012. The aging myostatin null phenotype: reduced adiposity, cardiac hypertrophy, enhanced cardiac stress response, and sexual dimorphism. J. Endocrinol. 213 (3), 263–275.

Jensen, M.D., 2008. Role of body fat distribution and the metabolic complications of obesity. J Clin. Endocrinol. Metab. 93 (11 Suppl 1), S57–S63.

Jin, T., Kim, O.Y., Shin, M.J., Choi, E.Y., Lee, S.S., Han, Y.S., et al., 2014. Fisetin up-regulates the expression of adiponectin in 3T3-L1 adipocytes via the activation of silent mating type information regulation 2 homologue 1 (SIRT1)-deacetylase and peroxisome proliferator-activated receptors (PPARs). J. Agric. Food Chem. 62 (43), 10468–10474.

Jung-Hynes, B., Reiter, R.J., Ahmad, N., 2010. Sirtuins, melatonin and circadian rhythms: building a bridge between aging and cancer. J. Pineal Res. 48 (1), 9–19.

Jung, U.J., Choi, M.S., 2014. Obesity and its metabolic complications: the role of adipokines and the relationship between obesity, inflammation, insulin resistance, dyslipidemia and nonalcoholic fatty liver disease. Int. J. Mol. Sci. 15 (4), 6184–6223.

Junnila, R.K., List, E.O., Berryman, D.E., Murrey, J.W., Kopchick, J.J., 2013. The GH/IGF-1 axis in ageing and longevity. Nat. Rev. Endocrinol. 9 (6), 366–376.

Kaeberlein, M., McVey, M., Guarente, L., 1999. The SIR2/3/4 complex and SIR2 alone promote longevity in Saccharomyces cerevisiae by two different mechanisms. Genes Dev. 13 (19), 2570–2580.

Kanfi, Y., Peshti, V., Gozlan, Y.M., Rathaus, M., Gil, R., Cohen, H.Y., 2008. Regulation of SIRT1 protein levels by nutrient availability. FEBS Lett. 582 (16), 2417–2423.

Kanfi, Y., Naiman, S., Amir, G., Peshti, V., Zinman, G., Nahum, L., et al., 2012. The sirtuin SIRT6 regulates lifespan in male mice. Nature 483 (7388), 218–221.

Kennaway, D.J., 2015. Are the proposed benefits of melatonin-rich foods too hard to swallow? Crit. Rev. Food Sci. Nutr.

Kim, D., Nguyen, M.D., Dobbin, M.M., Fischer, A., Sananbenesi, F., Rodgers, J.T., et al., 2007. SIRT1 deacetylase protects against neurodegeneration in models for Alzheimer's disease and amyotrophic lateral sclerosis. EMBO J. 26 (13), 3169–3179.

Kim, M.Y., Zhang, T., Kraus, W.L., 2005. Poly(ADP-ribosyl)ation by PARP-1: 'PAR-laying' NAD+ into a nuclear signal. Genes Dev. 19 (17), 1951–1967.

Kim, S.C., Kim, Y.H., Son, S.W., Moon, E.Y., Pyo, S., Um, S.H., 2015. Fisetin induces Sirt1 expression while inhibiting early adipogenesis in 3T3-L1 cells. Biochem. Biophys. Res. Commun. 467 (4), 638–644.

Korla, K., Mitra, C.K., 2014. Modelling the Krebs cycle and oxidative phosphorylation. J. Biomol. Struct. Dyn. 32 (2), 242–256.

Kornberg, H., 2000. Krebs and his trinity of cycles. Nat. Rev. Mol. Cell. Biol. 1 (3), 225–228.

Kotas, M.E., Gorecki, M.C., Gillum, M.P., 2013. Sirtuin-1 is a nutrient-dependent modulator of inflammation. Adipocyte 2 (2), 113–118.

Kraus, D., Yang, Q., Kong, D., Banks, A.S., Zhang, L., Rodgers, J.T., et al., 2014. Nicotinamide N-methyltransferase knockdown protects against diet-induced obesity. Nature 508 (7495), 258–262.

Kuningas, M., Putters, M., Westendorp, R.G., Slagboom, P.E., van Heemst, D., 2007. SIRT1 gene, age-related diseases, and mortality: the Leiden 85-plus study. J. Gerontol. A Biol. Sci. Med. Sci. 62 (9), 960–965.

Kwon, K.J., Kim, J.N., Kim, M.K., Lee, J., Ignarro, L.J., Kim, H.J., et al., 2011. Melatonin synergistically increases resveratrol-induced heme oxygenase-1 expression through the inhibition of ubiquitin-dependent proteasome pathway: a possible role in neuroprotection. J. Pineal Res. 50 (2), 110–123.

Lane, M.A., Baer, D.J., Rumpler, W.V., Weindruch, R., Ingram, D.K., Tilmont, E.M., et al., 1996. Calorie restriction lowers body temperature in rhesus monkeys, consistent with a postulated anti-aging mechanism in rodents. Proc. Natl. Acad. Sci. USA 93 (9), 4159–4164.

LaRocca, T.J., Gioscia-Ryan, R.A., Hearon Jr., C.M., Seals, D.R., 2013. The autophagy enhancer spermidine reverses arterial aging. Mech. Ageing Dev. 134 (7-8), 314–320.

Larson-Meyer, D.E., Heilbronn, L.K., Redman, L.M., Newcomer, B.R., Frisard, M.I., Anton, S., et al., 2006. Effect of calorie restriction with or without exercise on insulin sensitivity, beta-cell function, fat cell size, and ectopic lipid in overweight subjects. Diabetes Care 29 (6), 1337–1344.

Law, I.K., Liu, L., Xu, A., Lam, K.S., Vanhoutte, P.M., Che, C.M., et al., 2009. Identification and characterization of proteins interacting with SIRT1 and SIRT3: implications in the anti-aging and metabolic effects of sirtuins. Proteomics 9 (9), 2444–2456.

Lee, I.H., Cao, L., Mostoslavsky, R., Lombard, D.B., Liu, J., Bruns, N.E., et al., 2008. A role for the NAD-dependent deacetylase Sirt1 in the regulation of autophagy. Proc. Natl. Acad. Sci. USA 105 (9), 3374–3379.

Lee, I.H., Finkel, T., 2009. Regulation of autophagy by the p300 acetyltransferase. J. Biol. Chem. 284 (10), 6322–6328.

Lee, J., Bruce-Keller, A.J., Kruman, Y., Chan, S.L., Mattson, M.P., 1999. 2-Deoxy-D-glucose protects hippocampal neurons against excitotoxic and oxidative injury: evidence for the involvement of stress proteins. J. Neurosci. Res. 57 (1), 48–61.

Lee, S.H., Min, K.J., 2013. Caloric restriction and its mimetics. BMB Rep. 46 (4), 181–187.

Lefevre, M., Redman, L.M., Heilbronn, L.K., Smith, J.V., Martin, C.K., Rood, J.C., et al., 2009. Caloric restriction alone and with exercise improves CVD risk in healthy non-obese individuals. Atherosclerosis 203 (1), 206–213.

Levine, B., Kroemer, G., 2008. Autophagy in the pathogenesis of disease. Cell 132 (1), 27–42.

Li, Y., Bujo, H., Takahashi, K., Shibasaki, M., Zhu, Y., Yoshida, Y., et al., 2003. Visceral fat: higher responsiveness of fat mass and gene expression to calorie restriction than subcutaneous fat. Exp. Biol. Med. (Maywood) 228 (10), 1118–1123.

Li, Y., Wong, K., Giles, A., Jiang, J., Lee, J.W., Adams, A.C., et al., 2014. Hepatic SIRT1 attenuates hepatic steatosis and controls energy balance in mice by inducing fibroblast growth factor 21. Gastroenterology 146 (2), 539–549. e537.

Libert, S., Guarente, L., 2013. Metabolic and neuropsychiatric effects of calorie restriction and sirtuins. Annu. Rev. Physiol. 75, 669–684.

Lin, C.H., Lin, C.C., Ting, W.J., Pai, P.Y., Kuo, C.H., Ho, T.J., et al., 2014. Resveratrol enhanced FOXO3 phosphorylation via synergetic activation of SIRT1 and PI3K/Akt signaling to improve the effects of exercise in elderly rat hearts. Age (Dordr) 36 (5), 9705.

Lin, S.J., Ford, E., Haigis, M., Liszt, G., Guarente, L., 2004. Calorie restriction extends yeast life span by lowering the level of NADH. Genes Dev. 18 (1), 12–16.

Longo, V.D., Kennedy, B.K., 2006. Sirtuins in aging and age-related disease. Cell 126 (2), 257–268.

MacKay, D., Hathcock, J., Guarneri, E., 2012. Niacin: chemical forms, bioavailability, and health effects. Nutr. Rev. 70 (6), 357–366.

Madeo, F., Eisenberg, T., Buttner, S., Ruckenstuhl, C., Kroemer, G., 2010. Spermidine: a novel autophagy inducer and longevity elixir. Autophagy 6 (1), 160–162.

Madeo, F., Pietrocola, F., Eisenberg, T., Kroemer, G., 2014. Caloric restriction mimetics: towards a molecular definition. Nat. Rev. Drug Discov. 13 (10), 727–740.

Mai, V., Colbert, L.H., Berrigan, D., Perkins, S.N., Pfeiffer, R., Lavigne, J.A., et al., 2003. Calorie restriction and diet composition modulate spontaneous intestinal tumorigenesis in Apc(Min) mice through different mechanisms. Cancer Res. 63 (8), 1752–1755.

Marino, G., Pietrocola, F., Eisenberg, T., Kong, Y., Malik, S.A., Andryushkova, A., et al., 2014. Regulation of autophagy by cytosolic acetyl-coenzyme A. Mol. Cell 53 (5), 710–725.

Marshall, S., Yamasaki, K., Okuyama, R., 2005. Glucosamine induces rapid desensitization of glucose transport in isolated adipocytes by increasing GlcN-6-P levels. Biochem. Biophys. Res. Commun. 329 (3), 1155–1161.

Masri, S., 2015. Sirtuin-dependent clock control: new advances in metabolism, aging and cancer. Curr. Opin. Clin. Nutr. Metab. Care 18 (6), 521–527.

Mattison, J.A., Roth, G.S., Beasley, T.M., Tilmont, E.M., Handy, A.M., Herbert, R.L., et al., 2012. Impact of caloric restriction on health and survival in rhesus monkeys from the NIA study. Nature 489 (7415), 318–321.

Mattson, M.P., 2000. Neuroprotective signaling and the aging brain: take away my food and let me run. Brain Res. 886 (1-2), 47–53.

McCay, C.M., Crowell, M.F., Maynard, L.A., 1935. The effect of retarded growth upon the length of the life span and upon the ultimate body size. J. Nutr. 10, 63–70.

McKnight, L.L., Flickinger, E.A., France, J., Davenport, G.M., Shoveller, A.K., 2014. Mannoheptulose has differential effects on fasting and postprandial energy expenditure and respiratory quotient in adult Beagle dogs fed diets of different macronutrient contents. J. Nutr. Sci. 3, e17.

Meana, C., Rubin, J.M., Bordallo, C., Suarez, L., Bordallo, J., Sanchez, M., 2016. Correlation between endogenous polyamines in human cardiac tissues and clinical parameters in patients with heart failure. J. Cell Mol. Med. 20 (2), 302–312.

Menon, V., Zhi, X., Hossain, T., Bartke, A., Spong, A., Gesing, A., et al., 2014. The contribution of visceral fat to improved insulin signaling in Ames dwarf mice. Aging Cell 13 (3), 497–506.

Miller, R.A., Harrison, D.E., Astle, C.M., Baur, J.A., Boyd, A.R., de Cabo, R., et al., 2011. Rapamycin, but not resveratrol or simvastatin, extends life span of genetically heterogeneous mice. J. Gerontol. A Biol. Sci. Med. Sci. 66 (2), 191–201.

Minois, N., 2014. Molecular basis of the 'anti-aging' effect of spermidine and other natural polyamines - a mini-review. Gerontology 60 (4), 319–326.

Minois, N., Carmona-Gutierrez, D., Bauer, M.A., Rockenfeller, P., Eisenberg, T., Brandhorst, S., et al., 2012. Spermidine promotes stress resistance in Drosophila melanogaster through autophagy-dependent and -independent pathways. Cell. Death Dis. 3, e401.

Minois, N., Carmona-Gutierrez, D., Madeo, F., 2011. Polyamines in aging and disease. Aging (Albany NY) 3 (8), 716–732.

Mitchell, S.E., Tang, Z., Kerbois, C., Delville, C., Konstantopedos, P., Bruel, A., et al., 2015. The effects of graded levels of calorie restriction: I. impact of short term calorie and protein restriction on body composition in the C57BL/6 mouse. Oncotarget 6 (18), 15902–15930.

Mitchell, S.J., Martin-Montalvo, A., Mercken, E.M., Palacios, H.H., Ward, T.M., Abulwerdi, G., et al., 2014. The SIRT1 activator SRT1720 extends lifespan and improves health of mice fed a standard diet. Cell Rep. 6 (5), 836–843.

Morselli, E., Marino, G., Bennetzen, M.V., Eisenberg, T., Megalou, E., Schroeder, S., et al., 2011. Spermidine and resveratrol induce autophagy by distinct pathways converging on the acetylproteome. J. Cell Biol. 192 (4), 615–629.

Moschen, A.R., Wieser, V., Gerner, R.R., Bichler, A., Enrich, B., Moser, P., et al., 2013. Adipose tissue and liver expression of SIRT1, 3, and 6 increase after extensive weight loss in morbid obesity. J. Hepatol. 59 (6), 1315–1322.

Mouchiroud, L., Houtkooper, R.H., Moullan, N., Katsyuba, E., Ryu, D., Canto, C., et al., 2013. The NAD(+)/Sirtuin pathway modulates longevity through activation of mitochondrial UPR and FOXO signaling. Cell 154 (2), 430–441.

Muzumdar, R., Allison, D.B., Huffman, D.M., Ma, X., Atzmon, G., Einstein, F.H., et al., 2008. Visceral adipose tissue modulates mammalian longevity. Aging Cell 7 (3), 438–440.

Nishimura, K., Shiina, R., Kashiwagi, K., Igarashi, K., 2006. Decrease in polyamines with aging and their ingestion from food and drink. J. Biochem. 139 (1), 81–90.

Noh, J.S., Kim, H.Y., Park, C.H., Fujii, H., Yokozawa, T., 2010. Hypolipidaemic and antioxidative effects of oligonol, a low-molecular-weight polyphenol derived from lychee fruit, on renal damage in type 2 diabetic mice. Br. J. Nutr. 104 (8), 1120–1128.

Ou, X., Lee, M.R., Huang, X., Messina-Graham, S., Broxmeyer, H.E., 2014. SIRT1 positively regulates autophagy and mitochondria function in embryonic stem cells under oxidative stress. Stem Cells 32 (5), 1183–1194.

Park, S.K., Seong, R.K., Kim, J.A., Son, S.J., Kim, Y., Yokozawa, T., et al., 2016. Oligonol promotes anti-aging pathways via modulation of SIRT1-AMPK-Autophagy Pathway. Nutr. Res. Pract. 10 (1), 3–10.

Pearson, K.J., Baur, J.A., Lewis, K.N., Peshkin, L., Price, N.L., Labinskyy, N., et al., 2008. Resveratrol delays age-related deterioration and mimics transcriptional aspects of dietary restriction without extending life span. Cell Metab. 8 (2), 157–168.

Peeters, A.V., Beckers, S., Verrijken, A., Mertens, I., Roevens, P., Peeters, P.J., et al., 2008. Association of SIRT1 gene variation with visceral obesity. Hum. Genet. 124 (4), 431–436.

Pedersen, P.L., 2007. Warburg, me and Hexokinase 2: Multiple discoveries of key molecular events underlying one of cancers' most common phenotypes, the "Warburg Effect," i.e., elevated glycolysis in the presence of oxygen. J. Bioenergy Biomembr. 39 (3), 211–222.

Pedersen, S.B., Olholm, J., Paulsen, S.K., Bennetzen, M.F., Richelsen, B., 2008. Low Sirt1 expression, which is upregulated by fasting, in human adipose tissue from obese women. Int J Obes (Lond) 32 (8), 1250–1255.

Pfluger, P.T., Herranz, D., Velasco-Miguel, S., Serrano, M., Tschop, M.H., 2008. Sirt1 protects against high-fat diet-induced metabolic damage. Proc. Natl. Acad. Sci. USA 105 (28), 9793–9798.

Picard, F., Guarente, L., 2005. Molecular links between aging and adipose tissue. Int. J. Obes. (Lond) 29 (Suppl 1), S36–S39.

Picard, F., Kurtev, M., Chung, N., Topark-Ngarm, A., Senawong, T., Machado De Oliveira, R., et al., 2004. Sirt1 promotes fat mobilization in white adipocytes by repressing PPAR-gamma. Nature 429 (6993), 771–776.

Pietrocola, F., Lachkar, S., Enot, D.P., Niso-Santano, M., Bravo-San Pedro, J.M., Sica, V., et al., 2015. Spermidine induces autophagy by inhibiting the acetyltransferase EP300. Cell Death Differ. 22 (3), 509–516.

Piskunova, T.S., Yurova, M.N., Ovsyannikov, A.I., Semenchenko, A.V., Zabezhinski, M.A., Popovich, I.G., et al., 2008. Deficiency in poly(ADP-ribose) polymerase-1 (PARP-1) accelerates aging and spontaneous carcinogenesis in mice. Curr. Gerontol. Geriatr. Res., 754190.

Prado, C.M., Wells, J.C., Smith, S.R., Stephan, B.C., Siervo, M., 2012. Sarcopenic obesity: A Critical appraisal of the current evidence. Clin. Nutr. 31 (5), 583–601.

Purushotham, A., Schug, T.T., Xu, Q., Surapureddi, S., Guo, X., Li, X., 2009. Hepatocyte-specific deletion of SIRT1 alters fatty acid metabolism and results in hepatic steatosis and inflammation. Cell Metab. 9 (4), 327–338.

Pyo, J.O., Yoo, S.M., Ahn, H.H., Nah, J , Hong, S.H., Kam, T.I., et al., 2013. Overexpression of Atg5 in mice activates autophagy and extends lifespan. Nat. Commun. 4, 2300.

Qiang, L., Wang, H., Farmer, S.R., 2007. Adiponectin secretion is regulated by SIRT1 and the endoplasmic reticulum oxidoreductase Ero1-L alpha. Mol. Cell Biol. 27 (13), 4698–4707.

Qiang, L., Wang, L., Kon, N., Zhao, W., Lee, S., Zhang, Y., et al., 2012. Brown remodeling of white adipose tissue by SirT1-dependent deacetylation of Ppargamma. Cell 150 (3), 620–632.

Qiao, L., Shao, J., 2006. SIRT1 regulates adiponectin gene expression through Foxo1-C/enhancer-binding protein alpha transcriptional complex. J. Biol. Chem. 281 (52), 39915–39924.

Ramis, M.R., Esteban, S., Miralles, A., Tan, D.X., Reiter, R.J., 2015. Caloric restriction, resveratrol and melatonin: Role of SIRT1 and implications for aging and related-diseases. Mech. Ageing Dev. 146-148, 28–41.

Ravikumar, B., Sarkar, S., Davies, J.E., Futter, M., Garcia-Arencibia, M., Green-Thompson, Z.W., et al., 2010. Regulation of mammalian autophagy in physiology and pathophysiology. Physiol. Rev. 90 (4), 1383–1435.

Ravussin, E., Redman, L.M., Rochon, J., Das, S.K., Fontana, L., Kraus, W.E., et al., 2015. A 2-year randomized controlled trial of human caloric restriction: feasibility and effects on predictors of health span and longevity. J. Gerontol. A Biol. Sci. Med. Sci. 70 (9), 1097–1104.

Reiter, R.J., Tan, D.X., Rosales-Corral, S., Manchester, L.C., 2013. The universal nature, unequal distribution and antioxidant functions of melatonin and its derivatives. Mini Rev. Med. Chem. 13 (3), 373–384.

Rodgers, J.T., Lerin, C., Haas, W., Gygi, S.P., Spiegelman, B.M., Puigserver, P., 2005. Nutrient control of glucose homeostasis through a complex of PGC-1alpha and SIRT1. Nature 434 (7029), 113–118.

Romashkan, S.V., Das, S.K., Villareal, D.T., Ravussin, E., Redman, L.M., Rochon, J., et al., 2016. Safety of two-year caloric restriction in non-obese healthy individuals. Oncotarget.

Rongvaux, A., Andris, F., Van Gool, F., Leo, O., 2003. Reconstructing eukaryotic NAD metabolism. Bioessays 25 (7), 683–690.

Roth, G.S., Ingram, D.K., Lane, M.A., 1999. Calorie restriction in primates: will it work and how will we know? J. Am. Geriatr. Soc. 47 (7), 896–903.

Sakurai, T., Kitadate, K., Nishioka, H., Fujii, H., Ogasawara, J., Kizaki, T., et al., 2013. Oligomerised lychee fruit-derived polyphenol attenuates cognitive impairment in senescence-accelerated mice and endoplasmic reticulum stress in neuronal cells. Br. J. Nutr. 110 (9), 1549–1558.

Sale, S., Verschoyle, R.D., Boocock, D., Jones, D.J., Wilsher, N., Ruparelia, K.C., et al., 2004. Pharmacokinetics in mice and growth-inhibitory properties of the putative cancer chemopreventive agent resveratrol and the synthetic analogue trans 3,4,5,4'-tetramethoxystilbene. Br. J. Cancer 90 (3), 736–744.

Salek, R.M., Maguire, M.L., Bentley, E., Rubtsov, D.V., Hough, T., Cheeseman, M., et al., 2007. A metabolomic comparison of urinary changes in type 2 diabetes in mouse, rat, and human. Physiol. Genomics 29 (2), 99–108.

Santana, A., Santamarina, A., Souza, G., Mennitti, L., Okuda, M., Venancio, D., et al., 2015. Decaffeinated green tea extract rich in epigallocatechin-3-gallate improves insulin resistance and metabolic profiles in normolipidic diet--but not high-fat diet-fed mice. J. Nutr. Biochem. 26 (9), 893–902.

Sauve, A.A., Youn, D.Y., 2012. Sirtuins: NAD(+)-dependent deacetylase mechanism and regulation. Curr. Opin. Chem. Biol. 16 (5-6), 535–543.

Schmeisser, K., Mansfeld, J., Kuhlow, D., Weimer, S., Priebe, S., Heiland, I., et al., 2013. Role of sirtuins in lifespan regulation is linked to methylation of nicotinamide. Nat. Chem. Biol. 9 (11), 693–700.

Schroeder, S., Pendl, T., Zimmermann, A., Eisenberg, T., Carmona-Gutierrez, D., Ruckenstuhl, C., et al., 2014. Acetyl-coenzyme A: a metabolic master regulator of autophagy and longevity. Autophagy 10 (7), 1335–1337.

Senf, S.M., Sandesara, P.B., Reed, S.A., Judge, A.R., 2011. p300 Acetyltransferase activity differentially regulates the localization and activity of the FOXO homologues in skeletal muscle. Am. J. Physiol. Cell Physiol. 300 (6), C1490–C1501.

Shi, L., Tu, B.P., 2015. Acetyl-CoA and the regulation of metabolism: mechanisms and consequences. Curr. Opin. Cell Biol. 33, 125–131.

Shimoyama, Y., Suzuki, K., Hamajima, N., Niwa, T., 2011. Sirtuin 1 gene polymorphisms are associated with body fat and blood pressure in Japanese. Transl. Res. 157 (6), 339–347.

Shokolenko, I.N., Wilson, G.L., Alexeyev, M.F., 2014. Aging: A mitochondrial DNA perspective, critical analysis and an update. World J. Exp. Med. 4 (4), 46–57.

Slominski, A., Pisarchik, A., Semak, I., Sweatman, T., Wortsman, J., Szczesniewski, A., et al., 2002. Serotoninergic and melatoninergic systems are fully expressed in human skin. FASEB J. 16 (8), 896–898.

Smith, J.J., Kenney, R.D., Gagne, D.J., Frushour, B.P., Ladd, W., Galonek, H.L., et al., 2009. Small molecule activators of SIRT1 replicate signaling pathways triggered by calorie restriction in vivo. BMC Syst. Biol. 3, 31.

Smoliga, J.M., Baur, J.A., Hausenblas, H.A., 2011. Resveratrol and health--a comprehensive review of human clinical trials. Mol. Nutr. Food Res. 55 (8), 1129–1141.

Soda, K., Dobashi, Y., Kano, Y., Tsujinaka, S., Konishi, F., 2009. Polyamine-rich food decreases age-associated pathology and mortality in aged mice. Exp. Gerontol. 44 (11), 727–732.

Sohal, R.S., Weindruch, R., 1996. Oxidative stress, caloric restriction, and aging. Science 273 (5271), 59–63.

Someya, S., Yu, W., Hallows, W.C., Xu, J., Vann, J.M., Leeuwenburgh, C., et al., 2010. Sirt3 mediates reduction of oxidative damage and prevention of age-related hearing loss under caloric restriction. Cell 143 (5), 802–812.

Song, Y.S., Lee, S.K., Jang, Y.J., Park, H.S., Kim, J.H., Lee, Y.J., et al., 2013. Association between low SIRT1 expression in visceral and subcutaneous adipose tissues and metabolic abnormalities in women with obesity and type 2 diabetes. Diabetes Res. Clin. Pract. 101 (3), 341–348.

Song, J., Ke, S.F., Zhou, C.C., Zhang, S.L., Guan, Y.F., Xu, T.Y., et al., 2014. Nicotinamide phosphoribosyltransferase is required for the calorie restriction-mediated improvements in oxidative stress, mitochondrial biogenesis, and metabolic adaptation. J. Gerontol. A Biol. Sci. Med. Sci. 69 (1), 44–57.

Stewart, T.M., Bhapkar, M., Das, S., Galan, K., Martin, C.K., McAdams, L., et al., 2013. Comprehensive Assessment of Long-term Effects of Reducing Intake of Energy Phase 2 (CALERIE Phase 2) screening and recruitment: methods and results. Contemp. Clin. Trials 34 (1), 10–20.

Sun, C., Zhang, F., Ge, X., Yan, T., Chen, X., Shi, X., et al., 2007. SIRT1 improves insulin sensitivity under insulin-resistant conditions by repressing PTP1B. Cell Metab. 6 (4), 307–319.

Swerdlow, R.H., Bothwell, R., Hutfles, L., Burns, J.M., Reed, G.A., 2016. Tolerability and pharmacokinetics of oxaloacetate 100mg capsules in Alzheimer's subjects. BBA Clin. 5, 120–123.

Tatar, M., Bartke, A., Antebi, A., 2003. The endocrine regulation of aging by insulin-like signals. Science 299 (5611), 1346–1351.

Tchkonia, T., Thomou, T., Zhu, Y., Karagiannides, I., Pothoulakis, C., Jensen, M.D., et al., 2013. Mechanisms and metabolic implications of regional differences among fat depots. Cell Metab. 17 (5), 644–656.

Tenenbaum, D. 2014. "Monkey caloric restriction study shows big benefit; contradicts earlier study " Retrieved 20 April 2016, 2016, from <http://news.wisc.edu/monkey-caloric-restriction-study-shows-big-benefit-contradicts-earlier-study/>.

Tsang, A.W., Escalante-Semerena, J.C., 1998. CobB, a new member of the SIR2 family of eucaryotic regulatory proteins, is required to compensate for the lack of nicotinate mononucleotide:5,6-dimethylbenzimidazole phosphoribosyltransferase activity in cobT mutants during cobalamin biosynthesis in Salmonella typhimurium LT2. J. Biol. Chem. 273 (48), 31788–31794.

Turner, R.S., Thomas, R.G., Craft, S., van Dyck, C.H., Mintzer, J., Reynolds, B.A., et al., 2015. A randomized, double-blind, placebo-controlled trial of resveratrol for Alzheimer disease. Neurology 85 (16), 1383–1391.

Venigalla, M., Sonego, S., Gyengesi, E., Sharman, M.J., Munch, G., 2016. Novel promising therapeutics against chronic neuroinflammation and neurodegeneration in Alzheimer's disease. Neurochem. Int. 95, 63–74.

Walford, R.L., Harris, S.B., Gunion, M.W., 1992. The calorically restricted low-fat nutrient-dense diet in Biosphere 2 significantly lowers blood glucose, total leukocyte count, cholesterol, and blood pressure in humans. Proc. Natl. Acad. Sci. USA 89 (23), 11533–11537.

Waller, K.L., Mortensen, E.L., Avlund, K., Fagerlund, B., Lauritzen, M., Gammeltoft, S., et al., 2016. Melatonin and cortisol profiles in late midlife and their association with age-related changes in cognition. Nat. Sci. Sleep 8, 47–53.

Wang, Y., 2014. Molecular Links between Caloric Restriction and Sir2/SIRT1 Activation. Diabetes Metab. J. 38 (5), 321–329.

Wang, J., Vanegas, S.M., Du, X., Noble, T., Zingg, J.M., Meydani, M., et al., 2013. Caloric restriction favorably impacts metabolic and immune/inflammatory profiles in obese mice but curcumin/piperine consumption adds no further benefit. Nutr. Metab. (Lond) 10 (1), 29.

Wang, P., Xu, T.Y., Guan, Y.F., Tian, W.W., Viollet, B., Rui, Y.C., et al., 2011. Nicotinamide phosphoribosyltransferase protects against ischemic stroke through SIRT1-dependent adenosine monophosphate-activated kinase pathway. Ann. Neurol. 69 (2), 360–374.

Wang, T.A., Zhang, X.D., Guo, X.Y., Xian, S.L., Lu, Y.F., 2016. 3-Bromopyruvate and sodium citrate target glycolysis, suppress survivin, and induce mitochondrial-mediated apoptosis in gastric cancer cells and inhibit gastric orthotopic transplantation tumor growth. Oncol. Rep. 35 (3), 1287–1296.

Wang, Y., Xu, C., Liang, Y., Vanhoutte, P.M., 2012. SIRT1 in metabolic syndrome: where to target matters. Pharmacol. Ther. 136 (3), 305–318.

Weindruch, R., 1996. The retardation of aging by caloric restriction: studies in rodents and primates. Toxicol. Pathol. 24 (6), 742–745.

Weindruch, R., Sohal, R.S., 1997. Seminars in medicine of the Beth Israel Deaconess Medical Center. Caloric intake and aging. N Engl J Med 337 (14), 986–994.

Wellen, K.E., Hatzivassiliou, G., Sachdeva, U.M., Bui, T.V., Cross, J.R., Thompson, C.B., 2009. ATP-citrate lyase links cellular metabolism to histone acetylation. Science 324 (5930), 1076–1080.

Wenzel, E., Somoza, V., 2005. Metabolism and bioavailability of trans-resveratrol. Mol. Nutr. Food Res. 49 (5), 472–481.

White, A.T., McCurdy, C.E., Philp, A., Hamilton, D.L., Johnson, C.D., Schenk, S., 2013. Skeletal muscle-specific overexpression of SIRT1 does not enhance whole-body energy expenditure or insulin sensitivity in young mice. Diabetologia 56 (7), 1629–1637.

Wilkins, H.M., Harris, J.L., Carl, S.M., E, L., Lu, J., Eva Selfridge, J., et al., 2014. Oxaloacetate activates brain mitochondrial biogenesis, enhances the insulin pathway, reduces inflammation and stimulates neurogenesis. Hum. Mol. Genet. 23 (24), 6528–6541.

Wilkins, H.M., Koppel, S., Carl, S.M., Ramanujan, S., Weidling, I., Michaelis, M.L., et al., 2016. Oxaloacetate enhances neuronal cell bioenergetic fluxes and infrastructure. J. Neurochem. 137 (1), 76–87.

Williams, D.S., Cash, A., Hamadani, L., Diemer, T., 2009. Oxaloacetate supplementation increases lifespan in Caenorhabditis elegans through an AMPK/FOXO-dependent pathway. Aging Cell 8 (6), 765–768.

Witte, A.V., Fobker, M., Gellner, R., Knecht, S., Floel, A., 2009. Caloric restriction improves memory in elderly humans. Proc. Natl. Acad. Sci. USA 106 (4), 1255–1260.

Witte, A.V., Kerti, L., Margulies, D.S., Floel, A., 2014. Effects of resveratrol on memory performance, hippocampal functional connectivity, and glucose metabolism in healthy older adults. J. Neurosci. 34 (23), 7862–7870.

Xu, C., Bai, B., Fan, P., Cai, Y., Huang, B., Law, I.K., et al., 2013. Selective overexpression of human SIRT1 in adipose tissue enhances energy homeostasis and prevents the deterioration of insulin sensitivity with ageing in mice. Am. J. Transl. Res. 5 (4), 412–426.

Xu, C., Cai, Y., Fan, P., Bai, B., Chen, J., Deng, H.B., et al., 2015. Calorie restriction prevents metabolic aging caused by abnormal SIRT1 function in adipose tissues. Diabetes 64 (5), 1576–1590.

Yamada, M., Moriguch, Y., Mitani, T., Aoyama, T., Arai, H., 2014. Age-dependent changes in skeletal muscle mass and visceral fat area in Japanese adults from 40 to 79 years-of-age. Geriatr Gerontol Int. 14 (Suppl 1), 8–14.

Yang, H., Yang, T., Baur, J.A., Perez, E., Matsui, T., Carmona, J.J., et al., 2007. Nutrient-sensitive mitochondrial NAD+ levels dictate cell survival. Cell 130 (6), 1095–1107.

Ye, J., Keller, J.N., 2010. Regulation of energy metabolism by inflammation: a feedback response in obesity and calorie restriction. Aging (Albany NY) 2 (6), 361–368.

Yoshino, J., Mills, K.F., Yoon, M.J., Imai, S., 2011. Nicotinamide mononucleotide, a key NAD(+) intermediate, treats the pathophysiology of diet- and age-induced diabetes in mice. Cell Metab. 14 (4), 528–536.

Yoshizaki, T., Milne, J.C., Imamura, T., Schenk, S., Sonoda, N., Babendure, J.L., et al., 2009. SIRT1 exerts anti-inflammatory effects and improves insulin sensitivity in adipocytes. Mol. Cell Biol. 29 (5), 1363–1374.

Yuan, Y., Cruzat, V.F., Newsholme, P., Cheng, J., Chen, Y., Lu, Y., 2016. Regulation of SIRT1 in aging: Roles in mitochondrial function and biogenesis. Mech. Ageing Dev. 155, 10–21.

Zhang, J., Feng, X., Wu, J., Xu, H., Li, G., Zhu, D., et al., 2014. Neuroprotective effects of resveratrol on damages of mouse cortical neurons induced by beta-amyloid through activation of SIRT1/Akt1 pathway. Biofactors 40 (2), 258–267.

Zhu, H., Guo, Q., Mattson, M.P., 1999. Dietary restriction protects hippocampal neurons against the death-promoting action of a presenilin-1 mutation. Brain. Res. 842 (1), 224–229.

CHAPTER

23

Nutraceuticals for Healthy Skin Aging

Elaine Cristina Faria Abrahão Machado[1], *Letícia Ambrosano*[1], *Renan Lage*[1], *Beatrice Martinez Zugaib Abdalla*[2] *and Adilson Costa*[1]

[1]Catholic University of Campinas, Campinas, SP, Brazil [2]ABC School of Medicine, Santo Andre, SP, Brazil

INTRODUCTION

Skin aging is a multifactorial process related to the continuous reduction of size and the number and physiological functions of cells at the molecular level (Ramos-e-Silva and Carneiro, 2001). This process involves intrinsic (genetic and hormonal) and environmental factors (e.g., exposure to sunlight and pollution) as well as lifestyle factors (Rexbye et al., 2006).

A *nutraceutical* is a food or part thereof that provides health benefits, including prevention and treatment of diseases. Nutraceuticals can be isolated nutrients, dietary supplements, herbal products, or processed foods such as cereals, soups, and beverages, or even capsules, tablets, and powders (Kwak and Jukes, 2001). A related category, *nutricosmetics*, has products that meet the concepts of nutrition, health, and beauty. The active form of a nutraceutical is administered orally (Tabor and Blair, 2009).

Skin cells are constantly exposed to harmful processes that are mediated by reactive oxygen species (ROS) and oxidative stress, inflammation, and photodamage (Indo et al., 2015).

OXIDATIVE STRESS

Oxidative stress is damage caused by reduction–oxidation products and an increase in the number of free radicals—molecules with unpaired electrons—that associated with a reduction in the number of antioxidants (Powers and Jackson, 2008). The most important types of free radicals are the ROS, such as peroxide, superoxide anions, radical oxygen, and singlets (Wu and Cederbaum, 2003).

Lipid oxidation by ROS may damage cell structures and result in premature cell death because mitochondria are the main source of ROS in the cells; this process can be prevented by antioxidant action (Anderson et al., 2014). Over time, levels of antioxidants naturally decrease, which may lead to accumulated oxidative damage, which manifests as aging that affects different tissues (Kruk and Duchnik, 2014).

The exact role of ROS and mitochondrial dysfunction in the aging process remains unknown, but oxidative stress is evident in various diseases, including dermatological, neurological, and cardiovascular conditions (Adly, 2010).

Due to the exacerbation of such external stressors as ultraviolet radiation (UVR), pollution, and lifestyles, people began to supplement their diets with exogenous antioxidants. However, their misuse can alter the balance between the process of oxidation and natural oxidation, and thus should be prescribed cautiously based on knowledge of their actions (Cornelli, 2009).

Antioxidants are classified according to their functions (Cornelli, 2009):

- *Membrane* or *lipophilic antioxidants* are active primarily in collagen fibers, elastin, and cellular structures. Examples include vitamins A and E, and beta-carotene.

Nutrition and Functional Foods for Healthy Aging.
DOI: http://dx.doi.org/10.1016/B978-0-12-805376-8.00023-X

- *Circulating* or *hydrophilic antioxidants* are present at the microcirculatory level and in the extracellular matrix. Examples include vitamin C, polyphenols, flavonoids, and amino acids.
- *Intracytoplasmic* or *cytosolic antioxidants* are mainly active in the cytoplasm of epidermal cells. Examples include coenzyme Q10, lipoic acid, and squalene.
- *System antioxidants* act in the epidermis and in the elastic and collagen fibers of the dermis, at the microcirculatory level, and in the cells of the epidermis and dermis. Examples include zinc, selenium, and some amino acids (Costa, 2012).

In this chapter, the main nutraceuticals used in dermatology will be addressed. These have the potential to prevent and treat diseases related to intrinsic and extrinsic aging and inflammation and aid in the treatment of some cancers.

BETA-CAROTENE

Beta-carotene, the most abundant and efficient precursor of vitamin A, is a liposoluble antioxidant whose main activity occurs in collagen and elastin fibers (Wertz et al., 2005). It is a carotenoid derived from natural food sources such as carrots, tomatoes, spinach, sweet potato, other yellow and green vegetables, fruits, and seaweeds (Bayerl, 2008). It is a sunscreen agent and inhibits the peroxidation of lipids induced by free radicals. However, in those who smoke tobacco, it can increase the risk of lung cancer (Evans and Johnson, 2010).

Beta-carotene is used for the prevention of sunburns and photodamage, erythropoietic protoporphyria, psoriasis, vitiligo, and hairy leukoplakia in doses of 6–15 mg per day in adults. Separate dosages are used in erythropoietic protoporphyria—150–180 mg per day—and prevention of sunburns: 25 mg per day (Costa, 2012).

BIOTIN

Biotin is a hydrophilic vitamin that is also known as vitamin B_7 or vitamin H. Found in yeast, brown rice, fruits, nuts, eggs, meat, and milk, it is a coenzyme in carboxylation reactions, where it acts as a carrier of activated carbon dioxide. It is a cofactor in the metabolism of fatty acids, amino acids, and gluconeogenesis (Fiume, 2001).

Biotin is indicated in cases of androgenetic alopecia, alopecia areata, poliosis, onychorexis, onycholysis, palmoplantar pustulosis, atopic dermatitis, seborrheic dermatitis, palmoplantar keratodermia, and chronic cutaneous lupus erythematosus (Costa, 2012). The suitable dose for adults is 30 mcg, but for most of the diseases and nails doses of 2500–3000 mg per day are used (Fiume, 2001).

COENZYME Q10 OR UBIQUINONE

Coenzyme Q10 is present in all living cells of the body where it acts as an important antioxidant and is also active in the mitochondrial respiratory chain. However, the endogenous production of coenzyme Q10 decreases after age 20 and is reduced in myocardial cells (Sanoobar et al., 2014).

Coenzyme Q10 acts on oxidative stress and is indicated for prevention and treatment of fine lines and wrinkles, but it also aids in the treatment of heart failure and fibromyalgia (De Luca et al., 2016).

There is an important interrelationship between selenium and coenzyme Q10 because selenium is required to process the active form of coenzyme Q10 (Xia et al., 2003).

The oral absorption is limited due to its high molecular weight and because it is fat-soluble, the recommendation is to ingest it with food at a dose of 30–200 mg per day (Costa, 2012).

CITRULLINE–ARGININE

Citrulline–arginine is a component of marine biomass originating from a red algae, *Chondrus crispus*, which is found along the shores of the northern Atlantic Ocean. It is a stable dipeptide that improves the bioavailability of the arginine by increasing skin energy levels, encouraging cell growth and metabolism, and protecting the skin. In addition, it releases arginine and citrulline, amino acids that are important sources of nitrogen and essential for protein and collagen synthesis (Bidri and Choay, 2003).

Citrulline-arginine is indicated for the prevention and improvement of skin aging. It acts as a skin protector in extreme conditions such as cold and dry climates, pollution, and air conditioning. It also aids wound healing. The recommended dose is 100–1000 mg per day (Zhu et al., 2008).

ISOFLAVONE SOY BEANS

The best-known isoflavones are genistein, glycitein, and daidzein. They inhibit carcinogenesis and photocarcinogenesis through their antioxidant and antiproliferative effects and have also proven effective in reducing the formation of erythema induced by UVR (Wright et al., 2006). They unite and activate the alpha and beta estrogen receptors. They are widely used as preventive supplements for some types of cancer such as breast cancer and are also indicated for the prevention of osteoporosis (Pop et al., 2008). According to the North American Menopause Society, the doses range from 25 to 100 mg per day (Wright et al., 2006).

L-CARNOSINE

L-carnosine is a dipeptide composed of two amino acids—β-alanine and L-histidine—and is naturally found in muscle and heart tissues, the brain, and the liver. It has a powerful antioxidant function and protects and stabilizes cell membranes by preventing oxidative stress caused by free radicals. It also acts as a metal chelator and has a buffer effect on lactic acid in the muscle, including cases of intensive exercise (Prokopieva et al., 2016). The recommended dose is 500–2000 mg per day (Eades, 1994).

LYCOPENE

Lycopene is a liposoluble carotenoid and a powerful antioxidant found in some red foods such as tomatoes and their products, guava, watermelon, papaya, and cherry (Krinsky, 2001). It has a strong ability to attach to singlet oxygen, being suggested for the prevention of carcinogenesis and atherogenesis and to protect molecules such as lipids, low-density lipoproteins (LDLs), proteins, and DNA (Agarwal and Rao, 2000). Oxidation of lipids by reactive oxygen species can damage cell structures, and their high levels contribute to aging and carcinogenisis. Oxidative stress induced by ROS can be prevented by lycopene's antioxidant action (Kandola et al., 2015). It also has protective properties against erythema induced by UVR and photoaging mediated by oxidative stress (Rizwan et al., 2011). The average daily recommended intake of lycopene is about 35 mg (Agarwal and Rao, 2000).

LUTEIN

Lutein belongs to the group of carotenoids along with beta-carotene and lycopene. While the beta-carotene accumulates in the skin to provide a golden-yellow color, lutein accumulates preferentially in the macula lutea, protecting the retina from oxidative damage from UVR (Scarmo et al., 2010). It has antioxidant, anti-inflammatory, photoprotection, and anticarcinogenic properties and also acts to improve skin elasticity (Woodside et al., 2015).

The main natural sources of lutein are vegetables and green vegetables such as kale, spinach, chicory, celery, lettuce, fresh herbs, and egg yolk (Nachtigall et al., 2007). The oral and topical administration of lutein associated with zeaxanthin provided greater antioxidant functions and better hydration for severe skin compared to isolated treatments (Anunciato and Filho, 2012).

MELATONIN

Melatonin is a hormone released by the pineal gland and an important regulator of the circadian cycle with rhythmic production during both night and day but peak production at night (Hardeland, 2013). It also acts as an immunomodulator, modifies endocrine activity, and protects against UVR-induced damage (Fischer et al., 2008). An interrupted circadian clock can be an initial factor for the development of cutaneous diseases associated with oxidative stress. Melatonin and its metabolites act as local antioxidants, reducing mitochondrial damage and protecting skin from free radicals and thus act against skin aging (Kleszczynski and Fischer, 2012).

Melatonin is used for patients with insomnia, photoaging, protection against UVR-induced skin damage, and skin cancer and aids in the treatment of neurodegenerative diseases such as Alzheimer's (Ndiaye et al., 2014). The indicated initial dose is similar to physiological production of 0.3 mg per day and 1–3 mg per day is recommended for insomnia (Desotelle et al., 2012).

OMEGA-3

Omega-3 is a long-chain polyunsaturated fatty acid found mainly in fish such as salmon, tuna, cod, and dogfish (Raatz et al., 2013). It acts on cycloxygenase and lipoxygenase and in leukotrienes having a positive effect on blood flow (Alestas et al., 2006) and anti-inflammatory and antioxidant properties (Humbert et al., 2011). It also acts as a regulator of physiological functions of the skin such as inflammatory responses, platelet aggregation, vasodilation, and cell proliferation (Jung et al., 2014). It has been used in conventional treatments of various diseases such as cardiovascular disease, hypertriglyceridemia, atopic dermatitis, psoriasis, and acne vulgaris (Jeengar et al., 2015). The recommended daily dose is from 1.0 to 5.0 g (Koch et al., 2008).

POLYPHENOLS

Polyphenols are plant-derived micronutrients from diet that are important in preventing and improving the outcome of diseases. Since bioavailability differs greatly from one to another polyphenol, not necessarily the most abundant polyphenol in our diet has one the highest concentration of active metabolites in target tissues (Manach et al., 2005).

Polyphenols must go through two important phases to be absorbed and utilized systemically. The first phase is oxidation, reduction, and hydrolysis of polyphenol to increase its affinity for water. When added or exposed to a functional group with hydroxyl it transitions to phase two. During the second phase, new combinations occur to the polyphenols to make them more soluble in water and polarized, facilitating their transport and eventual elimination from the body (Scheepens et al., 2010).

There are several known groups of polyphenols. In this chapter, we will address those most closely related to the pathology of the skin and appendages.

Green Tea Polyphenols (*Camellia sinensis*)

The polyphenols of green tea are largely monomeric catechins, which include catechin, gallocatechin, epicatechin, epigallocatechin, gallate epicatechin, and epigallocatechin-3-gallate, the last being the most abundant and accounting for about 60% of catechins (Chow et al., 2001). They act as antioxidants, capturing ROS by transferring electrons to them so that are stable by becoming free radicals with one flavinic radical (Senger et al., 2011).

Epigallocatechin-3-Gallate

Epigallocatechin-3-gallate has potent antioxidant, antiinflammatory, and anticarcinogenic properties. It acts on matrix metalloproteinases, which are responsible for remodeling the extracellular matrix, and contributes to the structural integrity of tissue (Philips et al., 2007). It also prevents immunosuppression induction of interleukin-12 (IL-12). It also promotes the seizure and apoptosis of melanoma cells (Katiyar et al., 2007). It is also indicated for the prevention and treatment of photodamage and some types of cancer, including melanoma and squamous cell carcinoma. The recommended dosage is 200–800 mg per day fasting because it has low bioavailability (Costa, 2012).

Pycnogenol

Pycnogenol is a hydrosoluble flavinoid extracted from the bark of French *Pinus pinaster*. It is a potent antioxidant, recycles vitamin C, and regenerates vitamin E (Pinto et al., 2015). It inhibits gene expression of proinflammatory cytokines IL-1 and IL-2 and also inhibits matrix metalloproteinases and nitric oxide (Cho et al., 2001). It is indicated for the treatment of melasma and postinflammatory hyperpigmentation, traveler thrombosis, and chronic venous insufficiency, among others (Rohdewald, 2002). The recommended dose is 60–300 mg per day (Pinto et al., 2015).

Resveratrol

Resveratrol is a natural polyphenol found in more than 70 species of plants such as grapes (*Vitis vinifera*), cranberry (*Vaccinium macrocarpon*), and peanut (*Arachis hypogaea*). It acts by decreasing the vasoactive peptides, inhibits the oxidation of LDLs and the neurotoxicity of beta-amyloid. It increases the expression of glutathione peroxidase, which has a protective effect against oxidative stress (Perez and Gomez, 2015).

Resveratrol is suitable for preventing and improving skin aging and prevents photodamage. It also helps prevent some cancers such as breast, prostate, and colorectal cancer (Kennedy et al., 2010). There is no recommended daily dose but is safely used with dose of between 500 and 2000 mg per day. They should not be prescribed to women with a history of estrogen-dependent cancer. It can change the bioavailability of some drugs since it interacts with the cytochrome P450 (Perez and Gomez, 2015).

Polypodium leucotomos

Polypodium leucotomos is derived from a native tropical fern from Central and South America. It possesses beneficial properties attributed to the presence of numerous compounds with photoprotective and antioxidant properties (Nestor et al., 2014). It is able to eliminate free radicals and ROS, prevents the depletion of Langerhans cells, and inhibits mast cells in the skin (Nestor et al., 2014). Treatment use is indicated in photosensitivity, systemic lupus erythematosus, psoriasis, and vitiligo at a dose of 240 mg per day (Schalka et al., 2014).

PREBIOTICS

Prebiotics are nondigestible oligosaccharides, however fermentable, with the function of changing the activity and composition of the intestinal microbiota. They stimulate the growth of endogenous microbial populations (Blaut, 2002). They modulate key physiological functions such as absorption of calcium, lipid metabolism, modulation of intestinal microbiota, and reduced risk for colon carcinoma (Roberfroid, 2002). The indications are similar to those of probiotics as well as the doses.

PROBIOTICS

Probiotics are live microorganisms, mostly bacteria, that can be added to diets and confer a health benefit to the host when consumed in adequate amounts. They improve immunity and prevent some cancers such as colorectal and myeloid leukemia (Saad, 2006). The oral administration may regulate proinflammatory skin cytokines with specific decrease in IL-1α. They are indicated in the treatment of acne, seborrheic dermatitis, atopic dermatitis, and urticaria. The indicated doses are 5–10 million colony-forming units (CFUs) in children and 10–20 million CFUs in adults (Folster-Holst, 2010).

SELENIUM

Selenium is an essential micronutrient related to the action of glutathione peroxidase and thioredoxin reductase, enzymes involved in defending against oxidative stress (Schrauzer, 2000). It acts as an endogenous antioxidant in tissue oxygenation and protects against lipid peroxidation and neutrophils' phagocytic activity and is active in the regulation of thyroid hormones, DNA synthesis, and cell proliferation (Heyland et al., 2005). The indications are still controversial but suggested as a sunscreen because it protects against cytotoxicity induced by ultraviolet B radiation and wound healing (Bronsnick et al., 2014). The recommended daily dose for adults is 55 μg and is believed to contribute to the reduction of circulating antibodies in Hashimoto's thyroiditis when used at a dose of 200 mg (Costa, 2012).

SILICON

The largest source of silicon is foods with a high concentration of fiber such as vegetables and whole grains. It plays a vital role in human health by regulating the metabolism of various tissues, such as bone, cartilage, and connective tissue. One main function is the synthesis of collagen type I and its performance in the activity of prolyl hydroxylase enzyme (Reffit et al., 2003).

The skin plays an important structural role by connecting with glycosaminoglycans. In association with vitamin C, silicon stimulates the synthesis of hyaluronic acid and proteoglycan, increasing the affinity of water with glycosaminoglycans and reducing the destruction process of the dermal matrix produced by matrix metalloproteinases. It has also an active role in neutralizing free radicals (Calomme and Vanden-Berghe, 1997).

Silicon absorption in the gastrointestinal tract is inversely proportional to age, decreasing by the rate of 0.1 mg for every year of life. With aging, the amount of water in the dermis tends to decrease, and the presence of silicon in optimal quantities allows the connection of this water to dermal structures. It is used to prevent and improve skin aging and to improve the healing of wounds, burns, acne, eczema, psoriasis, and osteoporosis. The recommended dosage is 2–5 mg per day (Jugdaohsingh et al., 2004).

VITAMIN C

Vitamin C is a hydrophilic vitamin that is commonly consumed in large doses through its addition to many food products with the purpose of inhibiting the formation of carcinogenic nitrous metabolites (Bianchi and Antunes, 1999). It acts as an antioxidant, neutralizing ROS that are produced by cells of the dermis and epidermis, protecting the intracellular structures from oxidative stress (Manach et al., 2005).

It is also a cofactor for the production of collagen fibers and participates in the inhibition of the biosynthesis of elastin in fibroblasts, preventing its accumulation, highly present in photodamaged skin (Costa, 2012). When used with vitamin E, it acts synergistically working with its mechanism of transformation. (Eberlein-Koning et al., 1998).

It is indicated in the prevention and treatment of photodamage. For women, the recommended dose is 75 mg per day for men and 90 mg per day, and smokers should increase to 35 mg intake for those suffering increased oxidative stress. The maximum intake limit is 2000 mg per day, and it may cause side effects such as diarrhea (Amaya et al., 2001).

VITAMIN E

Vitamin E is the main lipophilic antioxidant and is found in the form of tocopherols. It is an important binder of paroxil radicals, preventing lipid peroxidation of polyunsaturated fatty acids. It is secreted by sebaceous glands, and the highest concentration of vitamin E is where fat production is greatest (Shils et al., 1999). It is indicated for preventing photodamage, sunburn, chronic cutaneous lupus erythematosus, granuloma annular, and atopic dermatitis (Costa, 2012). The recommended dose is 400–1000 mg per day for men and women. The maximum tolerated dose without adverse effects is 1000 mg per day (Eberlein-Koning et al., 1998) and should be used for at least 2–3 weeks to achieve its protective effect. Since it inhibits platelet aggregation, its use should be discontinued before any surgical procedure (Costa, 2012).

ZINC

Zinc is an essential element of the human body, and the skin is rich in zinc (Reeve et al., 1999). It serves as a catalyst for the enzymes responsible for DNA replication, gene transcription, and protein synthesis to neutralize free radicals (Vallee and Falchuk, 1993). Similar to selenium, it participates in the endogenous antioxidant system and plays an important physiological role in the immune response and wound healing. In studies with human fibroblasts, zinc performed its protective function against the cytotoxicity induced by UVR and lipid peroxidation (Leccia et al., 1999). It is indicated for treatment of acne, telogen effluvium, and periodontitis and for its photoprotective effects on topical use (Pinnell, 2003). The recommended daily dose is 8 mg but varies according to specific diseases (Kurmis et al., 2013).

CONCLUSIONS

Today's growing market for healthy lifestyles in which people are more observant of their health and seek to improve it by consuming food and other natural sources that contribute to their well-being and reduce the damage caused by intrinsic and extrinsic factors. Healthy aging may be strongly associated with a balanced diet, healthy lifestyle, and proper supplementation of nutraceuticals. Oxidative stress can lead to damage to biological structures and contribute to the aging process, inflammation, and some cancers.

Because the effectiveness of nutraceuticals is already known and demonstrated in a growing number of studies, antioxidants, vitamins, minerals, fatty acids, and other dietary nutrients are indispensable for maintaining the health of skin and other tissues throughout the body.

References

Adly, A.A.M., 2010. Oxidative stress and disease: an updated review. Res. J. Immunol. 3, 129–145.

Agarwal, S., Rao, A.V., 2000. Tomato lycopene and its role in human health and chronic diseases, Canada. Can. Med. Assoc. J. 6, 739–744.

Alestas, T., Ganceviciene, R., Fimmel, S., Müller-Decker, K., Zouboulis, C., 2006. Enzymes involved in the biosynthesis of leukotriene B4 and prostaglandin E2 are active in sebaceous glands, Germany. J. Mol. Med. 84, 75–87.

Amaya, J.F., Domene, S.M.A., Padovani, R.M., 2001. DRI: síntese comentada das novas propostas sobre recomendações nutricionais para antioxidantes. Rev. Nutr. 14 (1), 71–78.

Anderson, A., Bowman, A., Boulton, S., Manning, P., Birch-Machin, M., 2014. A role for human mitochondrial complex II in the production of reactive oxygen species in human skin, UK. Redox Biol. 2, 1016–1022.

Anunciato, T.P., Filho, P.A.R., 2012. Carotenoids and polyphenols in nutricosmetics, nutraceuticals, and cosmeceuticals, Brazil. J. Cosmet. Dermatol. 11, 51–54.

Bayerl, Ch, 2008. Beta-carotene in dermatology: does it help? Germany. Acta Dermatoven. APA 17, 160–166.

Bianchi, M.L.P., Antunes, L.M.G., 1999. Free radicals and the main dietary antioxidants. Rev. Nutr. 12 (2), 123–130.

Bidri, M., Choay, P., 2003. La taurine: un aminoacide particulier aux fonctions multiples. Ann. Pharm. Fr. 61, 385–391.

Blaut, M., 2002. Relationship of prebiotics and food to intestinal microflora. Eur. J. Nutr v. 41 (supplement 1), 1–16.

Bruera A., 2012, Nutracêuticos. In: Tratado Internacional de Cosmecêuticos, primeira ed. Guanabara Koogan, Rio de Janeiro.

Bronsnick, T., Murzaku, E.C., Rao, B.K., 2014. Diet in dermatology: Part I. Atopic dermatitis, acne and nonmelanoma skin cancer, USA. J. Am. Acad. Dermatol. 71, 353.

Calomme, M.R., Vanden-Berghe, D., 1997. Suplementation of calves wif stabilized orthosilic acid. Biol. Trace Elen. v.56 (n.2), 153–165.

Cho, K.J., Yun, C.H., Packer, L., Chung, A.S., 2001. Inhibition mechanism of bioflavonoids extracted from the bark of Pinus maritime on the expression of proinflammatory cytokines. Ann. N. Y. Acad. Sci 928, 141–156.

Chow, H.H. Sherry, et al., 2001. Phase I pharmacokinetic study of tea polyphenols following single-dose administration of epigallocatechin gallate and polyphenon E. Cancer Epidemiol. Biomark. Prevent. 10 (1), 53–58.

Cornelli, U., 2009. Antioxidant use in nutraceuticals, USA. Clin. Dermatol. 27, 175–194.

Costa, A., 2012. Tratado Internacional de Cosmecêuticos, primeira ed. Guanabara Koogan, Rio de Janeiro.

De Luca, C., Mikhal'chik, E.V., Suprun, M.V., Papacharalambous, M., Truhanov, A.I., Korkina, L.G., 2016. Skin antiageing and systemic redox effects of supplementation with marine collagen peptides and plant-derived antioxidants: a single-blind case-control clinical study, Russia. Oxid. Med. Cell Long., 1–14.

Desotelle, J.A., Wilking, M.J., Ahmad, N., 2012. The circadian control of skin and cutaneous photodamage, USA. Photochem. Photobiol. 88, 1037–1047.

Eades, M.D., 1994. The Doctors Complete Guide to Vitamins and Minerals. Dell Publishing Group.

Eberlein-Koning, B., Placzek, M., Brzybylla, B., 1998. Protective effects against sunburn of combined systemic ascorbic acid (vitamin C) and D-α-tocopherol (vitamin E). L. Am. Acad. Dermatol. 38, 45–48.

Evans, J.A., Johnson, E.J., 2010. The role of phytonutrients in skin health, USA. Nutrients 2, 903–928.

Fischer, T.W., Slominski, A., Zmijewski, M.A., Reiter, R.J., Paus, R., 2008. Melatonin as a major skin protectant: From free radical scavenging to DNA damage repair, Germany. Exp. Dermatol. 17, 713–730.

Fiume, M., 2001. Final Report on the safety assessment of biotin, International. J. Toxicol. 20 (Suppl 4), 1–12.

Folster-Holst, R., 2010. Probiotics in the treatment and prevention of atopic dermatitis. Ann. Nutr. Metab. 57, 16–19.

Hardeland, R., 2013. Chronobiology of melatonin beyond the feedback to the suprachiasmatic nucleus-consequences to melatonin dysfunction. Int. J. Mol. Sci. 14, 5817–5841.

Heyland, D.K., Dhaliwal, R., Suchner, U., Berger, M.M., 2005. Antioxidant nutrients: a systematic review of trace elements and vitamins in the critically ill patient. Canada. Intensive Care Med. 31, 327–337.

Humbert, P., Binda, D., Robin, S., Krutmann, J., 2011. Beauty from inside: nutrition-based strategies in cosmetic dermatology Nutrition for Healthy Skin, vol. 1. Springer, Berlin Heidelberg. pp.189–196.

Indo, H.P., Yen, H.C., Nakanishi, I., Matsumoto, K., Tamura, M., Nagano, Y., et al., 2015. A mitochondrial superoxide theory for oxidative stress diseases and aging, Japan. J. Clin. Biochem. Nutr. 56, 1–7.

Jeengar, M.K., Kumar, P.S., Thummuri, D., Shrivastava, S., Guntuku, L., Sistla, R., et al., 2015. Review on emu products for use as complementary and alternative medicine, India. Nutrition 31, 21–27.

Jugdaohsingh, R., et al., 2004. Dietary silicon intake is positively associated with bone mineral density in menand premenopausal women of the Framingham Offspring cohort. J. Bone Miner. Res. v.19 (n.2), 297–307.

Jung, J.Y., Kwon, H.H., Hong, J.S., Yoon, J.Y., Park, M.S., Jang, M.Y., et al., 2014. Effect of dietary supplementation with omega-3 fatty acid and gamma-linolenic acid on acne vulgaris: a randomized, double-blind, controlled trial, Korea. Acta Dermatol. Venereol. 94, 521–525.

Kandola, K., Bowman, A., Birch-Machin, M.A., 2015. Oxidative stress – a key emerging impact factor in health, ageing, lifestyle and aesthetics, UK. Int. J. Cosmet. Sci. 37, 1–8.

Katiyar, S., Elmets, C., Katiyar, S., 2007. Green tea and skin cancer: photoimmunology, angiogenesis and DNA repair. J. Nutr. Biol. 18 (5), 287–296.

Kennedy, D.O., Wightman, E.L., Reay, J.L., Lietz, G., Okello, E.J., Wilde, A., et al., 2010. Effects of resveratrol on cerebral blood flow variables and cognitive performance in humans: a double-blind, placebo-controlled, crossover investigation. Am. J. Clin. Nutr. 91 (6), 1590–1597.

Kleszczynski, K., Fischer, T.W., 2012. Melatonin and human skin aging, Germany. Dermatoendocrinology 4, 245–252.

Koch, C., Dolle, S., Metzger, M., Rasche, C., Jungclas, H., Ruhl, R., et al., 2008. Docosahexaenoic acid (DHA) supplementation in atopic eczema: a randomized, double-blind, controlled trial, Germany. Br. J. Dermatol. 158, 786–792.

Krinsky, N.I., 2001. Carotenoids as antioxidants, USA. Nutrition 17, 815–817.

Kruk, J., Duchnik, E., 2014. Oxidative stress and skin diseases: possible role of physical activity, Poland. Asian Pac. J. Cancer Prev. 15, 561–568.

Kurmis, R., Aromataris, E., Greenwood, J., 2013. The effectiveness of trace element supplementation following severe burn injury: a systematic review protocol, Australia. JBI Database Syst. Rev. Implement. Rep. 11, 44–53.

Kwak, N., Jukes, D., 2001. Part 1: the development of a regulatory concept, UK. Food Control. 12, 99–107.

Leccia, M.T., Richard, M.J., Favier, A., Béani, J.C., 1999. Zinc protects against ultraviolet A1-induced DNA damage and apoptosis in cultured human fibroblasts, France. Biol. Trace Elem. Res. 69, 177–190.

Manach, C., Williamson, G., Morand, C., Scalbert, A., Remesy, C., 2005. Bioavailability and bioefficacy of polyphenols in humans. I. Review of 97 bioavailability studies. Am. J. Clin. Nutr. 81, 230–242.

Nachtigall, A.M., Stringheta, P.C., Fidelis, P.C., Nachtigall, F.M., 2007. Determinação do teor de luteína em hortaliças, Brazil. B Ceppa 25, 181–192.

Ndiaye, M.A., Nihal, M., Wood, G.S., Ahmad, N., 2014. Skin, reactive oxygen species and circadian clocks, USA. Antioxid. Redox Signal. 20, 2982–2996.

Nestor, M., Bucay, V., Callender, V., Cohen, J.L., Sadick, N., Waldorf, H., 2014. Polypodium leucotomos as an adjunct treatment of pigmentary disorders. J. Clin. Aesthetic Dermatol. 7 (3), 13–17.

Philips, N., Keller, T., Hendrix, C., Hamilton, S., Arena, R., Tuason, M., et al., 2007. Regulation of the extracellular matrix remodeling by lutein in dermal fibroblasts, melanoma cells, and ultraviolet radiation exposed fibroblasts, USA. Arch. Dermatol. Res. 299, 373–379.

Pinnell, S.R., 2003. Cutaneous photodamage, oxidative stress, and topical antioxidant protection, USA. J. Am. Acad. Dermatol. 48, 1–22.

Pinto, C.A.S., Delfes, M.F.Z., Reis, L.M., Garbers, L.E., 2015. Passos PCVR, Torre DS. The use of pycnogenol in the treatment of melasma. Surg. Cosmet. Dermatol. 7 (3), 218–222.

Pop, E., Fischer, L., Coan, A., Gitzinger, M., Nakamura, J., Zeisel, S., 2008. Effects of a high dose of soy isoflavones on DNA damage, apoptosis and estrogenic outcomes in healthy, postmenopausal women-a phase I clinical trial. Menopause 15, 684–692.

Powers, S.K., Jackson, M.J., 2008. Exercise induced oxidative stress: cellular mechanisms and impact on muscle force production, USA. Physiol. Rev. 88, 1243–1276.

Prokopieva, V.D., Yarygina, E.G., Bokhan, N.A., Ivanova, S.A., 2016. Use of carnosine for oxidative stress reduction in different pathologies. Oxid. Med. Cell Longiv. 2016, 2939087.

Raatz, S.K., Rosenberger, T.A., Johnson, L.K., Wolters, W.W., Burr, G.S., Picklo, M.J., 2013. Dose-dependent consumption of farmed Atlantic Salmon (*Salmo salar*) increases plasma Phospholipid n-3 fatty acids differentially, USA. J. Acad. Nutr. Diet 113, 282–287.

Ramos-e-Silva, M.D., Carneiro, S.C.S., 2001. Cosmetics for the elderly, Brazil. Clin. Dermatol. 19, 413–423.

Reeve, V.E., Nishimura, N., Bosnic, M., Choo, A.K.H., Michalska, A.E., 1999. Dietary zinc, photoimmunosuppression and metallothionein (MT). In: Klassen C (ed), Metallothionein IV. Advances in Life Science, Switzerland, pp. 445–449.

Reffit, D., Ogston, N., Jugdaohsingh, R., Cheug, H.F.J., Evans, B.A.J., Thompson, R.P.H., et al., 2003. Orthosilicic acid stimulates collagen type i synthesis and osteoblast differentiation in human osteoblast-like cells in vitro. Bone 32, 127–135.

Rexbye, H., Petersen, I., Johansens, M., Klitkou, L., Jeune, B., Christensen, K., 2006. Influence of environmental factors on facial ageing, Denmark. Age Aging 35, 110–115.

Rizwan, M., Rodriguez-Blanco, I., Harbottle, A., Birch-Machin, M.A., Watson, R.E., Rhodes, L.E., 2011. Tomato paste rich in lycopene protects against cutaneous photodamage in humans in vivo: a randomized controlled trial. Br. J. Dermatol. 164, 154–162.

Roberfroid, M., 2002. Functional food concept and its application to prebiotics. Dig. Liver Dis v. 34 (Suppl. 2), 105–110.

Rohdewald, P.J., 2002. A review of the French maritime pine bark extract (Pycnogenol), a herbal medication with a diverse clinical pharmacology. Int. J. Clin. Pharmacol. Ther. 40 (4), 158–168.

Saad, S.M.I., 2006. Probióticos e prebióticos: o estado da arte. Rev. Brasileira de Ciências Farmacêuticas v. 42 (n.1), 1–16.

Sanoobar, M., Eghtesadi, S., Azimi, A., Khalili, M., Khodadadi, B., Jazayeri, S., et al., 2014. Coenzyme Q10 supplementation ameliorates inflammatory markers in patients with multiple sclerosis: a double blind, placebo, controlled randomized clinical trial. Nutr. Neurosci. 18, 169–176.

Scarmo, S., Cartmel, B., Lin, H., Leffell, D.J., Welch, E., Bhosale, P., et al., 2010. Significant correlations of dermal total carotenoids and dermal lycopene with their respective plasma levels in healthy adults, USA. Arch. Biochem. Biophys. 504, 34–39.

Scheepens, A., Tank, A., Paxton, J., 2010. Improving the oral bioavailability of benefitial polyphenols through designed synergies. Genes Nutr. 5, 75–87.

Schrauzer, G.N., 2000. Selenomethionine: a review of its nutritional significance, metabolism and toxicity, USA. J. Nutr. 130, 1653–1656.

Senger, A.E., Schawanke, C.H., Gottlieb, M.G., 2011. Green tea (*Camellia sinensis*) and its functionals properties on transmissible chronic diseases. Sci. Med. 20 (4), 292–300.

Shils, M., Olson, J., Shike, M., Ross, A., 1999. Modern Nutrition in Health and Disease, 9th ed Williams & Wilkins, Baltimore.

Tabor, A., Blair, R., 2009. Nutritional cosmetics, primeira ed. Elsevier, UK.

Vallee, B.L., Falchuk, K.H., 1993. The biochemical basis of zinc physiology, USA. Physiol. Rev. 73, 79–118.

Wertz, K., Hunziker, P.B., Seifert, N., Riss, G., Neeb, M., Steiner, G., et al., 2005. Beta-Carotene interferes with ultraviolet light A-induced gene expression by multiple pathways, Switzerland. J. Investig. Dermatol. 124, 428–434.

Woodside, J.V., McGrath, A.J., Lyner, N., McKinley, M.C., 2015. Carotenoids and health in older people, UK. Maturitas Elsevier 80, 63–68.

Wright, T., Spencer, J., Flowers, F., 2006. Chemoprevention of nonmelanoma skin câncer. J. Am. Acad. Dermatol. 54 (6), 933–946.
Wu, D., Cederbaum, A.I., 2003. Alcohol, oxidative stress, and free radical damage, USA. Alcohol Res. Health 27, 277–284.
Xia, L., Nordman, T., Olsson, J.M., Damdimopoulos, A., Bjorkhem-Bergman, L., Nalvarte, I., et al., 2003. The mammalian cytosolic selenoenzyme thioredoxin reductase reduces ubiquinone. A novel mechanism for defense against oxidative stress, Sweden. J. Biol. Chem. 278, 2141–2146.
Zhu, H., Wei, X., Bian, K., Murad, F., 2008. Effects of nitric oxide on skin burn wound healing. J. Burn. Care Res. 29 (5), 804–814.

Further Reading

Arab, L., Steck, S., 2000. Lycopene and cardiovascular disease, USA. Am. J. Clin. Nutr. 71 (6), 1691–1695.
Ascenso, A., Pedrosa, T., Pinho, S., Pinho, F., Oliveira, J.M.P.F., Marques, H.C., et al., 2016. The effect of lycopene preexposure on UV-B-Irradiated human keratinocytes, Portugal. Oxid. Med. Cell. Long. 1–15.
Barcelos, R.C.S., Mello-Sampayo, C., Antoniazzi, C.T.D., Segat, H.J., Silva, H., Veit, J.C., et al., 2015. Oral supplementation with fish oil reduces dryness and pruritus in the acetone-induced dry skin rat model, Br. J. Dermatol. Sc. 79, 298–304.
Cefali, L.C., Souza-Moreira, T.M., Corrêa, M.A., Salgado, H.R.N., Isaac, V.L.B., 2015. Development and evaluation of an emulsion containing lycopene for combating acceleration of skin aging, Brazil. Braz. J. Pharm. Sci. 51, 579–590.
Claustrat, B., Leston, J., 2015. Melatonin: physiological effects in humans, France. Neurochirurgie 61, 77–84.
Di Mascio, P., Kaiser, S., Sies, S., 1989. Lycopene as the most efficiente biological carotenoid singlet oxygen quencher, Germany. Arch. Biochem. Biophys. 274 (2), 532–538.
Godic, A., Poljšak, B., Adamic, M., Dahmane, R., 2014. The role of antioxidants in skin cancer prevention and treatment, Slovenia. Oxid. Med. Cell. Long. 1–6.
Ito, M.K., 2015. Long-chain omega-3 fatty acids, fibrates and niacin as therapeutic options in the treatment of hypertriglyceridemia: A review of the literature, USA. Atherosclerosis Elsevier 242, 647–656.
Karim, A.A., Azlan, A.A., Ismail, A., Hashim, P., Gani, S.S.A., Zainudin, B.H., et al., 2014. Phenolic composition, antioxidant, anti-wrinkles and tyrosinase inhibitory activities of cocoa pod extract, Malaysia. BMC Complement. Alternat. Med. 14, 381–394.
Katta, R., Desai, S.P., 2014. Diet in dermatology: The role of dietary intervention in skin disease (Review), USA. J. Clin. Aesthetic Dermatol. 7, 46–51.
Kim, T.K., Lin, Z., Tidwell, W.J., Li, W., Slominski, A.T., 2015. Melatonin and its metabolites accumulate in the human epidermis in vivo and inhibit proliferation and tyrosinase activity in epidermal malanocytes in vitro, USA. Mol. Cell. Endocrinol. 404, 1–8.
Marseglia, L., D'Angelo, G., Manti, S., Salpietro, C., Arrigo, T., Barberi, I., et al., 2014. Melatonin and atopy: role in atopic dermatitis and asthma, Italy. Int. J. Mol. Sci. 15, 13482–13493.
Perez, L.A.M., Gomez, M.R., 2016. Resveratrol inhibition of cellular respiration: new paradigm for an old mechanism. Int. J. Mol. Sci. 17, 368.
Pilkington, S.M., Massey, K.A., Bennett, S.P., Al-Aasswad, N.M., Roshdy, K., Gibbs, N.K., et al., 2013. Randomized controlled trial of oral omega-3 PUFA in solar-simulated radiation-induced suppression of human cutaneous immune responses, USA. Am. J. Clin. Nutr. 97, 646–652.
Ramos-e-Silva, M.D., Carneiro, S.C.S., 2007. Elderly skin and its rejuvenation: products and procedures for the aging skin, Brazil. J. Cosmet. Dermatol. 6, 40–50.
Reiter, R., J., 1993. The melatonin rhythm: both a clock and a calendar, USA. Experientia 49, 654–664.
Rinnerthaler, M., Bischof, J., Streubel, M.K., Trost, A., Richter, K., 2015. Review oxidative stress in aging human skin, Austria. Biomol 5, 545–589.
Rivera, S., Canela, R., 2012. Influence of sample processing on the analysis of carotenoids in Maize, Spain. Molecules 17, 11255–11268.
Roberts, J.E., Dennison, J., 2015. The photobiology of lutein and zeaxanthin in the eye, USA. J Ophthalmol, 1–8.
Rona, C., Berardesca, E., 2008. Aging skin and food supplements: the myth and the truth, Italy. Clin. Dermatol. 26, 641–647.
Safavi, S.M., Adeloo, A.H., 2015. The effect of dietary and supplementation of Omega-3 and Omega-6 fatty acids on healing of skin, gastrointestinal and diabetic wounds, Iran. J. Isfahan Med. School 33, 1–11.
Schalka, S., Vitale-Villarejo, M.A., Agelune, C.M., Bombarda, P.C.P., 2014. The benefits of using a compound containing a Polypodium leucotomos extract for reducing erythema and pigmentation resulting from ultraviolet radiation. Surg. Cosmet. Dermatol. 6 (4), 344–348.
Shami, N.J.I.E., Moreira, E.A.M., 2004. Licopeno como agente antioxidante, Brazil. Rev. Nutr. 17, 227–236.
Slominski, A., Tobin, D.J., Zmijewski, M.A., Wortsman, J., Paus, R., 2008. Melatonin in the skin: Synthesis, metabolism and functions, Germany. Trends Endocrinol. 19, 17–24.
Vranesic, D., 2010. The role of nutraceuticals in anti-aging medicine, Croatia. Acta Clin. Croatica 49, 537–544.

CHAPTER

24

Effects of Resveratrol on Cognitive Functions

Sebastian Huhn[1,2] *and A. Veronica Witte*[1,2]

[1]Max Planck Institute for Human Cognitive and Brain Sciences, Leipzig, Germany

[2]University of Leipzig, Leipzig, Germany

INTRODUCTION

The polyphenol resveratrol (RSV) is probably best known for its crucial role in the so-called French paradox. This concept aims to explain the paradoxical epidemiological observation that the French, despite a diet rich in saturated fatty acids, have a relatively low incidence of cardiovascular complications (Catalgol et al., 2012; Kulkarni and Canto, 2015). As integral ingredient of red wine, RSV is among the components of the French diet that are suspected to positively affect coronary health (Catalgol et al., 2012; Kulkarni and Canto, 2015). Furthermore, the moderate consumption of red wine has been linked to lower incidence of age-related neurological disorders, strokes, and cognitive deficits (Bastianetto et al., 2015).

This chapter starts with a brief overview of the sources, pharmacokinetics, and metabolism of RSV to provide the reader with a better understanding of the physiological processes in the context of RSV administration. In the following section, we provide a review of available animal and human studies on the effects of RSV on cognitive functions followed by a discussion of possible underlying mechanisms. The chapter closes with a discussion about the translation and interpretation of these findings in order to put the current research into a wider framework and point out implications for future studies.

BACKGROUND: SOURCES AND PHARMACOKINETICS OF RESVERATROL

The dietary sources of RSV include blueberries, red currants, and peanuts, although red grapes and red wine are the most substantial sources in the human diet (Baur and Sinclair, 2006; Ingram et al., 2006; Smoliga et al., 2011). The naturally occurring variance in concentration depends not only on the specific source but also on environmental factors such as weather and exposure to stressors (Gambini et al., 2015). An extensive overview of the specific polyphenol content in foods is provided in the online database Phenol-Explorer: Database on Polyphenol Content in Foods (for details, see Rothwell et al., 2013). Within plants, RSV acts as a phytoalexin, meaning it is characterized by low molecular weight and is involved in counteracting certain stressors (Gambini et al., 2015). Those stressors include parasites, fungi, ultraviolet radiation, excessive sunlight, and chemical substances (Carrizzo et al., 2013; Gambini et al., 2015).

Human intake of RSV occurs via the consumption of RSV-containing foods or via dietary supplements. In the intestine, RSV is absorbed by passive diffusion or after forming complexes with membrane transporters (Gambini et al., 2015). Absorption rate is supposed to be approximately 75%, which is rather high for a dietary polyphenol, but it also varies between different food items and ways of consumption (Gambini et al., 2015; Pangeni et al., 2014;

Nutrition and Functional Foods for Healthy Aging.
DOI: http://dx.doi.org/10.1016/B978-0-12-805376-8.00024-1

Vitaglione et al., 2005; Walle, 2011). For example, RSV absorption is lower after a high-fat breakfast compared to after overnight fasting (la Porte, 2010; Robinson et al., 2015; Vaz-da-Silva et al., 2008).

Once RSV reaches the bloodstream, it is present either in free form as glucuronide or as sulfate (Gambini et al., 2015). Usually RSV is quickly metabolized in phase II in the liver or duodenal cells and thus has low bioavailability (Davinelli et al., 2012). Emerging products are sulfates, glucuronides, and as many as five different urinary products (Gambini et al., 2015). This high rate of metabolism could be counteracted by the administration of RSV in combination with other chemicals such as quercetin that inhibit its sulfation and glucuronidation in the liver and duodenal tissue (De Santi et al., 2000; Gambini et al., 2015). However, others could not confirm these effects (la Porte, 2010), so the underlying mechanisms of how quercetin enhances the bioavailability of RSV remains somewhat unclear. The free form of RSV is characterized by a low water solubility, and more than 90% of free RSV binds to plasma lipoproteins (Gambini et al., 2015). Glucuronides and sulfates are either excreted or converted again to free RSV in target organs such as the liver (Gambini et al., 2015; Park and Pezzuto, 2015). Notably, RSV crosses the blood–brain barrier (Davinelli et al., 2012; Turner et al., 2015) and is thought to exert neuroprotective effects within the brain. For example, RSV was found to attenuate neuronal damage caused by a high-fat diet in mice and to protect against apoptotic insults (Chang et al., 2014).

In humans, supplementary RSV intake is considered to be safe and well tolerated up to 5 g per day (Almeida et al., 2009; Anton et al., 2014; Boocock et al., 2007; Brown et al., 2010; Cottart et al., 2014; la Porte, 2010; Patel et al., 2011; Turner et al., 2015). Minor adverse effects appeared at doses higher than 0.5 g RSV per day over long periods, starting from several weeks and up to one year (Cottart et al., 2014). These were described as mainly affecting the abdomen (e.g., flatulence, mild diarrhea) and remaining moderate and reversible (Cottart et al., 2014). Note that all of these observations are based on supplementary RSV products with a high level of purification and lack of contamination (Virmani et al., 2013). Furthermore, interactions with therapeutic products should be addressed in future studies, even though these have been considered to be marginal, to rule out negative consequences of RSV on pharmacotherapy (MacDonald et al., 2009). In addition, future studies should address the effects of RSV derivatives and analogs, as well as the development of methods that could slow down the rapid metabolism of RSV to eventually increase RSV bioavailability (Cottart et al., 2014).

ANIMAL STUDIES

Using various animal models, previous research investigated the use of RSV on a multitude of diseases and their underlying mechanisms. For example, improved outcomes in cardiovascular diseases and diabetes have been highly investigated and linked with positive effects of RSV not only on inflammation and oxidative stress but also on cancer (e.g., for reviews, see Knutson and Leeuwenburgh, 2008; Kundu and Surh, 2008; Das and Das, 2007).

Considering cognitive functions, a treatment with RSV was associated with improved spatial learning and memory as well as mood proxies in aged rodents (Abraham and Johnson, 2009; Casadesus et al., 2004; Kodali et al., 2015). The animals received RSV by either consuming blueberries or dietary supplements for at least four weeks. Moreover, findings were similar concerning pharmacologically induced learning deficits in rats (Gacar et al., 2011; Yazir et al., 2015) and in diabetic rats (Schmatz et al., 2009).

In addition, these and other studies (Galli et al., 2006; Liu et al., 2014) reported neuroprotective effects of RSV on the hippocampus, a key area involved in memory and spatial navigation in association with the preservation of cognitive functions. This was also accompanied with improvements in the brain's microvasculature in the RSV-treated rats compared to control animals (Oomen et al., 2009).

Getting closer to humans, the French RESTRIKAL study investigated the effects of RSV and caloric restriction (CR) in nonhuman primates. The study assessed the effect of an 18-month RSV-supplementation in 33 lemurs in comparison to control or CR subjects (Dal-Pan et al., 2011a; Dal-Pan et al., 2011b). RSV supplementation as well as CR led to a significant improvement in working memory, while only RSV treatment significantly enhanced spatial memory performance (Dal-Pan et al., 2011a).

HUMAN STUDIES

RSV in human studies made its first appearance in the 1990s in context of the French paradox. Afterward many studies reported improved health outcomes regarding cardiovascular diseases in association with RSV intake. However, available data on cardiovascular disease is still in conflict and definite recommendations to the public cannot yet be made (Kakoti et al., 2015; Zordoky et al., 2015).

Since the early studies in the framework of the French paradox, more research was conducted to identify potential beneficial effects of RSV on other leading causes of death such as obesity, diabetes, and cancer. For all of those diseases, the observed findings are promising in animal models, but the data in humans are not consistent enough and too conflicting to draw final conclusions (de Ligt et al., 2015; Scapagnini et al., 2014; Singh et al., 2015). For example, Semba et al. (2014) could not find a positive effect of RSV, measured in urinary samples, on a population-based cohort of 783 community-dwelling older adults (>65 years of age) in Chianti (Italy). They argued that a typical Western diet does not contain enough RSV to affect outcomes such as inflammation, several diseases, and mortality. Data are, however, most convincing in type 2 diabetes research. Here RSV is considered a leading candidate to support conventional pharmacological management (Hausenblas et al., 2015; Szkudelski and Szkudelska, 2015). The improvements of glycemic control and insulin sensitivity after RSV seem especially crucial for positive health outcomes in diabetes (Brasnyo et al., 2011; Szkudelski and Szkudelska, 2015).

Considering neurodegenerative processes and related decreases in cognitive functions, RSV is currently under phase III clinical trials to determine the potential therapeutic usage (Davinelli et al., 2012). Recently, RSV was found to be a safe and well-tolerated substance in populations at risk for Alzheimer's disease (AD) (Turner et al., 2015). Indeed, over the last few years, evidence from high-quality studies concluded that polyphenols, including RSV, might have a protective role against AD and other neurodegenerative diseases (Davinelli et al., 2012; Pasinetti et al., 2015; Rege et al., 2014; Tellone et al., 2015). Especially in combination with other compounds (e.g., clioquinol), RSV seems to be a candidate in the process of developing new drugs for AD (Mao et al., 2014).

Taken together, previous evidence suggested that RSV exerts numerous positive effects on human health outcomes, especially in diabetes, and including cognitive decline. Many findings observed in animal studies, however, still need to be established in humans. Yet the translation of animal findings to clinical outcomes faces a variety of challenges that need to be tackled (Singh et al., 2015).

One crucially important issue is that human studies on RSV suffer from a wide heterogeneity in study design (Crichton et al., 2013). For example, concerning the sources of RSV, different foods such as red wine and blueberry juice have been investigated as has isolated RSV administration in the form of a dietary supplement. Therefore, it is difficult to compare the actual dosage each participant received. But also within supplementation trials, the dosage varied substantially, e.g., participants of Brasnyo et al. (2011) received 10 mg daily, while others were administered 250 or 500 mg per day (Kennedy et al., 2010). Furthermore, the designs ranged from cross-sectional studies over single-dose experiments to longitudinal studies that incorporated a daily supplementation for several months. However, only a few randomized controlled trials with limited sample sizes are available so far. In addition, the studied outcome measures such as behavioral and neuropsychological tests were considerably different, rendering a comparison between studies difficult. In sum, the heterogeneity in study design and lack of large-scale randomized controlled trials prevent any recommendation for RSV as a supplement in prevention or therapy of any disease, even though most studies provided promising results (reviewed, e.g., in Huhn et al., 2015; Novelle et al., 2015).

RSV and Cognitive Functions

Considering cognitive effects, most studies investigated RSV within food items, but also data from supplementation studies are available. Nurk et al. (2009) investigated the effects of flavonol-rich foods that are also rich in RSV (chocolate, red wine, and tea) on several cognitive outcomes in a cross-sectional study with 2031 participants aged 70–74 from the Hordaland Health Study in Norway. In that study, a diet high in flavonol-rich foods served over the course of one year was measured using a self-reported food frequency questionnaire and was associated with better abilities in several cognitive domains in a dose-dependent manner compared to a nonconsumer group (Nurk et al., 2009). Red wine in particular had the strongest beneficial effect on cognitive test performance (Nurk et al., 2009).

In another study, Krikorian et al. (2010) administered wild blueberry juice every day for 12 weeks to a small sample of nine older adults with early memory changes. They found improved learning and memory performance in comparison with a matched, placebo-controlled sample (Krikorian et al., 2010).

The impact of a proprietary formulation of blueberries as part of a pill-based nutraceutical was investigated by Small et al. (2014) in a double-blind clinical trial with 52 participants aged 65–85 years in comparison to a placebo ($N = 53$). After two months, the intervention group improved significantly on two measures of processing speed, whereas no other cognitive domain (episodic memory, verbal ability, working memory, executive functioning, or complex speed) was affected (Small et al., 2014).

Brickman et al. (2014) used a diet containing high amounts of cocoa-flavonol in comparison to a low cocoa-flavonol diet in a randomized study with 37 healthy 50- to 69-year-old subjects. After three months of intervention, they found that the high cocoa-flavonol group had significantly enhanced hippocampus-associated memory functions (Brickman et al., 2014). Using functional magnetic resonance imaging (fMRI), they further showed this was associated with higher cerebral blood volume in the dentate gyrus, a hippocampal region characterized by lifelong neurogenesis and known to correlate blood volume with task performance (Brickman et al., 2014).

In the studies using isolated RSV supplements, the group around Kennedy et al. (2010) was the first to report the acute effect of RSV on cerebral blood flow after oral administration of a single dose of either 250 or 500 mg of RSV in a placebo-controlled, randomized crossover design. The 22 healthy adults showed a dose-dependent increase in cerebral blood flow measured via near infrared spectroscopy while they performed several cognitive tasks (Kennedy et al., 2010). Wightman and colleagues from the same working group confirmed those findings in two papers (Wightman et al., 2014; Wightman et al., 2015). Notably, in the latter study, Wightman et al. (2015) did not find chronic changes of cerebral blood flow or cognitive effects after four weeks of RSV supplementation (500 mg/day). This might be explained by the young age of (healthy) participants (28–30 years) because ceiling effects could have masked potential benefits on blood flow and cognitive performance or because of the short duration of the intervention, which might have not been long enough to exert positive effects. Interestingly, blood levels of RSV biomarkers in that study suggested that chronic oral administration of RSV lead to cumulative plasma levels in healthy humans (Wightman et al., 2015).

In our own study with 46 healthy but overweight older individuals, a daily intake of 200 mg RSV (in a formula with quercetin) over 26 weeks significantly improved memory performance compared to placebo intake (Witte et al., 2014). In addition, glycated hemoglobin (HbA1c) in peripheral blood was significantly reduced after RSV treatment, and this reduction in HbA1c correlated with higher functional connectivity of the hippocampus as measured using resting-state fMRI in the same subjects. Notably, changes in functional connectivity were found to partially mediate the observed increases in memory, which points to ameliorated glucose metabolism as one underlying mechanism of the positive effects of RSV on cognition (Witte et al., 2014).

In sum, only a few studies on cognitive functions in humans are available, and their results are inconclusive. Still, older populations in particular might benefit from RSV treatment. Little is known about the possible effects in populations already affected by AD or its precursor, mild cognitive impairment.

MECHANISMS

Postulated mechanisms of RSV range from antioxidant and antiinflammatory effects to neuroprotection and mimicking of CR. RSV seems to act on so many different molecular pathways and binding partners that it was previously called a "promiscuous molecule" (Britton et al., 2015). However, this variety of pathways might also explain the diverse range of conditions in which RSV appears to be beneficial for health (Britton et al., 2015). The following section contains a summary of the most commonly discussed mechanisms and binding partners of RSV to explain its various actions.

Resveratrol and Oxidation

RSV is suggested to possess both direct and indirect antioxidant effects (Spanier et al., 2009). The direct effect is inherent to the chemical structure of RSV—that is, its polyphenolic characteristic. Polyphenols are secondary metabolites of plants and characterized by the chemical structure of hydroxyl groups on aromatic rings (Manach et al., 2004). These aromatic rings are capable of balancing electron inequalities and either act as electron or hydrogen donors to annihilate free radicals (Vlachogianni et al., 2015).

In contrast, the indirect antioxidant effects are more complex because RSV acts on different pathways. RSV downregulates pro-oxidative enzymes (e.g., nicotinamide adenine dinucleotide phosphate, or NADPH), while at the same time it upregulates antioxidant enzymes (e.g., SOD1, Gpx1) (Spanier et al., 2009). This effect might even be multiplied in combination with synergistic antioxidants such as quercetin or rutin (Iacopini et al., 2008; McAnulty et al., 2013). Even though most of the studies are conducted in vitro, some human studies also have rendered supporting evidence (Crichton et al., 2013; Pignatelli et al., 2006).

The antioxidant effects of RSV are especially interesting in the framework of the free radical theory of aging. Here it is stated that reactive oxygen species (ROS) and oxidative stress contribute to the physiological aging process by causing damage to important cellular targets (Liochev, 2013), and they might thereby be associated with cognitive decline (Droge and Schipper, 2007). ROS-associated damages include increased mutation rate, growth inhibition, and changes of the insulin-signaling pathway (Droge and Schipper, 2007; Liochev, 2013). Nevertheless, it is important to keep in mind that ROS not only are harmful but also lead to adaptive processes that are important and beneficial for the organism (Liochev, 2013). Notably, the antioxidant effects of RSV are also important with regard to cognition because a higher level of ROS was seen in animals to be associated with cognitive deficits (Bastianetto et al., 2015; Dumont and Beal, 2011).

Resveratrol and Inflammation

The antiinflammatory effect of RSV is well shown in vitro; for example, several pathways have been proposed that all lead to a lower activity of nuclear factor kappa B (NFκB) (Jimenez-Gomez et al., 2013; Poulsen et al., 2015). In animal studies, those findings and some of the pathways were confirmed and Wang et al. (2013) showed a dose-dependent effect. Despite quite promising in vitro and animal studies, the available clinical trials have yet to report contradictory findings. Thus, antiinflammatory effects of RSV in humans need to be verified in future studies (Poulsen et al., 2015).

Inflammation is important in terms of cognition. Several neurological diseases such as AD are accompanied by inflammatory processes (Wyss-Coray and Rogers, 2012). Even low-grade subclinical inflammation present, for example, in adiposity and being one characteristic of the metabolic syndrome could lead to neurodegeneration (Misiak et al., 2012; Wyss-Coray and Rogers, 2012). Therefore, RSV was discussed as a therapeutic option in inflammation-related neurological disorders (Zhang et al., 2010), yet results should be interpreted with caution due to various limitations in the available studies (Wyss-Coray and Rogers, 2012).

Resveratrol as Calorie Restriction Mimetic

In addition, RSV seems to mimic calorie restriction. CR is a dietary intervention to deliberately reduce total caloric intake while avoiding malnutrition (Baur, 2010). This intervention was found to delay or prevent age-related diseases and to even prolong life span in animal studies (Baur, 2010; Roth and Ingram, 2015; Wood et al., 2004).

RSV seems to mimic CR especially via the activation of sirtuins (Kulkarni and Canto, 2015). Probably the key mediators of CR, sirtuins are nicotinamide adenine dinucleotide (NAD^+)-dependent deacetylases and adenosine diphosphate (ADP)–ribosyltransferases and central to the body's response to diet and exercise (Baur, 2010; Hubbard and Sinclair, 2014). Sirtuins gained a lot of attention after findings that sirtuins in response to CR can extend life span in organisms ranging from yeast, worms, and flies up to mammals and nonhuman primates (Ingram and Roth, 2015; Russo et al., 2014).

In yeast and animals the sirtuin *sir2* is involved in the replicative aging process, the alteration of life span and acts as a metabolic sensor capable of adapting gene expression to the cell's metabolic state (Kulkarni and Canto, 2015). The association of sirtuins with energy homeostasis seems to apply to humans as well (Lagouge et al., 2006).

The human homologue to *sir2* is the sirtuin known as *silent mating type information regulation 2 homolog 1* (*Sirt1*), which has received the most research attention in this regard (Hubbard and Sinclair, 2014; Kim et al., 2007). *Sirt1* is involved in numerous vital signaling pathways such as in DNA repair, apoptosis, neurogenesis, and glucose–insulin homeostasis (Hubbard and Sinclair, 2014). Notably, negative alterations in neurogenesis and insulin signaling have been linked to deteriorations in cognitive functions (Cholerton et al., 2013; Couillard-Despres et al., 2011; Lazarov and Marr, 2013).

Also, the CR-mimicking effect of RSV could be beneficial for cognitive functions as CR itself was shown to improve memory performance in a sample of 50 healthy elderly subjects after 3 months of intervention (Witte et al., 2009). A more recent study found improved recognition memory in combination with alterations of the hippocampus after a 12-week CR intervention in 19 postmenopausal obese women (Prehn et al., 2016).

Neuroprotective Effects of Resveratrol

Besides the mechanisms already described that also affect cognition and therefore can be considered neuroprotective, RSV might also exert more directly positive effects on brain pathologies. Probably the most investigated pathology with regard to AD is beta-amyloid (Aβ) and tau pathology. Even though separate mechanisms for Aβ and tau have been discussed to cause toxicity within the brain, Aβ formation is supposed to be the crucial step regarding AD pathogenesis and associated with neuronal death (Bastianetto et al., 2015; Ittner and Gotz, 2011). RSV could counteract the formation of Aβ within this pathological pathway either through its antioxidant effects or via activation of sirtuins (Bastianetto et al., 2015; Davinelli et al., 2012).

Using rodent AD models, it was found that administration of RSV decreases Aß levels in the hippocampus (Kim et al., 2007; Zhao et al., 2015). RSV furthermore protected the integrity of the blood–brain barrier and prevented learning impairment (Kim et al., 2007; Zhao et al., 2015). This effect might be linked to the activation of proteasomal degradation of Aβ or the activation of protein kinase C (or both) (Davinelli et al., 2012; Han et al., 2004; Marambaud et al., 2005). Aβ-induced cell death is probably affected by RSV in a dose-dependent manner (Han et al., 2004). Whether RSV directly leads to those effects or an indirect pathway is activated remains to be elucidated (Bastianetto et al., 2015; Karuppagounder et al., 2009; Wang et al., 2014).

Another component of the neuroprotective effects of RSV is the inhibition of processes leading to neuroinflammation, such as the inhibition of cyclooxygenases (COXs) (Bastianetto et al., 2015). COXs are proinflammatory molecules contributing to neuronal cell death (Bastianetto et al., 2015). Another way to counteract neuro-inflammation is to act on the release of proinflammatory factors by acting on the cellular cascade signaling pathways involving NFκB and activator protein 1 (Bastianetto et al., 2015; Wang et al., 2014). Furthermore, it was shown that RSV has the capacity to modulate the expression of neurotrophic factors such as the nerve growth factor. Neurotrophic factors are related to the development and survival of nerve cells during development, as well as functional maintenance and survival of adult neurons (Anastacio et al., 2014). Thus, RSV might promote neuronal survival via the release of neurotrophic factors (Rahvar et al., 2011).

Taken together, these findings underline the hypothesis that RSV might prevent cognitive decline, because it not only exerts neuroprotective effects within the brain but also attenuates cognitive symptoms related to diseases such as AD (Hubbard and Sinclair, 2014).

Resveratrol and Other Possible Mechanisms

Many more possible mechanisms for the impact of RSV on cognition are debated. They involve, for example, the AMP-activated protein kinase, the PI3K/Akt signaling pathway, or estrogen receptors (Kulkarni and Canto, 2015; Simao et al., 2012). (For detailed reviews on mechanisms and RSV binding partners, see Bitterman and Chung, 2015; Britton et al., 2015; Granzotto and Zatta, 2014; Kulkarni and Canto, 2015.)

LIMITATIONS AND CHALLENGES FOR FUTURE STUDIES

RSV administration has led to promising results in animal studies, yet more studies are needed to establish these findings in humans. To allow proper translation from animal models to humans, future work especially address the limitations of previous studies such as flaws in study design and limited sample sizes and tackle challenges such as finding the most appropriate dosage. This might help to draw better conclusions about the impact of RSV on human cognitive functions.

Concerning the administration of RSV, it is important to conduct further studies with isolated RSV and investigate interactions and possible synergistic or antagonistic effects with other agents such as quercetin and piperine (Bigford and Del Rossi, 2014; Johnson et al., 2011; Kakoti et al., 2015; Skroza et al., 2015; Vang, 2015). To improve the in vivo bioavailability of RSV, it is important to get as close to the active dosage used in animal studies as possible to improve the translation of findings (Johnson et al., 2011; Smoliga and Blanchard, 2014). Therefore, one major target for future trials should be the design of novel analogs that are not metabolized as fast as RSV or to increase solubility or half-life in plasma (Granzotto and Zatta, 2014; Pangeni et al., 2014; Rege et al., 2014; Vang, 2015). With regard to cognitive functions, it is especially noteworthy that RSV can be formulated into a muco-adhesive nanocarrier and thus be directly delivered into the brain through the nasal route (Pangeni et al., 2014).

Future animal studies should further address the different mechanisms underlying the effects of RSV to elucidate whether one or several points of action lead to the multitude of biological effects (Vang, 2015). Furthermore, it might be questioned if current animal models—those, e.g., regarding AD—are a good representation of disease-related processes in humans and if useful information can be extracted from using these models or if their use should be discontinued (Franco and Cedazo-Minguez, 2014).

To improve human studies and clinical trials, several variables must be targeted. Among them, sample size generally needs to be increased (Novelle et al., 2015). Within the studies, the large range of dosages makes it difficult to compare results. Also, more accurate tracing studies assessing RSV concentrations and associated metabolites within human plasma, tissue, and organs after RSV treatment would add knowledge about relevant in vivo dosages (Vang, 2015). The combination of novel encapsulation techniques might further help resolve the problem of solubility, stability, and bioavailability in humans (Davidov-Pardo and McClements, 2014). Besides that, it is also noteworthy to define the most accurate and meaningful biomarkers of RSV in human blood and tissues (Franco and Cedazo-Minguez, 2014). Moreover, the time of administration appears to significantly influence results because e.g., Almeida et al. (2009) found morning administration of RSV to have a higher bioavailability.

Future clinical trials should also carefully select the study population under investigation, as selection bias minimizes positive outcomes (Franco and Cedazo-Minguez, 2014; Smoliga et al., 2013). In this context, also the genetic background (including single-nucleotide polymorphisms) and gene expression, along with differences in age, sex, diet, and physical activity should be monitored (Smoliga et al., 2013). Eventually, only large-scale randomized controlled trials and long-term epidemiological studies together with meta-analyses will help to provide definitive answers on the effectiveness of RSV in humans (Smoliga et al., 2013).

CONCLUSION

After resveratrol first attracted research interest in the context of the French paradox, more studies were employed and found the supposed health benefits to be not only restricted to cardiovascular outcomes but also extended to diabetes, obesity, and even cancer. As our population is turning older and older, it is important to prolong life span as well as add healthy years to the life span (Hubbard and Sinclair, 2014). Therefore, RSV containing foods and red wine in moderate amounts should be recommended as part of a fruit- and vegetable-enriched diet (Carrizzo et al., 2013). Recent research also focused on the effects of RSV on neurodegenerative diseases and cognitive functions. Here the few randomized controlled studies in humans indicate that RSV administration is well tolerated and might enhance cognitive performance in older populations, yet definite conclusions cannot be drawn to date. However, despite all the limitations and considerations for improving future trials, RSV remains a powerful drug candidate with multispectrum therapeutic application that might provide beneficial health outcomes in future trials (Novelle et al., 2015; Pangeni et al., 2014).

References

Abraham, J., Johnson, R.W., 2009. Consuming a diet supplemented with resveratrol reduced infection-related neuroinflammation and deficits in working memory in aged mice. Rejuvenation Res. 12, 445–453.

Almeida, L., Vaz-da-Silva, M., Falcao, A., Soares, E., Costa, R., Loureiro, A.I., et al., 2009. Pharmacokinetic and safety profile of trans-resveratrol in a rising multiple-dose study in healthy volunteers. Mol. Nutr. Food Res. 53 (Suppl 1), S7–15.

Anastacio, J.R., Netto, C.A., Castro, C.C., Sanches, E.F., Ferreira, D.C., Noschang, C., et al., 2014. Resveratrol treatment has neuroprotective effects and prevents cognitive impairment after chronic cerebral hypoperfusion. Neurol. Res. 36, 627–633.

Anton, S.D., Embry, C., Marsiske, M., Lu, X., Doss, H., Leeuwenburgh, C., et al., 2014. Safety and metabolic outcomes of resveratrol supplementation in older adults: results of a twelve-week, placebo-controlled pilot study. Exp. Gerontol. 57, 181–187.

Bastianetto, S., Menard, C., Quirion, R., 2015. Neuroprotective action of resveratrol. Biochim. Biophys. Acta. 1852, 1195–1201.

Baur, J.A., 2010. Resveratrol, sirtuins, and the promise of a DR mimetic. Mech. Ageing Dev. 131, 261–269.

Baur, J.A., Sinclair, D.A., 2006. Therapeutic potential of resveratrol: the in vivo evidence. Nat. Rev. Drug Discov. 5, 493–506.

Bigford, G.E., Del Rossi, G., 2014. Supplemental substances derived from foods as adjunctive therapeutic agents for treatment of neurodegenerative diseases and disorders. Adv. Nutr. 5, 394–403.

Bitterman, J.L., Chung, J.H., 2015. Metabolic effects of resveratrol: addressing the controversies. Cell Mol. Life Sci. 72, 1473–1488.

Boocock, D.J., Faust, G.E., Patel, K.R., Schinas, A.M., Brown, V.A., Ducharme, M.P., et al., 2007. Phase I dose escalation pharmacokinetic study in healthy volunteers of resveratrol, a potential cancer chemopreventive agent. Cancer Epidemiol. Biomarkers Prev. 16, 1246–1252.

Brasnyo, P., Molnar, G.A., Mohas, M., Marko, L., Laczy, B., Cseh, J., et al., 2011. Resveratrol improves insulin sensitivity, reduces oxidative stress and activates the Akt pathway in type 2 diabetic patients. Br. J. Nutr. 106, 383–389.

Brickman, A.M., Khan, U.A., Provenzano, F.A., Yeung, L.K., Suzuki, W., Schroeter, H., et al., 2014. Enhancing dentate gyrus function with dietary flavanols improves cognition in older adults. Nat. Neurosci. 17, 1798–1803.

Britton, R.G., Kovoor, C., Brown, K., 2015. Direct molecular targets of resveratrol: identifying key interactions to unlock complex mechanisms. Ann. N. Y. Acad. Sci. 1348, 124–133.

Brown, V.A., Patel, K.R., Viskaduraki, M., Crowell, J.A., Perloff, M., Booth, T.D., et al., 2010. Repeat dose study of the cancer chemopreventive agent resveratrol in healthy volunteers: safety, pharmacokinetics, and effect on the insulin-like growth factor axis. Cancer Res. 70, 9003–9011.

Carrizzo, A., Forte, M., Damato, A., Trimarco, V., Salzano, F., Bartolo, M., et al., 2013. Antioxidant effects of resveratrol in cardiovascular, cerebral and metabolic diseases. Food Chem. Toxicol. 61, 215–226.

Casadesus, G., Shukitt-Hale, B., Stellwagen, H.M., Zhu, X., Lee, H.G., Smith, M.A., et al., 2004. Modulation of hippocampal plasticity and cognitive behavior by short-term blueberry supplementation in aged rats. Nutr. Neurosci. 7, 309–316.

Catalgol, B., Batirel, S., Taga, Y., Ozer, N.K., 2012. Resveratrol: French paradox revisited. Front. Pharmacol. 3, 141.

Chang, H.-C., Tai, Y.-T., Cherng, Y.-G., Lin, J.-W., Liu, S.-H., Chen, T.-L., et al., 2014. Resveratrol attenuates high-fat diet-induced disruption of the blood–brain barrier and protects brain neurons from apoptotic insults. J Agric. Food Chem. 62, 3466–3475.

Cholerton, B., Baker, L.D., Craft, S., 2013. Insulin, cognition, and dementia. Eur. J. Pharmacol. 719, 170–179.

Cottart, C.-H., Nivet-Antoine, V., Beaudeux, J.-L., 2014. Review of recent data on the metabolism, biological effects, and toxicity of resveratrol in humans. Mol. Nutr. Food Res. 58, 7–21.

Couillard-Despres, S., Iglseder, B., Aigner, L., 2011. Neurogenesis, cellular plasticity and cognition: the impact of stem cells in the adult and aging brain – a mini-review. Gerontology 57, 559–564.

Crichton, G.E., Bryan, J., Murphy, K.J., 2013. Dietary antioxidants, cognitive function and dementia – a systematic review. Plant Foods Hum. Nutr. 68, 279–292.

Dal-Pan, A., Pifferi, F., Marchal, J., Picq, J.L., Aujard, F., Consortium, R., 2011a. Cognitive performances are selectively enhanced during chronic caloric restriction or resveratrol supplementation in a primate. PLoS One 6, e16581.

Dal-Pan, A., Terrien, J., Pifferi, F., Botalla, R., Hardy, I., Marchal, J., et al., 2011b. Caloric restriction or resveratrol supplementation and ageing in a non-human primate: first-year outcome of the RESTRIKAL study in Microcebus murinus. Age (Dordr) 33, 15–31.

Das, S., Das, D., 2007. Anti-inflammatory responses of resveratrol. Inflamm. Allergy-Drug Targets 6, 168–173.

Davidov-Pardo, G., McClements, D.J., 2014. Resveratrol encapsulation: designing delivery systems to overcome solubility, stability and bioavailability issues. Trends Food Sci. Technol. 38, 88–103.

Davinelli, S., Sapere, N., Zella, D., Bracale, R., Intrieri, M., Scapagnini, G., 2012. Pleiotropic protective effects of phytochemicals in Alzheimer's disease. Oxid. Med. Cell. Longev. 2012, 386527.

de Ligt, M., Timmers, S., Schrauwen, P., 2015. Resveratrol and obesity: can resveratrol relieve metabolic disturbances? Biochim. Biophys. Acta 1852, 1137–1144.

De Santi, C., Pietrabissa, A., Spisni, R., Mosca, F., Pacifici, G.M., 2000. Sulphation of resveratrol, a natural compound present in wine, and its inhibition by natural flavonoids. Xenobiotica 30, 857–866.

Droge, W., Schipper, H.M., 2007. Oxidative stress and aberrant signaling in aging and cognitive decline. Aging Cell 6, 361–370.

Dumont, M., Beal, M.F., 2011. Neuroprotective strategies involving ROS in Alzheimer disease. Free Radic. Biol. Med. 51, 1014–1026.

Franco, R., Cedazo-Minguez, A., 2014. Successful therapies for Alzheimer's disease: why so many in animal models and none in humans? Front. Pharmacol. 5, 146.

Gacar, N., Mutlu, O., Utkan, T., Komsuoglu Celikyurt, I., Gocmez, S.S., Ulak, G., 2011. Beneficial effects of resveratrol on scopolamine but not mecamylamine induced memory impairment in the passive avoidance and Morris water maze tests in rats. Pharmacol. Biochem. Behav. 99, 316–323.

Galli, R.L., Bielinski, D.F., Szprengiel, A., Shukitt-Hale, B., Joseph, J.A., 2006. Blueberry supplemented diet reverses age-related decline in hippocampal HSP70 neuroprotection. Neurobiol. Aging 27, 344–350.

Gambini, J., Inglés, M., Olaso, G., Lopez-Grueso, R., Bonet-Costa, V., Gimeno-Mallench, L., et al., 2015. Properties of resveratrol: in vitroandin vivostudies about metabolism, bioavailability, and biological effects in animal models and humans. Oxid. Med. Cell. Longev. 2015, 1–13.

Goldberg, D.M., Yan, J., Soleas, G.J., 2003. Absorption of three wine-related polyphenols in three different matrices by healthy subjects. Clin. Biochem. 36, 79–87.

Granzotto, A., Zatta, P., 2014. Resveratrol and Alzheimer's disease: message in a bottle on red wine and cognition. Front. Aging Neurosci. 6, 95.

Han, Y.S., Zheng, W.H., Bastianetto, S., Chabot, J.G., Quirion, R., 2004. Neuroprotective effects of resveratrol against beta-amyloid-induced neurotoxicity in rat hippocampal neurons: involvement of protein kinase C. Br. J. Pharmacol. 141, 997–1005.

Hausenblas, H.A., Schoulda, J.A., Smoliga, J.M., 2015. Resveratrol treatment as an adjunct to pharmacological management in type 2 diabetes mellitus-systematic review and meta-analysis. Mol. Nutr. Food Res. 59, 147–159.

Hubbard, B.P., Sinclair, D.A., 2014. Small molecule SIRT1 activators for the treatment of aging and age-related diseases. Trends Pharmacol. Sci. 35, 146–154.

Huhn, S., Kharabian Masouleh, S., Stumvoll, M., Villringer, A., Witte, A.V., 2015. Components of a Mediterranean diet and their impact on cognitive functions in aging. Front. Aging Neurosci. 7, 132.

Iacopini, P., Baldi, M., Storchi, P., Sebastiani, L., 2008. Catechin, epicatechin, quercetin, rutin and resveratrol in red grape: content, in vitro antioxidant activity and interactions. J. Food Compos. Anal. 21, 589–598.

Ingram, D.K., Roth, G.S., 2015. Calorie restriction mimetics: can you have your cake and eat it, too? Ageing Res. Rev. 20, 46–62.

Ingram, D.K., Zhu, M., Mamczarz, J., Zou, S., Lane, M.A., Roth, G.S., et al., 2006. Calorie restriction mimetics: an emerging research field. Aging Cell 5, 97–108.

Ittner, L.M., Gotz, J., 2011. Amyloid-beta and tau – a toxic pas de deux in Alzheimer's disease. Nat. Rev. Neurosci. 12, 65–72.

Jimenez-Gomez, Y., Mattison, J.A., Pearson, K.J., Martin-Montalvo, A., Palacios, H.H., Sossong, A.M., et al., 2013. Resveratrol improves adipose insulin signaling and reduces the inflammatory response in adipose tissue of rhesus monkeys on high-fat, high-sugar diet. Cell. Metab. 18, 533–545.

Johnson, J.J., Nihal, M., Siddiqui, I.A., Scarlett, C.O., Bailey, H.H., Mukhtar, H., et al., 2011. Enhancing the bioavailability of resveratrol by combining it with piperine. Mol. Nutr. Food Res. 55, 1169–1176.

Kakoti, B.B., Hernandez-Ontiveros, D.G., Kataki, M.S., Shah, K., Pathak, Y., Panguluri, S.K., 2015. Resveratrol and Omega-3 Fatty acid: its implications in cardiovascular diseases. Front. Cardiovasc. Med. 2

Karuppagounder, S.S., Pinto, J.T., Xu, H., Chen, H.L., Beal, M.F., Gibson, G.E., 2009. Dietary supplementation with resveratrol reduces plaque pathology in a transgenic model of Alzheimer's disease. Neurochem. Int. 54, 111–118.

Kennedy, D.O., Wightman, E.L., Reay, J.L., Lietz, G., Okello, E.J., Wilde, A., et al., 2010. Effects of resveratrol on cerebral blood flow variables and cognitive performance in humans: a double-blind, placebo-controlled, crossover investigation. Am. J. Clin. Nutr. 91, 1590–1597.

Kim, D., Nguyen, M.D., Dobbin, M.M., Fischer, A., Sananbenesi, F., Rodgers, J.T., et al., 2007. SIRT1 deacetylase protects against neurodegeneration in models for Alzheimer's disease and amyotrophic lateral sclerosis. EMBO J. 26, 3169–3179.

Knutson, M.D., Leeuwenburgh, C., 2008. Resveratrol and novel potent activators of SIRT1: effects on aging and age-related diseases. Nutr. Rev. 66, 591–596.

Kodali, M., Parihar, V.K., Hattiangady, B., Mishra, V., Shuai, B., Shetty, A.K., 2015. Resveratrol prevents age-related memory and mood dysfunction with increased hippocampal neurogenesis and microvasculature, and reduced glial activation. Sci. Rep. 5, 8075.

Krikorian, R., Shidler, M.D., Nash, T.A., Kalt, W., Vinqvist-Tymchuk, M.R., Shukitt-Hale, B., et al., 2010. Blueberry supplementation improves memory in older adults. J. Agric. Food Chem. 58, 3996–4000.

Kulkarni, S.S., Canto, C., 2015. The molecular targets of resveratrol. Biochim. Biophys. Acta 1852, 1114–1123.

Kundu, J.K., Surh, Y.J., 2008. Cancer chemopreventive and therapeutic potential of resveratrol: mechanistic perspectives. Cancer Lett. 269, 243–261.

Lagouge, M., Argmann, C., Gerhart-Hines, Z., Meziane, H., Lerin, C., Daussin, F., et al., 2006. Resveratrol improves mitochondrial function and protects against metabolic disease by activating SIRT1 and PGC-1alpha. Cell 127, 1109–1122.

la Porte, C., 2010. Steady-state pharmacokinetics and tolerability of trans-resveratrol 2000mg twice daily with food, quercetin and alcohol (ethanol) in healthy human subjects. Clin. Pharmacokinet.

Lazarov, O., Marr, R.A., 2013. Of mice and men: neurogenesis, cognition and Alzheimer's disease. Front. Aging Neurosci. 5, 43.

Liochev, S.I., 2013. Reactive oxygen species and the free radical theory of aging. Free Radic. Biol. Med. 60, 1–4.

Liu, D., Zhang, Q., Gu, J., Wang, X., Xie, K., Xian, X., et al., 2014. Resveratrol prevents impaired cognition induced by chronic unpredictable mild stress in rats. Prog. Neuropsychopharmacol. Biol. Psychiatry 49, 21–29.

MacDonald, L., Foster, B.C., Akhtar, H., 2009. Food and therapeutic product interactions - a therapeutic perspective. J. Pharm. Pharm. Sci. 12, 367–377.

Manach, C., Scalbert, A., Morand, C., Remesy, C., Jimenez, L., 2004. Polyphenols: food sources and bioavailability. Am. J. Clin. Nutr. 79, 727–747.

Mao, F., Yan, J., Li, J., Jia, X., Miao, H., Sun, Y., et al., 2014. New multi-target-directed small molecules against Alzheimer's disease: a combination of resveratrol and clioquinol. Org. Biomol. Chem. 12, 5936–5944.

Marambaud, P., Zhao, H., Davies, P., 2005. Resveratrol promotes clearance of Alzheimer's disease amyloid-beta peptides. J. Biol. Chem. 280, 37377–37382.

McAnulty, L.S., Miller, L.E., Hosick, P.A., Utter, A.C., Quindry, J.C., McAnulty, S.R., 2013. Effect of resveratrol and quercetin supplementation on redox status and inflammation after exercise. Appl. Physiol. Nutr. Metab. 38, 760–765.

Misiak, B., Leszek, J., Kiejna, A., 2012. Metabolic syndrome, mild cognitive impairment and Alzheimer's disease--the emerging role of systemic low-grade inflammation and adiposity. Brain Res. Bull. 89, 144–149.

Novelle, M.G., Wahl, D., Dieguez, C., Bernier, M., de Cabo, R., 2015. Resveratrol supplementation: where are we now and where should we go? Ageing Res. Rev. 21, 1–15.

Nurk, E., Refsum, H., Drevon, C.A., Tell, G.S., Nygaard, H.A., Engedal, K., et al., 2009. Intake of flavonoid-rich wine, tea, and chocolate by elderly men and women is associated with better cognitive test performance. J. Nutr. 139, 120–127.

Oomen, C.A., Farkas, E., Roman, V., van der Beek, E.M., Luiten, P.G., Meerlo, P., 2009. Resveratrol preserves cerebrovascular density and cognitive function in aging mice. Front Aging Neurosci. 1, 4.

Pangeni, R., Sahni, J.K., Ali, J., Sharma, S., Baboota, S., 2014. Resveratrol: review on therapeutic potential and recent advances in drug delivery. Exp. Opin. Drug Deliv. 11, 1285–1298.

Park, E.J., Pezzuto, J.M., 2015. The pharmacology of resveratrol in animals and humans. Biochim. Biophys. Acta 1852, 1071–1113.

Pasinetti, G.M., Wang, J., Ho, L., Zhao, W., Dubner, L., 2015. Roles of resveratrol and other grape-derived polyphenols in Alzheimer's disease prevention and treatment. Biochim. Biophys. Acta 1852, 1202–1208.

Patel, K.R., Scott, E., Brown, V.A., Gescher, A.J., Steward, W.P., Brown, K., 2011. Clinical trials of resveratrol. Ann N. Y. Acad. Sci. 1215, 161–169.

Pignatelli, P., Ghiselli, A., Buchetti, B., Carnevale, R., Natella, F., Germano, G., et al., 2006. Polyphenols synergistically inhibit oxidative stress in subjects given red and white wine. Atherosclerosis 188, 77–83.

Poulsen, M.M., Fjeldborg, K., Ornstrup, M.J., Kjaer, T.N., Nohr, M.K., Pedersen, S.B., 2015. Resveratrol and inflammation: Challenges in translating pre-clinical findings to improved patient outcomes. Biochim. Biophys. Acta 1852, 1124–1136.

Prehn, K., Jumpertz von Schwartzenberg, R., Mai, K., Zeitz, U., Witte, A.V., Hampel, D., et al., 2016. Caloric restriction in older adults-differential effects of weight loss and reduced weight on brain structure and function. Cereb. Cortex.

Rahvar, M., Nikseresht, M., Shafiee, S.M., Naghibalhossaini, F., Rasti, M., Panjehshahin, M.R., et al., 2011. Effect of oral resveratrol on the BDNF gene expression in the hippocampus of the rat brain. Neurochem. Res. 36, 761–765.

Rege, S.D., Geetha, T., Griffin, G.D., Broderick, T.L., Babu, J.R., 2014. Neuroprotective effects of resveratrol in Alzheimer disease pathology. Front. Aging Neurosci. 6, 218.

Robinson, K., Mock, C., Liang, D., 2015. Pre-formulation studies of resveratrol. Drug Dev. Ind. Pharm. 41, 1464–1469.

Roth, G.S., Ingram, D.K., 2015. Calorie Restriction Mimetics: Progress and Potential. Nutrition, Exercise and Epigenetics: Ageing Interventions 2, 211–243.

Rothwell, J.A., Perez-Jimenez, J., Neveu, V., Medina-Remon, A., M'Hiri, N., Garcia-Lobato, P., et al., 2013. Phenol-Explorer 3.0: a major update of the Phenol-Explorer database to incorporate data on the effects of food processing on polyphenol content. Database (Oxford), 2013. bat070.

Russo, M., Sansone, L., Polletta, L., Runci, A., Rashid, M., Santis, E., et al., 2014. sirtuins and resveratrol-derived compounds: a model for understanding the beneficial effects of the mediterranean diet. Endocr. Metab. Immune Disorders-Drug Targets 14, 300–308.

Scapagnini, G., Davinelli, S., Kaneko, T., Koverech, G., Koverech, A., Calabrese, E.J., et al., 2014. Dose response biology of resveratrol in obesity. J. Cell Commun. Signal. 8, 385–391.

Schmatz, R., Mazzanti, C.M., Spanevello, R., Stefanello, N., Gutierres, J., Correa, M., et al., 2009. Resveratrol prevents memory deficits and the increase in acetylcholinesterase activity in streptozotocin-induced diabetic rats. Eur. J. Pharmacol. 610, 42–48.

Semba, R.D., Ferrucci, L., Bartali, B., Urpi-Sarda, M., Zamora-Ros, R., Sun, K., et al., 2014. Resveratrol levels and all-cause mortality in older community-dwelling adults. JAMA Intern. Med. 174, 1077–1084.

Simao, F., Matte, A., Pagnussat, A.S., Netto, C.A., Salbego, C.G., 2012. Resveratrol prevents CA1 neurons against ischemic injury by parallel modulation of both GSK-3beta and CREB through PI3-K/Akt pathways. Eur. J. Neurosci. 36, 2899–2905.

Singh, C.K., Ndiaye, M.A., Ahmad, N., 2015. Resveratrol and cancer: challenges for clinical translation. Biochim. Biophys. Acta 1852, 1178–1185.

Skroza, D., Generalić Mekinić, I., Svilović, S., Šimat, V., Katalinić, V., 2015. Investigation of the potential synergistic effect of resveratrol with other phenolic compounds: a case of binary phenolic mixtures. J. Food Compos. Anal. 38, 13–18.

Small, B.J., Rawson, K.S., Martin, C., Eisel, S.L., Sanberg, C.D., McEvoy, C.L., et al., 2014. Nutraceutical intervention improves older adults' cognitive functioning. Rejuvenation Res. 17, 27–32.

Smoliga, J., Blanchard, O., 2014. Enhancing the delivery of resveratrol in humans: if low bioavailability is the problem, what is the solution? Molecules 19, 17154–17172.

Smoliga, J.M., Baur, J.A., Hausenblas, H.A., 2011. Resveratrol and health--a comprehensive review of human clinical trials. Mol. Nutr. Food Res. 55, 1129–1141.

Smoliga, J.M., Colombo, E.S., Campen, M.J., 2013. A healthier approach to clinical trials evaluating resveratrol for primary prevention of age-related diseases in healthy populations. Aging (Albany NY) 5, 495–506.

Spanier, G., Xu, H., Xia, N., Tobias, S., Deng, S., Wojnowski, L., et al., 2009. Resveratrol reduces endothelial oxidative stress by modulating the gene expression of superoxide dismutase 1 (SOD1), glutathione peroxidase 1 (GPx1) and NADPH oxidase subunit (Nox4). J. Physiol. Pharmacol. 60 (Suppl 4), 111–116.

Szkudelski, T., Szkudelska, K., 2015. Resveratrol and diabetes: from animal to human studies. Biochim. Biophys. Acta 1852, 1145–1154.

Tellone, E., Galtieri, A., Russo, A., Giardina, B., Ficarra, S., 2015. Resveratrol: a focus on several neurodegenerative diseases. Oxid. Med. Cell. Longev. 2015, 1–14.

Turner, R.S., Thomas, R.G., Craft, S., van Dyck, C.H., Mintzer, J., Reynolds, B.A., et al., 2015. A randomized, double-blind, placebo-controlled trial of resveratrol for Alzheimer disease. Neurology.

Vang, O., 2015. Resveratrol: challenges in analyzing its biological effects. Ann. N. Y. Acad. Sci. 1348, 161–170.

Vaz-da-Silva, M., Loureiro, A.I., Falcao, A., Nunes, T., Rocha, J.F., Fernandes-Lopes, C., et al., 2008. Effect of food on the pharmacokinetic profile of trans-resveratrol. Int. J. Clin. Pharmacol. Ther. 46, 564–570.

Virmani, A., Pinto, L., Binienda, Z., Ali, S., 2013. Food, nutrigenomics, and neurodegeneration--neuroprotection by what you eat!. Mol. Neurobiol. 48, 353–362.

Vitaglione, P., Sforza, S., Galaverna, G., Ghidini, C., Caporaso, N., Vescovi, P.P., et al., 2005. Bioavailability of trans-resveratrol from red wine in humans. Mol. Nutr. Food Res. 49, 495–504.

Vlachogianni, I.C., Fragopoulou, E., Kostakis, I.K., Antonopoulou, S., 2015. In vitro assessment of antioxidant activity of tyrosol, resveratrol and their acetylated derivatives. Food Chem. 177, 165–173.

Walle, T., 2011. Bioavailability of resveratrol. Ann. N. Y. Acad. Sci. 1215, 9–15.

Wang, B., Sun, J., Li, X., Zhou, Q., Bai, J., Shi, Y., et al., 2013. Resveratrol prevents suppression of regulatory T-cell production, oxidative stress, and inflammation of mice prone or resistant to high-fat diet-induced obesity. Nutr. Res. 33, 971–981.

Wang, J., Bi, W., Cheng, A., Freire, D., Vempati, P., Zhao, W., et al., 2014. Targeting multiple pathogenic mechanisms with polyphenols for the treatment of Alzheimer's disease-experimental approach and therapeutic implications. Front. Aging Neurosci. 6, 42.

Wightman, E.L., Reay, J.L., Haskell, C.F., Williamson, G., Dew, T.P., Kennedy, D.O., 2014. Effects of resveratrol alone or in combination with piperine on cerebral blood flow parameters and cognitive performance in human subjects: a randomised, double-blind, placebo-controlled, cross-over investigation. Br. J. Nutr. 112, 203–213.

Wightman, E.L., Haskell-Ramsay, C.F., Reay, J.L., Williamson, G., Dew, T., Zhang, W., et al., 2015. The effects of chronic trans-resveratrol supplementation on aspects of cognitive function, mood, sleep, health and cerebral blood flow in healthy, young humans. Br. J. Nutr. 114, 1427–1437.

Witte, A.V., Fobker, M., Gellner, R., Knecht, S., Floel, A., 2009. Caloric restriction improves memory in elderly humans. Proc. Natl. Acad. Sci. USA 106, 1255–1260.

Witte, A.V., Kerti, L., Margulies, D.S., Floel, A., 2014. Effects of resveratrol on memory performance, hippocampal functional connectivity, and glucose metabolism in healthy older adults. J. Neurosci. 34, 7862–7870.

Wood, J.G., Rogina, B., Lavu, S., Howitz, K., Helfand, S.L., Tatar, M., et al., 2004. Sirtuin activators mimic caloric restriction and delay ageing in metazoans. Nature 2004, 686.

Wyss-Coray, T., Rogers, J., 2012. Inflammation in Alzheimer disease - a brief review of the basic science and clinical literature. Cold Spring Harb. Perspect. Med. 2, a006346.

Yazir, Y., Utkan, T., Gacar, N., Aricioglu, F., 2015. Resveratrol exerts anti-inflammatory and neuroprotective effects to prevent memory deficits in rats exposed to chronic unpredictable mild stress. Physiol. Behav. 138, 297–304.

Zhang, F., Liu, J., Shi, J.S., 2010. Anti-inflammatory activities of resveratrol in the brain: role of resveratrol in microglial activation. Eur. J. Pharmacol. 636, 1–7.

Zhao, H.F., Li, N., Wang, Q., Cheng, X.J., Li, X.M., Liu, T.T., 2015. Resveratrol decreases the insoluble Abeta1-42 level in hippocampus and protects the integrity of the blood-brain barrier in AD rats. Neuroscience 310, 641–649.

Zordoky, B.N., Robertson, I.M., Dyck, J.R., 2015. Preclinical and clinical evidence for the role of resveratrol in the treatment of cardiovascular diseases. Biochim. Biophys. Acta 1852, 1155–1177.

CHAPTER

25

North American Natural Health Products and Sexual Function in Aging Adults

Ruben Maya-Luevano, Jake Alexander Clor and Maria Pontes Ferreira

Wayne State University, Detroit, MI, United States

INTRODUCTION

Globally, the number of aging people 60 years and older is expected to more than double from 841 million people in 2013 to more than 2 billion by 2050 (United Nations, 2013). People in North America have among the highest life expectancies in the world (Rodrigues et al., 2012). Approximately 14% of people (one person in every seven) from the United States of America (US) is part of the older population (65 years and older). United States citizens in this age group have increased from 36 million in 2003 to 45 million in 2013 (a 25% increase), and their numbers are projected to more than double to 98 million in 2060 (US Department of Health and Human Services, 2014). In Canada, senior citizens make up the fastest-growing age group. In 2011, an estimated 5 million Canadians were in the age bracket of 65 years and older. That number is expected to double in the next 25 years to reach 10 million by 2036. It is projected that by 2051 about one in four Canadians will be 65 years or older (Employment and Social Development Canada, 2016).

From a global standpoint, the idea of "healthy aging" or "aging well" is a concept embraced by many older adults. Moreover, sexual dysfunction among aging adults is an important public health concern. In men, impotence is a major well-being concern and is associated with aging (Feldman et al., 2000). From 40% to 60% of older women in the US are affected by sexual dysfunction (Ambler et al., 2012). Older adults are inclined to use dietary supplements, also known as natural health products (NHPs), as a remedy for sexual dysfunction. As a class, NHPs include herbal preparations, vitamin and mineral supplements, and traditional and homeopathic medicines (Vohra et al., 2012).

Natural health products have been used in a variety of styles of medicine such as traditional Chinese medicine (TCM) and traditional Indian, or Ayurvedic, medicine. For example, *Panax ginseng* is an herbal aphrodisiac that has been used by the Chinese to increase libido in men (Chan, 2012). The use of NHPs in different traditional styles of medicine have encouraged scientists to further study their bioactive components (Chan, 2012). Unfortunately, traditional Native American medicine and derived natural health products from North American organisms are underappreciated. Thus, in this brief literature review, we will discuss possible therapeutic value of native North American bioactive organisms for sexual function, with a focus on aging adults.

To provide a sampling of native North American organisms or derived NHPs that may improve the sex lives of aging adults, we have separated this review into the five life kingdoms: Animalia, Plantae, Monera (Bacteria), Fungi, and Protista. We will discuss the topic of sexual dysfunction by introducing two different organisms per kingdom; each organism is discussed briefly in regards to traditional uses and followed by evidence-based studies.

Nutrition and Functional Foods for Healthy Aging.
DOI: http://dx.doi.org/10.1016/B978-0-12-805376-8.00025-3

KINGDOM ANIMALIA

Organisms belonging to the biological kingdom Animalia are eukaryotic and multicellular—that is, their tissues are made of cells and have a nucleus enclosed by a nuclear membrane. The cells have a cell membrane but lack rigid cell walls unlike members of the Plantae, Bacteria, and Fungi kingdoms. Animals are heterotrophs, meaning that they obtain their energy from feeding on other living organisms.

Caribou (*Rangifer tarandus*) Antler Velvet as a Sexual Stimulant

According to Save the Rhino International, someone who possesses a rhinoceros horn in countries such as China and Vietnam is seen as having elevated social status. Apart from the common image of the horn as a status symbol for elites, when powdered, the rhino horn is highly regarded as an ingestible sexual stimulant that can improve a man's sexual life (Puri, 2010). It is thus no surprise that rhinoceros poaching has become a big problem throughout the nations of southern Africa, driven by a growing demand for horns among Asian countries (Becker, 2012).

Despite a common Vietnamese belief that the rhino's horn has aphrodisiac properties, no scientific data support these claims (Puri, 2010). This folkloric reputation has contributed greatly to the endangerment of this species (Puri, 2010). Researchers from Save the Rhino International claim that when poachers from China and Vietnam tranquilize rhinos to cut their horns, they leave the animals to bleed to death.

Antler velvet from caribou (*Rangifer tarandus*), a North American reindeer, has been similarly used as a supplement by men and women to stimulate sexual desire (Caspari and Robbins, 2003). While the antler is still growing, a vascular skin known as *velvet* covers it (Hall, 2005), supplying nutrients and oxygen to the growing bone (Hall, 2005). Unlike rhinoceros horn, velvet and antlers can regenerate every year (Puri, 2010). Research has been conducted in Canada, New Zealand, Japan, Korea, and China showing that antler velvet from *R. tarandus* demonstrates androgenic and gonadotrophic effects that may help regulate the physiological processes of sex organs in men and women (Puri, 2010). For example, pantocrin is a natural product that can be extracted from velvet from *R. tarandus* antlers and consumed by people, purportedly to increase libido.

Not many studies have been done to find strong evidence that antler velvet actually functions as a sexual stimulant or is a possible remedy for sexual dysfunction (Puri, 2010), so it awaits further scientific determination of clinical efficacy regarding its potential as a sexual stimulant.

Blood Clam (*Scapharca broughtonii*) and Fertility

Bivalves are a class of shellfish common around the world. Their hinged two-part shells enclose all of their organs and muscles. These marine and coastal organisms have been important sources of protein for humans for thousands of years (Pauls, 2014). Shellfish meat, particularly that of oysters, has traditionally been described as having aphrodisiac properties that enhance sexual function. Like that of many bivalves, the meat of the blood clam, *Scapharca broughtonii*, can be eaten raw and prepared in dishes such as Japanese sushi (Sato et al., 1987).

S. broughtonii belongs to the family Arcidae and is found along East Asia's northwestern Pacific coast. It plays a commercially important role throughout East Asia (Yu et al., 2015). A common molecule found in the muscle extracts of *S. broughtonii* is *N*-Methyl-D-aspartic acid (NMDA). This blood clam is believed to be the first identified source containing NMDA (Sato et al., 1987). Moreover, D-aspartate, an amino acid, has been isolated from *S. broughtonii* (Tsesarskaia et al., 2009). This amino acid has been found to be present in numerous bivalves and snails (Shibata et al., 2001) (Figs. 25.1 and 25.2).

D-aspartate and NMDA are classified as amino acids and primary metabolites. Both are present in the neuroendocrine systems of vertebrates and invertebrates, where they contribute to the production and release of hormones (Tsesarskaia et al., 2009). NMDA is known as an agonist for some central nervous system glutamate receptors (Tarui et al., 2003). Lesser known, however, is the mechanism of action by which D-aspartate influences sexual function or the quality of spermatozoa (or both) (D'Aniello et al., 2012).

Studies have found that a correlation exists between supplementation of D-aspartate and semen concentration and semen quality in humans (D'Aniello et al., 2012). Oral doses of D-aspartate over the course of two to three months have been found to significantly improve spermatozoa count and mobility (D'Aniello et al., 2012). This in turn may improve human fertility. Due to limited populations of *S. broughtonii*, research into identifying new species containing D-aspartate and NMDA could be beneficial. Since bivalves have been found to be rich in D-aspartate, bivalves in the family Arcidae of North America's coastal regions could be studied as functional foods for sexual function promotion and fertility in men.

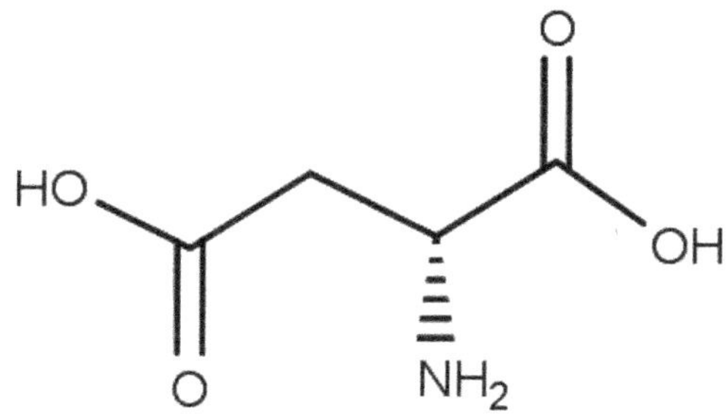

FIGURE 25.1 D-aspartate (aspartic acid) found in *Scapharca broughtonii*.

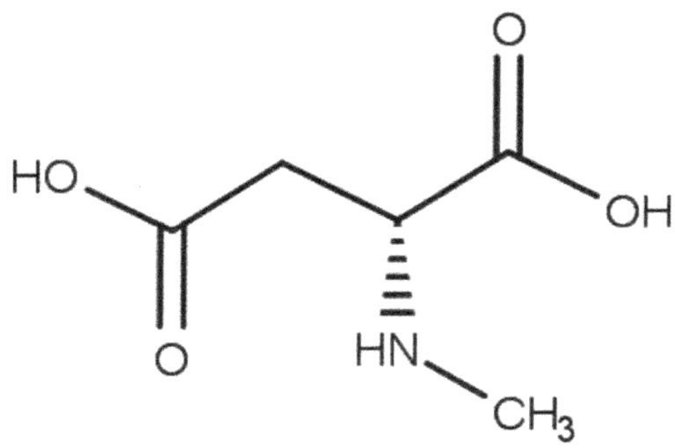

FIGURE 25.2 *N*-Methyl-D-aspartic acid found in *Scapharca broughtonii*.

KINGDOM PLANTAE

Plants are eukaryotes and belong to the kingdom Plantae. Unlike animal cells, plant cells have cell walls composed of a polysaccharide known as *cellulose*, the most common organic molecule on the planet. Plants use photosynthetic processes to create food energy, and are autotrophs. Most plants appear green due to the chlorophyll pigment found in chloroplasts.

Saw Palmetto (*Serenoa repens*) and Prostate Health

Serenoa repens, or saw palmetto, is a small shrublike palm native to the southern United States, including Florida, Mississippi, Georgia, South Carolina, and Louisiana (Anderson and Oakes, 2012). Growing in soil that is acidic, basic, moist, or dry (Anderson and Oakes, 2012), *S. repens* is the most abundant palm in the United States (Bennett and Hicklin, 1998). Its drupaceous fruit becomes ripe from August to October. Native Americans used multiple parts of the abundant *S. repens* plant. The leaves have traditionally been used to make thatched roofs and baskets (Bennett and Hicklin, 1998). In addition, various societies throughout the Americas have used palms in traditional medicine (Sosnowska and Balslev, 2009).

Focus has been increasing on using plant-based therapies to treat prostate disorders, with some of those therapies incorporating *S. repens* (Sosnowska and Balslev, 2009). Phytotherapeutic formulations prepared from the fruit of *S. repens* include liquid extracts, dried berries, powders, and tinctures (Penugonda and Lindshield, 2013). Two of the principal phytochemicals present in *S. repens* are its phytosterols and fatty acids (Penugonda and Lindshield, 2013). Phytosterols are found in plant cells and are cholesterol-like molecules (Ostlund, 2002). Phytosterols, particularly preparations of β-sitosterol, have been successfully used to treat symptoms of benign prostatic hyperplasia (BPH) (Higdon, 2007). The major fatty acids present in *S. repens* are lauric, myristic, palmitic, stearic, oleic, and linoleic (Penugonda and Lindshield, 2013) (Figs. 25.3 and 25.4).

Benign prostatic hyperplasia is a noncancerous enlargement of the prostrate. Fatty acids and phytosterols of *S. repens* may act to inhibit the enzyme 5α-reductase (De Monte et al., 2014). This enzyme may contribute to BPH by converting testosterone to dihydrotestosterone. Benign prostatic hyperplasia has been shown to be correlated with lower quality of life in men, which may include reduced sexual function such as by erectile dysfunction (Bruskewitz, 2003). Treatment of BPH could thus improve male sexual drive and erectile function. Although supplements and

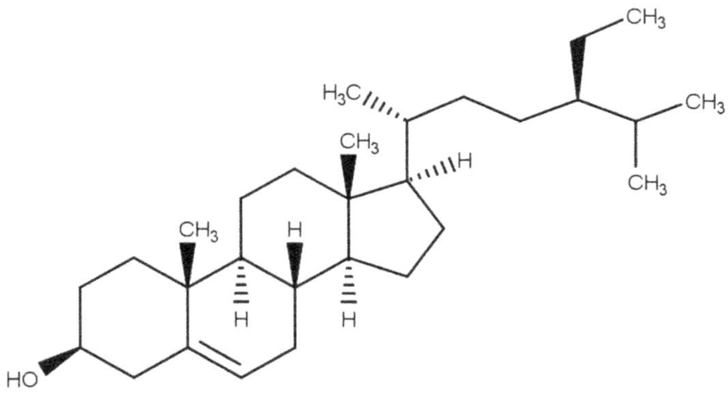

FIGURE 25.3 β-sitosterol, one of the major phytosterols present in *Serenoa repens*.

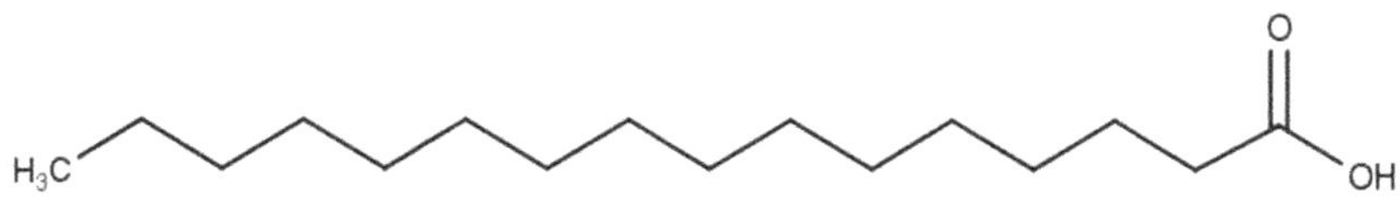

FIGURE 25.4 Palmitic acid, one of the major fatty acids present in *Serenoa repens*.

extracts from *S. repens* have been used in randomized clinical trials, relatively few studies have evaluated the composition of the different preparations used in the randomized clinical trials (Penugonda and Lindshield, 2013).

Studies have shown *S. repens* to have few side effects in treating BPH, while surgery and less invasive medical approaches can cause erectile and ejaculatory dysfunction (Orabi et al., 2011). Although few studies have evaluated the phytochemicals from various extracts of *S. repens*, the low reported side effects when using this botanical to treat BPH make it worthy of further study.

Damiana (*Turnera diffusa*) as an Herbal Aphrodisiac

Damiana (*Turnera diffusa*) has been used by both men and women as an herbal aphrodisiac since the ancient Mayan civilization (Balch and Bell, 2012). This small to medium-sized perennial plant is native to southwestern Texas in the United States and then southward through Mexico, Central America, the Caribbean, and South America (Everitt et al., 2002). *Turnera diffusa* can grow up to one to two meters tall, and its leaves are generally clustered (Everitt et al., 2002). Damiana leaves contain as much as 1% volatile oil consisting of 1,8-cineole, p-cymene, alpha and beta-pinene, thymol, alpha-copaene, and calamine (Kumar and Arora, 2013).

Damiana leaves are dried to make a tisane (herbal tea) or for smoking. In addition, *T. diffusa* is also available in capsules and as liquid extracts (tinctures) (Balch and Bell, 2012). Damiana is on the US Food and Drug Administration's so-called GRAS list (generally recognized as safe) and is often used as food flavoring (Kumar and Arora, 2013). The plant is found mainly in traditional herbal remedy products in combination with other botanicals such as *Cola nitida* (cola) and *Serenoa repens* (saw palmetto). Indigenous Mexican women currently make a natural herbal product by steeping 30 g of leaves into one liter of tequila for one week to obtain an aphrodisiac liquor that is reportedly consumed to enhance lovemaking (Porras, 2013).

Among various published studies on this botanical, one clinical study involving 1000 men in the United States and Europe showed that damiana can relieve erectile failure when a man attempts to repeat intercourse after an orgasm (Balch and Bell, 2012). In addition, taking a combination of damiana and the flowering plant muira puama (*Ptychopetalum olacoides*) has been associated with an increase of morning erections and sustained erection during intercourse (Balch and Bell, 2012). Of 77 participants in one double-blind placebo-controlled study, 34 women were given a nutritional supplement (Arginmax) containing damiana extract for four weeks, and 43 were given placebos. The women who received Arginmax showed an improvement in sexual desire, reduction in vaginal dryness, and improvement in clitoral sensation (Kumar et al., 2005). Unlike other uncontrolled studies evaluating damiana's efficacy in women, this study utilized a control group. Thus, the findings of this study are more suggestive of damiana's effectiveness in women who ingested this nutritional supplement.

Furthermore, an animal-based study was conducted in an effort to validate the traditional use of the plant for sexual dysfunction and impotence. A group of researchers in Italy administered a hydroalcoholic extract from the leaves of *T. diffusa* to sexually potent and sexually inactive or impotent rats (Arletti et al., 1999). This intervention study demonstrated that the extract had no effect on sexually potent rats but did improve the copulatory performance of the sexually inactive or impotent rats and increased the percentage of rats achieving ejaculation (Arletti et al., 1999).

Overall, however, scientific evidence that supports damiana's so-called aphrodisiac properties is lacking; these properties have not been demonstrated in humans. However, studies evaluating damiana's efficacy in male rats has indicated an improved sexual function (Edwards et al., 2015), making this botanical worthy of further research to better understand its use as a potential remedy for sexual dysfunction in aging humans.

KINGDOM BACTERIA

Bacteria fall into two different groupings: Bacteria and Archaea. The two species we have researched are from Kingdom Bacteria. These are single-celled prokaryotic organisms, meaning their DNA is not contained in a membrane-bound nucleus. Species of bacteria can be *heterotrophic* (requiring complex organic compounds of nitrogen and carbon) or *autotrophic* (requiring only carbon dioxide or carbonates as a source of carbon). Moreover, some species from the kingdom Bacteria are useful in industries such as food production and pharmaceuticals.

Lactic Acid Bacteria (*Lactobacillus*), Probiotics, and Vaginal Health

Portions of the human body in contact with the external environment—skin, mucous membranes, and gastrointestinal tract—are host to an extensive variety of microorganisms known as the *microbiota* (Petrova et al., 2015). Establishment of the human microbiome begins after birth and largely resembles that of an adult by two years of age (Luoto et al., 2013). The human microbiota can be supplemented with so-called good bacteria through the consumption of probiotic foods—that is, foods containing live microorganisms.

Throughout human history and across cultures, people have consumed probiotic foods. The diet of many indigenous Hawaiians contains a probiotic food called *poi* (Brown and Valiere, 2004). Poi is made from the underground stems of the taro plant (*Colocasia esculenta* L.), which are called *corms*. Once the corms are cooked and crushed, the resulting paste is fermented with lactic acid bacteria and yeasts that naturally occur on the plant's surface (Brown and Valiere, 2004). Poi preparations often contain several species of the genus *Lactobacillus*.

In recent years, the market for probiotic foods in the United States has noticeably expanded (Vanderhoof and Young, 2008). Yogurt and sauerkraut are examples of two probiotic foods common in Western cuisine. In North America, probiotics are commonly consumed as food or taken as dietary supplements to augment the gastrointestinal tract's health and function (Vanderhoof and Young, 2008). One of the common bioactive components of many probiotic foods and supplements are species of *Lactobacillus*, which are rod-shaped gram-positive bacteria (Schillinger, 1999). As lactic acid bacteria, they produce lactic acid from hexose sugars (Makarova et al., 2006). This acid contributes to the taste of many probiotic foods and can have important roles in human health.

Lactobacilli are the primary microbes present in the vaginal microbiota or flora (Barrons and Tassone, 2008). One way that these species regulate the vaginal ecosystem is by lowering pH. Maintaining a low vaginal pH is important to prevent the overgrowth of pathogenic bacteria leading to infections and bacterial vaginosis, the overgrowth of undesirable vaginal bacteria (Barrons and Tassone, 2008). The processes that maintain vaginal *Lactobacilli* growth and pH in reproductive-aged women are altered in postmenopausal women due partly to the thinning of the vaginal wall (Hoffmann et al., 2014). In a five-year study of postmenopausal women, Hoffmann et al. (2014) found that the prevalence of bacterial vaginosis increases with age.

Low levels of *Lactobacilli* in vaginal microbota can be treated with the help of probiotics. Many probiotic remedies are taken orally as food or supplements, although they can also be administered locally as vaginal suppositories, capsules, or tablets. Local administration (insertion of a vaginal suppository, capsule, or tablet) allows for direct colonization and increased control in probiotic remedies (Palmeira-de-Oliveira et al., 2015). Clinical data suggest that local administration of probiotics can help promote faster treatment of bacterial vaginosis and prevent recurrence (Palmeira-de-Oliveira et al., 2015). Since there are yet few remedies of this kind available, additional research is necessary to further develop topical probiotics for vaginal flora renewal.

Bartonella henselae and Regeneration of Blood Vessels

The prevalence of diabetes in aging US men (65 years and older) remains high at 26%, or 12 million seniors (American Diabetes Association, 2014). A meta-analysis by Agardh et al. (2011) estimates that diabetes will reach 300 million people worldwide by 2025. One complication of diabetes is vascular abnormalities that contribute to deficient blood flow into the penis and damaged blood vessels, which in turn serves as a possible explanation for the increased rate of erectile dysfunction among men with diabetes (Várkonyi and Kempler, 2014). Researchers at the Washington University School of Medicine in St. Louis have found a key mechanism that appears to contribute to the damage of blood vessels in diabetes (Dryden, 2007). Through studies utilizing rodent models, these researchers found two enzymes that have been linked to blood vessel damage: fatty acid synthase (FAS) and nitric oxide synthase (NOS) (Dryden, 2007).

These researchers conducted a study in which nondiabetic mice were genetically engineered to make FAS in all tissues except the endothelial cells lining the blood vessels (Dryden, 2007). These mice started to experience similar problems in their blood vessels as animals with diabetes. People with type 1 or type 2 diabetes have low levels of FAS or defects in the FAS enzyme (Wei et al., 2010).

Palmitoylation is the mechanism whereby NOS is modified to bind normally to endothelial cells (Dryden, 2007). In the absence of FAS, the genetically engineered mice lose NOS palmitoylation and are thus unable to modify NOS to normally interact with the endothelial cell membrane. This leads to blood vessel problems, further inhibiting angiogenesis in mice (Dryden, 2007).

Medical biologists seeking novel regenerative therapies discovered a bacterium (*Bartonella henselae*) that secretes a protein known as Bartonella adhesion (BadA) (Riess and Raddatz, 2007). Work is underway to study this as a potential remedy for erectile dysfunction due to the protein's ability to regenerate blood vessels in men. *Bartonella henselae* is a rod-shaped bacteria formerly known as *Rochalimaea henselae* (Brenner and O'Connor, 1993). BadA promotes the formation of blood vessels (angiogenesis), thus making *B. henselae* potentially useful for application in regeneration biology (Autenrieth, 2006). BadA achieves this effect by stimulating the formation and release of host growth factors such as vasculoendothelial growth factor (Autenrieth, 2006). Further study of this bacteria could provide scientists with information about its utility as a remedy for erectile dysfunction in diabetic men after damage to blood vessels.

KINGDOM FUNGI

Fungi are heterotrophic organisms that absorb nutrients from their surroundings, which means they are *saprotrophs* and feed off decaying matter. Thus, in the environment, fungi have an important role in breaking down organic materials. In addition, fungi are eukaryotic organisms that range from unicellular to multicellular. Edible fungi are consumed by people around the world and have a variety of applications beyond their role as food.

Brewer's Yeast (*Saccharomyces cerevisiae*) and Alcohol Consumption in Adult Humans

In the Western world, alcohol consumption has long been associated with alleged aphrodisiac properties such as increased sexual desire (Hernandez and Alfonso, 1997). Across cultures, alcohol has occupied a variety of important niches. The ingredients and methods of its production, however, have largely varied regionally and throughout time.

Production of beer began around 6000 years ago in what is now Iraq (Schneiter, 2004). Mesoamerican cultures also engaged in the production of alcoholic beverages such as pulque, a nondistilled fermentation of the sap of *Agave atrovirens*, *A. mapisaga*, or *A. salmiana* (Lappe-Oliveiras et al., 2008). Distilled spirits such as tequila and mescal can also be prepared from agave plants. North American native hops (*Humulus lupulus*) and grapes (*Vitis riparia*) are among the ingredients used to make beer and wine, respectively.

Alcoholic beverages served a significant role in the religion, rituals, divination, and healing of precontact Mesoamericans (Lappe-Oliveiras et al., 2008). Traditional fermentations of alcoholic beverages, including those prepared by Amerindians, occurred spontaneously without pure (single species) cultures of yeast (Lappe-Oliveiras et al., 2008). Yeasts first began to be cultivated in pure cultures during the 1800s, with *Saccharomyces cerevisiae* first being isolated in Denmark (Schneiter, 2004). *Saccharomyces cerevisiae* and related yeast strains are currently the most commercially important yeasts (Schneiter, 2004).

Ethanol is miscible in the lipids of cellular membranes, and its effects are associated with gamma aminobutyric acid receptors and NMDA receptors in cell membranes (Gilbert, 2014). The effects of alcohol on sexual behavior have been found to be influenced by both cognitive processes and physiological action in humans (Hernandez and

Alfonso, 1997). Moreover, studies have found that an individual's acquired expectations associated with alcohol consumption may have the largest influence on its effect (Hernandez and Alfonso, 1997). This is important because expectations may vary widely from person to person or across cultures, including expectations of alcohol's aphrodisiac properties.

Malatesta et al. (1982) found that for both men and women a positive correlation existed between blood alcohol level, orgasmic latency, and difficulty in achieving orgasm. With increased alcohol consumption, both men and women experience decreased orgasmic responsiveness both physiologically and behaviorally. However, women in an experimental study of alcohol's influence on orgasmic response reported greater cognitive sexual arousal and enjoyment as reported in a postmasturbation questionnaire (Malatesta et al., 1982). In their review of the literature on alcohol's influence on sexual functioning and sexual arousal, George and Gilmore (2013) concluded that the decreases in genital response are limited to acute consumption of alcohol in high doses and chronic consumption of alcohol, a finding similar to those of Malatesta et al. (1982). These findings suggest that consumption of alcohol that is not excessive or chronic may have positive effects on sexual desire. Moderate consumption of alcohol can be defined as approximately 15–45 g of ethanol per day for those aged 45–65 years and 15–30 g for those over 65 years (Ferreira and Weems, 2008). Ferreira and Weems (2008) define a standard drink as one that contains 15 g of ethanol. Further study into the effects of alcohol consumption in moderate doses and the effects of positive alcohol expectancies on sexual desire in older adults is needed.

Maitake Mushrooms (*Grifola frondosa*) as a Fungal Natural Remedy for Insulin Resistance

Diabetes is classified as either type 1 (insulin-dependent diabetes mellitus) or type 2 (noninsulin-dependent diabetes mellitus) (Hong et al., 2007). As people age, chances of being diagnosed with type 2 diabetes increase (American Diabetes Association, 2014). As previously stated, global incidence of diabetes is predicted to rise (Agardh et al., 2011). Erectile dysfunction is a common complication in men caused by type 2 diabetes (Várkonyi and Kempler, 2014), affecting between 35% and 75% of men (Várkonyi and Kempler, 2014). Type 2 diabetes also can have negative effects on orgasmic and ejaculatory function and libido in males (Várkonyi and Kempler, 2014).

Some NHPs may act as therapeutic agents to improve the lifestyle of men with type 2 diabetes. The use of these natural products over a prolonged period of time also could be safer than pharmaceuticals (Hong et al., 2007). *Grifola frondosa* (the maitake mushroom) is a fungus native to eastern North America and is typically found near oak trees (Fischer, 2011). It is also commonly referred to as the 'hen of the woods' (Fischer, 2011).

One study on the efficacy of maitakes in improving type 2 diabetes focused on the enhancement of insulin sensitivity by using an extract of a glycoprotein from *G. frondosa* known as SX Fraction in spontaneously hypertensive rats (Preuss et al., 2007). Oral consumption of SX Fraction showed enhanced sensitivity to exogenous insulin, thus suggesting that a glycoprotein extract from maitakes (SX Fraction) could be considered as an alternative method for improving insulin sensitivity. Moreover, reducing the insulin resistance associated with type 2 diabetes could improve its comorbidities (Preuss et al., 2007).

The results of this study and what we know about the association between type 2 diabetes and erectile dysfunction suggests a need for further research into the efficacy of *G. frondosa* as a nutraceutical.

KINGDOM PROTISTA

The colloquial definition of the Protista kingdom has often been described as being the collection of all organisms that do not fit into other life kingdoms. Protists can be heterotrophic or autotrophic. Protista contains widely diverse unicellular as well as multicellular organisms. Multicellular protists do not have differentiated tissues. In addition, protists are eukaryotic organisms that contain a nucleus. Protists are found throughout the world in moist environments.

Red Algae (*Chondrus crispus*), Carrageenan, and Sexual Lubricants

In a recent review, longitudinal studies have shown that diminished sexual function and vaginal dryness are commonly reported symptoms of postmenopausal women (Grant et al., 2015). Genitourinary syndrome of menopause (GSM) is a group of symptoms related to the decrease of estrogen and sex steroids in aging women and include genital dryness, irritation, and sexual dysfunction due to poor vaginal lubrication (Portman and Gass, 2014). Symptoms of GSM are undertreated because vulvovaginal health issues are typically not discussed by physicians with their patients (Goldstein et al., 2013). Poor vaginal lubrication can be treated with the use of sexual lubricants. A current area of research is in natural sexual lubricants derived from seaweed gels.

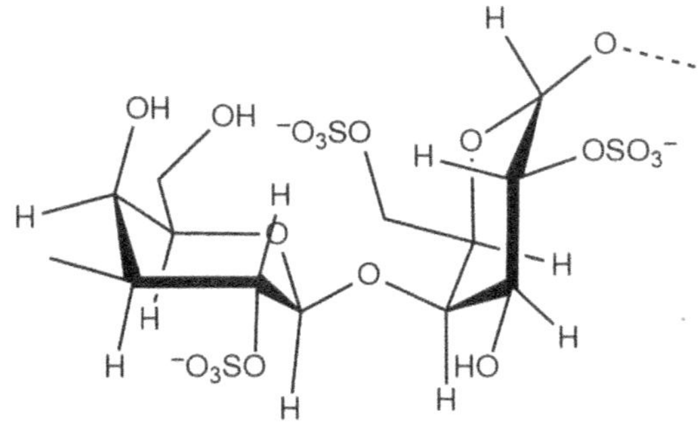

FIGURE 25.5 Skeletal structure of lambda carrageenan found in *Chondrus crispus*.

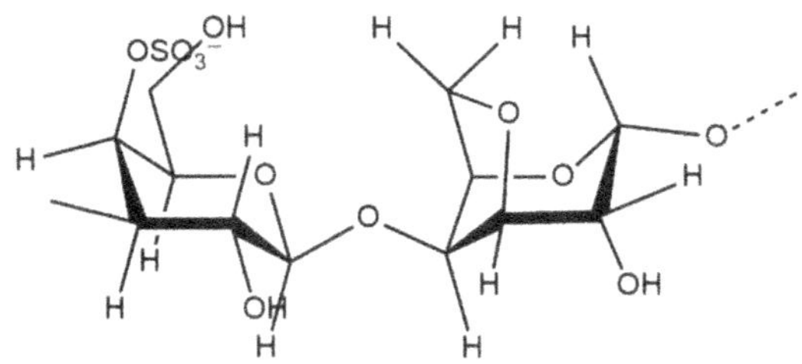

FIGURE 25.6 Skeletal structure of kappa carrageenan found in *Chondrus crispus*.

The earliest recorded uses of seaweed are described in Chinese literature. Seaweed-based lubricants were traditionally used for sexual intercourse. The Chinese harvested seaweed for medical use as long ago as 3000 B.C.E.; however, the practice of farming seaweed only originated within the last 400 years in Asia (Nash, 2011). Currently, red seaweeds have an economically important role throughout the world due to the presence of phycocolloids such as carrageenan (Pangestuti and Kim, 2014). Carrageenan has a variety of applications in food production as a thickener and stabilizer in dairy products, puddings, canned pet foods, imitation creams, and syrups (Buck et al., 2006; Rogers, 2011). In the United States and Canada, the red algae genus *Chondrus* is the primary source of carrageenans (Rogers, 2011). *Chondrus crispus* or irish moss, which can be found in the United States, contains kappa and lambda carrageenan (Prajapati et al., 2014) (Figs. 25.5 and 25.6).

A study in Thailand of the carrageenan-based lubricant Carraguard found that a majority of couples using this product reported increased sexual pleasure (Martin et al., 2010). The potential for carrageenan-based products to alleviate sexual dysfunction due to vaginal dryness in postmenopausal women is an avenue for research and development. Moreover, addressing the symptoms of GSM can positively influence the quality of life of postmenopausal women (Hyun-Kyung et al., 2015). An additional benefit of sexual lubricants made from the sulfated polysaccharide carrageenan is its use in preventing the transmission of disease (Buck et al., 2006). Carrageenan has been found to be inhibitory to papillomavirus infection in vitro and has potential for use as a microbicide (Buck et al., 2006). In a double-blind, randomized study, Marais et al. (2011) found that high-risk human papillomavirus prevalence was lower among compliant Carraguard users than among compliant placebo users. Carrageenan acts to inhibit viruses by preventing the entry of virions into cells and the binding of virions (Prajapati et al., 2014). Use of carrageenan-based lubricants to improve vaginal dryness and decrease infection make carrageenan an important focus for future research.

Brown Algae (*Laminaria digitata*) as a Source of Iodine for Thyroid Function

Thyroid dysfunction is a prevalent morbidity associated with aging in adults. Bensenor et al. (2012) state that treating and diagnosing hypothyroidism in aging adults is especially important because symptoms of thyroid dysfunction can be difficult to discern from the normal process of aging. More women experience thyroid issues than men, but its prevalence among all people older than 60 years was found to be 4.4% by the Framingham Heart Study (Sawin et al., 1985). Complications with thyroid function in aging adults can be associated with variations in levels of hormones that augment the function of the thyroid. Clinical diagnosis of thyroid disorders often entails measures of thyroid-stimulating hormone, triiodothyronine, and free thyroxine levels (Bensenor et al., 2012). Diagnosis of thyroid disorders among aging adults is important due to the comorbidities that are associated with thyroid dysfunction.

Many studies have found erectile dysfunction among men with thyroid dysfunctions (hypothyroidism or hyperthyroidism) to be elevated. A study designed to investigate the impact of thyroid dysfunction on sexual health by means of a Sexual Health Inventory for Males questionnaire found that men with thyroid dysfunctions were significantly more likely to have some degree of erectile dysfunction than those who did not have thyroid disorders (Krassas et al., 2008). Another study found that in the age group of 51–80 years, erectile dysfunction scores (as scored by questionnaire) were significantly better in those without thyroid disorders than in those with thyroid disorders (Veronelli et al., 2006). Although a relationship is present between thyroid disorders and erectile dysfunction, more research is necessary to determine the causes of the association.

Although not all thyroid disorders are caused by iodine deficiency, proper function of the thyroid requires optimal dietary iodine intake (Laurberg et al., 2010). Laurberg et al., (2010) also notes that severe iodine deficiency increases the risk of hypothyroidism, while moderate iodine deficiency increases the risk of both hypothyroidism and hyperthyroidism. This shows that a suboptimal intake of iodine can contribute to thyroid disorder and could potentially contribute to erectile dysfunction. A rich food source of iodine is seaweed, which concentrates iodine found in the ocean. In a study of 14 species of seaweed consumed by humans, Desideri et al. (2016) found that *Laminaria digitata* contained the highest concentration of iodine. *Laminaria digitata* is found in the northern Atlantic Ocean and is commonly distributed along the Atlantic coast of North America from Greenland to Cape Cod. This suggests that *L. digitata* should be further researched for use as an iodine-rich functional food. Further research could help to understand the connection between thyroid disorders and erectile dysfunction.

DISCUSSION

Natural health products derived from native North American organisms from the five biological kingdoms have the potential to improve a variety of conditions that inhibit sexual function in aging men and women. For example, erectile dysfunction has been shown to be potentially treatable by natural health products and derivative natural products. Moreover, several comorbidities associated with inhibited sexual function in older adults such as prostate health, vaginosis, and diabetes can be improved with natural health products. One weakness we discovered in our review of the current literature on natural health products for sexual function was in the paucity of clinical evidence for the efficacy of such agents. Further research is necessary to weigh the evidence as to whether compounds in organisms can influence sexual desire, for example. It is also important to understand the physiological mechanisms of the bioactive compounds that may have practical implications for the development of new therapies for sexual function and dysfunction in older adults.

Natural health products remain a commonly utilized—but understudied—source of complementary and integrative health treatments of morbidities in aging adults. The diversity of organisms in North America, including Greenland, is ideal for research into nutraceuticals that may improve sexual conditions associated with aging in adults. This ongoing research is important because of the growing proportion of older populations throughout the world, their proportionately higher rate of sexual dysfunctions, and their frequent use of natural health products alongside allopathic medications. Development of new therapies from natural health products may reduce undesirable side effects and costs in comparison with current pharmaceuticals. The bioactive compounds found in organisms may play an important role in drug discovery and thus should be a continued goal of medical research.

Acknowledgments

Thanks are due to Dr. Arul Chinnaiyan of the Department of Pathology at the University of Michigan Medical School and to Dr. Steven M. Firestine of the Department of Pharmaceutical Sciences in the Eugene Applebaum College of Pharmacy and Health Sciences at Wayne State University for their much appreciated help in critiquing earlier forms of this manuscript. All responsibility and accountability for this chapter rests solely upon the indicated authors. No funding was used to support this project.

References

Agardh, E., Allebeck, P., Hallqvist, J., Moradi, T., Sidorchuk, A., 2011. Type 2 diabetes incidence and socio-economic position: a systematic review and meta-analysis. Int. J. Epidemiol. 40 (3), 804–818.

Ambler, R.D., Bieber, J.E., Diamond, P.M., 2012. Sexual function in elderly women: a review of current literature. Obstet. Gynecol. 5 (1), 16–27.

American Diabetes Association., 2014. Age, race, gender & family history.

Anderson, M.K., Oakes, T., 2012. Plant guide for saw palmetto (Serenoa repens) USDA-Natural Resources Conservation Service. National Plants Data Team, Davis, California. 95616.

Arletti, R., Benelli, A., Cavazzuti, E., Scarpetta, G., Bertolini, A., 1999. Stimulating property of Turnera diffusa and Pfaffia paniculata extracts on the sexual-behavior of male rats. Psychopharmacol 143 (1), 15–19.

Autenrieth, B.I., 2006. Bacteria as the Basis for New Regenerative Therapies. ZRM.

Balch, A.P., Bell, S., 2012. Prescription for Herbal Healing, 2nd Edition: An Easy-to-Use A-to-Z Reference to Hundreds of Common Disorders and Their Herbal Remedies. Penguin. Print.

Barrons, R., Tassone, D., 2008. Use of Lactobacillus probiotics for bacterial genitourinary infections in women: a review. Clin. Ther. 30 (3), 453–468.

Becker, R., 2012. Medical Claims for Rhino Horn: You're Better on an Aspirin or Biting Your Nails. Africa Check. AFP Foundation. <https://africacheck.org/reports/medical-claims-for-rhino-horn-youre-better-on-an-aspirin-or-biting-your-nails/>.

Bennett, Bradley C., Hicklin, J.R., 1998. Uses of saw palmetto (Serenoa repens, Arecaceae) in Florida. Econ. Bot. 52 (4), 381–393.

Bensenor, I.M., Olmos, R.D., Lotufo, P.A., 2012. Hypothyroidism in the elderly: diagnosis and management. Clin. Intervent. Aging 7, 97–111.

Brown, A.C., Valiere, A., 2004. The medicinal uses of poi. Nutr. Clin. Care 7 (2), 69–74.

Brenner, D.J., O'Connor, P.S., 1993. Proposals to unify the genera bartonella and rochalimae, with descriptions of bartonella quintana comb. nov., bartonella visionii comb. nov., bartonella henselae comb. nov., and bartonella elizabathae comb. nov., and to remove the family bartonellaceae from the order rickettsiales. Int. J. Syst. Bacteriol. 43, 777–786.

Bruskewitz, R.C., 2003. Quality of Life and Sexual function in patients with benign prostatic hyperplasia. Rev. Urol. 5 (2), 72–80.

Buck, C.B., Thompson, C.D., Roberts, J.N., Müller, M., Lowy, D.R., Schiller, J.T., 2006. Carrageenan is a potent inhibitor of papillomavirus infection. PLoS Pathog. 2 (7), 671–680.

Caspari, E., Robbins, K., 2003. Animal life in nature, myth and dreams. Wilmette, IL: Chiron Publications. Print.

Chan, S.W., 2012. *Panax ginseng, Rhodiola rosea* and *Schisandra chinensis*. Int. J. Food Sci. Nutr. 63, 75–81.

D'Aniello, G., Ronsini, S., Notari, T., Grieco, N., Infante, V., D'Angelo, N., et al., 2012. D-Aspartate, a key element for the improvement of sperm quality. Adv. Sex. Med. 2, 47–53.

De Monte, C., Carradori, S., Granese, A., Di Pierro, G.B., Leonardo, C., De Nunzio, C., 2014. Modern extraction techniques and their impact on the pharmacological profile of Serenoa repens extracts for the treatment of lower urinary tract symptoms. BMC Urol. 14, 63.

Desideri, D., Cantaluppi, C., Ceccotto, F., Meli, M.A., Roselli, C., Feduzi, L., 2016. Essential and toxic elements in seaweed for human consumption. J. Toxicol. Environ. Health 79 (3), 112–122.

Dryden, J., 2007. Researchers discover root cause of blood vessel damage in diabetes. Washington University in St. Louis.

Edwards, E., Sarah., Rocha, I., Williamson, M.E., Heinrich, M., 2015. Phytopharmacy: An Evidence-based Guide to Herbal Medicinal Products, first ed. Wiley-Blackwell, Hoboken.

Employment and Social Development Canada., 2016. Canadians in context - Aging population. Indicators of Well-being in Canada.

Everitt, J.H., Drawe, D.L., Lonard, R.I., 2002. Damiana, Hierba Del Venado Trees, Shrubs & Cacti of South Texas. Texas Tech University Press, Lubbock.

Feldman, A.H., Johannes, B.C., Derby, A.C., Kleinman, P.K., Mckinlay, B.J., 2000. Erectile dysfunction and coronary risk factors: prospective results from the Massachusetts male aging study. Prev. Med. 30 (4), 328–338.

Ferreira, M.P., Weems, M.K.S., 2008. Alcohol consumption by aging adults in the United States: health benefits and detriments. J. Am. Dietetic Assoc. 108 (10), 1668–1676.

Fischer, D., 2011. Hen of the woods, Maitake or Sheepshead mushroom (Grifola frondosa).

George, W.H., Gilmore, A.K., 2013. Alcohol's effects on sexual arousal and sexual functioning. Comp. Addict. Behav. Disorders 1, 339–347.

Gilbert, S., 2014. Ethyl Alcohol. Toxipedia. Web. Accessed 21 January, 2016. <http://www.toxipedia.org/display/toxipedia/Ethyl+Alcohol>.

Goldstein, I., Dicks, B., Kim, N.N., Hartzell, R., 2013. Multidisciplinary overview of vaginal atrophy and associated genitourinary symptoms in postmenopausal women. Sex. Med. 1, 44–53.

Grant, M.D., Marbella, A., Wang, A.T., Pines, E., Hoag, J., Bonnell, C., et al., 2015. Menopausal symptoms: comparative effectiveness of therapies. Agency for Healthcare Research and Quality 147.

Hall, K.B., 2005. Bones and Cartilage: Developmental and Evolutionary Skeletal Biology. Elsevier Academic. Print, San Diego, CA.

Hernández, M., Alfonso, C.A., 1997. Psychoactive drugs and sexuality. Int. J. Mental Health 26 (1), 68–78.

Higdon, J., 2007. An evidence-based approach to dietary phytochemicals. Thieme Medical, Print, New York.

Hoffmann, J.N., You, H.M., Hedberg, E.C., Jordan, J.A., McClintock, M.K., 2014. Prevalence of bacterial vaginosis and Candida among postmenopausal women in the United States. J. Gerontol. B Psychol. Sci. Soc. Sci. 69 (8), 205–214.

Hong, L., Xun, M., Wutong, W., 2007. Anti-diabetic effect of an α-glucan from fruit body of maitake (grifola frondosa) on kk-ay mice. J. Pharmacy Pharmacol. 59, 575–582.

Hyun-Kyung, K., So-Yeon, K., Youn-Jee, C., Jang-Heub, K., Mee-Ran, K., 2015. The recent review of the genitourinary syndrome of menopause. J. Menopausal. Med. 21, 65–71.

Krassas, G.E., Tziomalos, K., Papadopoulou, F., Pontikides, N., Perros, P., 2008. Erectile dysfunction in patients with hyper- and hypothyroidism: how common and should we treat? J. Clin. Endocrinol. Metab. 93 (5), 1815–1819.

Kumar, A., Arora, R., 2013. Medicinal plants effective in treatment of sexual dysfunction: a review. J. Med. Plants Stud. 1 (1), 1–6.

Kumar, S., Taneja, R., Sharma, A., 2005. The genus Turnera: a review update. Pharmaceut. Biol. 43 (5), 383–391.

Lappe-Oliveiras, P., Moreno-Terrazas, R., Arrizón-Gaviño, J., Herrera-Suárez, T., García-Mendoza, A., Gschaedler-mathis, A., 2008. Yeasts associated with the production of Mexican alcoholic nondistilled and distilled agave beverages. Fed. Eur. Microbiol. Soc. Yeast 8, 1037–1052.

Laurberg, P., Cerqueira, C., Ovesen, L., Rasmussen, B.L., Perrild, H., Andersen, S., et al., 2010. Iodine intake as a determinant of thyroid disorders in populations. Best Practice & Research: Clinical Endocrinology & Metabolism. 24 (1), 13–27.

Luoto, R., Collado, M.C., Laitinen, K., Salminen, S., Isolauri, E., 2013. Metabolic syndrome and obesity in children In: Guarino, A. Quigley, E.M.M. Walker, W.A. (Eds.), Probiotic Bacteria and their effect on human health and well-being, vol. 107. World Rev Nutr Diet. Basel, Karger, pp. 95–102.

Makarova, K., Slesarev, A., Wolf, Y., Sorokin, A., Mirkin, B., Koonin, E., et al., 2006. Comparative genomics of the lactic acid bacteria. Proc. Natl. Acad. Sci USA 103 (42), 15611–15616.

Malatesta, V.J., Pollack, R.H., Crotty, T.D., Peacock, L.J., 1982. Acute alcohol intoxication and female orgasmic response. J. Sex. Res. 18 (1), 1–17.

Marais, D., Gawarecki, D., Allan, B., Ahmed, K., Altini, L., Cassim, N., et al., 2011. The effectiveness of Carraguard, a vaginal microbicide, in protecting women against high-risk human papillomavirus infection. Antiviral Therapy 16, 1219–1226.

Martin, S., Blanchard, K., Manopaiboon, C., Chaikummao, S., Schaffer, K., Friedland, B., et al., 2010. Carraguard acceptability among men and women in a couples study in Thailand. J. Womens Health 19 (8), 1561–1567.

Nash, C.E., 2011. The history of aquaculture. Blackwell Publishing, Iowa.

Orabi, H., Alberson, M., Lue, T.F., 2011. Association of lower urinary tract symptoms and erectile dysfunction: pathophysiological aspects and implications for clinical management. Int. J. Impotence Res. 23, 99–108.

Ostlund Jr, R., 2002. Phytosterols in human nutrition. Annu. Rev. 22, 533–549.

Palmeira-de-Oliveira, R., Palmeira-de-Oliveira, A., Martinez-de-Oliveira, J., 2015. New strategies for local treatment of vaginal infections. Adv. Drug Deliv. Rev. 92, 105–122.

Pangestuti, R., Kim, S.-K., 2014. Chapter Seven – Biological Activities of Carrageenan In: Kim, S.-K. (Ed.), Marine Carbohydrates: Fundamentals and Applications, Part A, Advances in Food and Nutritional Research, vol. 72. Elsevier Science, Amsterdam, pp. 113–124.

Pauls, E.P., 2014. *Encyclopedia Britannica*. "American Indian" Web.

Penugonda, K., Lindshield, B.L., 2013. Fatty acid and phytosterol content of commercial saw palmetto supplements. Nutrients 5, 3617–3633.

Petrova, M.I., Lievens, E., Malik, S., Imholz, N., Lebeer, S., 2015. Lactobacillus species as biomarkers and agents that can promote various aspects of vaginal health. Front. Physiol. 6, 81.

Porras, F., 2013. Afrodisíacos de origen Maya. Suite, 101.

Portman, D.J., Gass, M.L., 2014. Genitourinary syndrome of menopause: new terminology for vulvovaginal atrophy from the International Society for the Study of Women's Sexual Health and The North American Menopause Society. Climacteric 17 (5), 557–563.

Prajapati, V.D., Maheriya, P.M., Jani, G.K., Solanki, H.K., 2014. Carrageenan a natural seaweed polysaccharide and its applications. Carbohydrate Polymers 105, 97–112.

Preuss, G.H., Echard, B., Bagchi, D., Perricone, V.N., Zhuang, C., 2007. Enhanced insulin-hypoglycemic activity in rats consuming a specific glycoprotein extracted from Maitake mushroom. Mol. Cell Biochem. 306 (1-2), 105–113.

Puri, K.R., 2010. Chapter Six C Aphrodisiacs from the Animal Kingdom Deer Antler Natural Aphrodisiacs: Myth or Reality. Quest, LLC, Print, Columbia, MO.

Riess, T., Raddatz, G., 2007. Analysis of bartonella adhesin a expression reveals differences between various b. Henselae strains. Infect. Immun. 75, 35–43.

Rodrigues, R., Huber, M., Lamura, G., 2012. Facts and figures on healthy ageing and long-term care. European Centre for Social Welfare Policy and Research: Vienna.

Rogers, K., 2011. Fungi, algae, and protists. The Rosen Publishing Group, New York.

Sato, M., Inoue, F., Kanno, N., Sato, Y., 1987. The occurrence of N-methyl-D-aspartic acid in muscle extracts of the blood shell, Scapharca broughtonii. Biochem. J. 241 (1), 309–311.

Save the Rhino International Rhino Foundation, Poaching for Rhino Horn. n.d. Web. <https://www.savetherhino.org/about/mission_and_vision>.

Sawin, C.T., Castelli, W.P., Hershman, J.M., McNamara, P., Bacharach, P., 1985. The aging thyroid. Thyroid deficiency in the Framingham Study. Arch. Intern. Med. 145 (8), 1386–1388.

Schillinger, U., 1999. Isolation and identification of lactobacilli from novel-type probiotic and mild yoghurts and their stability during refrigerated storage. Int. J. Food Microbiol. 47, 79–87.

Schneiter, R., 2004. Genetics, molecular and cell biology of yeasts. Université de Fribourg Suisse, viewed 21 January, 2016. <https://www.unifr.ch/biochem/assets/files/schneiter/cours/Yeast/YeastGenetics.pdf>.

Shibata, K., Tarui, A., Todoroki, N., Kawamoto, S., Takahashi, S., Kera, Y., et al., 2001. Occurrence of N-methyl-L-aspartate in bivalves and its distribution compared with that of N-methyl-D-aspartate and D, L-aspartate. Comp. Biochem. Physiol. 130, 493–500.

Sosnowska, J., Balslev, H., 2009. American palm ethnomedicine: a meta-analysis. J. Ethnobiol. Ethnomed. 5 (43), 1.

Tarui A., Shibata, K., Takahshi., S., Kera, Y., Munegumi, T., Yamada, R., 2003. N-methyl-D-glutamate and N-methyl-L-glutamate in Scapharca broughtonii (Mollusca) and other invertebrates.

Tsesarskaia, M., Galindo, E., Szókan, G., Fisher, G., 2009. –HPLC determination of acidic D-amino acids and their N-methyl derivatives in biological tissues. Biomed. Chromatogr. 23 (6), 581–587.

US Department of Health and Human Services., 2014. A profile of older Americans: 2014. PsycEXTRA Dataset.

United Nations., 2013. World population ageing: 2013. Department of Economic and Social Affairs, Population Division (2013).

Vanderhoof, J.A., Young, R., 2008. Probiotics in the United States. Clin. Infect. Dis. 46 (2), 67–72.

Várkonyi, T., Kempler, P., 2014. Sexual dysfunction in diabetes. Diabetes and the Nervous System Handbook of Clinical Neurology, 223–232.

Veronelli, A., Masu, A., Ranieri, R., Rognoni, C., Laneri, M., Pontirolo, A.E., 2006. Prevalence of erectile dysfunction in thyroid disorders: comparison with control subjects and with obese and diabetic patients. Int. J. Impotence Res. 18, 111–114.

Vohra, S., Cvijovic, K., Boon, H., Foster, C.B., Jaeger, W., Legatt, D., et al., 2012. Study of natural health product adverse reactions (SONAR): active surveillance of adverse events following concurrent natural health product and prescription drug use in community pharmacies. PLoS ONE 7, 9.

Wei, X., Schneider, G.J., Shenouda, M.S., Lee, A., Towler, A.D., Chakravarthy, V.M., et al., 2010. De novo lipogenesis maintains vascular homeostasis through endothelial nitric-oxide synthase (enos) palmitoylation. J. Biol. Chem. 286 (4), 2933–2945.

Yu, H., Gao, S., Chen, A., Kong, L., Li, Q., 2015. Genetic diversity and population structure of the ark shell scapharca along the coast of China based on microsatellites. Biochem. Syst. Ecol 58, 235–241.

PART IV

PROTEIN AND ENERGY IN HEALTH AND GROWTH OF ELDERLY

CHAPTER

26

Physiological Aspects of Coenzyme Q_{10} in Plasma in Relationship with Exercise and Aging

Guillermo López-Lluch

Universidad Pablo de Olavide, Sevilla, Spain

OVERVIEW

Coenzyme Q (CoQ) is a lipophilic and active reduction–oxidation molecule located in all cell membranes and in blood lipoproteins (Ernster and Dallner, 1995; Ernster and Forsmark-Andree, 1993). It is composed of a quinone ring bound to a chain of isoprene units ranging from 6 to 10 units in length. The length of the isoprene chain determines the type of CoQ, which varies depending on the species. *Saccharomyces cerevisiae* has 6 units, *Candida maritima* has 7, *Escherichia coli* has 8, *Caenorhabditis elegans* and *Drosophila melanogaster* have 9, and rodents and humans have 10. CoQ cycles between its oxidized form and its reduced form, ubiquinone (oxCoQ) and ubiquinol (redCoQ), respectively, with redCoQ being the most abundant form in plasma and tissues. In fact, the ratio of redCoQ to oxCoQ is considered to be a marker of oxidative stress (Fig. 26.1) (Niklowitz et al., 2016).

In cells and tissues, CoQ's main role is to carry electrons in the mitochondrial electron transport chain (METC). METC transfers electrons from reduced molecules such as nicotinamide adenine dinucleotide (NADH) or succinate—which are produced during oxidation of glucose by glycolysis and by Kreb's cycle and by beta oxidation of lipids—to oxygen as the final electron acceptor with water as the product. During this process, the METC pumps protons from the matrix to the intermembrane space of mitochondria, inducing a gradient that is used by the mitochondrial ATPase to synthesize ATP from ADP + Pi (Fig. 26.2). In METC, CoQ is the only lipid directly involved in the transfer of electrons from complexes I or II to complex III (Lopez-Lluch et al., 2010). The importance of this lipid in the physiology of mitochondria is highlighted by the severity of rare diseases associated with deficiencies in CoQ synthesis that often produces a similar pathology than other mitochondria-associated rare diseases such as mitochondrial encephalomyopathy, lactic acidosis, and stroke-like episodes (MELAS) or myoclonic epilepsy with ragged red fibers (MERFF) (Yubero et al., 2015). CoQ molecules are also internal components of METC complex III, and its presence is essential for the stabilization of this complex (Santos-Ocana et al., 2002).

The role of CoQ in mitochondrial inner membrane is also associated with other essential activities in this organelle. CoQ is also involved in the transfer of electrons to the METC from beta oxidation, in the synthesis of purines by accepting electrons from dihydro-orotate dehydrogenase, in the control of the activity of uncoupling proteins, and the regulation of the permeability transition pore opening involved in mitochondrial swelling and apoptosis (Fig. 26.2) (Lopez-Lluch et al., 2010). Furthermore, redCoQ is a key lipid antioxidant in mitochondrial membranes as demonstrated many years ago (Takayanagi et al., 1980). Prevention of oxidative damage in mitochondrial membranes clearly depends on the amount of redCoQ through a direct antioxidant activity by recycling alpha-tocopherol to maintain its levels of the reduced form (Noack et al., 1994).

Nutrition and Functional Foods for Healthy Aging.
DOI: http://dx.doi.org/10.1016/B978-0-12-805376-8.00026-5

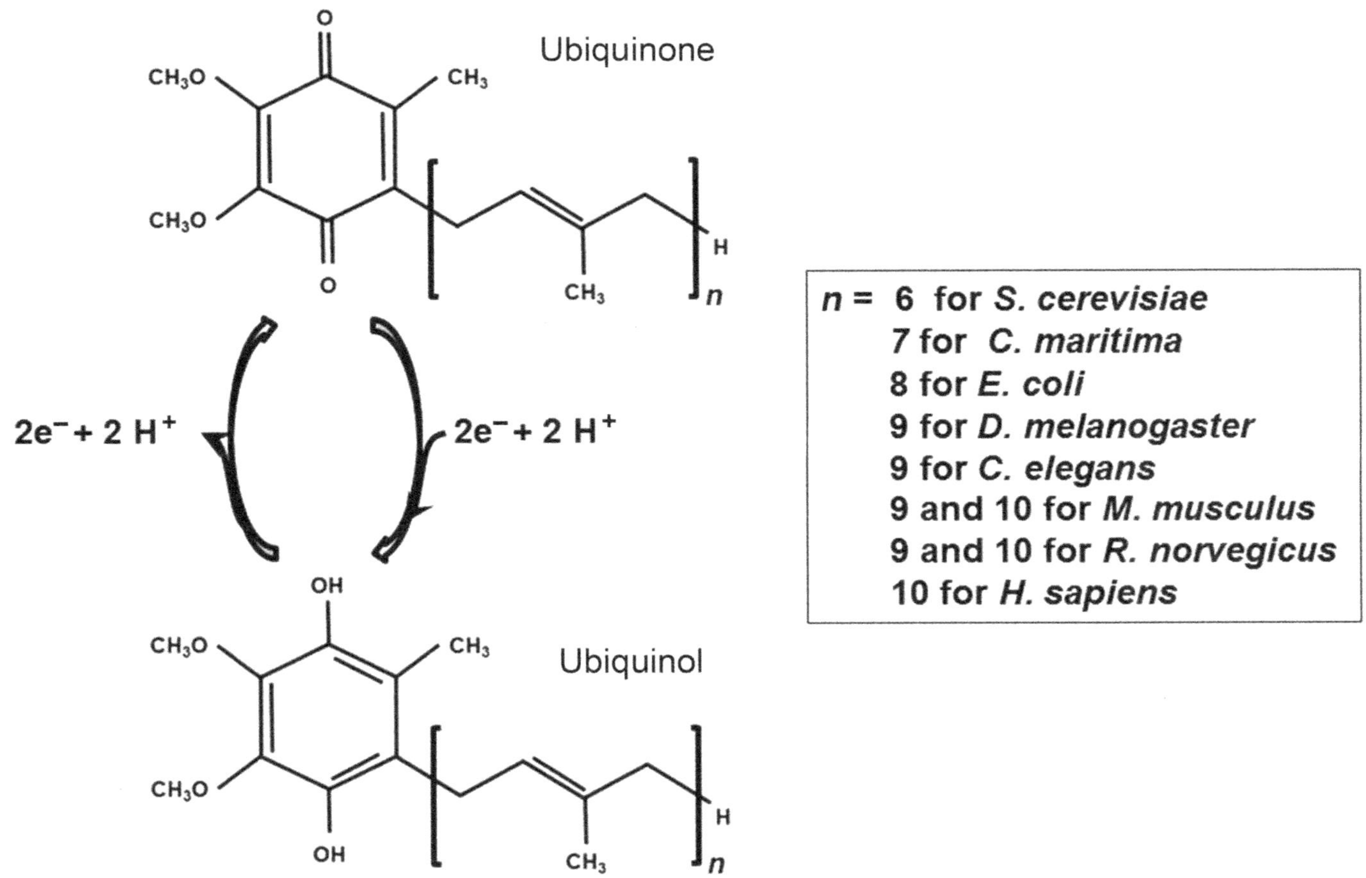

FIGURE 26.1 CoQ structure and redox cycle. CoQ is composed of a benzene ring linked to a isoprene chain. The chain confers its lipidic characteristics whereas the ring acts in the electron transferences. Oxidized CoQ is known as *ubiquinone*, whereas the reduced and active form is known as *ubiquinol*. The isoprene chain length changes in different organisms. The number of isoprene units is indicated for each species.

In other cell membranes, CoQ is involved in protecting the lipid bilayer against oxidative damage by maintaining alpha-tocopherol and vitamin C in their reduced and then active forms, respectively (Rodriguez-Aguilera et al., 2000). The maintenance of CoQ in its reduced form depends on different oxidoreductases that transfer electrons from nicotinamide adenine dinucleotide phosphate to the oxCoQ form reducing it (Villalba et al., 1997). To date, cytochrome b_5 reductase and NQO1 (DT-diaphorase) have been found as the main enzymes involved in CoQ recycling in cell membranes. However, other enzymes such as cytoplasmic NADH-Q reductase, thioredoxin reductase, lipoamide dehydrogenase, and glutathione reductase have been reported as electron transfer enzymes to CoQ in cells (Fig. 26.2) (Lopez-Lluch et al., 2010).

Apart from its role in cells, CoQ has an important presence in blood plasma. In humans, the range of CoQ_{10} in plasma is around 0.5–2nmol/mL (μM) (Lagendijk et al., 1996). CoQ is associated with lipoproteins that transfer cholesterol from the liver to other organs and from organs to the liver but is higher in low-density lipoprotein (LDL) particles than in high-density lipoprotein (HDL) particles (Bhagavan and Chopra, 2006). In fact, it has been considered that lipoproteins are the right carriers of CoQ in the circulation (Johansen et al., 1991; Laaksonen et al., 1995). Several studies have demonstrated the essential role of CoQ_{10} in the protection against oxidative damage of plasma lipoproteins. Higher levels of Q_{10} in lipoproteins are directly related to LDLs' higher resistance to initiation of lipid peroxidation (Mohr et al., 1992). In LDLs isolated from healthy volunteers supplemented with CoQ10, induction of lipid peroxidation with chemical initiators was delayed in comparison with nonsupplemented particles (Littarru et al., 1994). In contrast, lower CoQ_{10} levels in plasma have been associated with higher lipid peroxidation (Stocker et al., 1991). It has been also demonstrated that CoQ_{10} is more efficient than alpha-tocopherol in the protection of LDL against oxidation, being considered the primary lipid-soluble antioxidant in these particles (Stocker et al., 1991).

Other in vitro experiments with LDLs isolated from human blood demonstrated that these lipoproteins are protected against oxidative damage while CoQ_{10} levels remain in the particle. After oxidative stress, CoQ_{10} levels

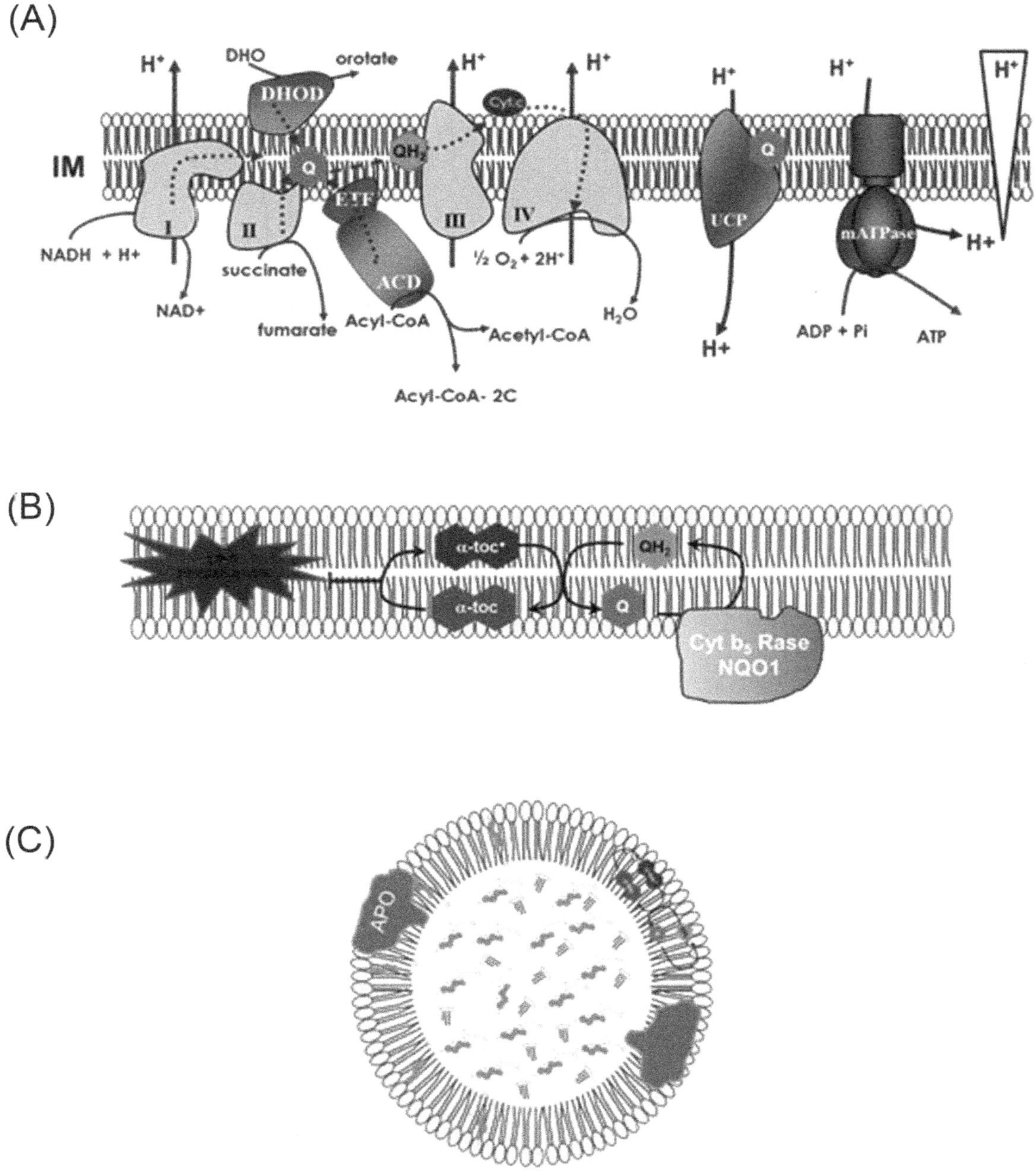

FIGURE 26.2 Function of CoQ in cell membranes and lipoproteins. (A) Function of CoQ in the inner mitochondrial membrane. CoQ is an essential component of the mitochondrial electron transfer chain, accepting electrons from complex I or complex II and giving them to complex III. CoQ can also receive electrons from beta oxidation of the fatty acids. This function is essential in the mitochondrial oxidative metabolism. CoQ also receive electrons from dihydro-orotate dehydrogenase acting as an essential component in the synthesis of pyridine nucleotides. Furthermore, the physiology of the mitochondria can be also regulated by CoQ, thus affecting the activity of uncoupling proteins and mitochondrial pores. (B) In cell membranes, including mitochondrial membranes, CoQ is essential for preventing lipoperoxidation by itself or maintaining alpha-tocopherol in its reduced state. In mitochondria, CoQ is reduced by the electron transport chain components, but in other membranes it is reduced by CoQ-dependent enzymes such as Cyt b_5 reductase and NQO1. (C) The presence of CoQ in lipoproteins has been associated with the prevention of lipid peroxidation of these particles. CoQ is associated with the particle's phospholipid external surface where, together with alpha-tocopherol, it protects the particle against lipid peroxidation.

decrease and the oxidation of lipids increases beyond the maintenance of alpha-tocopherol levels. Then cholesterol oxidation in LDLs starts only when almost all the CoQ_{10} is consumed. These experiments reinforce the idea that CoQ_{10} is the main antioxidant in human plasma lipoproteins (Yamamoto et al., 1991). This is critical because oxidized LDLs are key factors in the initiation and progression of atherosclerosis. This importance has been highlighted by the antiatherogenic effects of CoQ_{10} in apolipoprotein E knockout mice models (Witting et al., 2000). Furthermore, in a mice model of vitamin E deficiency associated with a high-fat diet, pharmacological doses of CoQ_{10} were capable of decreasing lipid peroxidation levels in atherosclerotic lesions probably by reducing the oxidation of LDLs (Littarru and Tiano, 2007). Among the positive cardiovascular effects of CoQ_{10}, its capability to antagonize the oxidation of plasma LDLs has been considered one of the most important (Belardinelli et al., 2006).

Due to its essential bioenergetic role or to its key function as lipid antioxidant, CoQ_{10} has also been associated with several human age-related chronic diseases such as diabetes, hypercholesterolemia, cardiac insufficiency, and neurodegenerative diseases (Lopez-Lluch et al., 2010; Quinzii et al., 2007).

In this chapter, we will focus on the activity of this essential molecule in aging and how physical activity or exercise can modify its levels and activity (Del Pozo-Cruz et al., 2014a; Del Pozo-Cruz et al., 2014b).

DO LEVELS OF CoQ DECREASE DURING AGING?

Being an essential factor in the bioenergetic machinery in cells and a key factor in the membrane and lipoproteins-associated antioxidant system, a putative role of CoQ in physiological decline and in increased age-related oxidative damage is feasible. However, it remains unclear how CoQ behaves during aging. Early studies demonstrate a peak of CoQ in organs such as the lung, heart, spleen, liver, kidney, pancreas, and adrenal gland at 20 years of age followed by a continuous decrease with further aging (Kalen et al., 1989). In humans, most of the studies about CoQ_{10} levels during aging have been performed using blood. Besides the early studies indicating a decrease in this essential lipid during aging, the results in plasma or blood are controversial. Some reports have shown a decrease of CoQ_{10} during aging (Ernster and Dallner, 1995), whereas other studies have shown that levels of CoQ_{10} in older people are higher than in young people (Kaikkonen et al., 1999). This can reflect the differences in populations and life styles. A recent interesting but brief report suggested that the redox status of CoQ_{10} in human plasma—that is, the percentage of oxCoQ_{10} in the total amount of CoQ_{10}—is greater in patients with geriatric diseases than in healthy patients (Wada et al., 2007).

Gender seems to be a factor that influences plasma levels of CoQ_{10}, with levels being higher in men than in women (Aejmelaeus et al., 1997). This fact was recently confirmed in a study that determined the levels of CoQ_{10} in the plasma of European adults (Niklowitz et al., 2016). In this work, authors show that levels of CoQ_{10} in plasma increase in people between ages 41 and 60 and decrease after 61. Levels of CoQ_{10} in men were higher than in women, which confirmed results published 20 years before (Aejmelaeus et al., 1997). When related to cholesterol levels, this age-dependent evolution was maintained when the levels of CoQ_{10} in μmol/mol of cholesterol were determined (Niklowitz et al., 2016). As in the article published previously by Wada et al. (2007), the authors conclude that the antioxidant capacity of CoQ_{10} impairs during aging because CoQ_{10} levels decrease when compared with levels in mature people and the proportion of oxidized CoQ_{10} increases in plasma, which indicates a higher use of the molecule in its antioxidant role or a decreased capacity to maintain CoQ_{10} in its reduced and active form (Niklowitz et al., 2016).

IMPORTANCE OF CoQ IN THE PREVENTION OF CARDIOVASCULAR DISEASE

Results from plasma indicate the importance of CoQ in the prevention of peroxidation in blood lipids and lipoproteins and in the progression of atherosclerosis. But CoQ_{10} is also an essential factor in several aspects of cardiovascular disease (CVD). The relationship between CoQ_{10} levels and cardiovascular disease was suggested in 1990 after a six-year study found that circulating levels of CoQ_{10} were significantly lower in patients suffering ischemic heart disease or dilated cardiomyopathy (Langsjoen et al., 1990). Some years before, Littarru and collaborators demonstrated that the concentrations of CoQ_{10} declined progressively in both blood and myocardial tissue with increasing severity of heart disease (Littarru et al., 1972).

A compilation of the mechanisms of CoQ_{10} against CVD was presented by Greenberg and Frishman in 1990 (Greenberg and Frishman, 1990). The positive effects of CoQ_{10} can be resumed in the improvement of cardiac bioenergetics, a higher antioxidant capacity, reduction of proinflammatory cytokines, and improvement of endothelial

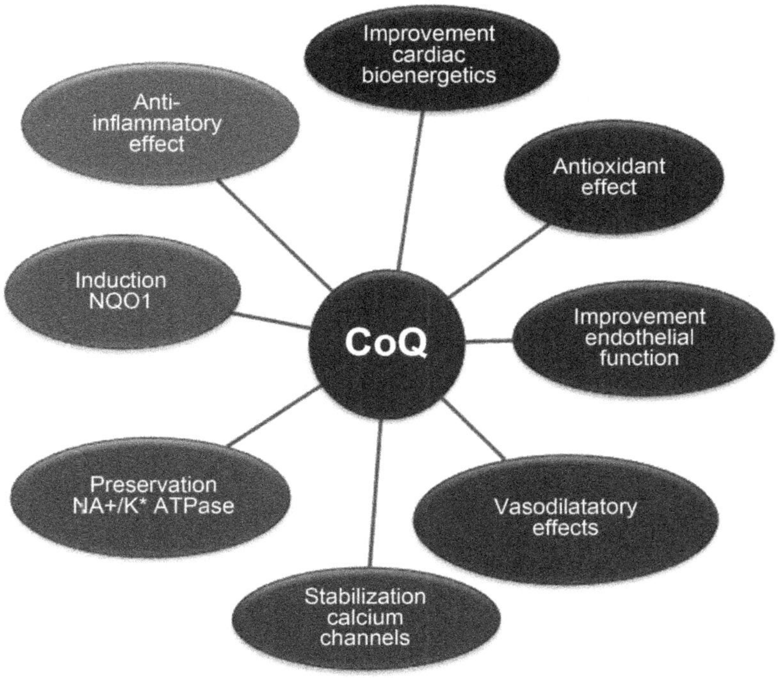

FIGURE 26.3 Functions of CoQ in the prevention of cardiovascular disease. CoQ has been associated with many positive effects in the prevention of cardiovascular disease and its progression. Apart from its antioxidant effects in muscle or lipoproteins, it also improves bioenergetics in the heart and endothelial functions and produces positive effects in vasodilatation and ion channel activities, as well as prevents proinflammatory processes.

function, including vasodilatory effects and the stabilization of calcium and sodium and potassium channels. All of these effects confirm the essential role of this lipid in the prevention of CVD in humans (Fig. 26.3).

Apart from these effects, there is also promising evidence of the beneficial effects of CoQ_{10} in the treatment of heart failure and hypertension (Pepe et al., 2007). Further, other studies have highlighted the important role of CoQ_{10} in CVD in general, reaching the conclusion that CoQ_{10} deficiency might be an important pathogenic mechanism involved in chronic heart failure (Littarru and Tiano, 2007). In fact, deficiency in plasma CoQ_{10} levels has been considered an independent predictor of mortality in patients suffering chronic heart failure (Molyneux et al., 2008). Further, in an interesting and recent paper, a negative relationship between the levels of redCoQ_{10} and the levels of N-terminal pro-brain natriuretic peptide (NT-proBNP), an indicator of the severity of heart failure, has been found. In heart failure patients, healthy subjects showed lower NT-proBNP levels, high redCoQ_{10} levels, and lower ratios of oxCoQ_{10} to redCoQ_{10}. Further, treatment with redCoQ10 in patients reduced the expression of genes related with NT-proBNP levels (Onur et al., 2015). All of these findings demonstrate the importance of CoQ_{10} in the initial phases and progression of CVD.

CoQ_{10} LEVELS CAN BE MODIFIED BY PHYSICAL ACTIVITY AND LIFESTYLE

CoQ_{10} levels in tissues are mainly the product of the compound's biosynthesis with probably a nonsignificant contribution from diet. However, we cannot discard a dietary effect because of the this lipid's long half-life in circulation. The major dietary sources of CoQ_{10} in humans are meat (including poultry), fish (sardines, tuna, and mackerel), some vegetables (broccoli and peanuts) and oils (olive, soy, and fish oils) (Kamei et al., 1986; Weber et al., 1997). The normal dietary intake has been considered to be between 2–5 mg/day. This concentration is not enough to reach a diary intake that is beneficial in pathological conditions, which require around 30–60 mg/day to prevent CoQ_{10} deficiency or 100–200 mg/day in therapeutic doses to treat heart disease (Kumar et al., 2009). However, due to accumulative effects and the direct effect of dietary CoQ_{10} in liver as the first organ receiving the compound, the positive effects of a balanced diet on the levels of CoQ_{10} in plasma during aging cannot be discarded.

Many different studies have demonstrated the positive effect or the practice of physical activity in the prevention of CVD and many other age-related diseases. We have been working on the effects of physical activity on endogenous antioxidant capacities in animal models and humans, and over the last years we have demonstrated that exercise in mice positively affects the activities of endogenous antioxidants in different tissues such as liver (Tung et al., 2014) and muscle (Rodriguez-Bies et al., 2015). The effect of exercise and other age-delaying factors such as calorie restriction or resveratrol depends on the organism's age (Rodriguez-Bies et al., 2015; Tung et al., 2014) and the tissue affected (Tung et al., 2015). Exercise increased CoQ_9 and CoQ_{10} levels in mice muscle with a higher effect in older than in younger animals. This effect was accompanied by the higher presence and activity of CoQ-dependent antioxidant enzymes, Cyt b_5 reductase, and NQO1 (Rodriguez-Bies et al., 2015). This effect was also found in liver, heart, and kidney tissues where NQO1 activity increased in exercised animals; whereas Cyt b_5 reductase was only affected in the kidney (Tung et al., 2015). Our results agree with the findings of Rinaldi and collaborators on rat heart, indicating that prolonged exercise can counterbalance the age-related effects in antioxidant systems in this organ (Rinaldi et al., 2006).

In humans, only data related to the levels of CoQ_{10} in plasma are available. Few studies show results about the effect of exercise on the levels of CoQ_{10} in human blood. In a recent publication of our group, we determined that higher levels of functional capacity (mostly cardiovascular and strength) are associated with higher levels of CoQ_{10} in blood. These higher levels of CoQ_{10} in plasma were associated with lower levels of oxidized lipids in plasma (Del Pozo-Cruz et al., 2014a; Del Pozo-Cruz et al., 2014b). As in the case of animals, the response to exercise in the elderly was higher than in young individuals (Del Pozo-Cruz et al., 2014a). In elderly people, we found that higher levels of CoQ_{10} were associated with better levels of cardiovascular performance, even when this parameter was normalized to cholesterol or triacylglycerides levels or analyzed separately in men and women, indicating that this effect was independent on the gender (Del Pozo-Cruz et al., 2014b). Our findings agree with other previous studies that have correlated the intensity of physical activity and other antioxidant parameters in human plasma (Aguilo et al., 2005; Aguilo et al., 2003).

In a study using a training protocol based on stretching exercise and cycling applied to sedentary individuals over 8 weeks, low changes in plasma CoQ_{10} levels were found (Belardinelli et al., 2006). Although the protocol applied is probably not enough to significantly increase CoQ_{10} levels, the effect of exercise tends to increase CoQ_{10} levels in plasma and increase the ratio of CoQ_{10} to LDL. In fact, the mean concentration of CoQ_{10} to LDL was 0.713 μg/mg in sedentary people and 0.813 μg/mg in exercised individuals. These results agree with our findings for people who maintain higher levels of physical activity over longer periods of time (Del Pozo-Cruz et al., 2014a).

It is interesting that exercise also increased the levels of plasma CoQ_{10} in people supplemented with 100 mg/day of CoQ_{10} in comparison with sedentary and supplemented people (Belardinelli et al., 2006). This increase was associated with marked improvements in cardiovascular parameters. This indicates that physical activity could act as an adjuvant of the protective effect of CoQ_{10} supplementation on CVD and other age-related diseases.

Other studies have tried to determine whether supplementation with CoQ_{10} can ameliorate physical capacity in humans. Supplementation with 300 mg/day of redCoQ_{10} neither increased exercise performance nor decreased oxidative stress (Bloomer et al., 2012), indicating that higher levels of CoQ_{10} obtained from supplements do not improve physical performance. However, in agreement with our findings, this study found that active subjects had already a baseline of total CoQ_{10} in plasma higher than the normal value found in typical populations (Bloomer et al., 2012).

Our finding about the positive relationship between CoQ_{10} levels in plasma and in LDLs and the lower lipoperoxidation degree in these conditions agrees with other studies that show a positive relationship between physical activity and lower lipid peroxidation levels in plasma (Leelarungrayub et al., 2011). In a cohort of sedentary women, six weeks of aerobic dance were enough to decrease lipid peroxide levels in plasma (Leelarungrayub et al., 2011). In another study carried out in men who undertook progressive resistance training, plasma levels of lipid peroxidation decreased in around 40% of them, whereas total antioxidant capacity and glutathione peroxidase activity only showed lower increases (Azizbeigi et al., 2013). Considering the low increase in CoQ_{10} levels found in sedentary people trained during 8 weeks (Belardinelli et al., 2006), it seems clear that physical activity produces modest increases in plasma's antioxidant capacity to protect cholesterol against oxidation and then to reduce CVD risk.

The increase of CoQ_{10} found in elderly people showing higher cardiovascular performance (Del Pozo-Cruz et al., 2014a,b) indicates higher protection not only against oxidative stress but also against the progression of cardiovascular disease.

PLASMA CoQ_{10} AND OBESITY

Sedentarism is one of the most important risk factors in several age-associated diseases, including hypercholesterolemia, diabetes, and hypertension. Sedentarism is directly associated with the pandemic of obesity seen around the world, and exercise has largely been proposed as therapy to reduce it (Warburton et al., 2006). High body mass index (BMI) has been suggested as significantly contributing to poor health as people age (Gomez-Cabello et al., 2012).

The relationship of CoQ_{10} to obesity is currently controversial. Different studies carried out with adult individuals have shown discrepancies in the relationship between BMI and CoQ_{10} levels. Some studies have shown similar, others increased, and still others decreased CoQ_{10} levels in obese people in comparison with nonobese individuals. A study demonstrated that plasma CoQ_{10} levels increased to a small degree in people showing metabolic syndrome (Miles et al., 2004). However, another study performed later did not show differences between people with BMIs around 54 and normal individuals around 28.5 (Mancini et al., 2008). However, when obese people were treated with biliopancreatic diversion, the reduction in BMI was accompanied by a drop in plasma CoQ_{10} reaching even lower levels than the group showing lower BMI. This indicates that the metabolic regulation after chirurgic reduction of the stomach was accompanied by changes in plasma CoQ_{10} levels (Mancini et al., 2008).

Our study has demonstrated that sedentarism and higher BMI are associated with decreased plasma CoQ_{10} levels and increased lipid peroxidation in elderly people (Del Pozo-Cruz et al., 2014b). There was a clear negative relationship between plasma total CoQ_{10} or its ratio with cholesterol (CoQ_{10}/cholesterol or CoQ_{10}/LDL) and BMI. This negative relationship was very clear in people showing a BMI higher than 30. In agreement with our findings, studies performed in other populations showed similar relationships. In Kenyans, plasma CoQ_{10} levels were higher and BMIs lower for people living in the countryside than people living in Nairobi, the capital, who showed higher BMIs (Theuri et al., 2013). These results also agree with the decrease of plasma CoQ_{10} levels found in young obese people age 25 in Missouri in the United States (Butler et al., 2003). However, similar determinations performed in children aged 11–12 years in Germany showed no differences in total plasma CoQ_{10} levels or in relationship with cholesterol or LDL between obese and normal individuals (Menke et al., 2004). These differences probably indicate the effect of the age in the amount of CoQ_{10} in plasma probably related with the deleterious effect of time on liver activity in obese people since assembly of CoQ_{10} and lipoproteins occurs in the liver.

Due to the controversial studies performed to date establishing the relationship between continuous exercise or obesity with CoQ_{10} levels and lipid peroxidation in human plasma, larger prospective cohort studies are required to confirm the importance of maintaining functional levels of CoQ_{10} in plasma. Longitudinal studies implementing programs designed to increase physical fitness (mainly cardiovascular capacity and muscle strength) will also clarify the relationships between the effects of such interventions on aging and on age-related disease biomarkers.

REGULATION OF CoQ_{10} LEVELS IN PLASMA

As already indicated, dietary sources of CoQ_{10} do not explain the variation of plasma levels of this molecule. Regulation of CoQ_{10} synthesis in the liver by exercise and other lifestyle choices such as caloric intake or the presence of bioactive compounds such as resveratrol can be important parameters to consider. Animal models indicate that the peroxisome proliferator-activated receptor (PPAR) plays a key role in the regulation of CoQ_{10} synthesis. In rodents, it has been demonstrated that several drugs alter hepatocellular organization. Treatment of rats with di(2-ethylhexyl)phthalate, an activator of PPAR, increases CoQ content in liver as well as in muscle, blood, and heart, which indicates that these factors are involved in the regulation of CoQ synthesis (Hruban et al., 1974). Furthermore, PPARα is required for the elevation of CoQ caused by peroxisomal inducers, although it is not required for its biosynthesis (Bentinger et al., 2008).

One recent paper showed that exercise increases the expression of PPARα in rat livers, an effect that improves whole body metabolism (Zhang et al., 2011). This would explain how exercise induces increases in CoQ levels in muscles of exercised mice (Rodriguez-Bies et al., 2015). In humans, the generation of PPARγ ligands by exercise activates PPARγ signaling affecting genes related to lipid metabolism (Thomas et al., 2012) in monocytes. This has been associated with the control of reverse cholesterol transport and antiinflammatory effects. Furthermore, the regulation of plasma lipids by PPARγ in liver has also been demonstrated in healthy adults. In this study, a significant increase in oxidized LDL in plasma was found in the exercised group before and after working out. However, the trend showed a biphasic response in time that increased after 4 weeks of exercise and decreased after that to reach normal levels at 8 weeks of exercise (Butcher et al., 2008). These results suggest that the duration of the practice of exercise is an important factor to consider in these studies. Our previous results and other interventions indicate that CoQ_{10} synthesis and levels can increase after the practice of exercise for more than eight weeks. How PPARs are activated and their role in CoQ_{10} synthesis and assembly to lipoproteins remains to be clarified but opens an interesting field in the prevention of atherosclerosis.

Selenium is another interesting factor in the synthesis of CoQ in the liver (Vadhanavikit and Ganther, 1994). Although no further research has been performed, a deficiency of selenium reduced the levels of CoQ_9 and CoQ_{10} in rat liver to around 50%, indicating an important effect of this oligo-element. The authors suggested that selenium preserves tissue against oxidative damage and is thus an integral part of the enzyme glutathione peroxidase (GPX) and preserves the capacity of cells to synthesize CoQ. Our research on mice demonstrate that age shows a clear decline in GPX and that exercise or resveratrol maintain higher levels of this enzyme during aging (Tung et al., 2015). However, the importance of GPX in CoQ_{10} synthesis and assembly with lipoproteins remain to be elucidated.

EFFECT OF STATINS ON CoQ_{10} LEVELS

Statins are widely used as anticholesterol drugs and mainly by older people who show high cholesterol levels as a chronic disease. As cholesterol, dolichol, prenylation, and CoQ share the same biosynthetic pathway, the inhibition of the first enzyme of this pathway, 3-hydroxy-3-methyl-glutaryl-coenzyme A reductase (HMG-CoA reductase), will also inhibit the synthesis of CoQ (Folkers et al., 1990). In the early 1990s, some studies demonstrated that CoQ_{10} decreases in human plasma due to the attenuation of CoQ_{10} synthesis (Folkers et al., 1990; Ghirlanda et al., 1993). When statins lower cholesterol, they simultaneously reduce serum CoQ_{10} by as much as 40% (Kumar et al., 2009). However, this effect has also been associated with the net decrease of cholesterol in blood, although some studies demonstrated that the decrease in plasma CoQ_{10} found in statin-treated individuals was also evident after adjusting to cholesterol levels (Kaikkonen et al., 1999). If we add the CoQ_{10} deficiency occurring with age to the chronic intake of statins to control cholesterol levels in an older population, the reduction of CoQ_{10} in plasma can aggravate the progression of atherosclerosis.

The side effects of statins appear to be a direct consequence of CoQ_{10} and short-chain isoprenoid depletion rather than cholesterol reduction (Littarru and Langsjoen, 2007). Supplementation of statin patients with CoQ_{10} shows conflicting results and thus far the beneficial aspects are not clear. However, in recent studies, significant CoQ_{10} depletion occurs secondary to statin therapy (Hargreaves et al., 2005). In this case, supplementation with CoQ_{10} is highly recommended. In fact, a study of 103 patients treated with statins and CoQ_{10} have demonstrated beneficial effects in dilated cardiomyopathy with decreasing side effects from the statins (Kumar et al., 2009). Furthermore, statins have been associated with myopathies. Supplementation with CoQ_{10} may decrease much of the pain associated with statin treatment (Caso et al., 2007).

Taking into consideration the long-term effects of statins and the common use of these drugs in an older population suffering hypercholesterolemia, a suitable alternative would be to increase physical activity. This would increase endogenous CoQ_{10} synthesis and reduce LDL oxidation and at least help to reduce the doses of these drugs and thus prevent their side effects.

CONCLUDING REMARKS

In many studies, only total cholesterol, LDL, HDL, and triglycerides are determined, but there is no parallel determination of lipid peroxidation or LDL oxidation levels. Probably, depending on an individual's lifestyle and level of exercise, the effect of CoQ_{10} in plasma can prevent LDL oxidation and reduce the risk of atherosclerosis even with moderate levels of cholesterol in blood. In fact, in a recent systematic review about supplementation with CoQ_{10} in humans, the authors concluded that CoQ_{10} has a potential to be a nutritional supplement to improve exercise capacity and reduce exercise-induced oxidative stress, muscle damage, and inflammation, although more studies are needed. The main problem is that the different CoQ_{10} formulations used in these studies, the timing of supplementation, and exercise tests make the interpretation of the data extremely difficult (Sarmiento et al., 2015).

Acknowledgments

The author is funded by the Andalusian Government grant BIO177 (FEDER funds of European Commission). Part of the research has been funded by the Spanish Ministry of Economy and Competitiveness grant DEP2012-39985. Author is also member of the CIBERER, Instituto Carlos III, of the Spanish Ministry of Health.

References

Aejmelaeus, R., Metsa-Ketela, T., Laippala, P., Solakivi, T., Alho, H., 1997. Ubiquinol-10 and total peroxyl radical trapping capacity of LDL lipoproteins during aging: the effects of Q-10 supplementation. Mol. Aspects. Med. 18 (Suppl), S113–S120.

Aguilo, A., Tauler, P., Pilar Guix, M., Villa, G., Cordova, A., Tur, J.A., et al., 2003. Effect of exercise intensity and training on antioxidants and cholesterol profile in cyclists. J. Nutr. Biochem. 14, 319–325.

Aguilo, A., Tauler, P., Fuentespina, E., Tur, J.A., Cordova, A., Pons, A., 2005. Antioxidant response to oxidative stress induced by exhaustive exercise. Physiol. Behav. 84, 1–7.

Azizbeigi, K., Azarbayjani, M.A., Peeri, M., Agha-alinejad, H., Stannard, S., 2013. The effect of progressive resistance training on oxidative stress and antioxidant enzyme activity in erythrocytes in untrained men. Int. J. Sport. Nutr. Exerc. Metab. 23, 230–238.

Belardinelli, R., Mucaj, A., Lacalaprice, F., Solenghi, M., Seddaiu, G., Principi, F., et al., 2006. Coenzyme Q10 and exercise training in chronic heart failure. Eur. Heart. J. 27, 2675–2681.

Bentinger, M., Tekle, M., Brismar, K., Chojnacki, T., Swiezewska, E., Dallner, G., 2008. Stimulation of coenzyme Q synthesis. Biofactors. 32, 99–111.

Bhagavan, H.N., Chopra, R.K., 2006. Coenzyme Q10: absorption, tissue uptake, metabolism, and pharmacokinetics. Free. Radic. Res. 40, 445–453.

Bloomer, R.J., Canale, R.E., McCarthy, C.G., Farney, T.M., 2012. Impact of oral ubiquinol on blood oxidative stress and exercise performance. Oxid. Med. Cell. Longev. 2012, 465020.

Butcher, L.R., Thomas, A., Backx, K., Roberts, A., Webb, R., Morris, K., 2008. Low-intensity exercise exerts beneficial effects on plasma lipids via PPARgamma. Med. Sci. Sports. Exerc. 40, 1263–1270.

Butler, M.G., Dasouki, M., Bittel, D., Hunter, S., Naini, A., DiMauro, S., 2003. Coenzyme Q10 levels in Prader-Willi syndrome: comparison with obese and non-obese subjects. Am. J. Med. Genet. A. 119A, 168–171.

Caso, G., Kelly, P., McNurlan, M.A., Lawson, W.E., 2007. Effect of coenzyme q10 on myopathic symptoms in patients treated with statins. Am. J. Cardiol. 99, 1409–1412.

Del Pozo-Cruz, J., Rodriguez-Bies, E., Ballesteros-Simarro, M., Navas-Enamorado, I., Tung, B.T., Navas, P., et al., 2014a. Physical activity affects plasma coenzyme Q10 levels differently in young and old humans. Biogerontology. 15, 199–211.

Del Pozo-Cruz, J., Rodriguez-Bies, E., Navas-Enamorado, I., Del Pozo-Cruz, B., Navas, P., Lopez-Lluch, G., 2014b. Relationship between functional capacity and body mass index with plasma coenzyme Q10 and oxidative damage in community-dwelling elderly-people. Exp. Gerontol. 52, 46–54.

Ernster, L., Dallner, G., 1995. Biochemical, physiological and medical aspects of ubiquinone function. Biochim. Biophys. Acta. 1271, 195–204.

Ernster, L., Forsmark-Andree, P., 1993. Ubiquinol: an endogenous antioxidant in aerobic organisms. Clin. Investig. 71, S60–S65.

Folkers, K., Langsjoen, P., Willis, R., Richardson, P., Xia, L.J., Ye, C.Q., et al., 1990. Lovastatin decreases coenzyme Q levels in humans. Proc. Natl. Acad. Sci. USA. 87, 8931–8934.

Ghirlanda, G., Oradei, A., Manto, A., Lippa, S., Uccioli, L., Caputo, S., et al., 1993. Evidence of plasma CoQ10-lowering effect by HMG-CoA reductase inhibitors: a double-blind, placebo-controlled study. J. Clin. Pharmacol. 33, 226–229.

Gomez-Cabello, A., Pedrero-Chamizo, R., Olivares, P.R., Hernandez-Perera, R., Rodriguez-Marroyo, J.A., Mata, E., et al., 2012. Sitting time increases the overweight and obesity risk independently of walking time in elderly people from Spain. Maturitas. 73, 337–343.

Greenberg, S., Frishman, W.H., 1990. Co-enzyme Q10: a new drug for cardiovascular disease. J. Clin. Pharmacol. 30, 596–608.

Hargreaves, I.P., Duncan, A.J., Heales, S.J., Land, J.M., 2005. The effect of HMG-CoA reductase inhibitors on coenzyme Q10: possible biochemical/clinical implications. Drug. Saf. 28, 659–676.

Hruban, Z., Gotoh, M., Slesers, A., Chou, S.F., 1974. Structure of hepatic microbodies in rats treated with acetylsalicylic acid, clofibrate, and dimethrin. Lab. Investig. 30, 64–75.

Johansen, K., Theorell, H., Karlsson, J., Diamant, B., Folkers, K., 1991. Coenzyme Q10, alpha-tocopherol and free cholesterol in HDL and LDL fractions. Ann. Med. 23, 649–656.

Kaikkonen, J., Nyyssonen, K., Tuomainen, T.P., Ristonmaa, U., Salonen, J.T., 1999. Determinants of plasma coenzyme Q10 in humans. FEBS Lett. 443, 163–166.

Kalen, A., Appelkvist, E.L., Dallner, G., 1989. Age-related changes in the lipid compositions of rat and human tissues. Lipids. 24, 579–584.

Kamei, M., Fujita, T., Kanbe, T., Sasaki, K., Oshiba, K., Otani, S., et al., 1986. The distribution and content of ubiquinone in foods. Int. J. Vitam. Nutr. Res. 56, 57–63.

Kumar, A., Kaur, H., Devi, P., Mohan, V., 2009. Role of coenzyme Q10 (CoQ10) in cardiac disease, hypertension and Meniere-like syndrome. Pharmacol. Ther. 124, 259–268.

Laaksonen, R., Riihimaki, A., Laitila, J., Martensson, K., Tikkanen, M.J., Himberg, J.J., 1995. Serum and muscle tissue ubiquinone levels in healthy subjects. J. Lab. Clin. Med. 125, 517–521.

Lagendijk, J., Ubbink, J.B., Vermaak, W.J., 1996 Measurement of the ratio between the reduced and oxidized forms of coenzyme Q10 in human plasma as a possible marker of oxidative stress. J. Lipid. Res. 37, 67–75.

Langsjoen, P.H., Langsjoen, P.H., Folkers, K., 1990. A six-year clinical study of therapy of cardiomyopathy with coenzyme Q10. Int. J. Tissue. React. 12, 169–171.

Leelarungrayub, D., Saidee, K., Pothongsunun, P., Pratanaphon, S., YanKai, A., Bloomer, R.J., 2011. Six weeks of aerobic dance exercise improves blood oxidative stress status and increases interleukin-2 in previously sedentary women. J. Bodyw. Mov. Ther. 15, 355–362.

Littarru, G.P., Langsjoen, P., 2007. Coenzyme Q10 and statins: biochemical and clinical implications. Mitochondrion. 7 (Suppl), S168–S174.

Littarru, G.P., Tiano, L., 2007. Bioenergetic and antioxidant properties of coenzyme Q10: recent developments. Mol. Biotechnol. 37, 31–37.

Littarru, G.P., Ho, L., Folkers, K., 1972. Deficiency of coenzyme Q 10 in human heart disease. II. Int. J. Vitam. Nutr. Res. 42, 413–434.

Littarru, G.P., Battino, M., Tomasetti, M., Mordente, A., Santini, S., Oradei, A., et al., 1994. Metabolic implications of coenzyme Q10 in red blood cells and plasma lipoproteins. Mol. Aspects. Med. 15 (Suppl), s67–s72.

Lopez-Lluch, G., Rodriguez-Aguilera, J.C., Santos-Ocana, C., Navas, P., 2010. Is coenzyme Q a key factor in aging? Mech. Ageing. Dev. 131, 225–235.

Mancini, A., Leone, E., Festa, R., Grande, G., Di Donna, V., De Marinis, L., et al., 2008. Evaluation of antioxidant systems (coenzyme Q10 and total antioxidant capacity) in morbid obesity before and after biliopancreatic diversion. Metabolism. 57, 1384–1389.

Menke, T., Niklowitz, P., de Sousa, G., Reinehr, T., Andler, W., 2004. Comparison of coenzyme Q10 plasma levels in obese and normal weight children. Clin. Chim. Acta. 349, 121–127.

Miles, M.V., Morrison, J.A., Horn, P.S., Tang, P.H., Pesce, A.J., 2004. Coenzyme Q10 changes are associated with metabolic syndrome. Clin. Chim. Acta. 344, 173–179.

Mohr, D., Bowry, V.W., Stocker, R., 1992. Dietary supplementation with coenzyme Q10 results in increased levels of ubiquinol-10 within circulating lipoproteins and increased resistance of human low-density lipoprotein to the initiation of lipid peroxidation. Biochim. Biophys. Acta. 1126, 247–254.

Molyneux, S.L., Florkowski, C.M., George, P.M., Pilbrow, A.P., Frampton, C.M., Lever, M., et al., 2008. Coenzyme Q10: an independent predictor of mortality in chronic heart failure. J. Am. Coll. Cardiol. 52, 1435–1441.

Niklowitz, P., Onur, S., Fischer, A., Laudes, M., Palussen, M., Menke, T., et al., 2016. Coenzyme Q10 serum concentration and redox status in European adults: influence of age, sex, and lipoprotein concentration. J. Clin. Biochem. Nutr.

Noack, H., Kube, U., Augustin, W., 1994. Relations between tocopherol depletion and coenzyme Q during lipid peroxidation in rat liver mitochondria. Free. Radic. Res. 20, 375–386.

Onur, S., Niklowitz, P., Jacobs, G., Lieb, W., Menke, T., Doring, F., 2015. Association between serum level of ubiquinol and NT-proBNP, a marker for chronic heart failure, in healthy elderly subjects. Biofactors. 41, 35–43.

Pepe, S., Marasco, S.F., Haas, S.J., Sheeran, F.L., Krum, H., Rosenfeldt, F.L., 2007. Coenzyme Q10 in cardiovascular disease. Mitochondrion. 7 (Suppl), S154–S167.

Quinzii, C.M., DiMauro, S., Hirano, M., 2007. Human coenzyme Q10 deficiency. Neurochem. Res. 32, 723–727.

Rinaldi, B., Corbi, G., Boccuti, S., Filippelli, W., Rengo, G., Leosco, D., et al., 2006. Exercise training affects age-induced changes in SOD and heat shock protein expression in rat heart. Exp. Gerontol. 41, 764–770.

Rodriguez-Aguilera, J.C., Lopez-Lluch, G., Santos-Ocana, C., Villalba, J.M., Gomez-Diaz, C., Navas, P., 2000. Plasma membrane redox system protects cells against oxidative stress. Redox. Rep. 5, 148–150.

Rodriguez-Bies, E., Navas, P., Lopez-Lluch, G., 2015. Age-dependent effect of every-other-day feeding and aerobic exercise in ubiquinone levels and related antioxidant activities in mice muscle. J. Gerontol. A. Biol. Sci. Med. Sci. 70, 33–43.

Santos-Ocana, C., Do, T.Q., Padilla, S., Navas, P., Clarke, C.F., 2002. Uptake of exogenous coenzyme Q and transport to mitochondria is required for bc1 complex stability in yeast coq mutants. J. Biol. Chem. 277, 10973–10981.

Sarmiento, A., Diaz-Castro, J., Pulido-Moranb, M., Kajarabille, N., Guisado, R., Ochoa, J.J., 2015. Coenzyme Q10 supplementation and exercise in healthy humans: a systematic review. Curr. Drug. Metab.

Stocker, R., Bowry, V.W., Frei, B., 1991. Ubiquinol-10 protects human low density lipoprotein more efficiently against lipid peroxidation than does alpha-tocopherol. Proc. Natl. Acad. Sci. USA. 88, 1646–1650.

Takayanagi, R., Takeshige, K., Minakami, S., 1980. NADH- and NADPH-dependent lipid peroxidation in bovine heart submitochondrial particles. Dependence on the rate of electron flow in the respiratory chain and an antioxidant role of ubiquinol. Biochem. J. 192, 853–860.

Theuri, G., Dallner, G., Brismar, K., Tekle, M., 2013. Effects of lifestyle on plasma levels of the IGF system and the antioxidants coenzyme Q10 and vitamin E in Kenyan rural and urban populations. Growth. Horm. IGF. Res. 23, 68–75.

Thomas, A.W., Davies, N.A., Moir, H., Watkeys, L., Ruffino, J.S., Isa, S.A., et al., 2012. Exercise-associated generation of PPARgamma ligands activates PPARgamma signaling events and upregulates genes related to lipid metabolism. J. Appl. Physiol. (1985) 112, 806–815.

Tung, B.T., Rodriguez-Bies, E., Ballesteros-Simarro, M., Motilva, V., Navas, P., Lopez-Lluch, G., 2014. Modulation of endogenous antioxidant activity by resveratrol and exercise in mouse liver is age dependent. J. Gerontol. A. Biol. Sci. Med. Sci. 69, 398–409.

Tung, B.T., Rodriguez-Bies, E., Thanh, H.N., Le-Thi-Thu, H., Navas, P., Sanchez, V.M., et al., 2015. Organ and tissue-dependent effect of resveratrol and exercise on antioxidant defenses of old mice. Aging. Clin. Exp. Res. 27, 775–783.

Vadhanavikit, S., Ganther, H.E., 1994. Selenium deficiency and decreased coenzyme Q levels. Mol. Aspects. Med. 15 (Suppl), s103–s107.

Villalba, J.M., Navarro, F., Gomez-Diaz, C., Arroyo, A., Bello, R.I., Navas, P., 1997. Role of cytochrome b5 reductase on the antioxidant function of coenzyme Q in the plasma membrane. Mol. Aspects. Med. 18 (Suppl), S7–13.

Wada, H., Goto, H., Hagiwara, S., Yamamoto, Y., 2007. Redox status of coenzyme Q10 is associated with chronological age. J. Am. Geriatr. Soc. 55, 1141–1142.

Warburton, D.E., Nicol, C.W., Bredin, S.S., 2006. Prescribing exercise as preventive therapy. CMAJ. 174, 961–974.

Weber, C., Bysted, A., Hllmer, G., 1997. The coenzyme Q10 content of the average Danish diet. Int. J. Vitam. Nutr. Res. 67, 123–129.

Witting, P.K., Pettersson, K., Letters, J., Stocker, R., 2000. Anti-atherogenic effect of coenzyme Q10 in apolipoprotein E gene knockout mice. Free. Radic. Biol. Med. 29, 295–305.

Yamamoto, Y., Kawamura, M., Tatsuno, K., Yamashita, S., Niki, E., Naito, C., 1991. Formation of lipid hydroperoxides in the cupric ion-induced oxidation of plasma and low density lipoprotein. In: Davies, K.J.A. (Ed.), Oxidative damage and repair. Chemical, biological and medical aspects. Pergamon Press, Elmsford.

Yubero, D., Montero, R., Armstrong, J., Espinos, C., Palau, F., Santos-Ocana, C., et al., 2015. Molecular diagnosis of coenzyme Q10 deficiency. Expert. Rev. Mol. Diagn. 15, 1049–1059.

Zhang, S., Liu, Y., Li, Q., Dong, X., Hu, H., Hu, R., et al., 2011. Exercise improved rat metabolism by raising PPAR-alpha. Int. J. Sports Med. 32, 568–573.

CHAPTER

27

Cellular and Physiological Effects of Arginine in Seniors

Vance L. Albaugh, Melissa K. Stewart and Adrian Barbul

Vanderbilt University School of Medicine, Nashville, TN, United States

INTRODUCTION

Arginine (2-amino-5-guanidinovaleric acid) is an alpha amino acid that has garnered significant research interest for its involvement in a several physiological and pathophysiological processes in human health and disease. Arginine was first shown to be a constituent of animal proteins in 1895 by Hedin (Rogers and Visek, 1985), which spurred interest in the compound's biologic actions. The discovery of arginine as the nitrogen source of nitric oxide (Palmer et al., 1988) has reinvigorated basic and clinical research on arginine and its potential uses as a nutraceutical or dietary supplement. Given its broad range of physiological actions, many of which are affected by normal physiological aging as well as pathological processes, the aim of this chapter is to review arginine's broad reach in human biology and identify the current state of research in many of these areas.

SOURCES OF ARGININE

Dietary Arginine and Nutritional Importance

Arginine is considered a "conditionally essential" amino acid, which means that its nutritional status (i.e., essential versus nonessential) depends on the health or developmental status of the organism. The human body has the ability to synthesize arginine de novo, but if arginine demand increases, the endogenous supply can be insufficient. Thus, during developmental periods or time of rapid growth and cellular turnover, arginine requirements are significantly increased and necessitate exogenous arginine supply. This need for additional arginine has been confirmed by numerous studies demonstrating that endogenous production is insufficient to meet the metabolic needs of growing infants and other neonates (e.g., piglets, young rats), of adults under highly catabolic conditions (e.g., sepsis, burn injury, trauma), or following extensive bowel resection (Wakabayashi et al., 1994).

Arginine has three potential sources in humans: (1) dietary arginine as a constituent of consumed protein, (2) recycled arginine from endogenous protein turnover, and (3) arginine synthesized de novo. Dietary arginine is available in a variety of foods but is most notably found in significant quantifies in seeds, nuts, seafood, algae, meats, rice protein concentrate, and soy protein isolate (Ros, 2015). In general, these foods have the highest per weight amounts of arginine (Hu et al., 1998; King et al., 2008). In addition to naturally occurring dietary sources, supplements are commercially available to consumers for several putative indications.

Like other dietary amino acids that are digested and liberated by intestinal peptidases, arginine is taken up in the diet through apical enterocyte membranes. Under normal conditions, approximately 40% (30–44%) of dietary arginine is extracted by the splanchnic tissues (Castillo et al., 1993), which is likely secondary to the relatively high arginase activity in the intestinal mucosa, a tissue with a high rate of cellular turnover. Dietary arginine uptake by

Nutrition and Functional Foods for Healthy Aging.
DOI: http://dx.doi.org/10.1016/B978-0-12-805376-8.00027-7

enterocytes uses several amino acid transporters. These transport systems continue to be identified and studied but include three major categories: system y^+(cationic amino acid-specific transporters), systems $B^{O,+}$ and $b^{O,+}$ (the sodium-dependent and sodium-independent broad-scope transporters, respectively), and the system y^+L (the cation-modulated broad-scope transporter). These transporters have been extensively reviewed elsewhere and continue to be characterized (for reviews, see Devés and Boyd, 1998). Although a discussion of these transporters is beyond the scope of this chapter, it is important to recognize that they are expressed on a variety of cell types in addition to enterocytes and determine the flux of arginine and other amino acids into and across cells and tissues, depending on the density of expression and cell polarity. Virtually all cells have the capacity for arginine transport across the plasma membrane, which facilitates its wide range of biologic uses (Devés and Boyd, 1998).

Endogenous Arginine and Whole-Body Arginine Flux

Arginine homeostasis, like that of most amino acids in the plasma, is a dynamic process. Typical arginine plasma concentrations in adult humans range from 80 to 120 μM, relative to the 2.5-mM concentration of total plasma amino acids (Brosnan, 2003). The half-life of arginine in humans and many other mammalian species is approximately one hour (Wu et al., 2007). Human whole-body arginine flux in the postabsorptive state is approximately 70 μM/h to 90 μM/kg/h (Castillo, 1996; Castillo et al., 1995). Thus, extrapolating that flux to a 24 h rate corresponds to approximately 15–20 g of arginine per day. Given that average daily dietary arginine consumption is only 4–6 g per day (Visek, 1986), a significant amount of recycling has to occur to meet basal arginine requirements.

Aside from exogenous dietary sources, baseline metabolic requirements for arginine are fulfilled by endogenous production. This occurs via three separate pathways with recycling from protein turnover being responsible for approximately 85% of available circulating arginine in humans (Castillo, 1996; Dejong et al., 1998). In addition to arginine recovery from protein turnover, arginine can be synthesized from other amino acid metabolites. In the adult human, de novo arginine synthesis can account for approximately 10–15% of arginine production (Luiking et al., 2012). This endogenous synthesis occurs from the conversion of proline, glutamate or glutamine, and citrulline, a nonproteinogenic amino acid that can be converted to arginine through organ-to-organ flux and metabolism by the intestine and kidney. The de novo synthesis of arginine from citrulline accounts for the largest amount of endogenously synthesized arginine (approximately 60–80%) (Curis et al., 2007; 2005). In fact, oral citrulline supplementation can be used to increase plasma arginine quite effectively, as citrulline has an exceedingly high bioavailability and virtually no citrulline is lost in the urine (Rougé et al., 2007; Urschel et al., 2006).

BIOCHEMISTRY OF ARGININE

Our understanding of the regulation of arginine metabolism has significantly increased over the last several decades. Arginine is well known for its role in maintaining long-term nitrogen balance as part of the urea cycle, and as the source of nitrogen in the synthesis of nitric oxide (NO). Our appreciation for arginine biochemistry and homeostasis continues to grow and includes a previously unrecognized organ-to-organ trafficking and subcellular localization of arginine-metabolizing enzymes. Each of these processes adds a number of layers of complexity to the role arginine plays in cellular metabolism. However, we have little knowledge of how the expression of catabolic or anabolic enzymes in these pathways changes with aging. We also do not know if arginine flux changes over an organism's or human's lifetime.

Arginine Catabolism

Several pathways degrade arginine for use in vital biologic processes. These enzymes have a wide tissue distribution, and the absence of any one of them can have detrimental effects. One of the most studied arginine-metabolizing enzymes is arginase, the final enzyme of the urea cycle that regenerates ornithine. Unlike the other urea cycle enzymes that exist as single isoforms, two human arginase isoforms are encoded by separate genes: arginase I (AI), which is cytosolic, and arginase II (AII), which localizes to the mitochondrion. (Note: K_m values for AI and AII isoforms are ~0.1 and ~5 mM, respectively (Moinard et al., 2015). Previously the AI and AII isoforms were referred to as *hepatic arginase* and *extrahepatic arginase*, respectively. Both arginase isoforms catalyze the hydrolysis of arginine to form ornithine and urea:

$$\text{arginine} + H_2O \rightarrow \text{ornithine} + \text{urea}$$

The AI gene was cloned in 1986 by Mori and colleagues (Haraguchi et al., 1987) and has a wide tissue distribution, including a high expression in the liver and, to a lesser extent, erythrocytes, gastrointestinal tract, thymus, skin, uterus, and sympathetic ganglia (Yu et al., 2001, 2003). The AII enzyme was discovered in a patient with known AI deficiency who was noted to have residual arginase activity. The AII gene includes a mitochondrial localization signal that targets it for the mitochondrial matrix. Unlike AI, the AII protein is a ubiquitously expressed enzyme (Morris, 2002) with its highest expression in the kidney, gastrointestinal tract, brain, and lactating mammary gland (Yu et al., 2003).

First discovered in the 1980s, nitric oxide synthase is another well studied enzyme that catalyzes the generation of NO and citrulline from arginine:

$$\text{arginine} + \text{NADPH} + O_2 + H^+ \rightarrow \text{NO} + \text{citrulline} + \text{NADP}^+$$

There are three isotypes of NOS: endothelial NOS (eNOS), inducible NOS (iNOS), and neuronal NOS (nNOS). NOS1 (neuronal NOS) and NOS3 (eNOS) are constitutive enzymes that are controlled by intracellular calcium and calmodulin (Luiking et al., 2012). NOS2 is inducible at the level of gene transcription, calcium independent, and expressed by macrophages and other tissues in response to (pro)inflammatory mediators (Luiking et al., 2012). From a functional perspective, the K_m values for arginine of the nNOS, eNOS, and iNOS enzymes are approximately 1.8, 3.6, and 12.5 μM, respectively (Gad, 2010).

The relationship between arginase and NOS, and their competition for available arginine, has led to a significant amount of investigation. The biological basis for the so-called arginine paradox remains unknown—that is, the K_m of NOS is in the micromolar range while the K_m of arginase is in the millimolar range. These enzymes appear to compete for arginine substrate, although biochemically this cannot be explained by K_m alone. Thus, the subcellular localization of these enzymes or local concentrations of arginine substrate (or both) must underlie the regulation of these two enzymes. Regardless, several studies have examined the possibilities of arginase contributing to the effects of aging such as endothelial dysfunction and hypertension. Exogenous arginine administration induces the expression of both the AI and AII enzymes and leads to early cellular senescence (Xiong et al., 2014). Increased arginase activity negatively influences eNOS efficiency in producing NO. This negative effect has been observed in hypertensive humans in whom exogenous arginine is ineffective in inducing vasodilation (Holowatz and Kenney, 2007). It is thought that increased arginase expression and activity leads to decreased availability of arginine for NO production. Consistent with this hypothesis, the ornithine produced by excessive arginase activity may be shunted to polyamine biosynthesis for vascular smooth muscle hypertrophy, further exacerbating vascular dysfunction with aging (Durante, 2013). Arginase expression is increased with aging in vascular smooth muscle cells, and this increased activity may decrease local arginine availability for vascular endothelial cells, thus decreasing NO biosynthesis. Not all NOS isoforms behave in the same manner, however, with iNOS actually promoting arginase activation as part of a negative feedback mechanism (Santhanam et al., 2007; Shin et al., 2012). Regardless, these cell-to-cell interactions between arginase and NOS affect each other's activity by decreasing arginine availability (Johnson et al., 2005; Kim et al., 2009).

Creatine, a molecule important in transient energy storage from high-energy phosphates of adenosine triphosphate (ATP), is a third molecule synthesized from arginine. The creatine synthetic pathway is important in tissues with fluctuating energy needs such as muscle but is important as a rapid source of ATP-derived energy in many other tissues, including the brain, retina, and spermatozoa (Wyss and Kaddurah-Daouk, 2000). Arginine is metabolized by the enzyme arginine:glycine amidinotransferase (K_m 9.2 mM) (Sipilä, 1980), which catalyzes the condensation of arginine and glycine in the following reaction to form a guanidino intermediate:

$$\text{arginine} + \text{glycine} \leftrightharpoons \text{guanidinoacetate} \rightarrow \text{creatine}$$

Production of this guanidinoacetate intermediate is the rate-limiting step in creatine production, an irreversible process. Creatine is also obtained from diet, so overall flux of arginine into this metabolic pathway is largely determined by the availability of dietary creatine. It is estimated that 20% of dietary intake of arginine is used for creatine phosphate synthesis (Brosnan and Brosnan, 2010). Significant amounts of dietary creatine can act as a feedback repressor of this enzyme to limit de novo creatine production from arginine (Stead et al., 2001; Wyss and Kaddurah-Daouk, 2000).

The fourth and last pathway that utilizes arginine as a direct precursor is the synthesis of agmatine, a compound involved in the synthesis of polyamines. The polyamines (i.e., putrescine, spermine, and spermidine) are vital to cellular proliferation; dysregulated polyamine synthesis is associated with cancer. Agmatine is an intermediate whose biologic functions have not been completely determined, but recent evidence suggests that it may play an inhibitory role on polyamine biosynthesis (Satriano, 2003). The enzyme that generates agmatine from arginine is arginine decarboxylase (K_m 0.75 mM) (Regunathan and Reis, 2000). As its name implies, it decarboxylates arginine to form agmatine and carbon dioxide:

$$\text{arginine} \leftrightharpoons \text{agmatine} + CO_2$$

The agmatine generated in this reaction can then be acted on by another enzyme, agmatinase (Iyer et al., 2002), which generates putrescine (a polyamine) and urea:

$$\text{agmatine} \leftrightharpoons \text{urea} + \text{putrescine}$$

The biologic actions of agmatine continue to be debated, as both the liver and kidney have high levels of arginine decarboxylase to produce agmatine, two tissues with high capacities for arginine biosynthesis (Lortie et al., 1996; Morrissey et al., 1995). There are conflicting reports on whether or not mammalian cells express significant arginine decarboxylase activity (Morris, 2004). The role of agmatine, agmatinase, and arginine decarboxylase continue to be an area of research and may potentially reveal further roles in mammals for this arginine-derived compound in the future.

Arginine Synthesis

Intestinal–Renal Axis

Arginine is synthesized endogenously through two related pathways. The first pathway is referred to as the *intestinal–renal axis*. First identified in the 1980s, it involves the coordinated actions of the intestine and kidneys in organ-to-organ metabolite shunting that culminates in de novo renal arginine synthesis and release (Fig. 27.1). Metabolic precursors of arginine are converted to citrulline, a common metabolic intermediate.

Cytosolic arginine can be hydrolyzed by arginase in the intestine to produce ornithine and urea:

$$\text{arginine} + H_2O \leftrightharpoons \text{urea} + \text{ornithine}$$

Of plasma arginine flux, 15% enters this extrahepatic arginase pathway that degrades arginine to ornithine and urea (Castillo, 1996). Similarly, proline, glutamine, and glutamate can also be metabolized to ornithine, which is subsequently converted to citrulline. Proline is first metabolized to pyrroline-5-carboxylate (P5C) via proline oxidase, and then ornithine aminotransferase coverts P5C to ornithine:

$$\text{proline} \leftrightharpoons \text{pyrroline} \sim 5 \sim \text{carboxylate} \leftrightharpoons \text{ornithine}$$

Glutamine can also be metabolized by glutaminase to form glutamate, which is then converted to P5C and ornithine via ornithine aminotransferase (similar to proline):

$$\text{glutamine} \rightarrow \text{glutamate} \rightarrow \text{pyrroline} \sim 5 \sim \text{carboxylate} \leftrightharpoons \text{ornithine}$$

Carbamoyl phosphate and ornithine are then finally condensed in a reaction catalyzed by ornithine transcarbamoylase:

$$\text{ornithine} + \text{carbamoyl phosphate} \leftrightharpoons \text{citrulline} + P_i$$

which generates citrulline in the mitochondria and is then transported to the cytosol ready for export. All of these enzymes that lead to the production of citrulline are expressed within the intestinal enterocytes and represent the expression of a partial urea cycle that exists within the small intestine. This partial urea cycle converts ornithine to citrulline before exporting it from the cell. In addition, dietary ornithine or amino acids that are degraded to ornithine can be recycled to arginine using the classical urea cycle enzymes.

After citrulline is produced by the intestinal enterocytes, it is released into the portal circulation and then recirculates via the arterial circulation to the kidneys. The kidneys efficiently extract the circulating citrulline and convert it to arginine (Fig. 27.1), which becomes available for the rest of the cells and tissues of the body. Experimental data have demonstrated that this de novo arginine synthesis via the intestinal–renal axis is tightly linked to citrulline availability (Luiking et al., 2012). This pathway of converting arginine precursors to a common nonarginine compound (i.e., citrulline) appears advantageous because the liver has virtually zero clearance of citrulline from the portal circulation (Morris, 2002). In stark contrast, the kidney efficiently clears circulating citrulline (Wu and Morris, 2003).

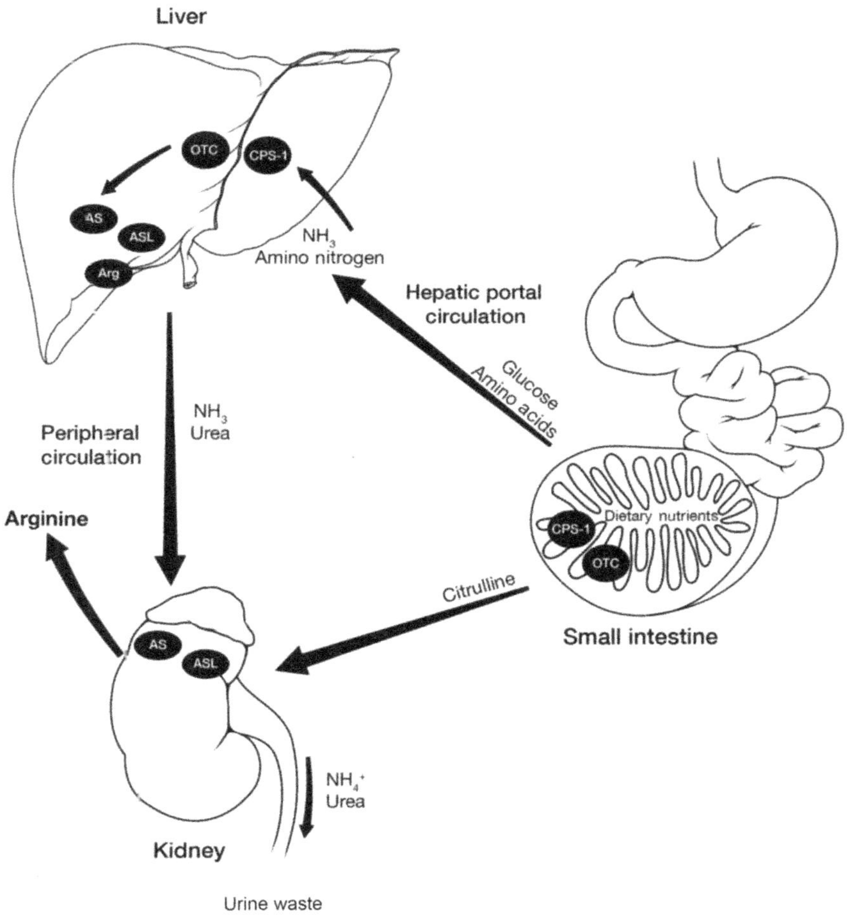

FIGURE 27.1 **The intestinal–renal axis of arginine synthesis.** Endogenous arginine synthesis involves a coordinated organ-to-organ trafficking of arginine precursors made possible by the expression of a partial urea cycle in the intestines and kidney, as well as a lack of hepatic citrulline clearance. The complete urea cycle consists of five enzymes: (1) carbamoyl phosphate synthetase 1, (2) ornithine transcarbamoylase (OTC), (3) argininosuccinate synthetase (AS), (4) argininosuccinate lyase (ASL), and (5) arginase (Arg). Dietary nutrients (e.g., amino acids, carbohydrates) are absorbed by CPS-1 and OTC-expressing intestinal enterocytes, which convert arginine precursors to citrulline. This conversion arginine precursors to bypass hepatic portal clearance, which is essentially zero for citrulline. This effectively shunts arginine precursors in the form of citrulline to the kidney. Once in the kidney, citrulline can be converted to arginine by the expression of AS and ASL, releasing arginine into circulation for use by peripheral tissues. Unlike arginine precursors and citrulline, other excess amino acid nitrogen is cleared in the hepatic portal circulation and converted to urea or NH_3, which is then excreted into the urine by the kidney.

Citrulline comes from several possible sources, including (1) diet; (2) arginine from the NOS pathway; (3) ornithine catabolism of proline, glutamate, or glutamine, and (4) asymmetric dimethyl arginine breakdown. In mice, and potentially humans, the predominant citrulline precursors in this situation are dietary arginine as well as citrulline (Marini, 2012).

Once in the kidney, two cytosolic enzymes that are classically expressed in the urea cycle allow for the conversion of ornithine to arginine. The first enzyme is argininosuccinate synthetase (AS), which condenses citrulline and aspartate to form argininosuccinate. Then the second enzyme, argininosuccinate lyase, generates arginine as well as fumarate as a by-product:

$$\text{citrulline} + \text{aspartate} \leftrightharpoons \text{argininosuccinate} \leftrightharpoons \text{arginine} + \text{fumarate}$$

Note that this is an energetically costly process to the cell, using two molar equivalents of ATP for the cycling process, although the benefit of shunting arginine around the liver appears to be desirable to provide sufficient arginine to the remaining tissues of the body.

Citrulline–Nitric Oxide Cycle

The citrulline–nitric oxide cycle is a theoretical pathway for which the magnitude of flux is inherently difficult to measure and not currently well appreciated. This pathway, however, seems to be active in cells with endogenous NOS activity, potentially as a way to ensure a continuous supply of arginine for NO production. Cells in which arginine would otherwise be limiting can recycle the citrulline produced as a by-product of NOS using Krebs cycle intermediates to continuously generate arginine (Wu and Morris, 2003). Similar to the intestinal–renal axis, the citrulline–NO cycle uses urea cycle enzymes. The citrulline that is produced through the activity of NOS is converted back to arginine via the action of the enzymes argininosuccinate synthase and argininosuccinate lyase. In the first reaction, argininosuccinate synthase condenses citrulline with aspartate:

$$\text{aspartate} + \text{citrulline} \leftrightharpoons \text{argininosuccinate}$$

Subsequently, argininosuccinate is converted back to arginine by the enzyme argininosuccinate lyase (ASL):

$$\text{argininosuccinate} \leftrightharpoons \text{arginine} + \text{fumarate}$$

Hypothetically, this citrulline–NO cycle could continuously generate arginine from citrulline as long as aspartate does not become a limiting factor. Thus, the other vital portion of this cycle is the continuous supply of aspartate. The beauty and simplicity of this cycle, however, is the pathway for the regeneration of aspartate and removal of fumarate that could otherwise build up significant concentrations. The cell appears to handle this via two routes. The first is by the actions of fumarase, which catalyzes the conversion of fumarate to malate, which then can be metabolized by malate dehydrogenase to form oxaloacetate:

$$\text{fumarate} \leftrightharpoons \text{malate} \leftrightharpoons \text{oxaloacetate}$$

Oxaloacetate can be subsequently acted on by the enzyme aspartate transaminase to regenerate aspartate:

$$\text{oxaloacetate} + \text{glutamate} \leftrightharpoons \alpha \sim \text{ketoglutarate} + \text{aspartate}$$

Alternatively, the fumarate can be converted to malate; then, instead of malate dehydrogenase, malic enzyme can convert the malate to pyruvate. Subsequently, pyruvate can be acted on by pyruvate carboxylase to reform oxaloacetate, which can eventually generate aspartate using the enzymatic conversions above:

$$\text{fumarate} \leftrightharpoons \text{malate} \leftrightharpoons \text{pyruvate} \leftrightharpoons \text{oxaloacetate}$$

As previously mentioned above, nearly all known cell types express AS and ASL. Thus, further studies are needed to determine the importance and flux rates of these processes in vivo (Morris, 2002). Regardless, experimental data from a number of investigators have suggested that this pathway is induced along with iNOS activity (Mori and Gotoh, 2000), which makes sense teleologically as a means to circumvent a potential arginine deficiency in a time of stress or need (e.g., infection and iNOS activity).

ARGININE PHYSIOLOGY AND BIOLOGICAL IMPORTANCE

As mentioned, arginine and its metabolites are important in numerous biologic processes. Arginine is most notable as a urea cycle intermediate and carrier of excretable nitrogen, as well as a precursor of NO that is important in vasodilation and the immune response. More recent studies continue to examine arginine and the arginases, which have critical importance in vascular pathology (Durante et al., 2007). Given our expanded understanding of the biologic actions of arginine, the physiologic effects of arginine supplementation have also been an area of intense investigation. How arginine metabolism changes over time and with aging of the body is less well understood and represent important areas for future research. Each of the aforementioned categories has a specific connection and interest to the aging population and will be broadly discussed in the following section.

Protein Synthesis and Degradation

Other important but less well recognized biological effects involving arginine are its role in targeting proteins for degradation as they come off the ribosome. This so-called *N*-end rule for protein degradation uses an amino terminal arginine as a marker for protein degradation, which may act as a quality control for cellular protein synthesis (Tasaki and Kwon, 2007; Varshavsky, 1996). Conversely, arginine is a potent stimulator as well as a substrate in protein synthesis. It is estimated that approximately 80% of arginine needed for protein translation comes from recycled arginine (Luiking et al., 2012). Moreover, arginine has been shown in several studies to stimulate the mammalian target of rapamycin (mTOR) pathway, a known regulator of protein translational initiation (Corl et al., 2008; Wang et al., 2012). This effect on protein translation via mTOR is independent of NO (Bauchart-Thevret et al., 2010). Specifically, arginine directly stimulates p70 S6 kinase and phosphorylation of eukaryotic initiation factor 4E binding protein-1 (Ban et al., 2004). In older individuals, evidence suggests that arginine may have protective effects on muscle wasting and could improve lean muscle mass. These studies, however, have examined arginine in combination therapies and not arginine supplementation alone (Clark et al., 2000; Flakoll et al., 2004; May et al., 2002). Overall, these studies have examined functional outcomes in groups with single or multiple amino acid supplements. The effects of these supplements may be either direct effects on skeletal muscle or indirect effects through other hormonal pathways such as growth hormone and insulin and insulin-like growth factor 1.

Acid–Base Homeostasis and the Urea Cycle

In addition to being an important anaplerotic precursor of the Krebs cycle through conversion to glutamate (Owen et al., 2002), arginine and its metabolism are vitally important in humans as an intermediate in the urea cycle. The final step in the pathway is catalysis of arginine by the enzyme arginase, which produces ornithine and urea, allowing the urea to be available for excretion and regenerating ornithine for the cycle to continue to function. It is important to note, as stressed by Morris, that many textbooks erroneously state that a significant amount of arginine comes from its synthesis from the urea cycle. This is far from the case, as virtually no net synthesis of arginine occurs in the liver (Morris, 2009).

Beyond its classic role in nitrogenous waste detoxification, arginine and the urea cycle also play an important role in acid–base homeostasis. This may be less well clinically appreciated, but the urea cycle is bicarbonate consuming (Häussinger, 1986) and critical in the maintenance of whole-body acid–base balance (Häussinger et al., 1984). Aside from the link between the urea cycle and acid–base homeostasis, recent evidence has demonstrated a role for sirtuins, a family of protein deacetylases, as a link between aging and the regulation of the urea cycle (Nakagawa and Guarente, 2009; Nakagawa et al., 2009).

Immunology

As the immune system ages, its capabilities decline and there is increased susceptibility to infection and cancer, with an increased incidence of autoimmune disorders (Agarwal and Busse, 2010). Given such, the use of arginine to prevent or overcome immunosenescence has received much attention.

The role of all amino acids in immunity, including arginine, has been well studied. Arginine is an essential determinant in immune cell metabolism. Specifically, arginine has been shown to be important in T-cell activation and proliferation, B-cell development, and cytokine production and activity (Bronte and Zanovello, 2005; Feldmeyer et al., 2012). Both enzymes of arginine metabolism, NOS and arginase, are felt to be responsible for its immunologic activity.

Absence of L-arginine in culture media results in significant reduction in proliferation of T lymphocytes in response to mitogens (Brittenden et al., 1994). The optimal L-arginine concentration in media for maximal T-lymphocyte proliferation is similar to those found in human plasma (Efron et al., 1991). Arginine is also required for the effective induction of cytotoxic T-cell function in vitro (Moriguchi et al., 1987). Jurkat T cells cultured in media lacking L-arginine manifest rapid reduction in the expression of the T-cell receptor (TCR), CD36ζ, caused by a short half-life of CD36ζ-mRNA(Rodriguez et al., 2002). It is important to note that CD36ζ phosphorylation is the rate-limiting step in the assembly and membrane expression of the TCR (Minami et al., 1987). Such reduction in mRNA decreases TCR internalization, thus leading to a decrease in total TCR cell membrane expression (Bronstein-Sitton et al., 1999; Valitutti et al., 1997).

Arginine has also been identified as being important in a specific stage of murine B-cell development (de Jonge et al., 2002a, b). The investigators engineered a transgenic mouse expressing arginase I under the control of the rat intestinal fatty-acid binding promoter and enhancer element. The mice demonstrated a 30–40% reduction of plasma arginine and showed a disruption in the B-cell development at the progenitor B to precursor B cell interface in the bone marrow. There were also decreased B cells in secondary lymphoid organs such as the spleen and Peyer's patches in the initial 3 weeks of the neonatal period. The defects were reversed with arginine supplementation (Fafournoux et al., 2000; LeBien, 2002).

Arginine is metabolized in macrophages and lymphocytes by two independent enzymatic pathways, NOS and arginase (Ochoa et al., 2001a). Several clinical conditions—including trauma (Munder et al., 1998), sepsis (Carraway et al., 2015; Witte, 2003), and liver transplantation (Ikemoto et al., 1998; Längle et al., 1995)—have been associated with increased arginase activity, leading to excessive catabolism and subsequent depletion of arginine. This coincides with decreased T-cell proliferation. Supplementation with L-arginine increases CD4+ cells (Kirk et al., 1992), suggesting that arginine may play an important role in reversing the immunosuppression observed during periods of stress (Bernstein, 1996). Specifically, trauma is associated with a greater than 10-fold increase in arginase activity (Ochoa et al., 2001b; 1991). In addition, increased arginase activity in the liver has been implicated in the increased tolerance of the liver to organ rejection (Callery et al., 1991; Schrempf Decker et al., 1983). Moreover, growing evidence suggests that arginine is also an important contributor to intestinal immune function (Li et al., 2007).

Following trauma or surgery, arginine-rich diets were found to reverse the alteration of T-cell function that was initially seen as secondary to the pathologic process. In addition, arginine supplementation in patients undergoing major abdominal operations for gastrointestinal malignancies resulted in increased in vitro immune responses, which correlated to decreased wound infections and decreased length of hospital stay (Daly et al., 1988). T-lymphocyte blastogenesis was also preserved and enhanced in moderately stressed intensive care unit patients given an enteral diet containing large amounts of arginine (Daly et al., 1988). Whether these effects translate into an improvement in clinical outcomes in critically ill patients remains unclear.

Of interest, arginine supplementation following vaccination against *Streptococcus pneumoniae* in people aged 60 and older resulted in increased neutrophil chemotaxis, natural killer cytotoxicity, and serum concentration of immunoglobulin G. These results suggest that arginine supplementation may enhance the immune response elicited by the pneumococcal vaccine in older people (Moriguti et al., 2005).

Wound Healing

In the United States, chronic wounds affect nearly 6.5 million patients and annually cost in excess of $25 to treat. This burden is expected to grow, in part due to an aging population (Sen et al., 2009). Much research has been focused on the prevention and treatment of wounds. Arginine supplementation has been investigated as a means of enhancing wound healing. Although a lot has been learned, much remains unknown.

Seifter and Levinson first postulated the role of arginine in wound healing in 1978. They demonstrated that arginine-deficient animals subjected to dorsal skin incision and closure had decreased wound breaking strength and wound collagen accumulation when compared to animals fed an normal arginine-containing diet (Seifter et al., 1978). Subsequent experiments revealed that chow-fed rats given a dietary supplement of 1% arginine had enhanced wound healing responses as assessed by wound breaking strength and collagen synthesis when compared to chow-fed controls. Likewise, parenteral fed rats given an amino acid mixture containing high doses of arginine (7.5 g/L) displayed superior wound healing via fresh wound strip breaking strength, fixed breaking strength, and collagen deposition (Barbul et al., 1985). In addition, mature rats fed diets supplemented with arginine and glycine had enhanced wound collagen deposition compared to controls (Chyun and Griminger, 1984).

Using a micromodel described by Goodson and Hunt that allows for studying fibroblastic responses and wound collagen deposition in human (Goodson and Hunt, 1982), 36 healthy human volunteers ages 25–35 years were given daily 17 g or 24.8 g of free arginine supplementation; this significantly increased the amount of hydroxyproline deposition at the wound site (an amino acid-specific for collagen) (Barbul et al., 1990). Subsequently, a study evaluated 30 volunteers > 70 years old who were given daily supplements of 17 g of free arginine and demonstrated significantly enhanced wound collagen accumulation. Arginine supplementation had no effect on the rate of epithelialization of a superficial skin defect, indicating that the predominant effect is on wound collagen deposition (Kirk et al., 1993). A more recent study demonstrated that arginine, in combination with other supplements, increases human wound collagen deposition (Williams et al., 2002).

No single theory can account for the observed effects of arginine on wound healing. Several possible mechanisms have been postulated to explain the effects and provide a framework for understanding (Fig. 27.2).

- Arginine supplementation provides a substrate for collagen synthesis at the wound site. Although free arginine makes up just a tiny amount of the collagen molecule, less than 5%, there could be utilization of arginine as substrate for proline through the following pathway:

$$\text{arginine} \rightarrow \text{ornithine} \rightarrow \text{glutamic semialdehyde} \rightarrow \text{proline}$$

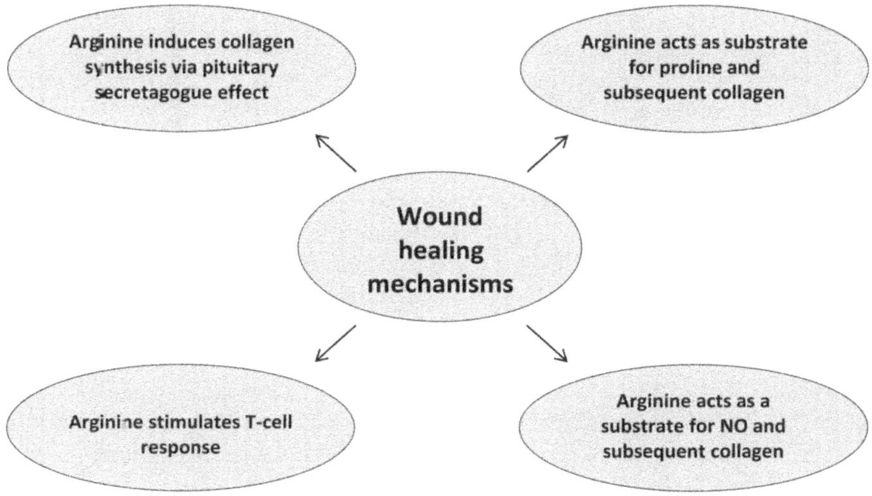

FIGURE 27.2 Wound healing and arginine: postulated mechanisms of action.

- Arginine levels are essentially nondetectable within the wound environment during the later phases of wound healing when fibroplasia predominates. While ornithine levels are higher in the wound than in the plasma, tracer isotope studies revealed that the rate of conversion of ornithine to proline in the wound is actually quite low, making this mechanism of arginine utilization unlikely (Albina et al., 2005).
- Arginine induces collagen synthesis via a pituitary secretagogue mechanism. The beneficial effects of supplemental arginine on wound healing are in many respects similar to those of growth hormone—namely, enhanced wound breaking strength and collagen deposition (Herndon et al., 1990; Jørgensen and Andreassen, 1988; Kowalewski and Yong, 1968). In support of such a mechanism, it has been noted that the effect of arginine on wound healing is abrogated in hypophysectomized animals (Barbul et al., 1983). In addition, arginine supplementation in doses that increase the wound healing response also induces elevations in plasma insulin-like growth factor, the peripheral mediator of growth hormone (Kirk et al., 1993).
- Arginine stimulates T-cell responses, thereby reducing the inhibitory effect of injury on T-cell function (Barbul et al., 1980a, b; Fabris and Mocchegiani, 1992). T lymphocytes are essential for normal wound healing as evidenced by decreased wound breaking strength in animals treated with monoclonal antibodies against T lymphocytes (Peterson et al., 1987). T lymphocytes are found immunohistochemically throughout the various phases of wound healing in distinct patterns (Fishel et al., 1987) and facilitating normal repair (Agaiby and Dyson, 1999).
- Arginine is the unique substrate for NO. Several studies suggest that NO plays a critical role in wound healing. Exogenous NO administration has been shown to increase collagen synthesis in cultured dermal fibroblasts (Schäffer et al., 1997). In contrast, inhibitors of NO have been shown to significantly impair healing of cutaneous incisional and colonic anastomotic healing in rodents (Efron, 1999; Schäffer et al., 1999). In models of impaired healing such as diabetes, NO synthesis is impaired together with decreased collagen accumulation, while administration of NO restores wound healing responses toward normal (Shi et al., 2003). Transfection of iNOS DNA into wounds results in supraphysiologic collagen deposition (Thornton et al., 1998). Conversely, mice lacking the iNOS gene have delayed the closure of excisional wounds, an impairment that is remedied by adenoviral transfer of the iNOS gene to the wound bed (Yamasaki et al., 1998). Strongly supporting this mechanism of action are findings that arginine does not stimulate wound healing in iNOS knockout mice, suggesting that the iNOS pathway is at least partially responsible for the enhancement of wound healing observed with the administration of arginine (Shi et al., 2000).

Cardiovascular Health

Cardiovascular disease, specifically heart disease, is the leading cause of death in the United States, accounting for more than 600,000 deaths per year (Xu et al., 2016). The role of arginine in cardiovascular health has been extensively studied at the basic science, translational, and clinical levels. Given that cardiovascular disease is a condition of aging, such discussion has implications for the elderly population.

As mentioned, arginine is the precursor for the endogenous synthesis of NO (Palmer et al., 1988; Schmidt et al., 1988). This pathway, although it only accounts for a small portion of arginine metabolism, has attracted much attention given the role of NO in vascular physiology and pathophysiology (Böger et al., 1996; Epstein et al., 1993). Normal plasma arginine concentrations are 80–120 μM, and the K_m for arginine as substrate for NOS is ~1–10 μM (Brosnan, 2003; Wu et al., 2007). Given such, it appears that there should be a surplus of substrate. Despite this logic, several studies indicate that administration of exogenous arginine increases the generation of NO, a phenomenon now termed the *arginine paradox*. When examining vascular endothelial function in a lysinuric protein intolerant patient who had a defect in a dibasic amino acid transporter, there was noted impaired uptake of exogenous arginine, leading to a 79% lower plasma concentration. Assessment of the NO-dependent endothelial function revealed 70% lower serum levels of NO. Moreover, the study revealed decreased flow-mediated brachial artery vasodilator response, elevated plasma fibrin degradation products, increased thrombin–antithrombin III complex, and reduced circulating platelet count. Parenteral infusion of arginine reversed all of these effects (Kamada et al., 2001).

Generated NO is an important messenger molecule with diverse function. Animal models of human disease—including hypercholesterolemic rabbits (Böger et al., 1997; 1995; Cooke et al., 1991), hyperlipidemic monkeys (Quillen et al., 1991), and hypertensive rats (Lüscher and Vanhoutte, 1986)—have shown that the biologic functions of endothelium-derived NO are impaired, leading to dysregulation of endothelial control of vascular tone and blood flow. In all of these models, arginine supplementation helped restore NO production and improve endothelial dysfunction.

Translated to the human population, a multitude of positive results in the prevention and management of cardiovascular disease and its downstream organ system effects have been reported. Examples include the following:

- 4–24 g/day of enteral arginine supplementation significantly lowered both systolic and diastolic blood pressure (Dong et al., 2011);
- 6.6 g/day of enteral arginine supplementation in patients with peripheral arterial disease resulted in a 66% increase in pain-free walking distance, 23% increase in total walking distance, and improved emotional and social functions per SF-36—effects that were initially noted at two weeks and were sustained at 10 weeks (Maxwell et al., 2000);
- 15 g/day of enteral arginine supplementation in patients with congestive heart failure led to improvement in glomerular filtration rate, natriuresis, and plasma endothelin levels at 5 days (Watanabe et al., 2000);
- 6.6 g/day of enteral arginine supplementation in a patient with type 1 diabetes with debilitating exertional angina pectoris resulted in complete amelioration of angina and normalized exercise capacity at 7 days (Schwartz, 2003);
- 8.4 g/day of enteral arginine supplementation in hypercholesterolemic humans showed modest attenuation of platelet reactivity and aggregation (Wolf et al., 1997); and
- 17 g/day of enteral arginine supplementation in a healthy, nonsmoking, elderly population revealed a decreased serum total cholesterol level with a reduction in low-density lipoprotein cholesterol but not high-density lipoprotein cholesterol. Thus, the ratio of low- to high-density lipoprotein fraction was increased (Hurson et al., 1995).

Despite the evidence supporting the use of arginine for cardiovascular health, other studies have failed to show any benefit. In one randomized clinic trial, there was no improvement in vascular stiffness measurements or ejection fraction with the addition of arginine in the acute postinfarction period (Schulman et al., 2006). Moreover, in men with stable angina, oral supplementation with 15 g/day of arginine was not associated with improvement in endothelium-dependent vasodilation, oxidative stress, or exercise performance (Walker et al., 2001). Lastly, oral supplementation of 6 g/day of arginine in patients with coronary artery disease did not affect exercise-induced changes in QT-interval duration, QT dispersion, or the magnitude of ST-segment depression (Bednarz et al., 2000).

Though the clinical and therapeutic benefit of arginine supplementation on mitigating cardiovascular disease varies, arginine supplementation may be favorable in at-risk patient populations. The possible role of arginine in maintaining or improving cardiac function prior to onset of severe disease merits further study.

Neurologic Function

Neurodegeneration is characterized by progressive deterioration in cognitive ability and capacity for independent living. The arising clinical syndrome—dementia—is typically a condition that affects older people and leads to disability and dependence (Prince et al., 2013). Given the rising epidemic secondary to population aging, much research has been undertaken on the topic.

Given its role in NO production via neuronal NOS, the function of arginine supplementation on neurologic function has yet to be fully investigated. However, studies exploring the importance of NO on memory and learning via synaptic plasticity is growing (Böhme et al., 1991; Susswein et al., 2004; Zhou and Zhu, 2009). In vitro experiments have shown that NO serves to increase glutamate release and increase synaptic effectiveness, an occurrence termed *potentiation* that is thought to improve memory (Epstein et al., 1993). In vivo, the same physiology is likely present, for studies reveal that inhibiting NO impairs learning behavior (Chapman et al., 1992). A few investigations have explored the role of arginine supplementation on age-related degenerative neurologic disorders, specifically senile dementia and Alzheimer's disease. The former study revealed improved cognitive function and reduced lipid peroxidation in 16 elderly patients following arginine supplementation (Ohtsuka and Nakaya, 2000). The latter concluded that arginine might provide a protective effect through the redox stress and inflammatory process and regulation of synaptic plasticity and neurogenesis (Yi et al., 2009).

Sexual Function

Sexual dysfunction is highly prevalent in both men and women and is a topic of particular importance to the elderly population because sexual dysfunction is clearly associated with advancing age (Laumann et al., 1999). Given the prevalence, a multitude of investigations have focused on sexual dysfunction, including a possible role for arginine supplementation. Thus far, there is no clear evidence of benefit. It is known that NO, through the synthesis of cyclic guanosine 5'-monophosphate, functions to initiate and maintain increased intracavernous pressure, penile vasodilatation, and penile erection. Thus, it is postulated that the production of NO via arginine, through the NOS pathway, may be of importance in sexual physiology.

In the 1950s, researchers first showed that adult men fed an arginine-deficient diet for nine days had an approximately 90% decreased sperm count and a 10-fold increase in the percentage of nonmotile sperm (Albanese, 1952). A subsequent study showed that supplementing infertile men with oral arginine for 6–8 weeks increased sperm counts and motility (Tanimura, 1967). The role of arginine in erectile dysfunction has also been studied. Studies in mice (Moody et al., 1997) and humans (Chen et al., 2001; Zorgniotti and Lizza, 1994) revealed improved erectile response and, in humans, subjective improvement in sexual function following arginine supplementation. A more robust study, however, utilizing a crossover design, failed to show benefit in arginine supplementation versus placebo in the management of impotence (Klotz et al., 1999). Despite the unclear benefit, arginine remains an active ingredient in most over-the-counter aphrodisiacs and sexual enhancement formulas.

Endocrinology

Endocrine disturbances are common in the aging population. A study in 2010 revealed that 9.6% of people 65 and older carried the diagnosis of diabetes mellitus (DM). An additional 9.3% of the population met clinical criteria for the disease but had not yet been diagnosed (Harris, 1990). Given such prevalence, the role of arginine on the endocrine system has been studied and will be discussed in the following.

Intravenous infusions of essential amino acids, specifically arginine, induce the release of insulin in humans (Floyd et al., 1966). Further, enteral intraduodenal arginine infusions result in sustained increases in plasma insulin levels (Dupre et al., 1969) with no observed hypoglycemic events. Later studies revealed that arginine supplementation also increases concentrations of glucagon (Palmer et al., 1976) and growth hormone (Merimee et al., 1965). The role of arginine in growth hormone secretion was further studied and revealed mixed results (Isidori et al., 1981). Arginine has also been found to stimulate the release of prolactin (Rakoff et al., 1973), pancreatic polypeptides, and somatostatin (Weir et al., 1978). Despite evidence of the endocrine-related actions of arginine, the underlying mechanism remains unclear. One proposed method is through arginine-derived NO (Schmidt et al., 1992).

Diabetes is associated with reduced levels of plasma arginine (Pieper et al., 1996) and elevated levels of the NOS inhibitor asymmetric dimethylarginine (Abbasi et al., 2001). Arginine supplementation may be an effective way to improve endothelial function and insulin sensitivity in DM (Giugliano et al., 1997; Wascher et al., 1997). Arginine also reduces microangiopathic complications of DM by counteracting lipid peroxidation (Lubec et al., 1997). A robust double-blind study revealed that oral administration of 9 g/day of arginine significantly improved peripheral and hepatic insulin sensitivity (Piatti et al., 2001). Again, the mechanisms remains unclear, but both NO-dependent (Schmidt et al., 1992) and NO-independent (Thams and Capito, 1999) pathways have been postulated to be operational.

ARGININE DOSING AND SUPPLEMENTATION

Throughout this chapter, we have discussed many putative effects of arginine based on the growing appreciation of arginine biochemistry and biology since the 1980s. The discovery of arginine as the precursor of nitric oxide led to increasing numbers of studies examining the potential effects in patients with coronary artery disease, peripheral artery disease, and other diseases that may benefit from increased NO production. However, many other conditions may also have therapeutic benefits, including wound healing and immunologic responses. Consumers have many over-the-counter supplements available to them, all of which are various formulations of arginine or arginine in combination with one or more other nutrients or compounds. Overall there is no good systematic data identifying which if any of these supplements might be beneficial. A number of studies examining oral arginine supplementation can be found in Table 27.1, which demonstrates the diversity in dosing and indications for arginine supplementation that have been examined in humans. When considering supplementation with arginine, an arginine-containing supplement, or any nutritional supplement, medical advice should always be obtained.

Pharmacokinetics of Arginine and Citrulline

The biologic effects of arginine appear to be influenced by its plasma concentration, and several studies have made kinetic measurements following single or multiple oral doses (Bode-Böger et al., 1998). More recently, the pharmacokinetics of citrulline have been investigated given the close relationship of arginine and citrulline (i.e., the citrulline–NO pathway), as well as the observation that citrulline increases circulating arginine via endogenous synthesis. For example, Moinard and colleagues found that citrulline supplementation increased plasma arginine concentrations without altering urea or urine urea nitrogen excretion, thus increasing nitrogen balance (Rougé et al., 2007).

The average plasma concentration of arginine in fasted humans is approximately 80–100 μM (Bode-Böger et al., 1998; Cynober, 2002; Tangphao et al., 1999), while citrulline concentration is significantly less at approximately 40 μM (Cynober, 2002). Two particular studies have reported both 6 g (Bode-Böger et al., 1998) or 10 g (Tangphao et al., 1999) oral supplementation of arginine leading to maximal concentrations of approximately 300 μM that are reached 60–90 min following ingestion. Maximal concentration is probably in this range for any single tolerated dose, given that increasing arginine concentration appears to plateau at greater administered amounts. When comparing arginine ingestion and citrulline ingestion at increasing doses, citrulline is actually more effective at increasing arginine concentration compared to supplemental arginine itself (Schwedhelm et al., 2008). As one might expect, this is consistent with the endogenous pathway of arginine synthesis mentioned previously in this chapter, which involves intestinal release of citrulline that completely bypasses the liver and is transported to the kidney, where citrulline is used for endogenous synthesis of arginine (Fig. 27.1) (Crenn et al., 2008).

The oral bioavailability of a single oral dose of arginine appears to plateau prior to a 6 g administration, as 6 g orally is associated with approximately 70% bioavailability (Bode-Böger et al., 1998) while 10 g appears to saturate transport and be only 20% bioavailable (Tangphao et al., 1999). In contrast to the bioavailability of arginine, however, citrulline bioavailability appears markedly increased, though there appears to be a lack of studies that fully evaluate the kinetics (Cynober, 2007). Regardless, no experiments appear to have used sufficient doses to saturate citrulline absorption by the gastrointestinal tract. The interesting finding is that citrulline lacks these common gastrointestinal (GI) side effects from similarly structural amino acids, indicating that the transport of citrulline does not appear to be limited (Breuillard et al., 2015; Schwedhelm et al., 2008).

Longevity of supplementation and risk of exposure to excess arginine or citrulline and its effect on long-term maintenance of metabolite concentrations remains unknown. It is important to note that most studies examine either acute (single dose) or subacute (days to weeks of treatment) dosing regimens and not chronic dosing (Schwedhelm et al., 2008). It is unknown how these different lengths of exposure affect the expression of metabolizing enzymes or other compensatory mechanisms given the increased arginine or citrulline delivered via supplementation. Also, it has yet to be elucidated whether the biologic effect could wane or subside with time or prolonged exposure.

Practical Considerations

There are several practical considerations regarding arginine supplementation. The obvious hurdle to overcome with increasingly larger doses of oral arginine supplementation is that arginine has an unpleasant taste, at least at doses of >7 g orally at a single administration (Evans et al., 2004). Larger doses (approximately 9 g per single oral dose and greater) tend to be poorly tolerated in terms of gastrointestinal cramping, bloating, and diarrhea. These GI

TABLE 27.1 Representative Studies Examining Oral Arginine Administration in Human Subjects on Clinical Endpoints

Study	Year	Subjects	Time Course	Total Daily Arginine Dose	Endpoints
Rector et al. (1996)	1996	Heart failure (*n*=15); crossover	6 weeks	5.6–12.6 g	Increased forearm blood flow
Wolf et al. (1997)	1997	Hypercholesterolemia (*n*=15 arginine, 8 placebo)	2 weeks	8.4 g	Decreased platelet aggregation
Ceremużyński et al. (1997)	1997	Prior MI; stable angina (*n*=12 arginine, 10 placebo)	3 days	6 g	Increased time to maximal ST depression during exercise; decreased maximal ST depression
Lerman et al., (1998)	1998	CAD (*n*=13 arginine, 13 placebo)	6 months	9 g	Increased acetylcholine-mediated coronary blood flow; improved symptom scores
Blum et al. (2000)	2000	CAD patients (*n*=30); crossover	1 months	9 g	Increased plasma arginine; no change in nitrogen oxides, flow-mediated brachial artery dilation, or vascular adhesion molecules
Mullen et al. (2000)	2000	Type 1 diabetes (ages 18–47; *n*=22 arginine, 22 placebo)	6 weeks	14 g	No change in endothelial dysfunction
Maxwell et al. (2000)	2000	PAD (intermittent claudication) (*n*=12/15 arginine, 14 placebo)	8 weeks	0, 3.3, 6.6 g	Increased pain-free walking and walking distance
Maxwell et al. (2002)	2002	CAD (chronic stale angina) (*n*=36); crossover	2 weeks	6 g (food sup)	Improved flow-mediated arterial dilation, increased treadmill exercise time
Lekakis et al. (2002)	2002	Essential hypertension (*n*=18 arg, 17 placebo)	1.5 h	6 g	Flow-mediated dilation of the brachial artery increased
Staff et al. (2004)	2004	Pre-eclampsia (*n*=15 arginine, 15 placebo)	5 days	12 g	No change in diastolic blood pressure
Oka et al. (2005)	2005	PAD (*n*=18 placebo, 18/17/19 arginine);	12 weeks	0, 9, 18, 27 g	Nonsignificant trends for increased speed and distance
VINTAGE MI Trial* (Schulman et al., 2006)	2006	60 years or older (*n*=78 arginine, 75 placebo); confirmed STEMI	6 months	9 g	No effect on vascular stiffness or ejection fraction; *trial halted for increased mortality in arginine group
NO-PAIN Study (Wilson et al., 2007)	2007	PAD; intermittent claudication (*n* = 67 placebo, 66 arginine)	6 months	3 g	No changes in nitrogen oxides, vascular reactivity, or walking distance
Ruel et al. (2008)	2008	Surgical three-vessel CAD (*n*=19 total, divided into 4 groups)	3 months	6 g vs. placebo (all patients receiving VEGF intraop)	Increased myocardial perfusion and contractility
Lucotti et al. (2009)	2009	Nondiabetic CAD (*n*=32 arginine, 32 placebo)	6 months	6.4 g	Increased insulin sensitivity; decreased IL-6, MCP-1

CAD, coronary arterial disease; *PAD*, peripheral arterial disease; *STEMI*, ST-elevation myocardial infarction; *MI*, myocardial infarction; *MCP-1*, monocyte chemotactic protein-1; *IL-6*, interleukin-6; *VEGF*, vasculoendothelial growth factor; *VINTAGE MI*, Vascular Interaction with Age in Myocardial Infarction.

effects are likely related to the osmotic effects of slow enterocyte uptake (Grimble, 2007), but there are data to suggest that these may be mediated by local increases in NO concentration in the enterocyte milieu as well. Note that supplementation is typically on a background dietary intake of arginine that typically ranges from 2.5 to 5 g/day (Gad, 2010). Despite previous studies reporting supplemental doses of up to 30 g/day (in split doses) being generally well tolerated, more recent studies suggest that nausea and diarrhea become nearly universal when single dosing is escalated—especially amounts of arginine from 15 to 30 g per single oral dose (Gad, 2010; Moinard et al., 2008).

As mentioned, the role of citrulline in arginine homeostasis has been studied, especially whether or not citrulline might be a more effective supplement compared to arginine. Citrulline is better tolerated based on the absence of reported gastrointestinal side effects (Moinard et al., 2008). Oral citrulline increases nitrogen balance and plasma arginine concentrations (Rougé et al., 2007). In fact, when the appearance of both citrulline and arginine in the plasma are measured following oral citrulline dosing, plasma arginine concentration increases in response to citrulline more than arginine supplementation. These results are consistent with the conversion of citrulline to arginine in the kidney being a saturable process (Moinard et al., 2008).

As previously mentioned, the GI side effects of arginine supplementation further make the potential for citrulline more attractive as a long-term, high-dose supplement. The intestinal dibasic amino acid transporter responsible for arginine absorption (as well as other amino acids) is a high-affinity and low-capacity system (Grimble, 2007). Arginine, ornithine, citrulline, and cystine share the same enterocyte transporter (Grimble, 2007), but citrulline remains free from many of these side effects associated with significant arginine intake. What is particularly interesting and currently unknown is why citrulline, but not the other metabolites sharing this transporter, lacks GI side effects.

Arginine Dosing and Aging

Whether or not aging affects how arginine dosing should or can be administered is not well studied. Moreover, the exact mechanisms of how aging affects the absorption of nutrients in general is not completely understood in human or animal models, and many questions remain (Holt, 2007; Keller and Layer, 2014; Schiller, 2009). Aging has a range of effects on macro- and micronutrient absorption, and it is likely that these effects could significantly vary between individuals. Clearly, many questions need to be answered about arginine metabolism in general as well as potentially innovative ways identified to take advantage of biology to augment endogenous responses to amino acids for therapeutic purposes. Could citrulline supplementation be a reasonable way to augment endogenous arginine availability? Could citrulline be advantageous in aged individuals or others with intrinsic intestinal pathology leading to poor GI absorption? These as well as many other questions are important but currently remain unanswered.

References

Abbasi, F., Asagmi, T., Cooke, J.P., Lamendola, C., McLaughlin, T., Reaven, G.M., et al., 2001. Plasma concentrations of asymmetric dimethylarginine are increased in patients with type 2 diabetes mellitus. Am. J. Cardiol 88, 1201–1203. <http://dx.doi.org/10.1016/S0002-9149(01)02063-X>.

Agaiby, A., Dyson, M., 1999. Immuno-inflammatory cell dynamics during cutaneous wound healing. J. Anat. 195, 531–542. <http://dx.doi.org/10.1046/j.1469-7580.1999.19540531.x>.

Agarwal, S., Busse, P.J., 2010. Innate and adaptive immunosenescence. Ann. Allergy Asthma Immunol. 104, 183–190. <http://dx.doi.org/10.1016/j.anai.2009.11.009>.

Albanese, A.A., 1952. The effects of amino acid deficiencies in man. Am. J. Clin. Nutr 1, 44–51.

Albina, J.E., Mahoney, E.J., Daley, J.M., Wesche, D.E., Morris Jr, S.M., Reichner, J.S., 2005. Macrophage arginase regulation by CCAAT/Enhancer-binding protein beta. Shock 23, 168–172. <http://dx.doi.org/10.1097/01.shk.0000148054.74268.e2>.

Ban, H., Shigemitsu, K., Yamatsuji, T., Haisa, M., Nakajo, T., Takaoka, M., et al., 2004. Arginine and Leucine regulate p70 S6 kinase and 4E-BP1 in intestinal epithelial cells. Int. J. Mol. Med. 13, 537–543. <http://dx.doi.org/10.3892/ijmm.13.4.537>.

Barbul, A., Wasserkrug, H.L., Seifter, E., Rettura, G., Levenson, S.M., Efron, G., 1980a. Immunostimulatory effects of arginine in normal and injured rats. J. Surg. Res. 29, 228–235. <http://dx.doi.org/10.1016/0022-4804(80)90165-1>.

Barbul, A., Wasserkrug, H.L., Sisto, D.A., Seifter, E., Rettura, G., Levenson, S.M., et al., 1980b. Thymic stimulatory actions of arginine. JPEN J. Parenter. Enteral. Nutr. 4, 446–449. <http://dx.doi.org/10.1177/014860718000400502>.

Barbul, A., Rettura, G., Levenson, S.M., Seifter, E., 1983. Wound healing and thymotropic effects of arginine: a pituitary mechanism of action. Am. J. Clin. Nutr 37, 786–794.

Barbul, A., Fishel, R.S., Shimazu, S., Wasserkrug, H.L., Yoshimura, N.N., Tao, R.C., et al., 1985. Intravenous hyperalimentation with high arginine levels improves wound healing and immune function. J. Surg. Res. 38, 328–334. <http://dx.doi.org/10.1016/0022-4804(85)90045-9>.

Barbul, A., Lazarou, S.A., Efron, D.T., Wasserkrug, H.L., Efron, G., 1990. Arginine enhances wound healing and lymphocyte immune responses in humans. Surgery 108, 336–337. 331–6– discussion.

Bauchart-Thevret, C., Cui, L., Wu, G., Burrin, D.G., 2010. Arginine-induced stimulation of protein synthesis and survival in IPEC-J2 cells is mediated by mTOR but not nitric oxide. AJP: Endocrinol. Metab. 299, E899–E909. <http://dx.doi.org/10.1152/ajpendo.00068.2010>.

Bednarz, B., Wolk, R., Chamiec, T., Herbaczyńska-Cedro, K., Winek, D., Ceremużyński, L., 2000. Effects of oral l-arginine supplementation on exercise-induced QT dispersion and exercise tolerance in stable angina pectoris. Int. J. Cardiol. 75, 205–210. <http://dx.doi.org/10.1016/S0167-5273(00)00324-7>.

Bernstein, L.H., 1996. The impact of immunonutrition. Gastroenterology 110, 1677–1678. <http://dx.doi.org/10.1053/gast.1996.v110.agast961677>.

Blum, A., Hathaway, L., Mincemoyer, R., Schenke, W.H., Kirby, M., Csako, G., et al., 2000. Oral L-arginine in patients with coronary artery disease on medical management. Circulation 101, 2160–2164.

Bode-Böger, S.M., Böger, R.H., Galland, A., Tsikas, D., Frölich, J.C., 1998. L-arginine-induced vasodilation in healthy humans: pharmacokinetic–pharmacodynamic relationship. Br. J. Clin. Pharmacol. 46, 489–497. <http://dx.doi.org/10.1046/j.1365-2125.1998.00803.x>.

Böger, R.H., Bode-Böger, S.M., Mügge, A., Kienke, S., Brandes, R., Dwenger, A., et al., 1995. Supplementation of hypercholesterolaemic rabbits with L-arginine reduces the vascular release of superoxide anions and restores NO production. Atherosclerosis 117, 273–284. <http://dx.doi.org/10.1016/0021-9150(95)05582-H>.

Böger, R.H., Bode-Böger, S.M., Frölich, J.C., 1996. The l-arginine—nitric oxide pathway: role in atherosclerosis and therapeutic implications. Atherosclerosis 127, 1–11. <http://dx.doi.org/10.1016/S0021-9150(96)05953-9>.

Böger, R.H., Bode-Böger, S.M., Brandes, R.P., Phivthong-ngam, L., Böhme, M., Nafe, R., et al., 1997. Dietary L-arginine reduces the progression of atherosclerosis in cholesterol-fed rabbits: comparison with lovastatin. Circulation 96, 1282–1290. <http://dx.doi.org/10.1161/01.CIR.96.4.1282>.

Böhme, G.A., Bon, C., Stutzmann, J.-M., Doble, A., Blanchard, J.-C., 1991. Possible involvement of nitric oxide in long-term potentiation. Eur. J. Pharmacol. 199, 379–381. <http://dx.doi.org/10.1016/0014-2999(91)90505-K>.

Breuillard, C., Cynober, L., Moinard, C., 2015. Citrulline and nitrogen homeostasis: an overview. Amino Acids 47, 685–691. <http://dx.doi.org/10.1007/s00726-015-1932-2>.

Brittenden, J., Heys, S.D., Ross, J., Park, K.G.M., Eremin, O., 1994. Nutritional pharmacology: effects of l-arginine on host defences, response to trauma and tumor growth. Clin. Sci. 86, 123–132. <http://dx.doi.org/10.1042/cs0860123>.

Bronstein-Sitton, N., Wang, L., Cohen, L., Baniyash, M., 1999. Expression of the T cell antigen receptor zeta chain following activation is controlled at distinct checkpoints. Implications for cell surface receptor down-modulation and re-expression. J. Biol. Chem. 274, 23659–23665. <http://dx.doi.org/10.1074/jbc.274.33.23659>.

Bronte, V., Zanovello, P., 2005. Regulation of immune responses by L-arginine metabolism. Nat. Rev. Immunol. 5, 641–654. <http://dx.doi.org/10.1038/nri1668>.

Brosnan, J.T., 2003. Interorgan amino acid transport and its regulation. J. Nutr 133, 2068S–2072S.

Brosnan, J.T., Brosnan, M.E., 2010. Creatine metabolism and the urea cycle. Mol. Genet. Metab. 100, S49–S52. <http://dx.doi.org/10.1016/j.ymgme.2010.02.020>.

Callery, M.P., Mangino, M.J., Flye, M.W., 1991. Arginine-specific suppression of mixed lymphocyte culture reactivity by kupffer cells - a basis of portal venous tolerance. Transplantation 51, 1076–1079. <http://dx.doi.org/10.1097/00007890-199105000-00028>.

Carraway, M.S., Piantadosi, C.A., Jenkinson, C.P., Huang, Y.-C.T., 2015. Differential expression of arginase and iNOS in the lung in sepsis. Exp. Lung Res. 24, 253–268. <http://dx.doi.org/10.3109/01902149809041533>.

Castillo, L., 1996. Whole body nitric oxide synthesis in healthy men determined from [15N]arginine-to-[15N]citrulline labeling. Proc. Natl. Acad. Sci. USA 93, 11460–11465.

Castillo, L., Chapman, T.E., Yu, Y.M., Ajami, A., Burke, J.F., Young, V.R., 1993. Dietary arginine uptake by the splanchnic region in adult humans. Am. J. Physiol 265, E532–E539.

Castillo, L., Sanchez, M., Vogt, J., Chapman, T.E., DeRojas-Walker, T.C., Tannenbaum, S.R., et al., 1995. Plasma arginine, citrulline, and ornithine kinetics in adults, with observations on nitric oxide synthesis. Am. J. Physiol. 268, E360–E367.

Ceremużyński, L., Chamiec, T., Herbaczyńska-Cedro, K., 1997. Effect of Supplemental Oral l-Arginine on Exercise Capacity in Patients With Stable Angina Pectoris. Am. J. Cardiol. 80, 331–333. <http://dx.doi.org/10.1016/S0002-9149(97)00354-8>.

Chapman, P.F., Atkins, C.M., Allen, M.T., Haley, J.E., Steinmetz, J.E., 1992. Inhibition of nitric oxide synthesis impairs two different forms of learning. Neuroreport 3, 567–570. <http://dx.doi.org/10.1097/00001756-199207000-00005>.

Chen, W., Chernichovsky, I., Sofer, M., 2001. Effect of oral administration of high-dose nitric oxide donor l-arginine in men with organic erectile dysfunction: results of a double-blind, randomized, placebo-controlled study. BJU Int. 83, 269–273. <http://dx.doi.org/10.1046/j.1464-410x.1999.00906.x>.

Chyun, J.H., Griminger, P., 1984. Improvement of nitrogen retention by arginine and glycine supplementation and its relation to collagen synthesis in traumatized mature and aged rats. J. Nutr 114, 1697–1704.

Clark, R., Feleke, G., Din, M., Yasmin, T., Singh, G., Khan, F., et al., 2000. Nutritional treatment for acquired immunodeficiency virus-associated wasting using beta-hydroxy beta-methylbutyrate, glutamine, and arginine: a randomized, double-blind, placebo-controlled study. JPEN J. Parenter. Enteral. Nutr. 24, 133–139. <http://dx.doi.org/10.1177/0148607100024003133>.

Cooke, J.P., Andon, N.A., Girerd, X.J., Hirsch, A.T., Creager, M.A., 1991. Arginine restores cholinergic relaxation of hypercholesterolemic rabbit thoracic aorta. Circulation 83, 1057–1062. <http://dx.doi.org/10.1161/01.CIR.83.3.1057>.

Corl, B.A., Odle, J., Niu, X., Moeser, A.J., Gatlin, L.A., Phillips, O.T., et al., 2008. Arginine activates intestinal p70(S6k) and protein synthesis in piglet rotavirus enteritis. J. Nutr 138, 24–29.

Crenn, P., Messing, B., Cynober, L., 2008. Citrulline as a biomarker of intestinal failure due to enterocyte mass reduction☆. Clin. Nutr. 27, 328–339. <http://dx.doi.org/10.1016/j.clnu.2008.02.005>.

Curis, E., Nicolis, I., Moinard, C., Osowska, S., Zerrouk, N., Bénazeth, S., et al., 2005. Almost all about citrulline in mammals. Amino acids 29, 177–205. <http://dx.doi.org/10.1007/s00726-005-0235-4>.

Curis, E., Crenn, P., Cynober, L., 2007. Citrulline and the gut. Curr. Opin. Clin. Nutr. Metab. Care 10, 620–626. <http://dx.doi.org/10.1097/MCO.0b013e32829fb38d>.

Cynober, L.A., 2002. Plasma amino acid levels with a note on membrane transport: characteristics, regulation, and metabolic significance. Nutrition 18, 761–766. <http://dx.doi.org/10.1016/S0899-9007(02)00780-3>.

Cynober, L., 2007. Pharmacokinetics of arginine and related amino acids. J. Nutr 137, 1646S–1649S.

Daly, J.M., Reynolds, J., Thom, A., Kinsley, L., Dietrick-Gallagher, M., Shou, J., et al., 1988. Immune and metabolic effects of arginine in the surgical patient. Ann. Surg 208, 512–523.

de Jonge, W.J., Hallemeesch, M.M., Kwikkers, K.L., Ruijter, J.M., de Gier-de Vries, C., van Roon, M.A., et al., 2002a. Overexpression of arginase I in enterocytes of transgenic mice elicits a selective arginine deficiency and affects skin, muscle, and lymphoid development. Am. J. Clin. Nutr. 76, 128–140. <http://dx.doi.org/10.1203/00006450-199804000-00002>.

de Jonge, W.J., Kwikkers, K.L., Velde te, A.A., van Deventer, S.J.H., Nolte, M.A., Mebius, R.E., et al., 2002b. Arginine deficiency affects early B cell maturation and lymphoid organ development in transgenic mice. J. Clin. Investig 110, 1539–1548. <http://dx.doi.org/10.1172/JCI16143>.

Dejong, C.H., Welters, C.F., Deutz, N.E., Heineman, E., Soeters, P.B., 1998. Renal arginine metabolism in fasted rats with subacute short bowel syndrome. Clin. Sci. 95, 409–418. <http://dx.doi.org/10.1042/cs0950409>.

Devés, R., Boyd, C.A., 1998. Transporters for cationic amino acids in animal cells: discovery, structure, and function. Physiol. Rev. 78, 487–545. <http://dx.doi.org/10.1016/0022-4804(91)90210-D>.

Dong, J.-Y., Qin, L.-Q., Zhang, Z., Zhao, Y., Wang, J., Arigoni, F., et al., 2011. Effect of oral l-arginine supplementation on blood pressure: a meta-analysis of randomized, double-blind, placebo-controlled trials. Am. Heart J. 162, 959–965. <http://dx.doi.org/10.1016/j.ahj.2011.09.012>.

Dupre, J., Curtis, J.D., Unger, R.H., Waddell, R.W., Beck, J.C., 1969. Effects of secretin, pancreozymin, or gastrin on the response of the endocrine pancreas to administration of glucose or arginine in man. J. Clin. Investig 48, 745–757. <http://dx.doi.org/10.1172/JCI106032>.

Durante, W., 2013. Role of Arginase in Vessel Wall Remodeling. Front. Immunol, 4. <http://dx.doi.org/10.3389/fimmu.2013.00111>.

Durante, W., Johnson, F.K., Johnson, R.A., 2007. Arginase: a critical regulator of nitric oxide synthesis and vascular function. Clin. Exp. Pharmacol. Physiol. 34, 906–911. <http://dx.doi.org/10.1111/j.1440-1681.2007.04638.x>.

Efron, D., 1999. Expression and function of inducible nitric oxide synthase during rat colon anastomotic healing. J. Gastrointest. Surg. 3, 592–601. <http://dx.doi.org/10.1016/S1091-255X(99)80080-8>.

Efron, D.T., Kirk, S.J., Regan, M.C., Wasserkrug, H.L., Barbul, A., 1991. Nitric oxide generation from L-arginine is required for optimal human peripheral blood lymphocyte DNA synthesis. Surgery 110, 327–334.

Epstein, F.H., Moncada, S., Higgs, A., 1993. The L-Arginine-Nitric Oxide Pathway. N. Engl. J. Med 329, 2002–2012. <http://dx.doi.org/10.1056/NEJM199312303292706>.

Evans, R.W., Fernstrom, J.D., Thompson, J., Morris Jr, S.M., Kuller, L.H., 2004. Biochemical responses of healthy subjects during dietary supplementation with L-arginine. J. Nutr. Biochem 15, 534–539. <http://dx.doi.org/10.1016/j.jnutbio.2004.03.005>.

Fabris, N., Mocchegiani, E., 1992. Arginine-containing compounds and thymic endocrine activity. Thymus 19 (Suppl 1), S21–S30.

Fafournoux, P., Bruhat, A., Jousse, C., 2000. Amino acid regulation of gene expression. Biochem. J 351, 1–12.

Feldmeyer, N., Wabnitz, G., Leicht, S., Luckner-Minden, C., Schiller, M., Franz, T., et al., 2012. Arginine deficiency leads to impaired cofilin dephosphorylation in activated human T lymphocytes. Int. Immunol. 24, 303–313. <http://dx.doi.org/10.1093/intimm/dxs004>.

Fishel, R.S., Barbul, A., Beschorner, W.E., Wasserkrug, H.L., Efron, G., 1987. Lymphocyte participation in wound healing. Morphologic assessment using monoclonal antibodies. Ann. Surg. 206, 25–29.

Flakoll, P., Sharp, R., Baier, S., Levenhagen, D., Carr, C., Nissen, S., 2004. Effect of β-hydroxy-β-methylbutyrate, arginine, and lysine supplementation on strength, functionality, body composition, and protein metabolism in elderly women. Nutrition 20, 445–451. <http://dx.doi.org/10.1016/j.nut.2004.01.009>.

Floyd Jr, J.C., Fajans, S.S., Conn, J.W., Knopf, R.F., Rull, J., 1966. Stimulation of insulin secretion by amino acids. J. Clin. Investig. 45, 1487–1502. <http://dx.doi.org/10.1172/JCI105456>.

Gad, M.Z., 2010. Anti-aging effects of l-arginine. J. Adv. Res. 1, 169–177. <http://dx.doi.org/10.1016/j.jare.2010.05.001>.

Giugliano, D., Marfella, R., Verrazzo, G., Acampora, R., Nappo, F., Ziccardi, P., et al., 1997. L-arginine for testing endothelium-dependent vascular functions in health and disease. Am. J. Physiol 273, E606–E612.

Goodson III, W.H., Hunt, T.K., 1982. Development of a new miniature method for the study of wound healing in human subjects. J. Surg. Res. 33, 394–401. <http://dx.doi.org/10.1016/0022-4804(82)90054-3 >.

Grimble, G.K., 2007. Adverse gastrointestinal effects of arginine and related amino acids. J. Nutr 137, 1693S–1701S.

Haraguchi, Y., Takiguchi, M., Amaya, Y., Kawamoto, S., Matsuda, I., Mori, M., 1987. Molecular cloning and nucleotide sequence of cDNA for human liver arginase. Proc. Natl. Acad. Sci. 84, 412–415.

Harris, M.I., 1990. Epidemiology of diabetes mellitus among the elderly in the United States. Clin. Geriatr. Med 6, 703–719.

Häussinger, D., 1986. Regulation of hepatic ammonia metabolism: the intercellular glutamine cycle. Adv. Enzyme Regul. 25, 159–180. <http://dx.doi.org/10.1016/0065-2571(86)90013-0>.

Häussinger, D., Gerok, W., Sies, H., 1984. Hepatic role in pH regulation: role of the intercellular glutamine cycle. Trends Biochem. Sci. 9, 300–302. <http://dx.doi.org/10.1016/0968-0004(84)90294-9>.

Herndon, D.N., Barrow, R.E., Kunkel, K.R., Broemeling, L., Rutan, R.L., 1990. Effects of recombinant human growth hormone on donor-site healing in severely burned children. Ann. Surg 212, 424–429. – discussion 430–1.

Holowatz, L.A., Kenney, W.L., 2007. Up-regulation of arginase activity contributes to attenuated reflex cutaneous vasodilatation in hypertensive humans. J. Physiol. 581, 863–872. <http://dx.doi.org/10.1113/jphysiol.2007.128959>.

Holt, P.R., 2007. Intestinal malabsorption in the elderly. Dig. Dis. 25, 144–150. <http://dx.doi.org/10.1159/000099479>.

Hu, F.B., Stampfer, M.J., Manson, J.E., Rimm, E.B., Colditz, G.A., Rosner, B.A., et al., 1998. Frequent nut consumption and risk of coronary heart disease in women: prospective cohort study. BMJ 317, 1341–1345. <http://dx.doi.org/10.1136/bmj.317.7169.1341>.

Hurson, M., Regan, M.C., Kirk, S.J., Wasserkrug, H.L., Barbul, A., 1995. Metabolic effects of arginine in a healthy elderly population. JPEN J. Parenter. Enteral. Nutr. 19, 227–230. <http://dx.doi.org/10.1177/0148607195019003227>.

Ikemoto, M., Tsunekawa, S., Tanaka, K., Tanaka, A., Yamaoka, Y., Ozawa, K., et al., 1998. Liver-type arginase in serum during and after liver transplantation: a novel index in monitoring conditions of the liver graft and its clinical significance. Clin. Chim. Acta 271, 11–23. <http://dx.doi.org/10.1016/S0009-8981(97)00226-X>.

Isidori, A., Monaco, Lo, A., Cappa, M., 1981. A study of growth hormone release in man after oral administration of amino acids. Curr. Med. Res. Opin. 7, 475–481. <http://dx.doi.org/10.1185/03007998109114287>.

Iyer, R.K., Kim, H.K., Tsoa, R.W., Grody, W.W., Cederbaum, S.D., 2002. Cloning and characterization of human agmatinase. Mol. Genet. Metab. 75, 209–218. <http://dx.doi.org/10.1006/mgme.2001.3277>.

Johnson, F.K., Johnson, R.A., Peyton, K.J., Durante, W., 2005. Arginase inhibition restores arteriolar endothelial function in Dahl rats with salt-induced hypertension. AJP: Regul. Integr. Comp. Physiol. 288, R1057–R1062. <http://dx.doi.org/10.1152/ajpregu.00758.2004>.

Jørgensen, P.H., Andreassen, T.T., 1988. Influence of biosynthetic human growth hormone on biomechanical properties of rat skin incisional wounds. Acta Chir. Scand. 154, 623–626.

Kamada, Y., Nagaretani, H., Tamura, S., Ohama, T., Maruyama, T., Hiraoka, H., et al., 2001. Vascular endothelial dysfunction resulting from l-arginine deficiency in a patient with lysinuric protein intolerance. J. Clin. Investig 108, 717–724. <http://dx.doi.org/10.1172/JCI11260>.

Keller, J., Layer, P., 2014. The Pathophysiology of Malabsorption. Visc. Med. 30, 150–154. <http://dx.doi.org/10.1159/000364794>.

Kim, J.H., Bugaj, L.J., Oh, Y.J., Bivalacqua, T.J., Ryoo, S., Soucy, K.G., et al., 2009. Arginase inhibition restores NOS coupling and reverses endothelial dysfunction and vascular stiffness in old rats. J. Appl. Physiol. 107, 1249–1257. <http://dx.doi.org/10.1152/japplphysiol.91393.2008>.

King, D.E., Mainous III, A.G., Geesey, M.E., 2008. Variation in L-arginine intake follow demographics and lifestyle factors that may impact cardiovascular disease risk. Nutr. Res. 28, 21–24. <http://dx.doi.org/10.1016/j.nutres.2007.11.003>.

Kirk, S.J., Regan, M.C., Wasserkrug, H.L., Sodeyama, M., Barbul, A., 1992. Arginine enhances T-Cell responses in athymic nude mice. JPEN J. Parenter. Enteral. Nutr. 16, 429–432. <http://dx.doi.org/10.1177/0148607192016005429>.

Kirk, S.J., Hurson, M., Regan, M.C., Holt, D.R., Wasserkrug, H.L., Barbul, A., 1993. Arginine stimulates wound healing and immune function in elderly human beings. Surgery 114, 155–159. – discussion 160.

Klotz, T., Mathers, M.J., Braun, M., Bloch, W., Engelmann, U., 1999. Effectiveness of oral L-arginine in first-line treatment of erectile dysfunction in a controlled crossover study. Urol. Int. 63, 220–223. <http://dx.doi.org/10.1159/000030454>.

Kowalewski, K., Yong, S., 1968. Effect of growth hormone and an anabolic steroid on hydroxyproline in healing dermal wounds in rats. Eur. J. Endocrinol. 59, 53–66. <http://dx.doi.org/10.1530/acta.0.0590053>.

Laumann, E.O., Paik, A., Rosen, R.C., 1999. Sexual dysfunction in the United States: prevalence and predictors. JAMA 281, 537–544. <http://dx.doi.org/10.1001/jama.281.6.537>.

Längle, F., Roth, E., Steininger, R., Winkler, S., Mühlbacher, F., 1995. Arginase release following liver reperfusion. Evidence of hemodynamic action of arginase infusions. Transplantation 59, 1542–1549.

LeBien, T.W., 2002. Arginine: an unusual dietary requirement of pre-B lymphocytes? J. Clin. Investig. 110, 1411–1413. <http://dx.doi.org/10.1172/JCI17210>.

Lekakis, J.P., Papathanassiou, S., Papaioannou, T.G., Papamichael, C.M., Zakopoulos, N., Kotsis, V., et al., 2002. Oral l-arginine improves endothelial dysfunction in patients with essential hypertension. Int. J. Cardiol. 86, 317–323. <http://dx.doi.org/10.1016/S0167-5273(02)00413-8>.

Lerman, A., Burnett, J.C., Higano, S.T., McKinley, L.J., Holmes, D.R., 1998. Long-term L-arginine supplementation improves small-vessel coronary endothelial function in humans. Circulation 97, 2123–2128. <http://dx.doi.org/10.1161/01.CIR.97.21.2123>.

Li, P., Yin, Y.-L., Li, D., Kim, S.W., Wu, G., 2007. Amino acids and immune function. Br. J. Nutr. 98, 237–252. <http://dx.doi.org/10.1017/S000711450769936X>.

Lortie, M.J., Novotny, W.F., Peterson, O.W., Vallon, V., Malvey, K., Mendonca, M., et al., 1996. Agmatine, a bioactive metabolite of arginine. Production, degradation, and functional effects in the kidney of the rat. J. Clin. Investig. 97, 413–420. <http://dx.doi.org/10.1172/JCI118430>.

Lubec, B., Hayn, M., Kitzmüller, E., Vierhapper, H., Lubec, G., 1997. l-Arginine reduces lipid peroxidation in patients with diabetes mellitus. Free Radic. Biol. Med 22, 355–357. <http://dx.doi.org/10.1016/S0891-5849(96)00386-3>.

Lucotti, P., Monti, L., Setola, E., La Canna, G., Castiglioni, A., Rossodivita, A., et al., 2009. Oral l-arginine supplementation improves endothelial function and ameliorates insulin sensitivity and inflammation in cardiopathic nondiabetic patients after an aortocoronary bypass. Metabolism 58, 1270–1276. <http://dx.doi.org/10.1016/j.metabol.2009.03.029>.

Luiking, Y.C., Have, Ten, G.A.M., Wolfe, R.R., Deutz, N.E.P., 2012. Arginine de novo and nitric oxide production in disease states. AJP: Endocrinol. Metab. 303, E1177–E1189. <http://dx.doi.org/10.1152/ajpendo.00284.2012>.

Lüscher, T.F., Vanhoutte, P.M., 1986. Endothelium-dependent contractions to acetylcholine in the aorta of the spontaneously hypertensive rat. Hypertension 8, 344–348. <http://dx.doi.org/10.1161/01.HYP.8.4.344>.

Marini, J.C., 2012. Arginine and ornithine are the main precursors for citrulline synthesis in mice. J. Nutr. 142, 572–580. <http://dx.doi.org/10.3945/jn.111.153825>.

Maxwell, A.J., Anderson, B.E., Cooke, J.P., 2000. Nutritional therapy for peripheral arterial disease: a double-blind, placebo-controlled, randomized trial of HeartBar®. Vasc. Med. 5, 11–19. <http://dx.doi.org/10.1177/1358836X0000500103>.

Maxwell, A.J., Zapien, M.P., Pearce, G.L., MacCallum, G., Stone, P.H., 2002. Randomized trial of a medical food for the dietary management of chronic, stable angina. J. Am. Coll. Cardiol. 39, 37–45. <http://dx.doi.org/10.1016/S0735-1097(01)01708-9>.

May, P.E., Barber, A., D'Olimpio, J.T., Hourihane, A., Abumrad, N.N., 2002. Reversal of cancer-related wasting using oral supplementation with a combination of β-hydroxy-β-methylbutyrate, arginine, and glutamine. Am. J. Surg. 183, 471–479. <http://dx.doi.org/10.1016/S0002-9610(02)00823-1>.

Merimee, T., Lillicrap, D., Rabinowitz, D., 1965. Effect of arginine on serum-levels of human growth-hormone. Lancet 286, 668–670. <http://dx.doi.org/10.1016/S0140-6736(65)90399-5>.

Minami, Y., Weissman, A.M., Samelson, L.E., Klausner, R.D., 1987. Building a multichain receptor: synthesis, degradation, and assembly of the T-cell antigen receptor. Proc. Natl. Acad. Sci. USA 84, 2688–2692.

Moinard, C., Nicolis, I., Neveux, N., Darquy, S., Bénazeth, S., Cynober, L., 2008. Dose-ranging effects of citrulline administration on plasma amino acids and hormonal patterns in healthy subjects: the Citrudose pharmacokinetic study. Br. J. Nutr. 99, 855–862. <http://dx.doi.org/10.1017/S0007114507841110>.

Moinard, C., Maccario, J., Walrand, S., Lasserre, V., Marc, J., Boirie, Y., et al., 2015. Arginine behavior after arginine or citrulline administration in older subjects. Br. J. Nutr, 1–6. <http://dx.doi.org/10.1017/S0007114515004638>.

Moody, J.A., Vernet, D., Laidlaw, S., Rajfer, J., Gonzalez-Cadavid, N.F., 1997. Effects of long-term oral administration of L-Arginine on the rat erectile response. J. Urol. 158, 942–947. <http://dx.doi.org/10.1016/S0022-5347(01)64368-4 > >.

Mori, M., Gotoh, T., 2000. Regulation of nitric oxide production by arginine metabolic enzymes. Biochem. Biophys. Res. Commun. 275, 715–719. <http://dx.doi.org/10.1006/bbrc.2000.3169>.

Moriguchi, S., Mukai, K., Hiraoka, I., Kishino, Y., 1987. Functional changes in human lymphocytes and monocytes after in vitro incubation with arginine. Nutr. Res. <http://dx.doi.org/10.1016/S0271-5317(87)80102-1 > >.

Moriguti, J.C., Ferriolli, E., Donadi, E.A., Marchini, J.S., 2005. Effects of arginine supplementation on the humoral and innate immune response of older people. Eur. J. Clin. Nutr. 59, 1362–1366. <http://dx.doi.org/10.1038/sj.ejcn.1602247>.

Morris, S.M., 2002. Regulation of enzymes of the urea cycle and arginine metabolism. Annu. Rev. Nutr. 22, 87–105. <http://dx.doi.org/10.1146/annurev.nutr.22.110801.140547>.

Morris, S.M., 2004. Enzymes of arginine metabolism. J. Nutr 134, 2743S–2747S. – discussion 2765S–2767S.

Morris Jr, S.M., 2009. Recent advances in arginine metabolism: roles and regulation of the arginases. Br. J. Pharmacol. 157, 922–930. <http://dx.doi.org/10.1111/j.1476-5381.2009.00278.x>.

Morrissey, J., McCracken, R., Ishidoya, S., Klahr, S., 1995. Partial cloning and characterization of an arginine decarboxylase in the kidney. Kidney Int. 47, 1458–1461. <http://dx.doi.org/10.1038/ki.1995.204>.

Mullen, M.J., Wright, D., Donald, A.E., Thorne, S., Thomson, H., Deanfield, J.E., 2000. Atorvastatin but not l-arginine improves endothelial function in type I diabetes mellitus: a double-blind study. J. Am. Coll. Cardiol. 36, 410–416. <http://dx.doi.org/10.1016/S0735-1097(00)00743-9> >.

Munder, M., Eichmann, K., Modolell, M., 1998. Alternative metabolic states in murine macrophages reflected by the nitric oxide synthase/arginase balance: competitive regulation by CD4+ T cells correlates with Th1/Th2 phenotype. J. Immunol. 160, 5347–5354. <http://dx.doi.org/10.1016/0167-5699(96)80606-2>.

Nakagawa, T., Guarente, L., 2009. Urea cycle regulation by mitochondrial sirtuin, SIRT5. Aging (Albany NY) 1, 578–581.

Nakagawa, T., Lomb, D.J., Haigis, M.C., Guarente, L., 2009. SIRT5 deacetylates carbamoyl phosphate synthetase 1 and regulates the urea cycle. Cell 137, 560–570. <http://dx.doi.org/10.1016/j.cell.2009.02.026>.

Ochoa, J.B., Udekwu, A.O., Billiar, T.R., Curran, R.D., Cerra, F.B., Simmons, R.L., et al., 1991. Nitrogen oxide levels in patients after trauma and during sepsis. Ann. Surg 214, 621–626.

Ochoa, J., Strange, J., Kearney, P., Gellin, G., Endean, E., Fitzpatrick, E., 2001a. Effects of L-arginine on the proliferation of T lymphocyte subpopulations. JPEN J. Parenter. Enteral. Nutr. 25, 23–29. <http://dx.doi.org/10.1177/014860710102500123>.

Ochoa, J.B., Bernard, A.C., O'Brien, W.E., Griffen, M.M., Maley, M.E., Rockich, A.K., et al., 2001b. Arginase I expression and activity in human mononuclear cells after injury. Ann. Surg. 233, 393–399.

Ohtsuka, Y., Nakaya, J., 2000. Effect of oral administration of L-arginine on senile dementia. Am. J. Med. 108, 439. <http://dx.doi.org/10.1016/S0002-9343(99)00396-4>.

Oka, R.K., Szuba, A., Giacomini, J.C., Cooke, J.P., 2005. A pilot study of l-arginine supplementation on functional capacity in peripheral arterial disease. Vasc. Med. 10, 265–274. <http://dx.doi.org/10.1191/1358863x05vm637oa>.

Owen, O.E., Kalhan, S.C., Hanson, R.W., 2002. The key role of anaplerosis and cataplerosis for citric acid cycle function. J. Biol. Chem. 277, 30409–30412. <http://dx.doi.org/10.1074/jbc.R200006200>.

Palmer, J.P., Benson, J.W., Walter, R.M., Ensinck, J.W., 1976. Arginine-stimulated acute phase of insulin and glucagon secretion in diabetic subjects. J. Clin. Investig. 58, 565–570. <http://dx.doi.org/10.1172/JCI108502>.

Palmer, R., Ashton, D.S., Moncada, S., 1988. Vascular endothelial cells synthesize nitric oxide from L-arginine. Nature 333, 664–666. <http://dx.doi.org/10.1038/333664a0>.

Peterson, J.M., Barbul, A., Breslin, R.J., Wasserkrug, H.L., Efron, G., 1987. Significance of T-lymphocytes in wound healing. Surgery 102, 300–305.

Piatti, P., Monti, L.D., Valsecchi, G., Magni, F., Setola, E., Marchesi, F., et al., 2001. Long-term oral L-Arginine administration improves peripheral and hepatic insulin sensitivity in Type 2 diabetic patients. Diabetes Care 24, 875–880. <http://dx.doi.org/10.2337/diacare.24.5.875>.

Pieper, G.M., Siebeneich, W., Dondlinger, L.A., 1996. Short-term oral administration of l-arginine reverses defective endothelium-dependent relaxation and cGMP generation in diabetes. Eur. J. Pharmacol. 317, 317–320. <http://dx.doi.org/10.1016/S0014-2999(96)00831-X>.

Prince, M., Bryce, R., Albanese, E., Wimo, A., Ribeiro, W., Ferri, C.P., 2013. The global prevalence of dementia: a systematic review and meta-analysis. Alzheimer's & Dementia 9, 63–75. <e2. doi:10.1016/j.jalz.2012.11.007>.

Quillen, J.E., Sellke, F.W., Armstrong, M.L., Harrison, D.G., 1991. Long-term cholesterol feeding alters the reactivity of primate coronary microvessels to platelet products. Arteriosclerosis Thrombosis Vasc. Biol. 11, 639–644. <http://dx.doi.org/10.1161/01.ATV.11.3.639>.

Rakoff, J.S., Siler, T.M., Sinha, Y.N., Yen, S.S.C., 1973. Prolactin and growth hormone release in response to sequential stimulation by arginine and synthetic TRF. J. Clin. Endocrinol. Metab. 37, 641–644. <http://dx.doi.org/10.1210/jcem-37-5-641>.

Rector, T.S., Bank, A.J., Mullen, K.A., Tschumperlin, L.K., Sih, R., Pillai, K., et al., 1996. Randomized, double-blind, placebo-controlled study of supplemental oral L-arginine in patients with heart failure. Circulation 93, 2135–2141. <http://dx.doi.org/10.1161/01.CIR.93.12.2135>.

Regunathan, S., Reis, D.J., 2000. Characterization of arginine decarboxylase in rat brain and liver: distinction from ornithine decarboxylase. J. Neurochem 74, 2201–2208.

Rodriguez, P.C., Zea, A.H., Culotta, K.S., Zabaleta, J., Ochoa, J.B., Ochoa, A.C., 2002. Regulation of T cell receptor CD3zeta chain expression by L-arginine. J. Biol. Chem. 277, 21123–21129. <http://dx.doi.org/10.1074/jbc.M110675200>.

Rogers, Q.R., Visek, W.J., 1985. Metabolic role of urea cycle intermediates: nutritional and clinical aspects. Introduction. J. Nutr 115, 505–508.

Ros, E., 2015. Nuts and CVD. Br. J. Nutr. 113 (Suppl 2), S111–S120. <http://dx.doi.org/10.1017/S0007114514003924>.

Rougé, C., Robert, Des, C., Robins, A., Le Bacquer, O., Volteau, C., et al., 2007. Manipulation of citrulline availability in humans. AJP: Gastrointest. Liver Physiol. 293, G1061–G1067. <http://dx.doi.org/10.1152/ajpgi.00289.2007>.

Ruel, M., Beanlands, R.S., Lortie, M., Chan, V., Camack, N., deKemp, R.A., et al., 2008. Concomitant treatment with oral L-arginine improves the efficacy of surgical angiogenesis in patients with severe diffuse coronary artery disease: the Endothelial Modulation in Angiogenic Therapy randomized controlled trial. J. Thorac. Cardiovasc. Surg. 135, 762–770. – 770.e1. doi:10.1016/j.jtcvs.2007.09.073.

Santhanam, L., Lim, H.K., Lim, H.K., Miriel, V., Brown, T., Patel, M., et al., 2007. Inducible NO synthase dependent S-nitrosylation and activation of arginase1 contribute to age-related endothelial dysfunction. Circul. Res. 101, 692–702. <http://dx.doi.org/10.1161/CIRCRESAHA.107.157727>.

Satriano, J., 2003. Agmatine: at the crossroads of the arginine pathways. Ann. N. Y. Acad. Sci 1009, 34–43. <http://dx.doi.org/10.1196/annals.1304.004>.

Schäffer, M.R., Efron, P.A., Thornton, F.J., Klingel, K., Gross, S.S., Barbul, A., 1997. Nitric oxide, an autocrine regulator of wound fibroblast synthetic function. J. Immunol. 158, 2375–2381.

Schäffer, M.R., Tantry, U., Thornton, F.J., Barbul, A., 1999. Inhibition of nitric oxide synthesis in wounds: pharmacology and effect on accumulation of collagen in wounds in mice. Eur. J. Surg. 165, 262–267. <http://dx.doi.org/10.1080/110241599750007153>.

Schiller, L.R., 2009. Diarrhea and malabsorption in the elderly. Gastroenterol. Clin. N. Am. 38, 481–502. <http://dx.doi.org/10.1016/j.gtc.2009.06.008>.

Schmidt, H.H.H.W., Nau, H., Wittfoht, W., Gerlach, J., Prescher, K.-E., Klein, M.M., et al., 1988. Arginine is a physiological precursor of endothelium-derived nitric oxide. Eur. J. Pharmacol. 154, 213–216. <http://dx.doi.org/10.1016/0014-2999(88)90101-X>.

Schmidt, H., Warner, T., Ishii, K., Sheng, H., Murad, F., 1992. Insulin secretion from pancreatic B cells caused by L-arginine-derived nitrogen oxides. Science 255, 721–723. <http://dx.doi.org/10.1126/science.1371193>.

Schrempf Decker, G.E., Baron, D.P., Brattig, N.W., Bockhorn, H., Berg, P.A., 1983. Biological and immunological characterization of a human liver immunoregulatory protein. Hepatology 3, 939–946. <http://dx.doi.org/10.1002/hep.1840030610>.

Schulman, S.P., Becker, L.C., Kass, D.A., Champion, H.C., Terrin, M.L., Forman, S., et al., 2006. L-Arginine therapy in acute myocardial infarction: the vascular interaction with age in myocardial infarction (VINTAGE MI) randomized clinical trial. JAMA 295, 58–64. <http://dx.doi.org/10.1001/jama.295.1.58>.

Schwartz, L., 2003. Amelioration of microvascular angina with arginine supplementation. Ann. Intern. Med. 138, 160. <http://dx.doi.org/10.7326/0003-4819-138-2-200301210-00027>.

Schwedhelm, E., Maas, R., Freese, R., Jung, D., Lukacs, Z., Jambrecina, A., et al., 2008. Pharmacokinetic and pharmacodynamic properties of oral L-citrulline and L-arginine: impact on nitric oxide metabolism. Br. J. Clin. Pharmacol. 65, 51–59. <http://dx.doi.org/10.1111/j.1365-2125.2007.02990.x>.

Seifter, E., Rettura, G., Barbul, A., Levenson, S.M., 1978. Arginine: an essential amino acid for injured rats. Surgery 84, 224–230.

Sen, C.K., Gordillo, G.M., Roy, S., Kirsner, R., Lambert, L., Hunt, T.K., et al., 2009. Human skin wounds: a major and snowballing threat to public health and the economy. Wound Repair Regen. 17, 763–771. <http://dx.doi.org/10.1111/j.1524-475X.2009.00543.x>.

Shi, H.P., Efron, D.T., Most, D., Tantry, U.S., Barbul, A., 2000. Supplemental dietary arginine enhances wound healing in normal but not inducible nitric oxide synthase knockout mice. Surgery 128, 374–378. <http://dx.doi.org/10.1067/msy.2000.107372>.

Shi, H.P., Most, D., Efron, D.T., Witte, M.B., Barbul, A., 2003. Supplemental L-arginine enhances wound healing in diabetic rats. Wound Repair Regen. 11, 198–203. <http://dx.doi.org/10.1046/j.1524-475X.2003.11308.x>.

Shin, W., Berkowitz, D.E., Ryoo, S., 2012. Increased arginase II activity contributes to endothelial dysfunction through endothelial nitric oxide synthase uncoupling in aged mice. Exp. Mol. Med. 44, 594–602. <http://dx.doi.org/10.3858/emm.2012.44.10.068>.

Sipilä, I., 1980. Inhibition of arginine-glycine amidinotransferase by ornithine. A possible mechanism for the muscular and chorioretinal atrophies in gyrate atrophy of the choroid and retina with hyperornithinemia. Biochim. Biophys. Acta 613, 79–84.

Staff, A.C., Berge, L., Haugen, G., Lorentzen, B., Mikkelsen, B., Henriksen, T., 2004. Dietary supplementation with l-arginine or placebo in women with pre-eclampsia. Acta Obstet. Gynecol. Scand. 83, 103–107. <http://dx.doi.org/10.1111/j.1600-0412.2004.00321.x>.

Stead, L.M., Au, K.P., Jacobs, R.L., Brosnan, M.E., Brosnan, J.T., 2001. Methylation demand and homocysteine metabolism: effects of dietary provision of creatine and guanidinoacetate. AJP: Endocrinol. Metab. 281, E1095–E1100.

Susswein, A.J., Katzoff, A., Miller, N., Hurwitz, I., 2004. Nitric oxide and memory. Neuroscientist 10, 153–162. <http://dx.doi.org/10.1177/1073858403261226>.

Tangphao, O., Grossmann, M., Chalon, S., Hoffman, B.B., Blaschke, T.F., 1999. Pharmacokinetics of intravenous and oral l-arginine in normal volunteers. Br. J. Clin. Pharmacol. 47, 261–266. <http://dx.doi.org/10.1046/j.1365-2125.1999.00883.x>.

Tanimura, J., 1967. Studies on arginine in human semen. II. The effects of medication with L-arginine-HCL on male infertility. Bull. Osaka Med. Sch. 13, 84–89.

Tasaki, T., Kwon, Y.T., 2007. The mammalian N-end rule pathway: new insights into its components and physiological roles. Trends Biochem. Sci. 32, 520–528. <http://dx.doi.org/10.1016/j.tibs.2007.08.010>.

Thams, P., Capito, K., 1999. L-arginine stimulation of glucose-induced insulin secretion through membrane depolarization and independent of nitric oxide. Eur. J. Endocrinol. 140, 87–93. <http://dx.doi.org/10.1530/eje.0.1400087>.

Thornton, F.J., Schäffer, M.R., Witte, M.B., Moldawer, L.L., MacKay, S.L.D., Abouhamze, A., et al., 1998. Enhanced collagen accumulation following direct transfection of the inducible nitric oxide synthase gene in cutaneous wounds. Biochem. Biophys. Res. Commun. 246, 654–659. <http://dx.doi.org/10.1006/bbrc.1998.8681>.

Urschel, K.L., Shoveler, A.K., Uwiera, R.R.E., Pencharz, P.B., Ball, R.O., 2006. Citrulline is an effective arginine precursor in enterally fed neonatal piglets. J. Nutr 136, 1806–1813.

Valitutti, S., Müller, S., Salio, M., Lanzavecchia, A., 1997. Degradation of T cell receptor (TCR)-CD3-zeta complexes after antigenic stimulation. J. Exp. Med. 185, 1859–1864.

Varshavsky, A., 1996. The N-end rule: functions, mysteries, uses. Proc. Natl. Acad. Sci. 93, 12142–12149.

Visek, W.J., 1986. Arginine needs, physiological state and usual diets. A reevaluation. J. Nutr 116, 36–46.

Wakabayashi, Y., Yamada, E., Yoshida, T., Takahashi, H., 1994. Arginine becomes an essential amino acid after massive resection of rat small intestine. J. Biol. Chem. 269, 32667–32671.

Walker, H.A., McGing, E., Fisher, I., Böger, R.H., Bode-Böger, S.M., Jackson, G., et al., 2001. Endothelium-dependent vasodilation is independent of the plasma L-arginine/ADMA ratio in men with stable angina. J. Am. Coll. Cardiol. 38, 499–505. <http://dx.doi.org/10.1016/S0735-1097(01)01380-8>.

Wang, Y., Zhang, L., Zhou, G., Liao, Z., Ahmad, H., Liu, W., et al., 2012. Dietary L-arginine supplementation improves the intestinal development through increasing mucosal Akt and mammalian target of rapamycin signals in intra-uterine growth retarded piglets. Br. J. Nutr. 108, 1371–1381. <http://dx.doi.org/10.1017/S0007114511006763>.

Wascher, T.C., Graier, W.F., Dittrich, P., Hussain, M.A., Bahadori, B., Wallner, S., et al., 1997. Effects of low-dose l-arginine on insulin-mediated vasodilatation and insulin sensitivity. Eur. J. Clin. Investig. 27, 690–695. <http://dx.doi.org/10.1046/j.1365-2362.1997.1730718.x>.

Watanabe, G., Tomiyama, H., Doba, N., 2000. Effects of oral administration of L-arginine on renal function in patients with heart failure. J. Hypertens. 18, 229–234.

Weir, G.C., Samols, E., Loo, S., Patel, Y.C., Gabbay, K.H., 1978. Somatostatin and pancreatic polypeptide secretion: effects of glucagon, insulin, and arginine. Diabetes 28, 35–40. <http://dx.doi.org/10.2337/diab.28.1.35>.

Williams, J.Z., Abumrad, N., Barbul, A., 2002. Effect of a specialized amino acid mixture on human collagen deposition. Ann. Surg 236, 369–374. discussion 374–5. doi:10.1097/01.SLA.0000027527.01984.00.

Wilson, A.M., Harada, R., Nair, N., Balasubramanian, N., Cooke, J.P., 2007. L-arginine supplementation in peripheral arterial disease: no benefit and possible harm. Circulation 116, 188–195. <http://dx.doi.org/10.1161/CIRCULATIONAHA.106.683656>.

Witte, M., 2003. Arginase acts as an alternative pathway of L-arginine metabolism in experimental colon anastomosis. J. Gastrointest. Surg. 7, 378–385. <http://dx.doi.org/10.1016/S1091-255X(02)00431-6>.

Wolf, A., Zalpour, C., Theilmeier, G., Wang, B.-Y., Ma, A., Anderson, B., et al., 1997. Dietary L-arginine supplementation normalizes platelet aggregation in hypercholesterolemic humans. J. Am. Coll. Cardiol. 29, 479–485. <http://dx.doi.org/10.1016/S0735-1097(97)00523-8>.

Wu, G., Morris Jr, S.M., 2003. Arginine metabolism in mammals. Metabolic and Therapeutic Aspects of Amino Acids in Clinical Nutrition, 153–161.

Wu, G., Bazer, F.W., Cudd, T.A., Jobgen, W.S., Kim, S.W., Lassala, A., et al., 2007. Pharmacokinetics and safety of arginine supplementation in animals. J. Nutr 137, 1673S–1680S.

Wyss, M., Kaddurah-Daouk, R., 2000. Creatine and creatinine metabolism. Physiol. Rev. 80, 1107–1213.

Xiong, Y., Fru, M.F., Yu, Y., Montani, J.-P., Ming, X.-F., Yang, Z., 2014. Long term exposure to L-arginine accelerates endothelial cell senescence through arginase-II and S6K1 signaling. Aging (Albany NY) 6, 369–379.

Xu, J., Murphy, S.L., Kochanek, K.D., Bastian, B.A., 2016. National Vital Statistics Reports [WWW Document]. cdc.gov. URL <http://www.cdc.gov/nchs/data/nvsr/nvsr64/nvsr64_02.pdf> (accessed 3.30.16).

Yamasaki, K., Edington, H.D., McClosky, C., Tzeng, E., Lizonova, A., Kovesdi, I., et al., 1998. Reversal of impaired wound repair in iNOS-deficient mice by topical adenoviral-mediated iNOS gene transfer. J. Clin. Investig. 101, 967–971. <http://dx.doi.org/10.1172/JCI2067>.

Yi, J., Horky, L.L., Friedlich, A.L., Shi, Y., Rogers, J.T., Huang, X., 2009. L-arginine and Alzheimer's disease. Int. J. Clin. Exp. Pathol. 2, 211–238.

Yu, H., Iyer, R.K., Kern, R.M., Rodriguez, W.I., Grody, W.W., Cederbaum, S.D., 2001. Expression of arginase isozymes in mouse brain. Journal of Neurosci. Res. 66, 406–422. <http://dx.doi.org/10.1002/jnr.1233>.

Yu, H., Yoo, P.K., Aguirre, C.C., Tsoa, R.W., Kern, R.M., Grody, W.W., et al., 2003. Widespread expression of arginase I in mouse tissues. Biochemical and physiological implications. J. Histochem. Cytochem. 51, 1151–1160. <http://dx.doi.org/10.1177/002215540305100905>.

Zhou, L., Zhu, D.-Y., 2009. Neuronal nitric oxide synthase: structure, subcellular localization, regulation, and clinical implications. Nitric Oxide 20, 223–230. <http://dx.doi.org/10.1016/j.niox.2009.03.001>.

Zorgniotti, A.W., Lizza, E.F., 1994. Effect of large doses of the nitric oxide precursor, L-arginine, on erectile dysfunction. Int. J. Impot. Res 6, 33–35. – discussion 36.

C H A P T E R

28

Late-Onset Caloric Restriction Alters Skeletal Muscle Metabolism: Mechanisms from Animal and Human Studies

Chiao-nan Chen

Chang Gung University, Taoyuan, Taiwan

Skeletal muscle is an organ that enables individuals to move, protecting and supporting the skeleton and regulating the whole body's glucose homeostasis. Energy-production systems in skeletal muscles are important in terms of skeletal muscle function because the generation of force and movement requires energy. In this chapter, we review skeletal muscle metabolism and its regulators. We discuss the changes in skeletal muscle metabolism with aging. The impacts and the mechanisms of the age-related metabolic changes in skeletal muscles are also discussed. Lastly, we show evidence from animal and human studies about the effects of caloric restriction on age-related changes in skeletal muscle metabolism. The impacts and mechanisms of changes related to calorie restriction (CR) in skeletal muscles are also discussed.

SKELETAL MUSCLE METABOLISM

Skeletal muscle is the largest organ in human. The key functions of skeletal muscle are force generation and movement, both of which require energy. Thus, energy-production systems in muscles not only are important for normal cellular maintenance but also critical for an individual's capacity for movement. Fuel metabolism and energy production in muscles are mainly regulated by anaerobic and aerobic metabolism. In anaerobic metabolism where oxygen is not required, glucose that is transported from the bloodstream into muscle cells, is broken down into a net of two units of adenosine triphosphate (ATP) and two lactates (Benard et al., 2010). In aerobic metabolism where oxygen is required, glucose is broken down into two pyruvates in cytoplasm. Pyruvates are then transported into the matrix of the mitochondria by mitochondrial pyruvate carrier, where it is transformed into acetyl-CoA. Acetyl-CoA is also generated in the mitochondrial matrix by β oxidation where fatty acids are broken down. Acetyl-CoA is the primary substrate that enters the tricarboxylic acid (TCA) cycle (also known as the *citric acid cycle* or *Krebs cycle*), where a series of chemical reactions happen and reducing equivalents (nicotinamide adenine dinucleotide and $FADH_2$) are produced. The reducing equivalents produced from the TCA cycle are oxidized by complexes in the electron-transport chain (ETC) on the mitochondrial inner membrane. Complexes I to IV transfer electrons and pump protons from the mitochondrial matrix into the intermembrane space, creating a proton gradient (an electrochemical gradient) across the mitochondrial inner membrane. As the protons flow back across the inner membrane through the ATP synthase (also called complex V), it drives ATP synthesis. The process happening on the

Nutrition and Functional Foods for Healthy Aging.
DOI: http://dx.doi.org/10.1016/B978-0-12-805376-8.00028-9

ETC is called *oxidative phosphorylation* (OXPHOS), because proton gradient created by oxidizing reduced cofactors is used to phosphorylate adenosine diphosphate (ADP) to ATP. The net energy production in aerobic metabolism is 36 ATP. Collectively, energy production in skeletal muscles is mainly through anaerobic metabolism and aerobic metabolism. Anaerobic metabolism contains fewer steps of reactions and is faster in generating ATP compared to aerobic metabolism. Thus, anaerobic metabolism is effective for high-intensity and short-duration activities. Aerobic metabolism generates greater amounts of ATP than anaerobic metabolism, but it takes longer. Energy provided from aerobic metabolism is critical for sustained activities.

The key player in the cellular aerobic metabolism is the mitochondrion. The number and efficiency of mitochondria determine the capacity of cellular aerobic metabolism. The number increases by mitochondrial biogenesis, which is upregulated in conditions of energy deprivation (Lopez-Lluch et al., 2008; Peterson et al., 2012). During energy deprivation, the ratio of adenosine monophosphate (AMP) to ATP increases. This increased ratio activates AMP-activated protein kinase (AMPK) (Canto and Auwerx, 2011). The activated AMPK activates another nutrient-sensing protein silent mating type information regulation 2 homolog 1 (SIRT-1). AMPK and SIRT-1 activate the key regulator of mitochondrial biogenesis peroxisome proliferator-activated receptor gamma coactivator 1α (PGC-1α) by phosphorylation and deacetylation, respectively (Canto and Auwerx, 2011). Activated PGC-1α translocates to the nucleus and activates several nuclear transcription factors involving in mitochondrial biogenesis, including nuclear respiratory factor-1 (NRF-1), NRF-2, and mitochondrial transcription factor A (TFAM) (Anderson et al., 2008) (Fig. 28.1).

Mitochondrial efficiency is another factor that influences the energy-production capacity of cells. It is affected by the coupling status between proton flux from the intermembrane space to the matrix and the phosphorylation of ADP. When there is uncoupling (e.g., protons move back to matrix without going through ATP synthases), the efficiency of ETC decreases (Bellanti et al., 2013). Uncoupling proteins are shown to contribute to the mitochondrial uncoupling in muscle tissues (Bellanti et al., 2013). In addition to the uncoupling between the proton flux and the phosphorylation, any impairment of complexes in ETC results in decreased enzymatic functions of complexes and thus decreases the efficiency of mitochondria.

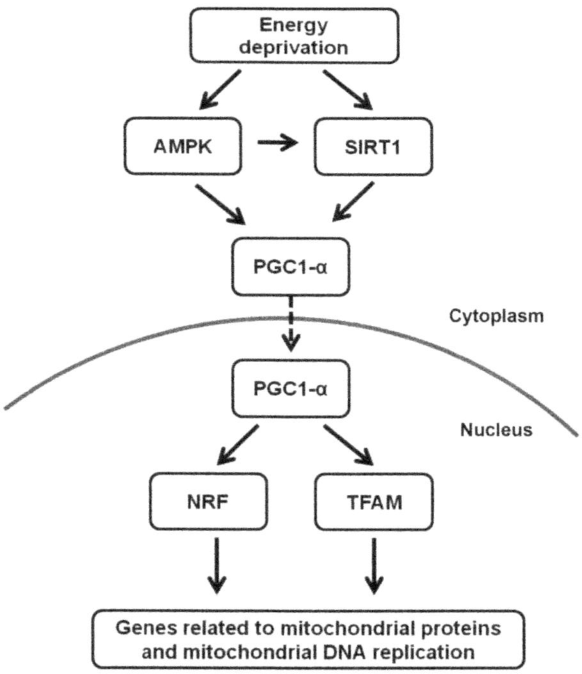

FIGURE 28.1 The regulation of mitochondrial biogenesis. *AMPK* AMP-activated protein kinase; *SIRT-1* silent mating type information regulation 2 homolog 1; *PGC-1α* peroxisome proliferator-activated receptor gamma c1α; *NRF* nuclear respiratory factor; *TFAM* mitochondrial transcription factor A.

SKELETAL MUSCLE METABOLISM CHANGES WITH AGING

Metabolism in skeletal muscles changes significantly with aging. The pattern of cellular metabolism is defined as the ratio of mitochondrial OXPHOS to glycolysis, which decreases with aging (Chen et al., 2015) **(Fig. 28.2A)**. This change suggests aging muscles shift energy metabolism away from mitochondrial respiration toward glycolysis. The metabolic shift was also reported in aging heart and liver cells, and in skeletal muscles with disuse atrophy (Bellanti et al., 2013, Stein and Wade, 2005). By assessing mitochondrial OXPHOS to glycolysis simultaneously, Chen et al. found that mitochondrial OXPHOS in muscles decreases significantly with aging but the glycolysis does not show significant changes with aging (Chen et al., 2015) **(Fig. 28.2B, C)**. These findings suggest that the decreased mitochondrial OXPHOS is the main contributor to the age-related changes of the metabolic pattern in skeletal muscles.

Many studies have demonstrated that muscle mitochondria change with aging. Morphologically, aging muscles have a greater percentage of muscle fibers with large deletion mutations in mitochondrial DNA and abnormal mitochondrial ETC enzymes (McKiernan et al., 2011). Mitochondria in aging muscles show lower variation in their shape, and the cristae are less visible and defined (Figueiredo et al., 2008). Mitochondrial content in skeletal muscles also decreases with aging (Gouspillou et al., 2014; Lanza et al., 2012; Miller et al., 2012). Genomic profiling reveals that genes that associate with glucose metabolism, TCA cycles, and oxidative phosphorylation are downregulated with aging. Proteomic analysis also indicated the expression of several mitochondrial proteins decreases with aging, including complexes in ETC. The activities of citrate syntheses and complexes in ETC were found to be decreased in aging muscles when normalized to muscle weight (Ibebunjo et al., 2013; Mansouri et al., 2006). The age-related changes of mitochondria in skeletal muscles observed in animals are also seen in humans. Using principle component analysis and parametric analysis of gene-set enrichment, Mercken et al. found that pathways associated with mitochondrial electron transport and oxidative phosphorylation are downregulated in middle-aged individuals with a Western diet compared to young individuals with a Western diet (Mercken et al., 2013). Taken together, muscles of old animals contain greater amounts of mitochondria with DNA large deletion mutations. Mitochondrial content and structure change consistently with aging. Mitochondrial content in muscles decreases with aging. The expression of mitochondrial proteins and enzyme activities in muscles also decreases with aging.

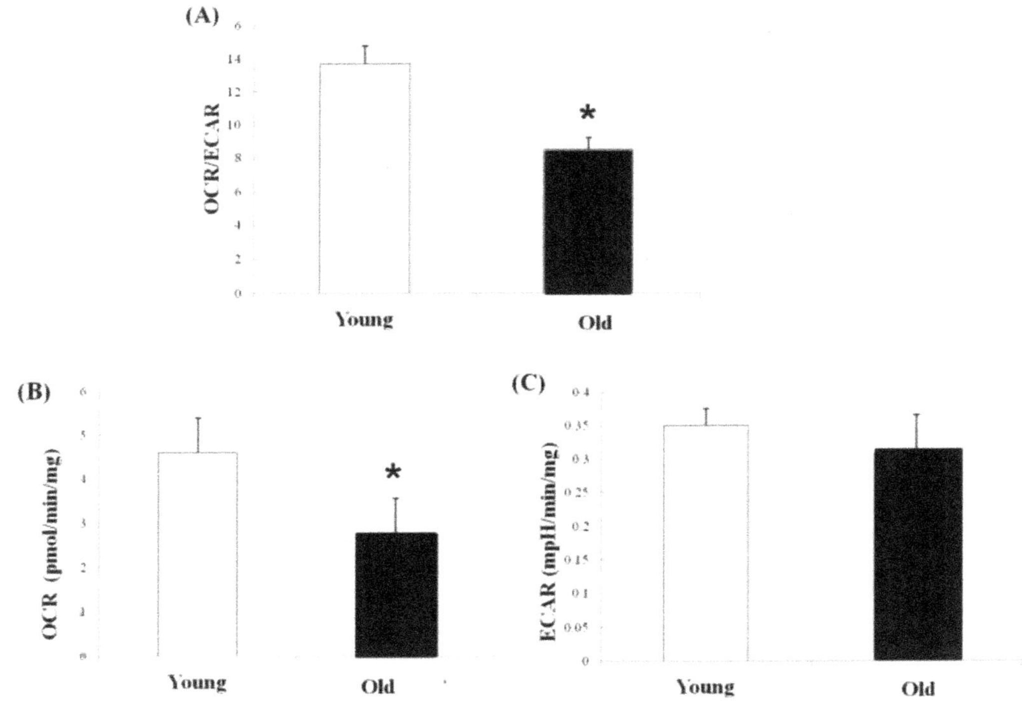

FIGURE 28.2 Effects of age on energy metabolism of muscle cells. (A) Ratio of oxygen consumption rate (OCR) to extracellular acidification rate (ECAR); (B) OCR, (C) ECAR. *<0.05 compared to young rats. *Modified from Chen, C.N., Lin, S.Y., Liao, Y.H., Li, Z.J., Wong, A.M., 2015. Late-onset caloric restriction alters skeletal muscle metabolism by modulating pyruvate metabolism. Am. J. Physiol. Endocrinol. Metab. 308, E942–E949.*

In addition to the changes in structure and composition, mitochondrial function in muscles decreases with aging. The research of Mansouri et al. reported that ATP production per milligram of protein in the muscles of 28-month-old rats is only 70% of that in muscles of seven-month-old rats (Mansouri et al., 2006). The mitochondrial oxygen consumption rate (OCR) was found to be decreased with aging in both slow-twitch and fast-twitch muscles in many experimental models, including isolated mitochondria, permeabilized muscle fibers, and intact muscles (Chen et al., 2015; Figueiredo et al., 2008; Hempenstall et al., 2012; Lanza et al., 2012). Research that evaluated human muscle mitochondrial function in vivo by nuclear magnetic resonance found that rates of mitochondrial OXPHOS in muscles of the elderly is 40% less compared with rates in young individuals with matched lean body mass and fat mass (Petersen et al., 2003). Mitochondrial efficiency defined as the amount of ATP produced per unit of consumed oxygen also decreased with aging (Lanza et al., 2012). Lanza et al. normalized the mitochondrial function with mitochondrial DNA copy numbers and indicated that the decreased mitochondrial content plays the key role in the age-related decrease of mitochondrial function in muscle cells (Lanza et al., 2012). Collectively, ATP generation capacity in muscles decreases with aging. The age-related decrease of energy generation capacity is associated with the decreases of mitochondrial number and efficiency, mitochondrial DNA mutations, downregulation of proteins in TCA cycles and ETC, and reduced mitochondrial respiration.

IMPACTS OF THE AGE-RELATED CHANGES IN SKELETAL MUSCLE METABOLISM

The age-related changes of skeletal muscle metabolism have multiple facets of influences on skeletal muscles, including skeletal muscle mass, exercise performance, fuel metabolism, and muscular insulin resistance. It has been shown that the cellular metabolic pattern associates with muscle mass. The greater the ratio of mitochondrial OXPHOS to glycolysis, the greater the muscle mass (Chen et al., 2015) (Fig. 28.3). Similarly, functional annotation analysis revealed that the downregulation of genes in the mitochondrial energy metabolic pathway (e.g., tricarboxylic acid cycle and oxidative phosphorylation) is associated with age-related muscle loss (Ibebunjo et al., 2013). Stein et al. also indicated that the shifts of muscle metabolism away from fat oxidation toward glycolysis contributes to disuse-induced loss of muscle mass because the metabolic changes precede the decrease of muscle mass (Stein and Wade, 2005). ATP deficiency likely mediates the metabolic shift and muscle atrophy. Glycolysis is less efficient than OXPHOS in terms of ATP generation, so muscles that depend more on glycolysis over OXPHOS may suffer ATP deficiency, which is a trigger for protein degradation and the inhibition of protein synthesis (Sandri, 2008). Another possible mechanism for the link between mitochondrial dysfunction and the loss of muscle mass is oxidative stress. Mitochondria are major sites of free radical generation; the dysfunction of mitochondria results in greater release of free radicals (Marzetti et al., 2013). The increased free radical generation can result in oxidative modification of proteins, which increases the susceptibility of proteins for degradation (Jackman and Kandarian, 2004).

Reduced exercise performance is another result of metabolic changes of skeletal muscles. Santanasto et al. investigated the relationship between skeletal muscle mitochondrial function and fatigability in the elderly during exercise. They found that individuals with higher fatigability during exercise have lower oxidative capacity in

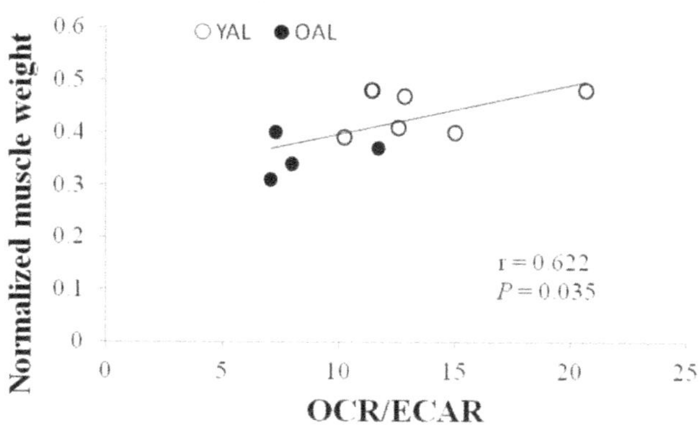

FIGURE 28.3 The relationship between metabolic pattern and normalized muscle weight (e.g., muscle weight divided by body weight). *OCR:ECAR* ratio of oxygen consumption rate to extracellular acidification rate; *YAL* young rats fed ad libitum; *OAL* old rats fed ad libitum. *Modified from Chen, C.N., Lin, S.Y., Liao, Y.H., Li, Z.J., Wong, A.M., 2015. Late-onset caloric restriction alters skeletal muscle metabolism by modulating pyruvate metabolism. Am. J. Physiol. Endocrinol. Metab. 308, E942–E949.*

their skeletal muscles (Santanasto et al., 2015). Similarly, Gouspillou et al. compared muscle energetics (e.g., the response of energy supply to the changes of energy demand) by modular control analysis and magnetic resonance spectroscopy measurements between young and old rats. They found that the increased energy supply in response to muscle contractions was significantly reduced in the muscles of old rats. Mitochondrial dysfunction is found to be the main contributor to the reduced energetics in aging muscles (Gouspillou et al., 2014). Collectively, mitochondria, being the powerhouses of skeletal muscles, influence the exercise performance of individuals. The impaired mitochondrial function and the metabolic shifts away from mitochondrial respiration toward glycolysis reduce the exercise performance of the elderly.

Shifts in fuel metabolism and increased muscular insulin resistance (e.g., reduced muscular glucose uptake during insulin stimulation) are the results of metabolic changes in skeletal muscles. It was found that mitochondria in the muscles of the elderly are impaired in their ability to shift the metabolism from lipid to glucose oxidation under insulin stimulation. The impairment in the shifting of substrate utilization may result in muscle insulin resistance and an increase of intramyocellular lipid content in the elderly (Petersen et al., 2015). In agreement with this, studies that assessed peripheral insulin resistance by hyperinsulinemic-euglycemic clamp reported that peripheral insulin resistance is greater in the elderly compared to young individuals with matched lean body mass and fat mass (Fink et al., 1983; Petersen et al., 2003). Using glucose and glycerol tracer infusions, Petersen indicated that skeletal muscle is the main tissue responsible for the increased peripheral body insulin resistance of the elderly (Petersen et al., 2003). Taken together, the changes of skeletal muscle metabolism with aging impair the glucose uptake of skeletal muscles and further influence the glucose homeostasis of the elderly.

MECHANISMS OF AGE-RELATED CHANGES IN SKELETAL MUSCLE METABOLISM

Increased oxidative stress and blunted mitochondrial biogenesis are the most proposed mechanisms underlying the age-related changes of skeletal muscle metabolism. Increased oxidative stress and mitochondrial DNA mutations contribute to the age-related mitochondrial dysfunction in skeletal muscles. It has been shown that the release of superoxide from mitochondria and the hydrogen peroxide level in mitochondria are greater in the muscles of old animals than those in young animals (Lanza et al., 2012; Mansouri et al., 2006; Xu et al., 2010). The accumulation of oxidative modified proteins and markers of DNA damage in muscles are also greater in older animals (Chen et al., 2008; Lanza et al., 2012; Li et al., 2012; Mansouri et al., 2006; Xu et al., 2010). Research that identified the specific mitochondrial proteins that are targets of oxidative modification found citrate synthase is one target of oxidants (Li et al., 2012). Oxidative modification impairs protein functions. For example, the activity of mitochondrial protein cytochrome c oxidase was found to be negatively correlated with oxidant 4-hydroxy-2-nonenal concentration (Chen et al., 2001). The ability to shift substrate utilization of mitochondria is also affected by oxidative stress. The study of Anderson et al. found that lowering the mitochondrial oxidative stress improved insulin resistance in animals fed a high-fat diet (Anderson et al., 2009). Upregulation of uncoupling proteins is a mechanism for aging muscles to protect mitochondria from oxidative damages (Bellanti et al., 2013). Uncoupling proteins, although it reduces the generation of ROS, increases the proton leak and reduces the mitochondrial efficiency of muscles (Anderson and Weindruch, 2010). Taken together, oxidative stress in skeletal muscles increases with aging. The increased oxidative stress results in dysfunctions of mitochondrial enzymes and mitochondrial function (Johnson et al., 2013; Peterson et al., 2012).

Regulators of mitochondrial biogenesis change with aging. The content of AMPK and phosphorylated AMPK in muscles is greater in middle-aged animals compared to young animals (Chen et al., 2015). The upregulation of AMPK in muscles of middle-aged animals is likely a compensatory adaptation for the impaired AMPK function. The compensatory adaptation observed in middle-aged animals disappears when animals are older. The levels of AMPK content and phosphorylation in muscles of old animals are shown significantly decreased than those in young animals (Koltai et al., 2012). In addition, the response of AMPK to stimuli is blunted in old animals. Reznick et al. compared muscle AMPK activity and its responsiveness between young and old animals. They found that basal AMPK activity in muscles is similar between young and old animals, but the responsiveness of AMPK in the muscles of old animals is significantly decreased than that of young animals. Muscle AMPK activity was found increased in young rats in response to acute stimulation by exercise and 5′-aminoimidazole-4-carboxamide-1-β-D-ribofuranoside (an activator of AMPK), however the AMPK activity in the muscles of old animals does not change in response to the acute stimuli (Reznick et al., 2007). Findings on the changes of PGC-1α in relation to aging are inconsistent. Some studies reported decreased PGC-1α expression in aging muscles (Hempenstall et al., 2012; Ibebunjo et al., 2013; Koltai et al., 2012), while other studies reported no changes (Chen et al., 2015). Hempenstall investigated the expression of PGC-1α in different cellular localization and found that the expression of total PGC-1α in muscles decreased with aging, but the level of PGC-1α in the nucleus is greater in old animals (Hempenstall et al., 2012). Because PGC-1α is translocated into nucleus under stress conditions (Anderson et al., 2008), the increased nuclear localization of PGC-1α in aging muscles suggests these muscles are under energy deficit.

CALORIC RESTRICTION ALTERS SKELETAL MUSCLE METABOLISM

Scientists have devoted much time to discover the "pill" that can extend both health span and life span. To date, caloric restriction is the only nonpharmaceutical and nongenetic strategy that has been shown to improve health, delay the onset of age-related pathologies on a range of model organisms, and possibly extend the life span of animals (Fontana et al., 2010).

One remarkable effect of CR is improving whole-body glucose homeostasis. Golman et al. reported that adult onset of caloric restriction lowered the incidence of impaired glucose homeostasis in rhesus monkeys (Colman et al., 2009). Similarly, Civitarese et al. found that 25% of CR for six months improved the whole-body insulin sensitivity of young overweight individuals (Civitarese et al., 2007). The improvement of whole-body glucose homeostasis is partly due to the CR-related changes of skeletal muscle metabolism. Insulin signaling of skeletal muscles in adult monkeys with four years of CR diet was found upregulated more than that in monkeys fed ad libitum, characterized by greater content and activation of the insulin receptor substrate (IRS), IRS-associated PI3-kinase, and glucose transporter GLUT4 (Wang et al., 2009). Together with the improvement of insulin sensitivity and glucose uptake, the metabolic pattern in skeletal muscles is also modified with CR. It has been shown that CR reprograms the cellular metabolism from glycolysis to OXPHOS in the muscles of middle-aged rats (Chen et al., 2015). This CR-induced metabolic reprogramming in skeletal muscles is likely a result of improved mitochondrial function that reverses the age-related increase of dependency on glycolysis as the energy source.

Mitochondrial function in skeletal muscles improves with CR. Morphologically, CR decreases the age-related increased number of muscle fibers with abnormal ETC enzymes (McKiernan et al., 2011). CR reduces the increased number of abnormal mitochondria in aging muscles (Jang et al., 2012; Lanza et al., 2012). Mitochondrial pyruvate carrier, a transmembrane protein responsible for the transportation of pyruvate from cytosol into the mitochondrial matrix, shows increased content in the muscles of middle-aged rats with CR than those in middle-aged rats fed ad libitum (Chen et al., 2015). Functionally, CR improves the age-related reduced oxidative capacity of mitochondria (Hempenstall et al., 2012; Lanza et al., 2012). In addition, CR improves decreased mitochondrial efficiency in aging muscles (Lanza et al., 2012). In human research, it was shown that 30% of CR reversed the age-related transcriptional changes of mitochondrial ETC and oxidative phosphorylation in the muscles of middle-aged individuals (Mercken et al., 2013).

CR-induced improvement of cellular metabolism not only enhances the insulin sensitivity of skeletal muscles but also benefits the size of skeletal muscles. CR was shown to attenuate age-related muscle loss in adult monkeys and rats (Colman et al., 2009; Kim et al., 2008; McKiernan et al., 2011). CR-induced decrease of protein degradation contributes to the beneficial effects of CR on muscle size. Adult monkeys with CR showed lower proteasome content and activity in skeletal muscles compared to monkeys fed ad libitum (Wang et al., 2009). In addition, apoptosis decreases in the muscles of animals with CR (Wang et al., 2009). The study of Chen et al. investigated the relationship between the cellular metabolic pattern and muscle mass. They found that the effects of CR on muscle mass are highly correlated with the effects of CR on cellular metabolism. Muscles that show greater increases in the ratio of the oxygen consumption rate to the cellular glycolytic rate have greater increases of muscle weight per body weight (Chen et al., 2015) (Fig. 28.4).

MECHANISMS OF THE CR-INDUCED ALTERATION IN SKELETAL MUSCLE METABOLISM

Increased antioxidant capacity and reduced oxidative stress are key mechanisms underlying the beneficial effects of CR on aging skeletal muscles. CR increases catalase activity and manganese superoxide dismutase (MnSOD) expression in the muscles of animals (Jang et al., 2012; Joseph et al., 2013; Lanza et al., 2012). Generation of mitochondrial reactive oxygen species (ROS) in skeletal muscles decreases with CR (Jang et al., 2012). Age-related increases of oxidative damage, including DNA damage and the accumulation of oxidative modified proteins, are shown to decrease with CR (Lanza et al., 2012; Li et al., 2012). The CR-induced upregulation of the protective system is likely via the activation of AMPK that activates forkhead box O (FOXO), a transcriptional factor that regulates a spectrum of stress-resistance genes, including antioxidants (Canto and Auwerx, 2011; Mercken et al., 2013). Mercken et al. compared the effect of

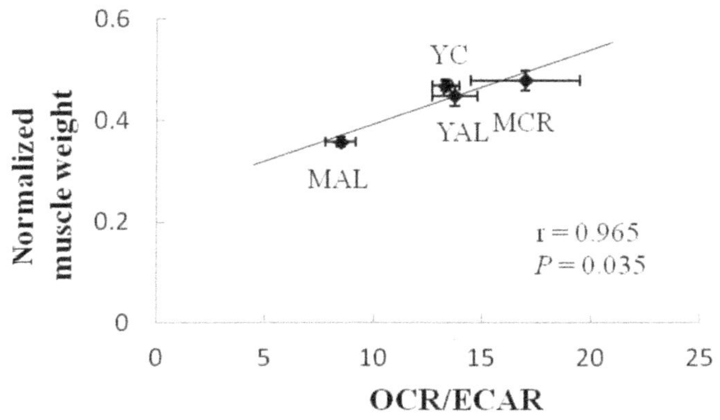

FIGURE 28.4 The relationship between the normalized muscle weight and the cellular metabolic pattern. *YAL* young rats fed ad libitum; *YCR* young rats with CR; *OAL* old rats fed ad libitum; *OCR* old rats with CR. *Used with permission from Chen, C.N., Lin, S.Y., Liao, Y.H., Li, Z.J., Wong, A.M., 2015. Late-onset caloric restriction alters skeletal muscle metabolism by modulating pyruvate metabolism. Am. J. Physiol. Endocrinol. Metab. 308, E942–E949.*

aging and chronic CR on skeletal muscles among young individuals with Western diets, middle-aged individuals with Western diet, and middle-aged individuals with 4–20 years of calorie-restricted diet. They found that CR upregulated the expression of FOXO (Mercken et al., 2013). The expression of MnSOD in muscles is also greater in middle-aged individuals with CR than in middle-aged individuals with Western diets (Mercken et al., 2013).

Regarding mitochondrial biogenesis, many studies found that CR upregulates the regulators of mitochondrial biogenesis (Civitarese et al., 2007; Hempenstall et al., 2012; Joseph et al., 2013; Mercken et al., 2013; Miller et al., 2012). The gene expressions of SIRT-1, AMPK, and PGC-1α in muscles were found upregulated in middle-aged individuals with CR than in middle-aged individuals with Western diets (Mercken et al., 2013). Similarly, Civitarese et al. found that gene expressions of TFAM, SIRT-1, and PGC-1α were upregulated in young overweight individuals receiving six months of 25% CR compared to that of the control group (Civitarese et al., 2007). Although most studies found that regulators of mitochondrial biogenesis increase with CR, the effects of CR on mitochondrial content is still being debated. For example, Hempenstall et al. found that even though total and nuclear protein content of PGC-1α increased in skeletal muscles with CR, mitochondrial content did not increase in muscles, irrespective of short-term (one month) or long-term (18 months) of CR (Hempenstall et al., 2012). The research of Civitarese et al., however, found that mitochondrial DNA content increased together with the increased expression of regulators of mitochondrial biogenesis (Civitarese et al., 2007). Because many studies found that CR improves mitochondrial functions but does not increase mitochondrial content in skeletal muscles (Hempenstall et al., 2012; Lanza et al., 2012), it is thought that CR-induced improvement of mitochondrial function is via the protection from oxidative damages but not the enhancement of mitochondrial biogenesis (Hancock et al., 2011; Hempenstall et al., 2012; Lanza et al., 2012).

CONCLUSION

Caloric restriction is a diet strategy for healthy aging. It delays the onset of many age-related pathologies, including diabetes and cardiovascular diseases. Regarding skeletal muscles, age-related muscle loss is partly due to increased oxidative stress and the shift of metabolic patterns away from mitochondrial respiration and toward glycolysis. Because metabolic reprogramming and the upregulation of cellular protective systems are important features of CR, evidence supports the beneficial effects of CR on aging skeletal muscles.

References

Anderson, R.M., Weindruch, R., 2010. Metabolic reprogramming, caloric restriction and aging. Trends Endocrinol. Metab. 21, 134–141.

Anderson, R.M., Barger, J.L., Edwards, M.G., Braun, K.H., O'Connor, C.E., Prolla, T.A., et al., 2008. Dynamic regulation of PGC-1alpha localization and turnover implicates mitochondrial adaptation in calorie restriction and the stress response. Aging Cell 7, 101–111.

Anderson, E.J., Lustig, M.E., Boyle, K.E., Woodlief, T.L., Kane, D.A., Lin, C.T., et al., 2009. Mitochondrial H2O2 emission and cellular redox state link excess fat intake to insulin resistance in both rodents and humans. J. Clin. Investig. 119, 573–581.

Bellanti, F., Romano, A.D., Giudetti, A.M., Rollo, T., Blonda, M., Tamborra, R., et al., 2013. Many faces of mitochondrial uncoupling during age: damage or defense? J. Gerontol. A Biol. Sci. Med. Sci. 68, 892–902.

Benard, G., Bellance, N., Jose, C., Melser, S., Nouette-Gaulain, K., Rossignol, R., 2010. Multi-site control and regulation of mitochondrial energy production. Biochim. Biophys. Acta 1797, 698–709.

Canto, C., Auwerx, J., 2011. Calorie restriction: is AMPK a key sensor and effector? Physiology (Bethesda) 26, 214–224.

Chen, C.N., Ferrington, D.A., Thompson, L.V., 2008. Carbonic anhydrase III and four-and-a-half LIM protein 1 are preferentially oxidized with muscle unloading. J. Appl. Physiol. (1985) 105, 1554–1561.

Chen, J., Henderson, G.I., Freeman, G.L., 2001. Role of 4-hydroxynonenal in modification of cytochrome c oxidase in ischemia/reperfused rat heart. J. Mol. Cell Cardiol. 33, 1919–1927.

Chen, C.N., Lin, S.Y., Liao, Y.H., Li, Z.J., Wong, A.M., 2015. Late-onset caloric restriction alters skeletal muscle metabolism by modulating pyruvate metabolism. Am. J. Physiol. Endocrinol. Metab. 308, E942–E949.

Civitarese, A.E., Carling, S., Heilbronn, L.K., Hulver, M.H., Ukropcova, B., Deutsch, W.A., et al., 2007. Calorie restriction increases muscle mitochondrial biogenesis in healthy humans. PLoS Med. 4, e76.

Colman, R.J., Anderson, R.M., Johnson, S.C., Kastman, E.K., Kosmatka, K.J., Beasley, T.M., et al., 2009. Caloric restriction delays disease onset and mortality in rhesus monkeys. Science 325, 201–204.

Figueiredo, P.A., Ferreira, R.M., Appell, H.J., Duarte, J.A., 2008. Age-induced morphological, biochemical, and functional alterations in isolated mitochondria from murine skeletal muscle. J. Gerontol. A Biol. Sci. Med. Sci. 63, 350–359.

Fink, R.I., Kolterman, O.G., Griffin, J., Olefsky, J.M., 1983. Mechanisms of insulin resistance in aging. J. Clin. Investig. 71, 1523–1535.

Fontana, L., Partridge, L., Longo, V.D., 2010. Extending healthy life span - from yeast to humans. Science 328, 321–326.

Gouspillou, G., Bourdel-Marchasson, I., Rouland, R., Calmettes, G., Biran, M., Deschodt-Arsac, V., et al., 2014. Mitochondrial energetics is impaired in vivo in aged skeletal muscle. Aging Cell 13, 39–48.

Hancock, C.R., Han, D.H., Higashida, K., Kim, S.H., Holloszy, J.O., 2011. Does calorie restriction induce mitochondrial biogenesis? A reevaluation. FASEB J. 25, 785–791.

Hempenstall, S., Page, M.M., Wallen, K.R., Selman, C., 2012. Dietary restriction increases skeletal muscle mitochondrial respiration but not mitochondrial content in C57BL/6 mice. Mech. Ageing Dev. 133, 37–45.

Ibebunjo, C., Chick, J.M., Kendall, T., Eash, J.K., Li, C., Zhang, Y., et al., 2013. Genomic and proteomic profiling reveals reduced mitochondrial function and disruption of the neuromuscular junction driving rat sarcopenia. Mol. Cell Biol. 33, 194–212.

Jackman, R.W., Kandarian, S.C., 2004. The molecular basis of skeletal muscle atrophy. Am. J. Physiol. Cell Physiol. 287, C834–C843.

Jang, Y.C., Liu, Y., Hayworth, C.R., Bhattacharya, A., Lustgarten, M.S., Muller, F.L., et al., 2012. Dietary restriction attenuates age-associated muscle atrophy by lowering oxidative stress in mice even in complete absence of CuZnSOD. Aging Cell 11, 770–782.

Johnson, M.L., Robinson, M.M., Nair, K.S., 2013. Skeletal muscle aging and the mitochondrion. Trends Endocrinol. Metab. 24, 247–256.

Joseph, A.M., Malamo, A.G., Silvestre, J., Wawrzyniak, N., Carey-Love, S., Nguyen, L.M., et al., 2013. Short-term caloric restriction, resveratrol, or combined treatment regimens initiated in late-life alter mitochondrial protein expression profiles in a fiber-type specific manner in aged animals. Exp. Gerontol. 48, 858–868.

Kim, J.H., Kwak, H.B., Leeuwenburgh, C., Lawler, J.M., 2008. Lifelong exercise and mild (8%) caloric restriction attenuate age-induced alterations in plantaris muscle morphology, oxidative stress and IGF-1 in the Fischer-344 rat. Exp. Gerontol. 43, 317–329.

Koltai, E., Hart, N., Taylor, A.W., Goto, S., Ngo, J.K., Davies, K.J., et al., 2012. Age-associated declines in mitochondrial biogenesis and protein quality control factors are minimized by exercise training. Am. J. Physiol. Regul. Integr. Comp. Physiol. 303, R127–R134.

Lanza, I.R., Zabielski, P., Klaus, K.A., Morse, D.M., Heppelmann, C.J., Bergen, H.R., et al., 2012. Chronic caloric restriction preserves mitochondrial function in senescence without increasing mitochondrial biogenesis. Cell Metab. 16, 777–788.

Li, X.D., Rebrin, I., Forster, M.J., Sohal, R.S., 2012. Effects of age and caloric restriction on mitochondrial protein oxidative damage in mice. Mech. Ageing Dev. 133, 30–36.

Lopez-Lluch, G., Irusta, P.M., Navas, P., de Cabo, R., 2008. Mitochondrial biogenesis and healthy aging. Exp. Gerontol. 43, 813–819.

Mansouri, A., Muller, F.L., Liu, Y., Ng, R., Faulkner, J., Hamilton, M., et al., 2006. Alterations in mitochondrial function, hydrogen peroxide release and oxidative damage in mouse hind-limb skeletal muscle during aging. Mech. Ageing Dev. 127, 298–306.

Marzetti, E., Calvani, R., Cesari, M., Buford, T.W., Lorenzi, M., Behnke, B.J., et al., 2013. Mitochondrial dysfunction and sarcopenia of aging: from signaling pathways to clinical trials. Int. J. Biochem. Cell Biol. 45, 2288–2301.

McKiernan, S.H., Colman, R.J., Lopez, M., Beasley, T.M., Aiken, J.M., Anderson, R.M., et al., 2011. Caloric restriction delays aging-induced cellular phenotypes in rhesus monkey skeletal muscle. Exp. Gerontol. 46, 23–29.

Mercken, E.M., Crosby, S.D., Lamming, D.W., JeBailey, L., Krzysik-Walker, S., Villareal, D.T., et al., 2013. Calorie restriction in humans inhibits the PI3K/AKT pathway and induces a younger transcription profile. Aging Cell 12, 645–651.

Miller, B.F., Robinson, M.M., Bruss, M.D., Hellerstein, M., Hamilton, K.L., 2012. A comprehensive assessment of mitochondrial protein synthesis and cellular proliferation with age and caloric restriction. Aging Cell 11, 150–161.

Petersen, K.F., Befroy, D., Dufour, S., Dziura, J., Ariyan, C., Rothman, D.L., et al., 2003. Mitochondrial dysfunction in the elderly: possible role in insulin resistance. Science 300, 1140–1142.

Petersen, K.F., Morino, K., Alves, T.C., Kibbey, R.G., Dufour, S., Sono, S., et al., 2015. Effect of aging on muscle mitochondrial substrate utilization in humans. Proc. Natl. Acad. Sci. USA 112, 11330–11334.

Peterson, C.M., Johannsen, D.L., Ravussin, E., 2012. Skeletal muscle mitochondria and aging: a review. J. Aging Res. 2012, 194821.

Reznick, R.M., Zong, H., Li, J., Morino, K., Moore, I.K., Yu, H.J., et al., 2007. Aging-associated reductions in AMP-activated protein kinase activity and mitochondrial biogenesis. Cell Metab. 5, 151–156.

Sandri, M., 2008. Signaling in muscle atrophy and hypertrophy. Physiology (Bethesda) 23, 160–170.

Santanasto, A.J., Glynn, N.W., Jubrias, S.A., Conley, K.E., Boudreau, R.M., Amati, F., et al., 2015. Skeletal Muscle Mitochondrial Function and Fatigability in Older Adults. J. Gerontol. A Biol. Sci. Med. Sci. 70, 1379–1385.

Stein, T.P., Wade, C.E., 2005. Metabolic consequences of muscle disuse atrophy. J. Nutr. 135, 1824S–1828S.

Wang, Z.Q., Floyd, Z.E., Qin, J., Liu, X., Yu, Y., Zhang, X.H., et al., 2009. Modulation of skeletal muscle insulin signaling with chronic caloric restriction in cynomolgus monkeys. Diabetes 58, 1488–1498.

Xu, X., Chen, C.N., Arriaga, E.A., Thompson, L.V., 2010. Asymmetric superoxide release inside and outside the mitochondria in skeletal muscle under conditions of aging and disuse. J. Appl. Physiol. 109, 1133–1139.

CHAPTER

29

Healthy Foods for Healthy Aging: The Case for Protein

Karen S. Kubena and W. Alex McIntosh

Texas A&M University, College Station, TX, Unites States

Aging results in the accumulation of damage to cellular macromolecules, including DNA, protein, and lipids (Mathers, 2015). While life expectancy has increased consistently in Western societies over the past 200 years, the challenge is to ensure that the additional time in those extra years is free from frailty and chronic poor health (Kirkwood, 2008). Thus, discussion about what has been called the healthy aging phenotype is occurring, a concept defined as "the condition of being alive while having highly preserved functioning metabolic, hormonal, and neuroendocrine control systems at the organ, tissue, and molecular levels" (Franco et al., 2009). The phenotype also results in resilience that minimizes the risk of cardiovascular disease (CVD) and dementia (Kiefte-de Jong et al., 2014).

The human body's expected life span is affected by the presence of specific genes and lifestyle characteristics that may decrease an individual's risk of chronic disease. These characteristics include adequate dietary intake that promotes healthy body weight, routine physical activity, adequate sleep, the avoidance of excess stress, and limited exposure to toxins (e.g., by smoking and alcohol). All of these affect chromosomes and likely long-term health (Passarino et al., 2016).

An active area of research involves dietary restriction as a means of increasing life span. Initially only targeting calorie restriction, research has now migrated to the modification of macronutrients. While too early to apply to current older adults, investigations into dietary balance as related to energy-sensing and nutrient-sensing signaling pathways may yield recommendations for modification of macronutrient intake (carbohydrate, protein, and fat) that can lengthen life span and improve health significantly (Fontana and Partridge, 2015). Santos et al. (2016) reviewed studies that suggest that altering proportions of protein and carbohydrate could result in significant changes in life span and perhaps decreased cancer development. Some data indicate that plant as compared to animal protein may be beneficial in suppressing the function of these signaling pathways and thus slow aging and the development of disease—hypertension, for example—while dietary fat seems to have no effect on the pathways (Santos et al., 2016). From a different perspective, Levine et al. (2014), reported that protein intake, either low or primarily of plant origin, was associated with reduced mortality in humans 50–65 years old and related to a reduction in growth hormone (insulin-like growth factor 1), while high protein intake by those 65 years and older reduced mortality (Levine et al., 2014).

A variety of nutrient modifications and, more recently, dietary patterns have been suggested to help individuals achieve the goal of healthy aging. Recommendations about dietary intake come from the federal government, health and professional organizations, and so on. Here we discuss two major federal sources that have focused on promoting Americans' overall health: Dietary Reference Intakes (DRIs) and Dietary Guidelines for Americans (DGA). We follow with a discussion on nutrients and foods, especially those of particular importance to the health of older adults, i.e., protein and protein-containing foods—and finally the what and why of good food choices. A word about the Mediterranean diet is also in order because this is a tried and true approach to healthy eating.

Nutrition and Functional Foods for Healthy Aging.
DOI: http://dx.doi.org/10.1016/B978-0-12-805376-8.00029-0

RECOMMENDATIONS: AN INSTRUCTION MANUAL FOR EATING TO ACHIEVE HEALTHY AGING

Dietary Reference Intakes

Recommendations for energy and nutrient intake for adults in the United States come from the DRIs and now the 2015–2020 DGA (the most recent edition). DRIs are the result of extensive reviews of data from studies on the minimum amount of nutrients needed to prevent deficiencies in nearly all healthy people of the respective gender and age group (Science, 2006). Each DRI is thus composed of several recommendations, including the Estimated Average Requirement (EAR), which estimates the needs of 50% of the population; Recommended Dietary Allowances (RDA), which estimates the needs of the mean plus two standard deviations or 97.5% of the population; Adequate Intakes (AI), which sets a recommended amount of intake although there is inadequate information to set an RDA; and the Tolerable Upper Intake Level, which is the highest level of daily intake of a nutrient not associated with adverse health effects.

Identifying the level of nutrient that meets the needs of healthy people in age-gender groups requires acceptance of the basis for these decisions by scientists, health professionals, and policy makers who use these resources. Protein is an example of a nutrient for which the RDA is the subject of much debate. Not only is the method of determining protein needs being scrutinized but so is the widespread acceptance of the RDA as the optimal level of protein. Wolfe and Miller questioned the use of nitrogen balance to determine protein needs since no physiologically relevant end point is measured (Wolfe and Miller, 2008). When less protein is consumed, the body adapts to conserve body protein, potentially resulting in less nitrogen excretion. The actual situation thus could be a gradual loss of lean body mass not detected by nitrogen balance (Volpi et al., 2013). In the original nitrogen balance studies for development of the protein RDA in 1943, almost all data came from college-aged men; no consideration was given to the increased needs of subgroups such as older adults (Wolfe and Miller, 2008). These researchers indicated that the RDA defines the level of protein required to avoid a deficiency, thus actually leading to a loss of body protein. That is not consistent with the customary concept of the RDA as the appropriate and often now recommended maximum intake of protein.

Within the DRI document is a discussion of acceptable macronutrient distribution range (AMDR) (National Academy of Sciences, 2005a). This concept addresses the question about division of calories among macronutrients because total calories from recommended levels of fat plus carbohydrate and protein totals only about one-third of the total energy recommended. As a component of discussion of the use of the DRIs for diet planning, a table is provided that indicates an appropriate range for dietary intake of macronutrients with the example of a 2000-kcal diet. The range of percentage of energy as protein is 10–35%, according to the AMDR. The calculation of dietary protein as a proportion of energy intake, using daily energy utilization for a 19-year-old sedentary man (76 kg and 1.76 m tall) was reported by Wolfe and Miller (2008). According to the DRI discussion of energy needs, the value in this case would be 37.8 kcal/kg/day. The range of protein intake for this man was then computed to be 0.95–3.3 g/kg or 10% and 35% kcal, respectively. The RDA of 0.8 g/kg is below even the lowest level of this range (National Academy of Sciences, 2005b; Wolfe and Miller, 2008).

Data from the National Health and Nutrition Examination Survey (NHANES) of 2001–10 of people 19 and older ($n = 23{,}876$) provided information on usual dietary intakes and the variables related to protein metabolism and dietary intake (Pasiakos et al., 2015). The average intake varied from 0.69 g/kg to 1.51 g/kg body weight, although the recommended level (RDA) is 0.8 g/kg. In all deciles, body mass index (BMI) and waist circumference, the latter a measure of abdominal obesity and a risk factor for CVD, were inversely related while the high-density lipoprotein (HDL) cholesterol level was directly related to protein intake. This is consistent with many other studies but contrary to recommendations from agencies and investigators who suggest that higher protein intake presents a risk for cardiometabolic health.

The Dietary Guidelines for Americans, 2015–2020

The 1990 National Nutrition Monitoring and Related Research Act requires release of a report providing information and guidelines about nutrition and diet for the general public every 5 years. The report, Dietary Guidelines for Americans, is a joint effort by the US Departments of Health and Human Services and Agriculture (Agriculture, 2015) and is based on previous guidelines and current research. The report is used to guide professionals and consumers in diet planning, to formulate health policies and programs at the federal level, and to guide nutrition education in federal education programs.

Another resource, one written to assist the formulation of the 2015–2020 DGA, is the *Scientific Report of the 2015 Dietary Guidelines Advisory Committee* (Committee, 2015). Within the report is a list of shortfall nutrients, those present at inadequate levels in the diets of a large number of people and dietary components that are overconsumed, i.e., sodium and saturated fats in particular. The 2015 scientific report also defines a healthy diet as one that includes among other things, low-fat and nonfat dairy. A diet also should include less red and processed meats. Concern has been expressed that adoption of the recommendations could adversely affect the intake of important nutrients in an effort to achieve the standard for dietary components such as type of dietary fat (Phillips et al., 2015).

The shortfall nutrients identified in the 2015 scientific report include vitamins A and D, calcium, magnesium, and potassium plus iron in some subgroups. Several of these nutrients are present in animal-source foods in highly bioavailable forms. The new dietary guidelines encourage the intake of many highly nutritious foods, including vegetables, fruits (especially whole fruits), and grains (at least half of which are whole grains), plus some animal proteins. This group includes fat-free or low-fat dairy, including milk, yogurt, and cheese and with the option to substitute soy beverages. Also, a variety of protein foods are recommended, including seafood, lean meats and poultry, and eggs. Again, plant-based foods are offered as options—in particular, nuts, seeds, and soy products.

For a variety of reasons, not the least of which is an interest in health, many people in developed countries have changed their attitudes about foods and their healthfulness and have adopted some level of vegetarianism from nonmeat eater to vegan. Consequently, consumption of some high-nutrient animal-source foods has decreased, including milk and dairy products, meat, poultry, fish, and eggs. Unfortunately, the foods chosen from the ever-changing array of food products may be nutrient dense, although the potential exists that substitutes also could be less nutrient dense and more energy dense. The FDA defined nutrient density as the amount of beneficial nutrients relative to a food's energy content (Drewnowski, 2005). The value of vegetables, fruits, whole grains, and many other plant-based foods for nutrition and health is not in question, but for those who eat animal-source foods, including appropriate milk and milk products, eggs, fish, poultry, and lean meat can promote nutritional adequacy, particularly with these short-fall nutrients. Aging adults who have consumed animal-source protein foods for many years may not be well served by being encouraged to abandon some of these foods in favor of plant-based foods, from which they could choose breads and desserts.

A 2014 report of trends in the dietary intake of older Americans using the NHANES data revealed that the primary source of energy for this age group, which had been red meat in the 1977–78 study, had been replaced in the 2005–10 NHANES report by breads followed by grain desserts, fruit, milk, and dairy desserts (Johnston et al., 2014). Absent in this ranking are nutritious plant-source foods such as vegetables and legumes and nutritious animal-source foods such as eggs, poultry, fish, and lean meat.

Table 29.1 includes the recommendations for inclusion of food groups by energy level for males and females (sedentary 51+ years): 2000 kcal and 1600 kcal, respectively.

DIETARY PROTEIN: THE FOUNDATION OF A HEALTHY BODY AND HEALTHY AGING

All Proteins Are Not Created Equal

Dietary proteins vary not only in the quantities of amino acids in them but also which ones are included. Essential or indispensable amino acids are those that cannot be synthesized in the body at the level needed to sustain normal function; dispensable amino acids are produced in quantities as needed from fats, carbohydrates, or other amino acids. Evaluation of protein quality is based on the presence of essential amino acids and the balance between them, as well as on digestibility. Dietary proteins vary markedly in amino acid composition but also in the presence or absence of compounds such as matrix components, including fiber and antinutritional factors such as trypsin inhibitor, which usually decreases the use of amino acids (Gilani et al., 2005; Schaafsma, 2005).

Identifying the most appropriate scoring method for proteins is an ongoing project since no system has yet been universally accepted. One system under consideration is the Protein Digestibility-Corrected Amino Acid Score (PDCAAS), which includes an evaluation of amino acid composition and digestibility. However, it does not correct for the presence of antinutritional factors, and scoring (0–1.0) is truncated at 1.0 (Millward et al., 2008). Another system that has been used for many years is the protein efficiency ratio (PER), which is based on animal growth. Protein quality rankings for some foods by these two systems follow (food, PER, and PDCAAS): egg = 3.9, 1.00; beef = 3.9, 0.92; milk = 2.5, 1.00; soy protein = 2.2, 1.00; peanuts = 1.8, 0.52; black beans = n/a, 0.75; and wheat gluten = 0.8, 0.25 (Hoffman and Falvo, 2004). As these data indicate, animal proteins are generally categorized

TABLE 29.1 Recommended Amounts of Foods by Day or Week in the 2015–2020 Dietary Guidelines for Americans for Adults Age 51+ and Sedentary[a]

Food Group	Female: 1600 kcal[b]	Male: 2000 kcal	Frequency
Vegetables (c-eq)[c]	*2*	*2.5*	***Daily***
Dark green	1.5	1.5	Weekly
Red and orange	4	5.5	Weekly
Legumes	1	1.5	Weekly
Starchy vegetables	4	5	Weekly
Other vegetables	3.5	4	Weekly
Fruits (c-eq)	*1.5*	2	**Daily**
Grains (oz-eq)	*5*	*6*	***Daily***
Whole grains	3	3	Weekly
Refined grains	2	3	Weekly
Dairy (c-eq)	*3*	*3*	***Daily***
Protein foods (oz-eq)	*5*	*5.5*	***Daily***
Seafood	8	8	Weekly
Meats, poultry, eggs	23	26	Weekly
Nuts, seeds, soy products	4	5	Weekly
Oils (g)	*22*	*27*	***Daily***
Other (kcal)	***130***	***270***	***Daily***

[a]*Appendix 3. USDA Food Patterns: Healthy U.S.-Style Eating Pattern (Agriculture, 2015).*
[b]*Appendix 7. Nutritional Goals for Age-Sex Groups Based on Dietary Reference Intakes and Dietary Guidelines Recommendations (Agriculture, 2015).*
[c]*Abbreviations: c–eq, cup equivalent; oz-eq, ounce equivalent.*

as higher quality than plant proteins. Soy protein is an exception and is considered to be a good-quality protein. Complementation of proteins, which vegans routinely do and formulators of animal feeds do when designing grains for animals, can improve a mixture's protein quality. Pencharz et al. expressed concern about this option for older adults since a higher intake of complementary proteins is required to provide needed essential amino acids compared to the amount needed from animal protein (Pencharz et al., 2016). Sarcopenia (the loss of lean body mass) and obesity are both concerns for older adults.

How Much Is Enough?

In 1943, requirements for protein by nonpregnant nonlactating healthy adults were determined to be 0.8 g/kg body weight; the requirements had the goal of helping troops in World War II meet the nutritional needs of a fighting force (Wolfe, 2015; Wolfe and Miller, 2008). Protein intake by older adults from NHANES 2003–2004 as reported by Fulgoni was below the RDA level (0.8 g/kg) by 10–25% with 5–9% below the EAR for protein (0.66 g/kg) (Fulgoni, 2008). The body adapts to a change in homeostasis—in this case, low protein intake—by decreasing the metabolism of protein so that the level of nitrogen excretion also decreases. In nitrogen balance, if less nitrogen is excreted when less nitrogen is ingested, nitrogen balance data could be interpreted as being closer to normal than what actually occurs (Volpi et al., 2013). Other concerns about the use of nitrogen balance to determine protein needs expressed by Pencharz et al. include the need for at least 3 days of data and a 7- to 10-day adaptation period between tests of levels of intake (Pencharz et al., 2016). Complete collection and analysis of nitrogen excretion (primarily urine and feces) is a challenge. Finally, calculating nitrogen balance is associated with wide variability because of large numbers for nitrogen intake and nitrogen excretion but small differences between them (nitrogen balance) (Pencharz et al., 2016).

Recent investigations of older adults' protein needs were conducted with the method now recommended by the Institute of Medicine: indicator amino acid oxidation (IAAO). Utilization of amino acids as measured with the use of stable isotopes is a noninvasive and fairly rapid method with short adaptation between tests (Pencharz et al., 2016). Use of the IAAO to determine protein needs in men 65 and older resulted in an estimated EAR and RDA of 0.94 g/

kg/day and 1.24 g/kg/day, respectively (Rafii et al., 2016). The authors concluded that both the current EAR and RDA were underestimated by 30%. These results mimic those of a previous investigation in women 65 and older (Rafii et al., 2015). In that study, the EAR and RDA were found to be 0.96 and 1.29 g/kg/day, about 30–40% higher than the current recommendations.

Evidence of benefits to older adults from higher protein intake has been reported in many areas. Frailty is a clinical syndrome that involves unintentional loss of lean body mass (10 lb/year), which leads to low grip strength, slow walking, exhaustion, and low physical activity (Fried et al., 2001). The presence of the syndrome in a cohort study of 1822 individuals 60 and older was found to be inversely related to dietary intake of total protein, animal protein, and monounsaturated fatty acids (Sandoval-Insausti et al., 2016). A 3-year observation of lean mass in older adults concluded that lower protein intake was associated with large losses of lean body mass (Houston et al., 2008). A case-control study of healthy elderly individuals revealed unhealthy weight loss in subjects with low protein intake (<0.8 g/kg) in comparison to those with a high protein intake (>1.2 g/kg) (Gray-Donald et al., 2014). In another report, supplemental protein provided to elderly people six times a day on a weight-loss diet resulted in higher lean body mass and decreased abdominal fat than those on a more traditional protein level (Arciero et al., 2013).

Myofibrillar protein synthesis in the healthy elderly has been reported to require a higher protein-synthesis response to dietary protein in comparison to younger men (Moore, 2014). Wall et al. suggested that aging results in muscle anabolic inflexibility, a key factor in the development of sarcopenia (Wall et al., 2015). Loss of lean body mass during weight loss while fat mass is essentially maintained is called *sarcopenic obesity*. Research indicates that decreased muscle mass results in loss of muscle strength (sarcopenia) and is significantly related to increased mortality (Li and Heber, 2012; Reginster et al., 2016). Treatment of this type of obesity requires exercise (preferably resistance), modest energy restriction, and protein supplementation (Han et al., 2011).

NHANES data from 2011 to 2012 illustrate that the prevalence of obesity in people 60 and older is 35.4% (BMI > 30) (Ogden et al., 2014). Obesity is a concern in older adults, one that increases risk of developing and worsening chronic diseases such as type 2 diabetes, hypertension, heart failure, and physical disability (Han et al., 2011). Recommendations to reduce body weight modestly (5–10 kg) have been shown to be effective in controlling these problems but not necessarily as much as in younger groups (Han et al., 2011). Consequently, the use of waist circumference rather than only BMI is recommended to assess the prevalence of adipocytes of visceral abdominal fat, adipokines from which are more likely to be related to inflammation, insulin insensitivity, and so on (Ouchi et al., 2011).

Concerns about older individuals' increased dietary protein involved previous reports that high protein intake even with calcium supplementation was associated with increased urinary calcium, a concern for bone mineral density (BMD). However, BMD and bone strength were not measured in these studies. Zhu et al. provided a high-protein (30 g whey) or placebo drink (2.1 g protein) and 600 mg calcium to healthy women 70–80 years of age for 2 years (Zhu et al., 2011). Urinary calcium was slightly higher in the whey group, but volumetric BMD and femoral neck strength were not significantly different at the end of the study. High protein intake has been reported to increase calcium absorption with possible long-term effects on bone (Tang et al., 2014).

Other changes in nutrient utilization occur with aging. For instance, requirements for vitamin D increase in older adults because of a potential decreased ability to form vitamin D_3 with ultraviolet B light or hydroxylate vitamin D to its hormonal form (Holick, 2014). Also, impaired intestinal absorption related to less secretion of the intrinsic factor required for vitamin B_{12} absorption due to achlorhydria suggests an increased need for this nutrient (Allen, 2009). Since less energy is used by the body for normal function due to a loss of lean body mass (decrease of as much as 50% by ages 75–80) and there is lower physical activity, nutrient density is a major concern (Kalyani et al., 2014). Therefore, food choice is important; and functional foods work.

MILK: A NATURAL FUNCTIONAL FOOD FOR A STRONG AND HEALTHY BODY

Because of the extraordinary food human infants receive right after birth, which includes all of the nutrients they need and a plethora of bioactive substances to help them safely grow, it is not a surprise that even after heat treatment, milk for calves is quite excellent for humans as well.

Part of the Scientific Report for the Dietary Guidelines Dietary Advisory Committee focused on nutrient intake in less than needed levels for a significant component of the population of the United States (Committee, 2015). These were called *shortfall nutrients* because of underconsumption in comparison to the EAR, which meets the needs of 50% of the US population. Of the eight nutrients categorized as shortfall, dairy is considered an important food source for five of them. Each food group included in the dietary guidelines was evaluated to assess its contribution of nutrients and energy across all calorie levels (Appendix E-3.2 Table 29.1 (Committee, 2015)). Information on dairy intake is not specific for older adults; however, data over all calorie levels indicate that dairy foods provide the following nutrients (% EAR): calcium = 67%, vitamin D = 64%, potassium = 21%, magnesium = 17%, and vitamin A = 32%. A total of 28% of recommended high-quality protein (PER 2.5, PDCAAS 1.0) is provided as well.

Bioactive peptides in milk include calcium, vitamin D, casein, whey, metabolites of milk proteins, and many more that are still being identified. The most active seems to be whey protein, which increases satiety and controls appetite in part by increasing the secretion of anorectic hormones cholecystokinin, leptin, and glucagon-like-peptide 1 and by decreasing the orexigenic hormone ghrelin (Sousa et al., 2012). In addition, whey apparently has a beneficial effect on glucose metabolism in diabetics and obese patients, weight reduction, and maintenance of muscle mass. Levels of cerebral glutathione were observed to increase in older adults as dairy intake increased. This antioxidant is vital for the brain's capacity to scavenge reactive oxygen species (ROS) and free radicals in oxidative stress (Choi et al., 2015).

Fermented dairy products, cheese, and yogurt have a record of reducing the risk of diabetes while transpalmitoleic acid, a fatty acid in milk, might also be involved (Visioli and Strata, 2014). Tripeptides formed from the action of the microbiota on milk protein have angiotensin-converting enzyme (ACE)-inhibiting activity. ACE inhibitors are potent antihypertensive medications (Phelan and Kerins, 2011). Investigations focusing on cheese illustrated reductions of triglyceride and increased HDL cholesterol. Favorable effects may come from metabolism by the microbiota of indigestible carbohydrates in cheese and other substances found in cheese that resulted in different effects on lipid metabolism of cheese as compared to butter, another high-fat dairy food (Visioli and Strata, 2014). Zjeng et al. suggested that products of microbial metabolism and increased fecal fat output related to cheese intake might play a role in the French paradox (Zheng et al., 2015). Bioactive peptides from milk have been shown to positively affect several aspects of the metabolic syndrome (Ricci-Cabello et al., 2012).

Interest in inflammation as a factor in chronic disease is increasing along with evidence that milk's bioactivity prevents inflammation (Da Silva and Rudkowska, 2015). Suppression of inflammatory markers, including tumor necrosis factor alpha and interleukin 6, and the downregulation of gene encoding for proinflammatory cytokines has been linked to the intake of dairy products with potential roles for naturally occurring trans fatty acids, milk proteins, and minerals (Kim et al., 2013; McGregor and Poppitt, 2013; Siriwardhana et al., 2013). The recommendation that older adults include two cups of low-fat or fat-free milk each day is beneficial in spite of evidence that high-fat dairy may be more effective than low-fat dairy (Zheng et al., 2015).

Lactose intolerance occurs with a deficiency of the enzyme lactase with symptoms following lactose (the primary carbohydrate in milk) ingestion. The importance of dairy as previously outlined indicates that management of the symptoms rather than avoidance of lactose is needed. Blinded studies illustrated that almost all patients with self-reported lactose intolerance can ingest at least 12 g lactose (one cup milk) without symptoms if taken with other food (Deng et al., 2015). Lactase supplements and low-lactose milk and dairy products if needed usually are effective.

EGGS: A NUTRITIOUS FOOD WITH BIG HEALTH BENEFITS

Visual impairment with potential blindness is most often related to cataracts (51%), glaucoma (8%), and age-related macular degeneration (AMD) (5%) (Abdel-Aal et al., 2013; Poh et al., 2016). Considered to be partly an oxidative process, AMD was the focus of investigations on slowing the disease's progression through dietary components (Age-Related Eye Disease Study (AREDS) and Age-Related Eye Disease Study 2 (AREDS 2)) (Broadhead et al., 2015). Evidence was encouraging and resulted in the development of supplements using the study formulations. The AREDS 2 formula replaces beta-carotene (risk of lung cancer in smokers) with the antioxidants eicosapentaneoic acid (EPA) and docosahexaenoic acid (DHA) and the carotenoids lutein and xeazanthin. The latter substances have been identified as being beneficial because of their involvement in the formation of the macular membrane, which protects the eye from ROS damage associated with macular degeneration and cataracts (Blesso et al., 2013b; Meagher et al., 2013).

While dietary intake of eggs was discouraged for decades, that philosophy is slowly changing. Egg consumption has been shown to be associated with an increase in HDL cholesterol and larger HDL cholesterol particles (Fernandez, 2010). Since HDL transports lutein and zeaxanthin to the retina of the eye, higher HDL levels means more of these antioxidants can be delivered to the macula (Blesso, 2013b). The egg yolk content of lutein and zeaxanthin was found to be 292 mcg/g and 213 mcg/g, respectively (Handelman et al., 1999), and the bioavailability of zeaxanthin was shown to be higher from eggs than from other foods (Thurnham, 2007). Data from the NHANES 2003–2004 indicate that dietary intake of lutein and zeaxanthin by adults 71 and older was approximately 1000 mcg/day and 107 mcg/day, respectively (Johnson et al., 2010). The Institute of Medicine's Panel on Dietary Antioxidants and Related Compounds, Food and Nutrition Board, stated that data were not available to allow development of recommended intakes of lutein and zeaxanthin (National Academy of Sciences, 2000).

The relationship between dietary intake and coronary artery disease (CAD) was identified through studies that began in the 1940s and included the Seven Countries Study led by Ancel Keyes. Initial findings implicated the effect of saturated fat on total serum cholesterol in cohorts in the United States, Japan, and five European countries (Willett, 2006). From feeding trials conducted by Keyes and others, along with another large prospective study in Framingham, Massachusetts, evidence of the beneficial effect of polyunsaturated fat emerged, resulting in early recommendations to reduce saturated fat, including eggs, and increase polyunsaturated fat in the diet. Evidence from a vast amount of subsequent research on diet and CAD over the last 60 years explained many of the complexities of lipid metabolism and thus the impact of dietary factors on development of CAD. A Harvard egg study was a massive prospective investigation using 118,000 subjects from the Health Professional Follow-Up Study (1986–94) and the Nurses' Health Study (1980–94) (Hu et al., 1999). The frequency of egg consumption (<1/week to >1/day) was evaluated with the development of cardiac events (myocardial infarction, fatal coronary heart disease, and stroke). Results of the study indicated that consumption of as much as 1 egg/day was not related to increased risk of occurrence of cardiac events, although some concern existed about the response of diabetic subjects (Hu et al., 1999). Concern about the response of diabetic or glucose intolerant subjects continues. Studies continue to reveal that egg consumption by nondiabetics is not related to increased cardiovascular risk and may lower risk. Once again, diabetics have some additional risk and should use eggs with caution (Li et al., 2013; Rong et al., 2013; Shin et al., 2013; Tran et al., 2014). Egg consumption results in increased LDL levels for most people, although two good outcomes continue to be reported—increases in LDL particle size and HDL levels increase. Also, the ratio between LDLs and HDLs is unchanged, so the end result is a less atherogenic profile (Blesso et al., 2013a; Herron et al., 2004).

Egg is a source of the highest-quality protein and the shortfall nutrients vitamin D and vitamin A. In addition, vitamin E, riboflavin, and vitamin B_{12} are provided. Cholesterol content is 186 mg/egg (USDA ARS Beltsville Human Nutrition Research Center, 2012), but concern about direct associations between cholesterol in foods and CVD has decreased. The list of dietary components about which there is concern about overconsumption in the *Scientific Report for the 2015 Dietary Guidelines for Americans* (Committee, 2015) does not include cholesterol. Recent studies of egg consumption as related to chronic disease resulted in the conclusion that egg consumption of less than two per day by older men was associated with a reduced risk of type 2 diabetes (Djousse et al., 2016; Virtanen et al., 2015). Griffin stated that consensus has been achieved that a relatively small effect of dietary cholesterol, primarily from eggs, on LDL cholesterol and the risk of CVD exists in comparison to other diet and lifestyle factors (Griffin, 2016).

One key recommendation for Healthy Eating Patterns in Chapter 1 of the 2015–2020 Dietary Guidelines for Americans states, "A healthy eating pattern includes: A variety of protein foods, including seafood, lean meats and poultry, eggs, legumes (beans and peas), and nuts, seeds, and soy products." Recommendations to include eggs in the diet as shown in Table 29.1 is as a part of the protein foods group and a total of 23 and 26 ounce-equivalents (oz-eq)/week for females and males, respectively. That converts to a daily recommendation of 3.3 and 3.7 oz-eq/day for females and males, respectively, for meat, poultry, and eggs (1 egg = 1 oz-eq). Based on research, eggs should be a part of the diet of nondiabetic older adults, especially in consideration of AMD.

Eggs are a valuable resource for feeding hungry people. Research will provide the answers to a few unanswered questions.

SEAFOOD: POWERFUL HELP FOR HEALTHY AGING

The recommendation for inclusion of seafood in the diet (see Table 29.1) is the equivalent of eight ounces per week for older females and males. Such strong support for seafood intake comes from the research base that is particularly applicable to older adults. Nutritional composition of fish in general includes high-quality protein and significant amounts of two shortfall nutrients, vitamins D and B_{12}. However, the most famous attribute of fish these days, especially high-fat fish, is the fatty acid content.

Marine oils docosahexanoic (22:6n-3) and eicosapentanoic (20:5n-3), generally from fish from northern waters (plus catfish), are considered to be highly beneficial for human health from pregnancy through old age. Research reports support their role in preventing CVD, including decreased triglycerides, platelet aggregation, inflammation, and oxidative stress (Mozaffarian and Wu, 2012). Also, the particle sizes for both LDL cholesterol and HDL cholesterol were reported to increase with DHA, a positive change in these lipoproteins; and the fatty acids have been known for some time to be effective for arrhythmias. Nevertheless, a high-fish diet for 8 weeks by older Australians did not positively impact inflammatory cytokines, blood pressure, or lipids (Grieger et al., 2014). Two studies, one in

Greece and the other in countries in the Americas, China, and India, were conducted to assess relationships between fish intake and depression (Albanese et al., 2012; Bountziouka et al., 2009). Results from the first observational study of 1190 people were so positive that the authors were suggesting causation, while the 15,122 subjects in the second study were studied for different types of depression and showed varying results, depending on several variables, not the least of which was country. However, in response to early research, DHA was added quickly to preterm infant formulas to promote neural development (Richard et al., 2016). Further evidence of the involvement of fish oils in brain function comes from studies of cognitive decline in older adults such as the study by Qin et al. (2014). The prospective cohort study of 1566 adults 55 and older continued for 5.3 years and revealed a relationship between fish consumption and slowing cognitive change as well as a positive effect on memory in those 65 and older.

BMD of the hip as related to the intake of fish and polyunsaturated fatty acids (PUFAs) was studied in older adults in the Framingham Osteoporosis Study over a 4-year period. Hip bone density was maintained in those who had higher fish intakes (Harris et al., 2015). Fracture risks in early life, midlife, and later life were related to fish and PUFA intake differently in men and women and were positively associated with lower risk later in life in men and in midlife in women. Choi and Park (2016) observed that consumption of seafood was associated with less risk of osteoporosis in Koreans but not in Americans, perhaps because the Koreans ate four to five times as much fish as the Americans.

The effectiveness of DHA and EPA on cardiovascular risk, cognitive function, and bone health suggests that older adults should strictly adhere to the recommendation for seafood.

MEAT AND POULTRY: A JUICY ISSUE

Keep It Lean and Keep It Fresh, Not Processed

The DGA recommendation for lean meat and poultry is combined with eggs to total 3.3 and 3.7 oz-eq/day for females and males, respectively, plus 1 and 1.5 c-eq for legumes (total 4.3 and 4.7 oz/c-eq). Nutritional contribution of meat for older adults includes high-quality protein (Wyness, 2015). Asp et al. (2012), demonstrated that consumption of moderate amounts of lean beef was positively associated with muscle mass in a group of older adults. The fatty acid content of meats varies by species, breed, age, and type of feed, among other factors. About half of saturated fatty acids is stearic acid, which is quickly converted in the liver to oleic acid, a monounsaturated fatty acid, which has a neutral if not positive effect on total and LDL cholesterol. Micronutrients in beef include iron, mostly in the heme form, which is far more absorbable (20–30%) than nonheme iron (5–15%) but usually not a concern for older adults. Vitamin B_{12}, a shortfall nutrient, is present in significant amounts (Wyness, 2015). Bioactive peptides make up another component of meat and include peptides that are antihypertensive (ACE inhibition), antithrombotic, or antioxidant (Huang et al., 2013).

Using the Women's Health Study data, Song et al. (2004) found that women who consumed greater amounts of total red meat in 1993, especially processed meat, tended to be diagnosed with type 2 diabetes 8.8 years later. A review of the relationship between the intake of red and processed meat and the risk of coronary heart disease was reported by Micha et al. (2010). Red meat consumption was not associated with the presence of these cardiometabolic problems, but the intake of processed meat resulted in an increased risk of coronary heart disease and type 2 diabetes. Differences could be related to the high sodium or nitrate content of processed forms (Micha et al., 2010). A meta-analysis of randomized controlled trials on the influence of beef, poultry, and fish on lipoprotein levels conducted between 1950 and 2010 reported no significant differences (Maki et al., 2012). Two large prospective cohort studies in Shanghai investigated differences in total and cause-specific mortality. Red meat intake (95% pork) as compared to poultry was related to both higher total mortality and risk of ischemic heart disease mortality in men but not in women (Takata et al., 2014).

Meat intake, particularly beef, has been associated with health benefits but also risks. Bradlee et al. (2014) reported that the inclusion of lean beef in the diet of adolescent girls was associated with a slight reduction in LDL cholesterol (Bradlee et al., 2014). A 2012 randomized control trial compared the effect of 141 g red meat/day as compared to 28 g/day (DASH diet) on lipoprotein metabolism (Roussell et al., 2012). Total cholesterol and LDL cholesterol were reduced to the same degree in both diets. Using blood lipids and food-intake data, researchers found that beef intake had a negative relationship with total cholesterol and HDL cholesterol but was not related to LDL cholesterol or triglycerides (Asp et al., 2012). Intake of red meat was associated with an increased hazard ratio (HR) for stroke in the prospective cohort study, the Atherosclerosis Risk in Communities Study (quartiles of red meat intake and HR follow: 1.13, 1.44, 1.33, and 1.47) (Haring et al., 2015).

Recently, concerns have been expressed about the association of red meat with the development of cancer. The relationship between red meat intake and the risk of colorectal cancer (CRC) was evaluated with a pooled analysis of 11 studies (Ananthakrishnan et al., 2015). Results indicated that high use of red meat was associated with increased risk of CRC from retrospective case-control studies. A meta-analysis of prospective cohort studies with risk assessments of all-cause, cardiovascular, and cancer mortality by red or processed meat intakes was performed (Wang et al., 2016) Results indicated that higher consumptions of total red and processed meat were related to increased risks of total, cardiovascular, and cancer mortality. Carr et al. (2016) performed a systematic review of prospective studies on associations between red meat subtypes and the risk of CRC that reported risk estimates with colorectal, colon, or rectal cancer or the risk of colorectal adenoma (Carr et al., 2016). Beef consumption was positively associated with an increased risk of CRC and colon cancer, and lamb was associated with a higher risk of CRC. Questions existed about the pork studies, but no association with cancer was found for poultry.

Poultry has also been shown to contain bioactive peptides just like beef and pork (Haring et al., 2015; Huang et al., 2013). Little information is available on the health effects of poultry, although a study of longitudinal changes in BMI related to changes in meat consumption included a significant trend toward decreased BMI in those with the highest intake of chicken as compared to the lowest (Gilsing et al., 2012). Poultry without skin has been designated as a nutrient-dense food by the 2005 DGA (Nicklas et al., 2014). Results suggest that lean red meat and poultry are high-nutrient protein sources that can be included in a healthy diet. As far as processed meats go, the advice is to "cut the baloney."

FOOD CHOICES FOR THE ELDERLY: ARE THESE GOOD FOR HEALTHY AGING?

Food intake by individuals varies with gender, education, age, and other sociodemographic characteristics. Using data from the 2005–2006 NHANES study, Berner et al. examined the intake of animal protein by animal source by age group and gender (Berner et al., 2013). Beginning with the total percentage of protein from animal sources by women, those between the ages of 51 and 70 got 63.8% of their protein from animal sources, and those older than 70 got 60.7%. The percentages for men in these two age groups were 66.9% and 62.3%, respectively. The authors observed that overall protein consumption appears to have declined since 1988–91. Males and females in the Berner et al., study ate greater amounts of protein foods at dinner time; more than 65% of this protein came from animals (Berner et al., 2013). Red meats served as the greatest source of animal protein for both age groups for men; for women, the greatest source, again regardless of age group, was dairy products. Fish contributed between 4.1% of protein for men 71 and older and 5.9% for women 51–70; eggs accounted for 3.8% of protein for women 71 and older and 5.5% for men 71 and older. A similar study using 2002–2003 NHANES data focused on differences in "dietary adequacy components" (e.g., milk) and "dietary moderation components" (e.g., saturated fat) based on the Healthy Eating Index (Hiza et al., 2013). Those 75 and older had diets that were more adequate in terms of milk; they tended to consume an amount of calories from saturated fat more closely to recommended amounts than did the 65–74 year olds. Among those 65 and older, milk intake was considered more adequate for non-Hispanic whites than blacks, as was women's intake compared to men in this age group. College-educated seniors consumed more moderate amounts of saturated fat than those who had less than a high school education. Similarly, the calories from saturated fat of those 65 and older who were college educated was considered more moderate than that of both those with some education or an associate's degree or with less than high school educations. College-educated elderly consumed more total fruits and vegetables than those with less education.

Eating out contributed to beef intake among the elderly as demonstrated in What We Eat in America, NHANES 2011–2012. Daily intake of beef stood at 40 g for women ages 60–69 and 37 g for those 70 and older (Bowman et al., 2013). Men consumed higher quantities than women; intakes of 74 g and 53 g by group, respectively. A comparison study of eight countries found cholesterol intakes ranged from 354 mg in Belgium to 214 mg in Portugal (Haveman-Nies et al., 2001). The amount of fats and oils consumed was highest in Belgium (59 g) and lowest in the United States (6 g). Milk intake was highest in the Netherlands and lowest in both Belgium and Italy. The elderly in the United States and Spain had the highest score on the Greek Mediterranean diet compared of that of the other countries (Haveman-Nies, et al., 2001).

Gille et al. found that more than 90% of middle-aged and elderly Swiss citizens indicated that eating healthily was important to them, but only 71% were familiar with the Swiss Food Pyramid (Gille et al., 2016). Of this group, only 38% said they adhered to this in their food choices. Among all respondents, 3% failed to consumed the recommended servings of dairy (including milk); 68% failed to meet guidelines for the intake of eggs, meat, or fish; and similarly high percentages of respondents consumed less from the cereals, fruits, and vegetable food groups. Men's consumption of eggs, meat, and fish exceeded that of women's; women tended to consume more from the cereal, legumes, and potatoes groups. Studies are lacking regarding the consequences of elderly persons' knowledge of the dietary guidelines in the United States.

Some studies have focused on differences in protein sources by race. Elderly white males consumed 12 g less of meats, poultry, and fish than elderly black males, but this difference was not significant (Bowman, 2009). By contrast, elderly white males consumed a great deal more milk and dairy products than elderly black males. This accounted for 12% of daily energy intake for elderly white males compared to only 7.2% for elderly black males. A similar difference between elderly black women was found. An earlier study of elderly black men and women found that both males and females consumed 330% of the RDA for cholesterol while consuming slightly higher recommended servings of meat, poultry, and fish but eating insufficient servings of milk and cheese (Lee et al., 1998).

Institutional residence also appears to affect the foods the elderly consume. Spanish elderly in institutional settings received more milk products than any other food group, followed by potatoes and sweets and pastries (Mila et al., 2012). These and other high-energy dense foods such as fats and sauces provided much of their energy intake. Fruit and vegetable intake was considered insufficient. A study of low-income elderly living in "sheltered housing" found that many foods were eaten only a few times a week. Of those who only ate certain foods a few days a week, 50% did so for meat, 20% for eggs, 34% for cheese, 23% for yogurt, and 18% for milk (Caughey et al., 1995). Quandt et al. (2009) performed research on low-income elderly in rural counties of Kentucky, indicating that the most frequent breakfast pattern involved bacon, ham, or sausage, eggs, and biscuits. Lunch and dinner tended to include a mixed dish and "starchy" sides. Mixed dishes may have included meat.

Some elderly also exhibit food "pickiness"; some of this may have more to do with eating difficulties rather than dislike (Maitre et al., 2014). This French study found that elderly who indicated a high level of pickiness tended to be malnourished and pickiness had a stronger association than eating difficulties with malnutrition, but those who experienced both difficulty and pickiness were worse off. Donini et al. (2013) studied elderly people suffering from anorexia of the elderly, finding that such persons tended to consume fewer foods than recommended from all food groups, but especially those such as "meat, fish, eggs" and "fruits and vegetables" (Donini et al., 2013).

Kant et al. (2004) used data from the National Health Interview Surveys 1987 and 1992 to study the link between a scale rating healthy eating habits (e.g., eating lean meat, low-fat dairy products, not eating fat from red meat, eating a number of kinds of fruit and vegetables) and mortality, finding that both men and women ages 45 and older were less at risk of dying over time if they made more healthy food choices (Kant et al., 2004). Kant et al. (2009) replicated this study using the National Institutes of Health and American Association of Retired Persons study of adults 65 and older, finding that the risk of mortality was lower for those in the highest quintile of the healthy diet scale (Kant et al., 2009). Both men and women were more likely found in the highest quintile on the healthy diet scale, and healthy eating practices were highest among those with higher income and greater education.

Using NHANES data for the time period 2001–04, Krebs-Smith et al. (2010) found that compared to recommended amounts of MyPyramid food groups, most age groups fell short of meeting those amounts. Far more than half of individuals aged 51–70 consumed insufficient amounts of meat and beans, milk, oils, fruits, whole fruits, total vegetables, dark green vegetables, orange vegetables, legumes, other vegetables, total grains, and whole grains. Slightly fewer of those respondents 71 and older consumed insufficient amounts from these food groups than did those 51–70. In addition, persons in this age group tended to overconsume added sugars and solid fats. More elderly males consumed the recommended amounts of meat and beans than females did of these foods but were more likely to consume less than the recommended amounts total fruits and whole fruits. Older females tended to consume more added sugars than their male counterparts.

One study followed elderly participants over a 5-year period, measuring their food intake and risk factors (Jankovic et al., 2014). Consumption of high-fat meat, high-fat milk, and egg and egg products declined over the period while fruit intake increased; however, these changes appeared to have little effect on the risk factors associated with CVD. Efforts to link a healthy diet to mortality from CVD and CHD found that those with a more healthy diet were less likely to have died from either of these two causes (Stefler et al., 2014). A US study of individuals older than 75 found several dietary patterns. The most frequent dietary pattern (named "sweets and dairy") consisted of sweets and dairy products ("baked goods, milk, sweetened coffee and tea, and dairy-based deserts") and the lowest intake of poultry (Hsiao et al., 2013). The second most frequent pattern (named "health-conscious") consisted of greater intakes of pastas, rice, whole fruits, vegetables, and fish and lower intakes of eggs, bread, fried vegetables, and fats. The final pattern (dubbed "the Western") consisted of high intakes of eggs, bread, fried vegetables, and fats with less fruit and milk intake. Of interest, red meat was found to be part of all three patterns. Individuals in the group whose pattern followed the "sweets and dairy" tended to have higher rates of hypertension than those in the "health-conscious" group.

SOCIAL INFLUENCES, VALUES, ATTITUDES, AND MEAT: BEHIND THE SCENES OF FOOD CHOICES

Studies have found that many people in many countries have come to believe that eating meat is unhealthy and have either reduced or eliminated meat from their diets. Zey and McIntosh (1992) found that women in Texas were more likely to indicate their intention to eat less meat in the future if their husbands or boyfriends supported this intention (Zey and McIntosh, 1992). Respondents who believe that eating meat was good for their health were less likely to intend to consume less meat. No difference was found by age. A similar study performed in Australia found that age was associated with attitudes about meat; elderly respondents were more likely to perceive eating meat as necessary for health and that it caused no risk to health and was not fattening (Lea and Worsley, 2001).

Recently a series of studies have focused on values and morality and meat. One study found that values such as universalism (protecting humans, animals, and the natural environment) and security ("prioritizing personal health, community safety, and protection of resources") tended to lead these value holders to consume less red meat (Hayley et al., 2015). Those who valued power ("attainment of social status, prestige, and dominance") tended to consume more red meat. Another study reported that meat eaters expressed fewer concerns for animal health while vegetarians expressed more concern (De Backer and Hudders, 2015). A similar study of red and processed meat found that those who held positive attitudes about animal welfare tended to eat less meat and those with such attitudes tended to be over age 60 (Clonan et al., 2015). However, those more than 60 years of age were no more likely to eat less red meat than those of younger ages. Others have examined disgust as a motivation for excluding meat from their diets; several studies found the greater this reaction, the lower the consumption of meat, but this association was more prevalent among adolescents and young adults than among older adults (Kubberod et al., 2008; Ruby and Heine, 2012). Others have studied what they consider the "meat paradox"—that is, while some people enjoyed eating meat, they experience concerns when they consider how animals are treated. While many spend little time attempting to reconcile these potentially conflicting views, others have adhered to rationales in order to avoid feeling guilty (Piazza et al., 2015). Those who do consume meat drew on arguments that eating meat is natural, normal, necessary, and nice (Piazza et al., 2015). As yet, these researchers have not reported on associations with age and other sociodemographic variables.

CULTURE, PERCEPTIONS OF FOOD CHOICES, AND EATING HABITS: PERCEPTION IS REALITY

Schifflett and McIntosh (1986–1987) studied 805 elderly found in 13 nutrition sites (congregate meal programs) in order to examine the relationship between perceived age-appropriate food choices and future time perspectives. Future time perspective has to do with elderly persons' views that they cannot plan what they may be doing in the next several years or that they only plan to maintain current activities (a more negative time perspective) versus maintain current activities plus adding new ones (a more positive time perspective). Five patterns of changes or maintenance of their eating habits were identified, including (1) maintaining lifelong eating habits, (2) changing food intake to follow a physician-prescribed diet, (3) following self-prescribed diets that involve fewer sweets and less fat and salt in order to avoid illness, (4) reducing food intake because of lower levels of physical activity, and (5) changing food choices because of taste abilities, social isolation, or reduced income. Those who had a more positive outlooks regarding the future were more likely to change to follow a diet or maintain their food choices than those who had negative outlooks about the future. Those who changed their diet because of their lessened ability to taste food or because they lived alone tended to have a more negative view of the future. These two patterns were stronger for males than for females. Similarly, those who either living with a spouse or alone tended to make more health-related changes rather than negative changes in their diets compared with others who lived with someone else who was not their spouse. Having a low income increased the likelihood that a respondent saw a bleaker future and made food habit changes based on changing taste ability or social isolation, but those who perceived their health had worsened tended make more positive changes in their food choices.

Life satisfaction and perceptions of satisfaction with various aspects of people's lives change as they age. This occurs because of fewer resources, changes in their connections to significant others, and difficulties in shopping for, preparing, and eating foods. Dean et al. (2008) argue that the more closely tied between the resources available to the individual and the goals they have for "food-related" aspects of their lives, the greater their satisfaction with their food lives. The researchers found that those with greater income, good storage facilities for food, social support, transportation, and abilities to taste and smell as well as a higher congruence between their level and the relevance of their resources were more likely to enjoy a greater level of food-related life satisfaction. Some foods the elderly preferred consisted of foods eaten in the past, which helped them maintain connection with their past (Fjellstrom et al., 2001). In addition to the generation in which the person was born when it comes to food choices, so did the stage of life an individual finds her- or himself. These authors note that those growing up in the 1970s developed a preference for "one-hand food, eaten on the run" but found no particular patterns for earlier generations (Fjellstrom et al., 2001).

THE MEDITERRANEAN DIET: FAST-FOOD ADVICE

The Mediterranean diet is a hot topic and the focus of a vast number of research reports in peer-reviewed journals and discussions in all types of media. The relationship between dietary intake and CAD was first identified through studies that began in the 1940s, including the Seven Countries Study led by Ancel Keyes. Initial findings implicated the effects of saturated fat on total serum cholesterol in cohorts in the United States, Japan, and five European countries (Willett, 2006). From feeding trials conducted by Keyes and others, along with another large prospective study in Framingham, Massachusetts, evidence of the beneficial effect of polyunsaturated fat emerged, resulting in early recommendations to reduce saturated fats and increase polyunsaturated fats in the diet. Evidence from a massive amount of subsequent research on diet and CAD over the last 60 years has explained many of the complexities of lipid metabolism and thus the impact of dietary factors on the development of CAD.

Dietary recommendations to promote cardiovascular health are plentiful, although one particular dietary pattern is enjoying considerable support in developed countries: the Mediterranean diet. This diet was considered to be responsible for a significant component of the variation in the incidence of CAD among the seven countries more than 60 years ago. Participating countries in which the traditional diet was reported surrounded the Mediterranean Sea—Italy, Greece, and countries of the former Yugoslavia. The fundamentals of the diet include a significant amount of olive oil, plant-based foods, fish, and wine. Bach-Faig et al. (2011) described the Mediterranean diet as followed primarily by poor rural societies in the Mediterranean area in the 1960s and including plant foods (cereals, fruits, vegetables, legumes, tree nuts, seed, and olives); olive oil as a major source of fat in the diet; relatively high intakes of fish and seafood; moderate intakes of eggs, poultry, and dairy (cheese and yogurt); and low consumption of red meat. A moderate amount of wine (alcohol) is included as well. The diet's healthfulness arises from a variety of foods included to prevent deficiencies and culinary methods that capitalize on the components of the diet, especially olive oil (Bach-Faig et al., 2011). Calibriso et al. (2016) reported that polyphenols in olive oil and serum metabolites may result in reduced oxidative stress and inflammatory angiogenic responses that are found in chronic degenerative diseases. Modification of gene expression by these phenolic compounds to protect proteins in cellular mechanisms involved in resistance to oxidative stress and inflammation has been reported (Silva et al., 2015).

Adherence to this food pattern has been reported to have a beneficial effect on chronic inflammation and endothelial dysfunction, conditions related to metabolic syndrome, type 2 diabetes, and CVD (Garcia-Fernandez et al., 2014; Meydani, 2005). Gotsis et al. (2015) reviewed results of studies over a 5-year period in which positive effects of the Mediterranean diet were reported for cancer at several sites (European Prospective Study into Cancer and Nutrition), chronic kidney disease, dyslipidemia, hypertension, type 2 diabetes, obesity, atherosclerosis, nonalcoholic fatty liver disease, and respiratory problems, including asthma and sleep apnea. Protection from cognitive decline associated with use of the Mediterranean diet was reported in a study of an elderly population in Athens (Trichopoulou et al., 2015).

Telomeres are protective sequences of nucleotides at the end of chromosomes that preserve genome stability by permitting normal cell division to take place (Boccardi et al., 2016). Telomere length decreases with each cell division until the telomeres are unable to function normally; this is the point when cell senescence occurs. The enzyme telomerase can repair damage to telomeres and restore cell viability. Oxidative stress and inflammation, which are known to play a role in obesity and cardiometabolic disease, are related to lower telomerase activity. Characteristics of an unhealthy lifestyle are associated with oxidative stress and shorter telomeres (Boccardi, et al., 2016). Investigation into the role of the Mediterranean diet in protecting telomere length in the Prevención con Dieta Mediterránea randomized trial in Navarra, Spain, resulted in stabilization of telomere length after 5 years (Garcia-Calzon et al., 2015). A cross-sectional study of an African American and Hispanic population in Washington Heights, New York City, demonstrated that increasing adherence to a Mediterranean diet was associated with longer telomere length (Gu et al., 2015).

The conclusion that can be derived from these studies is that diet can promote healthy aging. Considering the extensive research on the need for protein in the diet of older adults, increasing the amount of eggs, dairy, and cheese will make the Mediterranean diet one that can be adopted by older adults and anyone else who is on a quest for healthy aging.

CONCLUSIONS

The modern human life span has increased greatly over the past 200 years. To ensure that the extra time is spent in health and not in disease, optimal food choices are needed. DRIs and DGAs are good starts, and the Mediterranean diet is available with an arsenal of strong research for encouragement. More eggs, milk, and cheese for older adults will be helpful because without enough protein, the body could be headed for unhealthy aging.

References

Abdel-Aal, El-S.M., Akhtar, H., Zaheer, K., Ali, R., 2013. Dietary sources of lutein and zeaxanthin carotenoids and their role in eye health. Nutrients 5, 1169–1185.

Agriculture, U.S.D.o.H.a.H.S.a.U.S.D.o., 2015. 2015-2020 dietary guidelines for Americans. <http://health.gov/dietaryguidelines/2015/guidelines/>.

Albanese, E., Lombardo, F.L., Dangour, A.D., Guerra, M., Acosta, D., Huang, Y., et al., 2012. No association between fish intake and depression in over 15,000 older adults from seven low and middle income countries--the 10/66 study. PLoS One 7, e38879.

Allen, L.H., 2009. How common is vitamin B-12 deficiency? Am. J. Clin. Nutr. 89, 693S–696S.

Ananthakrishnan, A.N., Du, M., Berndt, S.I., Brenner, H., Caan, B.J., Casey, G., et al., 2015. Red meat intake, NAT2, and risk of colorectal cancer: a pooled analysis of 11 studies. Cancer Epidemiol. Biomarkers Prev. 24, 198–205.

Arciero, P.J., Ormsbee, M.J., Gentile, C.L., Nindl, B.C., Brestoff, J.R., Ruby, M., 2013. Increased protein intake and meal frequency reduces abdominal fat during energy balance and energy deficit. Obesity (Silver Spring) 21, 1357–1366.

Asp, M.L., Richardson, J.R., Collene, A.L., Droll, K.R., Belury, M.A., 2012. Dietary protein and beef consumption predict for markers of muscle mass and nutrition status in older adults. J. Nutr. Health Aging 16, 784–790.

Bach-Faig, A., Berry, E.M., Lairon, D., Reguant, J., Trichopoulou, A., Dernini, S., et al., 2011. Mediterranean diet pyramid today. Science and cultural updates. Public Health Nutr. 14, 2274–2284.

Berner, L.A., Becker, G., Wise, M., Doi, J., 2013. Characterization of dietary protein among older adults in the United States: amount, animal sources, and meal patterns. J. Acad. Nutr. Diet. 113, 809–815.

Blesso, C.N., Andersen, C.J., Barona, J., Volek, J.S., Fernandez, M.L., 2013a. Whole egg consumption improves lipoprotein profiles and insulin sensitivity to a greater extent than yolk-free egg substitute in individuals with metabolic syndrome. Metabolism 62, 400–410.

Blesso, C.N., Andersen, C.J., Bolling, B.W., Fernandez, M.L., 2013b. Egg intake improves carotenoid status by increasing plasma HDL cholesterol in adults with metabolic syndrome. Food Funct. 4, 213–221.

Boccardi, V., Paolisso, G., Mecocci, P., 2016. Nutrition and lifestyle in healthy aging: the telomerase challenge. Aging 8, 12–15.

Bountziouka, V., Polychronopoulos, E., Zeimbekis, A., Papavenetiou, E., Ladoukaki, E., Papairakleous, N., et al., 2009. Long-term fish intake is associated with less severe depressive symptoms among elderly men and women: the MEDIS (MEDiterranean ISlands Elderly) epidemiological study. J. Aging Health 21, 864–880.

Bowman, S.A., 2009. Socioeconomic characteristics, dietary and lifestyle patterns, and health and weight status of older adults in NHANES, 1999-2002: a comparison of Caucasians and African American. J. Nutr. Elder. 28, 30–46.

Bowman, S.A., Martins, C.L., Clemens, J., Carlson, J., Lin, B.-H., Moshfegh, A.J., 2013. Retail Food Commodity Intakes: Mean Amounts of Retail Commodities per Individual, 2007-08. US Department of Agriculture, ARS & ERS, Washington, DC.

Bradlee, M.L., Singer, M.R., Moore, L.L., 2014. Lean red meat consumption and lipid profiles in adolescent girls. J. Hum. Nutr. Diet. 27 (Suppl 2), 292–300.

Broadhead, G.K., Grigg, J.R., Chang, A.A., McCluskey, P., 2015. Dietary modification and supplementation for the treatment of age-related macular degeneration. Nutr. Rev. 73, 448–462.

Calabriso, N., Massaro, M., Scoditti, E., D'Amore, S., Gnoni, A., Pellegrino, M., et al., 2016. Extra virgin olive oil rich in polyphenols modulates VEGF-induced angiogenic responses by preventing NADPH oxidase activity and expression. J. Nutr. Biochem. 28, 19–29.

Carr, P.R., Walter, V., Brenner, H., Hoffmeister, M., 2016. Meat subtypes and their association with colorectal cancer: systematic review and meta-analysis. Int. J. Cancer 138, 293–302.

Caughey, P., Seaman, C.E.A., Parry, D.A., 1995. What do people eat? An investigation of the dietary req uirements of elderly people. Br. Food J. 97, 9–12.

Choi, I.Y., Lee, P., Denney, D.R., Spaeth, K., Nast, O., Ptomey, L., et al., 2015. Dairy intake is associated with brain glutathione concentration in older adults. Am. J. Clin. Nutr. 101, 287–293.

Choi, E., Park, Y., 2016. The association between the consumption of fish/shellfish and the risk of osteoporosis in men and postmenopausal women aged 50 years or older. Nutrients 8, 113–123.

Clonan, A., Wilson, P., Swift, J.A., Leibovici, D.G., Holdsworth, M., 2015. Red and processed meat consumption and purchasing behaviors and attitudes: impacts for human health, animal welfare and environmental sustainability. Public Health Nutr. 18, 2446–2456.

Dietary Guidelines Advisory Committee, 2015. Scientific Report of the 2015 Dietary Guidelines Advisory Committee. Washington, D.C.:U.S. Department of Agriculture and U.S. Department of Health and Human Services. https://health.gov/dietaryguidelines/2015-scientific-report/PDFs/Scientific-Report-of-the-2015-Dietary-Guidelines-Advisory-Committee.pdf.

Da Silva, M.S., Rudkowska, I., 2015. Dairy nutrients and their effect on inflammatory profile in molecular studies. Mol. Nutr. Food Res. 59, 1249–1263.

De Backer, C.J.S., Hudders, L., 2015. Meat morals: relationship between meat consumption consumer attitudes towards human and animal welfare and moral behavior. Meat Sci. 99, 68–74.

Dean, M., Grunert, K.G., Raats, M.M., Asger-Nielson, N., Lumbers, M., 2008. The impact of personal resources and their goal relevance on satisfaction with food-related life among the elderly. Appetite 50, 308–315.

Deng, Y., Misselwitz, B., Dai, N., Fox, M., 2015. Lactose Intolerance in Adults: Biological Mechanism and Dietary Management. Nutrients 7, 8020–8035.

Djousse, L., Khawaja, O.A., Gaziano, J.M., 2016. Egg consumption and risk of type 2 diabetes: a meta-analysis of prospective studies. Am. J. Clin. Nutr. 103, 474–480.

Donini, L.M., Poggiogalle, E., Piredda, M., Pinto, A., Barbagallo, M., Cucinotta, D., et al., 2013. Anorexia and eating patterns in the elderly. PLoS One 8, e63539.

Drewnowski, A., 2005. Concept of a nutritious food toward a nutrient density score. Am. J. Clin. Nutr. 82, 721–732.

Fernandez, M.L., 2010. Effects of eggs on plasma lipoproteins in healthy populations. Food Funct. 1, 156–160.

Fjellstrom, C., Sidenvall, B., Nydahl, M., 2001. Food intake and the elderly – social aspects. In: Frewer, L., Risvik, E., Schifferstein, H. (Eds.), Food, People and Society: A European Perspective of Consumers' Food Choices. Springer-Verlag, Berlin, pp. 197–210.

Fontana, L., Partridge, L., 2015. Promoting health and longevity through diet: from model organisms to humans. Cell 161, 106–118.

Franco, O.H., Karnik, K., Osborne, G., Ordovas, J.M., Catt, M., van der Ouderaa, F., 2009. Changing course in ageing research: the healthy ageing phenotype. Maturitas 63, 13–19.

Fried, L.P., Tangen, C.M., Walston, J., Newman, A.B., Hirsch, C., Gottdiener, J., et al., 2001. Frailty in older adults: evidence for a phenotype. J. Gerontol. A Biol. Sci. Med. Sci. 56, M146–M156.

Fulgoni III, V.L., 2008. Current protein intake in America: analysis of the National Health and Nutrition Examination Survey, 2003-2004. Am. J. Clin. Nutr. 87, 1554S–1557S.

Garcia-Calzon, S., Zalba, G., Ruiz-Canela, M., Shivappa, N., Hebert, J.R., Martinez, J.A., et al., 2015. Dietary inflammatory index and telomere length in subjects with a high cardiovascular disease risk from the PREDIMED-NARARRA study: cross-sectional and longitudinal analyzes over 5 y. Am. J. Clin. Nutr. 102, 897–904.

Garcia-Fernandez, E., Rico-Cabanas, L., Rosgaard, N., Estruch, R., Bach-Faig, A., 2014. Mediterranean diet and cardiodiabesity: a review. Nutrients 6, 3474–3500.

Gilani, G.S., Cockell, K.A., Sepehr, E., 2005. Effects of antinutritional factors on protein digestibility and amino acid availability in foods. J. AOAC Int. 88, 967–987.

Gille, D., Butikofer, U., Chollet, M., Schmid, A., Altintzoglou, T., Honkanen, P., et al., 2016. Nutrition behavior of the middle-aged and elderly: compliance with dietary recommendations of the food pyramid. Clin. Nutr. 35, 638–644.

Gilsing, A.M., Weijenberg, M.P., Hughes, L.A., Ambergen, T., Dagnelie, P.C., Goldbohm, R.A., et al., 2012. Longitudinal changes in BMI in older adults are associated with meat consumption differentially, by type of meat consumed. J. Nutr. 142, 340–349.

Gotsis, E., Anagnostis, P., Mariolis, A., Vlachou, A., Katsiki, N., Karagiannis, A., 2015. Health benefits of the Mediterranean Diet: an update of research over the last 5 years. Angiology 66, 304–318.

Gray-Donald, K., St-Arnaud-McKenzie, D., Gaudreau, P., Morais, J.A., Shatenstein, B., Payette, H., 2014. Protein intake protects against weight loss in healthy community-dwelling older adults. J. Nutr. 144, 321–326.

Grieger, J.A., Miller, M.D., Cobiac, L., 2014. Investigation of the effects of a high fish diet on inflammatory cytokines, blood pressure, and lipids in healthy older Australians. Food Nutr. Res. 58.

Griffin, B.A., 2016. Eggs: good or bad? Proc. Nutr. Soc. 75, 259–264.

Gu, Y., Honig, L.S., Schupf, N., Lee, J.H., Luchsinger, J.A., Stern, Y., et al., 2015. Mediterranean diet and leukocyte telomere length in a multi-ethnic elderly population. Age (Dordr). 37, 24.

Han, T.S., Tajar, A., Lean, M.E., 2011. Obesity and weight management in the elderly. Br. Med. Bull. 97, 169–196.

Handelman, G.J., Nightingale, Z.D., Lichtenstein, A.H., Schaefer, E.J., Blumberg, J.B., 1999. Lutein and zeaxanthin concentrations in plasma after dietary supplementation with egg yolk. Am. J. Clin. Nutr. 70, 247–251.

Haring, B., Misialek, J.R., Rebholz, C.M., Petruski-Ivleva, N., Gottesman, R.F., Mosley, T.H., et al., 2015. Association of Dietary Protein Consumption With Incident Silent Cerebral Infarcts and Stroke: The Atherosclerosis Risk in Communities (ARIC) Study. Stroke 46, 3443–3450.

Harris, T.B., Song, X., Reinders, I., Lang, T.F., Garcia, M.E., Siggeirsdottir, K., et al., 2015. Am. J. Clin. Nutr. 101, 947–955.

Haveman-Nies, A., Tuker, K.L., de Groot, L.C.P.G.M., Wilson, P.W.F., van Starern, W.A., 2001. Evaluation of dietary quality in relationship to nutritional and lifestyle factors in elderly people of the US Framingham Heart Study and the European SENECA study. Eur. J. Clin. Nutr. 55, 870–880.

Hayley, A., Zinkiewicz, L., Hardiman, K., 2015. Values, attitudes, and frequency of meat consumption: predicting meat-reduced diet in Australians. Appetite 84, 98–106.

Herron, K.L., Lofgren, I.E., Sharman, M., Volek, J.S., Fernandez, M.L., 2004. High intake of cholesterol results in less atherogenic low-density lipoprotein particles in men and women independent of response classification. Metabolism 53, 823–830.

Hiza, H.A.B., Casavale, K.O., Guenther, P.M., Davis, C., 2013. Diet quality of Americans differs by age, sex, race'/ethnicity, income, and education level. J. Acad. Nutr. Diet. 113, 297–306.

Hoffman, J.R., Falvo, M.J., 2004. Protein - which is best? J. Sports Sci. Med. 3, 118–130.

Holick, M.F., 2014. Sunlight, ultraviolet radiation, vitamin D and skin cancer: how much sunlight do we need? Adv. Exp. Med. Biol. 810, 1–16.

Houston, D.K., Nicklas, B.J., Ding, J., Harris, T.B., Tylavsky, F.A., Newman, A.B., et al., 2008. Dietary protein intake is associated with lean mass change in older, community-dwelling adults: the Health, Aging, and Body Composition (Health ABC) Study. Am. J. Clin. Nutr. 87, 150–155.

Hsiao, P.Y., Mitchell, D.C., Coffman, D.L., Allman, R.M., Locher, J.L., Sawyer, P., et al., 2013. Dietary patterns and diet quality among diverse older adults: the University of Alabama at Birmingham Study of Aging. J. Nutr. Health Aging 17, 19–25.

Hu, F.B., Stampfer, M.J., Rimm, E.B., Manson, J.E., Ascherio, A., Colditz, G.A., et al., 1999. A prospective study of egg consumption and risk of cardiovascular disease in men and women. JAMA 281, 1387–1394.

Huang, W.Y., Davidge, S.T., Wu, J., 2013. Bioactive natural constituents from food sources-potential use in hypertension prevention and treatment. Crit. Rev. Food Sci. Nutr. 53, 615–630.

Jankovic, N., Geelen, A., Streppel, M.T., de Groot, L.C., Orfanos, P., van den Hooven, E.H., et al., 2014. Adherence to a healthy diet according to the World Health Organization guidelines and all-cause mortality in elderly adults from Europe and the United States. Am. J. Epidemiol. 180, 978–988.

Johnson, E.J., Maras, J.E., Rasmussen, H.M., Tucker, K.L., 2010. Intake of lutein and zeaxanthin differ with age, sex, and ethnicity. J. Am. Diet. Assoc. 110, 1357–1362.

Johnston, R., Poti, J.M., Popkin, B.M., 2014. Eating and aging: trends in dietary intake among older Americans from 1977-2010. J. Nutr. Health Aging 18, 234–242.

Kalyani, R.R., Corriere, M., Ferrucci, L., 2014. Age-related and disease-related muscle loss: the effect of diabetes, obesity, and other diseases. Lancet Diabetes Endocrinol. 2, 819–829.

Kant, A.K., Graubard, B.I., Schatzkin, A., 2004. Dietary patterns predict mortality in a national cohort: the National Health Interviews Surveys, 1987 and 1992. J. Nutr. 134, 1793–1799.

Kant, A.K., Leitzmann, M.F., Park, Y., Hollenbeck, A., Shatzkin, A., 2009. Patterns of recommended dietary behaviors predict subsequent risk of mortality in a large cohort of men and women in the United States. J. Nutr. 139, 1374–1380.

Kiefte-de Jong, J.C., Mathers, J.C., Franco, O.H., 2014. Nutrition and healthy ageing: the key ingredients. Proc. Nutr. Soc. 73, 249–259.

Kim, Y., Kelly, O.J., Ilich, J.Z., 2013. Synergism of alpha-linolenic acid, conjugated linoleic acid and calcium in decreasing adipocyte and increasing osteoblast cell growth. Lipids 48, 787–802.

Kirkwood, T.B., 2008. A systematic look at an old problem. Nature 451, 644–647.

Krebs-Smith, S.M., Guenther, P.M., Subar, A.F., Kirkpatrick, S.I., Dodd, K.W., 2010. Americans do not meet federal dietary recommendations. J. Nutr. 140, 1832–1838.

Kubberod, E., Oydis, G.I., Dingstad, E.R., Henjes, I.J., 2008. The effects of animality in the consumption experience – An experiment. J. Food Prod. Market. 44, 103–124.

Lea, E., Worsley, A., 2001. Influences on meat consumption in Australia. Appetite 36, 127–136.

Lee, C.J., Templeton, S.B., Marlette, M., Walker, R.S., Fahm, E.G., 1998. Dietary quality and nutrient intakes of Black southern rural elderly. J. Nutr. Elder. 27, 1–15.

Levine, M.E., Suarez, J.A., Brandhorst, S., Balasubramanian, P., Cheng, C.W., Madia, F., et al., 2014. Low protein intake is associated with a major reduction in IGF-1, cancer, and overall mortality in the 65 and younger but not older population. Cell Metab. 19, 407–417.

Li, Y., Zhou, C., Zhou, X., Li, L., 2013. Egg consumption and risk of cardiovascular diseases and diabetes: a meta-analysis. Atherosclerosis 229, 524–530.

Li, Z., Heber, D., 2012. Sarcopenic obesity in the elderly and strategies for weight management. Nutr. Rev. 70, 57–64.

Maitre, I., Van Wymelbeke, V., Amand, M., Vigeau, E., Issanchou, S., Sulmont-Rossé, C., 2014. Food pickiness in the elderly: relationship with dependency and malnutrition. Food Qual. Prefer. 32, 145–151.

Maki, K.C., Van Elswyk, M.E., Alexander, D.D., Rains, T.M., Sohn, E.L., McNeill, S., 2012. A meta-analysis of randomized controlled trials that compare the lipid effects of beef versus poultry and/or fish consumption. J. Clin. Lipidol. 6, 352–361.

Mathers, J.C., 2015. Impact of nutrition on the ageing process. Br. J. Nutr. 113 (Suppl), S18–S22.

McGregor, R.A., Poppitt, S.D., 2013. Milk protein for improved metabolic health: a review of the evidence. Nutr. Metab. (Lond.) 10, 46.

Meagher, K.A., Thurnham, D.I., Beatty, S., Howard, A.N., Connolly, E., Cummins, W., et al., 2013. Serum response to supplemental macular carotenoids in subjects with and without age-related macular degeneration. Br. J. Nutr. 110, 289–300.

Meydani, M., 2005. A Mediterranean-style diet and metabolic syndrome. Nutr. Rev. 63, 312–314.

Micha, R., Wallace, S.K., Mozaffarian, D., 2010. Red and processed meat consumption and risk of incident coronary heart disease, stroke, and diabetes mellitus: a systematic review and meta-analysis. Circulation 121, 2271–2283.

Mila, R., Abellana, R., Padro, L., Basulto, J., Farran, A., 2012. High consumption foods and their influence on energy intake in institutionalized older adults. J. Nutr. Health Aging 16, 115–122.

Millward, D.J., Layman, D.K., Tome, D., Schaafsma, G., 2008. Protein quality assessment: impact of expanding understanding of protein and amino acid needs for optimal health. Am. J. Clin. Nutr. 87, 1576S–1581S.

Moore, D.R., 2014. Keeping older muscle "young" through dietary protein and physical activity. Adv. Nutr. 5, 599S–607S.

Mozaffarian, D., Wu, J.H., 2012. (n-3) fatty acids and cardiovascular health: are effects of EPA and DHA shared or complementary? J. Nutr. 142, 614S–625S.

National Academy of Sciences, F.a.N.B., Institute of Medicine, 2000. Dietary Reference Intakes for Vitamin C, Vitamin E, Selenium, and Carotenoids. National Academy Press, Washington, DC.325–382

National Academy of Sciences, F.a.N.B., Institute of Medicine, 2005a. Dietary Reference Intakes for Energy, Carbohydrate, Fiber, Fat, Fatty Acids, Cholesterol, Protein, and Amino Acids. National Academies Press, Washington, DC.107–264

National Academy of Sciences, F.a.N.B., Institute of Medicine, 2005b. Dietary Reference Intakes for Energy, Carbohydrate, Fiber, Fat, Fatty Acids, Cholesterol, Protein, and Amino Acids. National Academies Press, Washington, DC.936–967

Nicklas, T.A., Drewnowski, A., O'Neil, C.E., 2014. The nutrient density approach to healthy eating: challenges and opportunities. Public Health Nutr. 17, 2626–2636.

Ogden, C.L., Carroll, M.D., Kit, B.K., Flegal, K.M., 2014. Prevalence of childhood and adult obesity in the United States, 2011-2012. JAMA 311, 806–814.

Ouchi, N., Parker, J.L., Lugus, J.J., Walsh, K., 2011. Adipokines in inflammation and metabolic disease. Nat. Rev. Immunol. 11, 85–97.

Pasiakos, S.M., Lieberman, H.R., Fulgoni III, V.L., 2015. Higher-protein diets are associated with higher HDL cholesterol and lower BMI and waist circumference in US adults. J. Nutr. 145, 605–614.

Passarino, G., De Rango, F., Montesanto, A., 2016. Human longevity: Genetics or Lifestyle? It takes two to tango. Immun. Ageing 13, 12.

Pencharz, P.B., Elango, R., Wolfe, R.R., 2016. Recent developments in understanding protein needs - how much and what kind should we eat? Appl. Physiol. Nutr. Metab. 41, 577–580.

Phelan, M., Kerins, D., 2011. The potential role of milk-derived peptides in cardiovascular disease. Food Funct. 2, 153–167.

Phillips, S.M., Fulgoni 3rd, V.L., Heaney, R.P., Nicklas, T.A., Slavin, J.L., Weaver, C.M., 2015. Commonly consumed protein foods contribute to nutrient intake, diet quality, and nutrient adequacy. Am. J. Clin. Nutr. 101, 1346S–1352S.

Piazza, J., Ruby, M.B., Loughnan, S., Luong, M., Kulik, J., Watkins, H.M., et al., 2015. Rationalizing meat consumption: the 4Ns. Appetite 91, 114–128.

Poh, S., Mohamed Abdul, R.B., Lamoureux, E.L., Wong, T.Y., Sabanayagam, C., 2016. Metabolic syndrome and eye diseases. Diabetes Res. Clin. Pract. 113, 86–100.

Qin, B., Plassman, B.L., Edwards, L.J., Popkin, B.M., Adair, L.S., Mendez, M.A., 2014. Fish intake is associated with slower cognitive decline in Chinese older adults. J. Nutr. 144, 1579–1585.

Quandt, S.A., Chen, H., Bell, R.A., Anderson, A.M., Savoca, M.R., Kohrman, T., et al., 2009. Disparities in oral health status between older adults in a multiethnic rural community: the rural nutrition and oral health study. J. Am. Geriatr. Soc. 57, 1369–1375.

Rafii, M., Chapman, K., Elango, R., Campbell, W.W., Ball, R.O., Pencharz, P.B., et al., 2016. Dietary Protein Requirement of Men >65 Years Old Determined by the Indicator Amino Acid Oxidation Technique Is Higher than the Current Estimated Average Requirement. J. Nutr. 146, 681–687.

Rafii, M., Chapman, K., Owens, J., Elango, R., Campbell, W.W., Ball, R.O., et al., 2015. Dietary protein requirement of female adults >65 years determined by the indicator amino acid oxidation technique is higher than current recommendations. J. Nutr. 145, 18–24.

Reginster, J.Y., Cooper, C., Rizzoli, R., Kanis, J.A., Appelboom, G., Bautmans, I., et al., 2016. Recommendations for the conduct of clinical trials for drugs to treat or prevent sarcopenia. Aging Clin. Exp. Res. 28, 47–58.

Ricci-Cabello, I., Herrera, M.O., Artacho, R., 2012. Possible role of milk-derived bioactive peptides in the treatment and prevention of metabolic syndrome. Nutr. Rev. 70, 241–255.

Richard, C., Lewis, E.D., Field, C.J., 2016. Evidence for the essentiality of arachidonic and docosahexaenoic acid in the postnatal maternal and infant diet for the development of the infant's immune system early in life. Appl. Physiol. Nutr. Metab. 41, 461–475.

Rong, Y., Chen, L., Zhu, T., Song, Y., Yu, M., Shan, Z., et al., 2013. Egg consumption and risk of coronary heart disease and stroke: dose-response meta-analysis of prospective cohort studies. BMJ 346, e8539.

Roussell, M.A., Hill, A.M., Gaugler, T.L., West, S.G., Heuvel, J.P., Alaupovic, P., et al., 2012. Beef in an optimal lean diet study: effects on lipids, lipoproteins, and apolipoproteins. Am. J. Clin. Nutr. 95, 9–16.

Ruby, M.B., Heine, S.J., 2012. Too close to home: factors predicting meat avoidance. Appetite 59, 47–52.

Sandoval-Insausti, H., Perez-Tasigchana, R.F., Lopez-Garcia, E., Garcia-Esquinas, E., Rodriguez-Artalejo, F., Guallar-Castillon, P., 2016. Macronutrients Intake and Incident Frailty in Older Adults: A Prospective Cohort Study. J. Gerontol. A Biol. Sci. Med. Sci. 71, 1329–1334.

Santos, J., Leitao-Correia, F., Sousa, M.J., Leao, C., 2016. Dietary Restriction and Nutrient Balance in Aging. Oxid. Med. Cell. Longev. 2016, 4010357.

Schaafsma, G., 2005. The Protein Digestibility-Corrected Amino Acid Score (PDCAAS)--a concept for describing protein quality in foods and food ingredients: a critical review. J. AOAC Int. 88, 988–994.

Science, I.o.M.o.t.N.A.o., 2006. Dietary Reference Intakes: The Essential Guide to Nutrient Requirements. National Academies Press, Washington, DC.

Shifflett, P.A., McIntosh, W.A., 1986–1987. Food habits and future time: an exploratory study of age-appropriate food habits among the elderly. Int. J. Aging. Hum. Dev. 24, 1–17.

Shin, J.Y., Xun, P., Nakamura, Y., He, K., 2013. Egg consumption in relation to risk of cardiovascular disease and diabetes: a systematic review and meta-analysis. Am. J. Clin. Nutr. 98, 146–159.

Silva, S., Combet, E., Figueira, M.E., Koeck, T., Mullen, W., Bronze, M.R., 2015. New perspectives on bioactivity of olive oil: evidence from animal models, human interventions and the use of urinary proteomic biomarkers. Proc. Nutr. Soc. 74, 268–281.

Siriwardhana, N., Kalupahana, N.S., Cekanova, M., LeMieux, M., Greer, B., Moustaid-Moussa, N., 2013. Modulation of adipose tissue inflammation by bioactive food compounds. J. Nutr. Biochem. 24, 613–623.

Song, Y., Manson, J.E., Buring, J.E., Liu, S., 2004. A prospective study of red meat consumption and type 2 diabetes in middle-aged and elderly women: the women's health study.. Diabetes Care 27, 2108–2115.

Sousa, G.T., Lira, F.S., Rosa, J.C., de Oliveira, E.P., Oyama, L.M., Santos, R.V., et al., 2012. Dietary whey protein lessens several risk factors for metabolic diseases: a review. Lipids Health Dis. 11, 67.

Stefler, D., Pikhart, H., Kubinova, R., Pajak, A., Malyutina, S., Siminova, G., et al., 2014. Healthy diet indicator sand mortality in Eastern European populations: prospective evidence from the HAPIEE cohort. Eur. J. Clin. Nutr. 68, 1346–1352.

Takata, Y., Ansai, T., Soh, I., Awano, S., Nakamichi, I., Akifusa, S., et al., 2014. Serum total cholesterol concentration and 10-year mortality in an 85-year-old population. Clin. Interv. Aging 9, 293–300.

Tang, M., O'Connor, L.E., Campbell, W.W., 2014. Diet-induced weight loss: the effect of dietary protein on bone. J. Acad. Nutr. Diet. 114, 72–85.

Thurnham, D.I., 2007. Macular zeaxanthins and lutein -- a review of dietary sources and bioavailability and some relationships with macular pigment optical density and age-related macular disease. Nutr. Res. Rev. 20, 163–179.

Tran, N.L., Barraj, L.M., Heilman, J.M., Scrafford, C.G., 2014. Egg consumption and cardiovascular disease among diabetic individuals: a systematic review of the literature. Diabetes Metab. Syndr. Obes. 7, 121–137.

Trichopoulou, A., Kyrozis, A., Rossi, M., Katsoulis, M., Trichopoulos, D., La Vecchia, C., et al., 2015. Mediterranean diet and cognitive decline over time in an elderly Mediterranean population. Eur. J. Nutr. 54, 1311–1321.

USDA ARS Beltsville Human Nutrition Resesarch Center, F.S.R.G., 2012. Breakfast in America, 2001-2002. <http://www.ars.usad.gov/SP2UserFiles/pdfDBrief/1_Breakfast_2001-2002.pdf>.

Virtanen, J.K., Mursu, J., Tuomainen, T.P., Virtanen, H.E., Voutilainen, S., 2015. Egg consumption and risk of incident type 2 diabetes in men: the Kuopio Ischaemic Heart Disease Risk Factor Study. Am. J. Clin. Nutr. 101, 1088–1096.

Visioli, F., Strata, A., 2014. Milk, dairy products, and their functional effects in humans: a narrative review of recent evidence. Adv. Nutr. 5, 131–143.

Volpi, E., Campbell, W.W., Dwyer, J.T., Johnson, M.A., Jensen, G.L., Morley, J.E., et al., 2013. Is the optimal level of protein intake for older adults greater than the recommended dietary allowance? J. Gerontol. A Biol. Sci. Med. Sci. 68, 677–681.

Wall, B.T., Gorissen, S.H., Pennings, B., Koopman, R., Groen, B.B., Verdijk, L.B., et al., 2015. Aging Is Accompanied by a Blunted Muscle Protein Synthetic Response to Protein Ingestion. PLoS One 10, e0140903.

Wang, X., Lin, X., Ouyang, Y.Y., Liu, J., Zhao, G., Pan, A., et al., 2016. Red and processed meat consumption and mortality: dose-response meta-analysis of prospective cohort studies. Public Health Nutr. 19, 893–905.

Willett, W.C., 2006. The Mediterranean diet: science and practice. Public Health Nutr. 9, 105–110.

Wolfe, R.R., 2015. Update on protein intake: importance of milk proteins for health status of the elderly. Nutr. Rev. 73 (Suppl 1), 41–47.

Wolfe, R.R., Miller, S.L., 2008. The recommended dietary allowance of protein: a misunderstood concept. JAMA 299, 2891–2893.

Wyness, L., 2015. The role of red meat in the diet: nutrition and health benefits. Proc. Nutr. Soc. 75, 227–232.

Zey, M., McIntosh, W.A., 1992. Predicting the intent to consume beef among women. Rural Soc. 57, 250–255.

Zheng, H., Yde, C.C., Clausen, M.R., Kristensen, M., Lorenzen, J., Astrup, A., et al., 2015. Metabolomics investigation to shed light on cheese as a possible piece in the French paradox puzzle. J. Agric. Food Chem. 63, 2830–2839.

Zhu, K., Meng, X., Kerr, D.A., Devine, A., Solah, V., Binns, C.W., et al., 2011. The effects of a two-year randomized, controlled trial of whey protein supplementation on bone structure, IGF-1, and urinary calcium excretion in older postmenopausal women. J. Bone Miner. Res. 26, 2298–2306.

Index

Note: Page numbers followed by "*f*" and "*t*" refer to figures and tables, respectively.